AF624952

The Oxford Handbook of Digital Technologies and Mental Health

Oxford Library of Psychology

Area Editors:

Clinical Psychology
David H. Barlow

Cognitive Neuroscience
Kevin N. Ochsner and Stephen M. Kosslyn

Cognitive Psychology
Daniel Reisberg

Counseling Psychology
Elizabeth M. Altmaier and Jo-Ida C. Hansen

Developmental Psychology
Philip David Zelazo

Health Psychology
Howard S. Friedman

History of Psychology
David B. Baker

Methods and Measurement
Todd D. Little

Neuropsychology
Kenneth M. Adams

Organizational Psychology
Steve W. J. Kozlowski

Personality and Social Psychology
Kay Deaux and Mark Snyder

OXFORD LIBRARY OF PSYCHOLOGY

The Oxford Handbook of Digital Technologies and Mental Health

Edited by

Marc N. Potenza, Kyle A. Faust, and
David Faust

OXFORD
UNIVERSITY PRESS

2020

OXFORD
UNIVERSITY PRESS

Oxford University Press is a department of the University of Oxford. It furthers the University's objective of excellence in research, scholarship, and education by publishing worldwide. Oxford is a registered trade mark of Oxford University Press in the UK and certain other countries.

Published in the United States of America by Oxford University Press
198 Madison Avenue, New York, NY 10016, United States of America.

© Oxford University Press 2020

All rights reserved. No part of this publication may be reproduced, stored in a retrieval system, or transmitted, in any form or by any means, without the prior permission in writing of Oxford University Press, or as expressly permitted by law, by license, or under terms agreed with the appropriate reproduction rights organization. Inquiries concerning reproduction outside the scope of the above should be sent to the Rights Department, Oxford University Press, at the address above.

You must not circulate this work in any other form and you must impose this same condition on any acquirer.

Library of Congress Cataloging-in-Publication Data
Names: Potenza, Marc N., 1965– editor. | Faust, Kyle A., editor. | Faust, David, 1952– editor.
Title: The Oxford handbook of digital technologies and mental health / edited by Marc N. Potenza, Kyle A. Faust, and David Faust.
Description: New York, NY : Oxford University Press, [2020] |
Summary: "This book provides an academically oriented and scientifically based description of how technological advances may have contributed to a wide range of mental health outcomes, covering the spectrum from problems and maladies to improved and expanded healthcare services"—Provided by publisher.
Identifiers: LCCN 2020021147 (print) | LCCN 2020021148 (ebook) |
ISBN 9780190218058 (hardback) | ISBN 9780190670023 (epub)
Subjects: LCSH: Internet addiction. | Video game addiction. |
Internet in psychotherapy. | Internet in medicine.
Classification: LCC RC569.5.I54 O94 2929 (print) | LCC RC569.5.I54 (ebook) | DDC 616.85/84—dc23
LC record available at https://lccn.loc.gov/2020021147
LC ebook record available at https://lccn.loc.gov/2020021148

9 8 7 6 5 4 3 2 1

Printed by Integrated Books International, United States of America

From Marc N. Potenza:

To my parents Janet and Joseph for the care and opportunities they provided to me; to my brother Michael for his support and camaraderie; to my children Nicolas and Elise for the joy that they have brought to me; and to my wonderful wife Gretchen, the true love of my life. With much gratitude and wishes for good health and wellness.

From Kyle Faust:

To my parents, Pam and David,
To all of my grandparents,
To my siblings and sister-in-law, Jordan, Sasha, and Fontanna,
To my Niece and Nephews: Tay Leigh, Kingston, and Benjamin,
Thank you all for being such a wonderful and supportive family.

From David Faust:

Once again to my loving family, for whom I will be forever grateful:
my wife Pamela and my children Kyle, Jordan, and Sasha;

and to whom I now happily add my daughter-in-law, Fontanna Faust, and my grandchildren:

Tay Leigh, Kingston, Benjamin Faust, and others to come, with all my
love and optimism for a future that fulfills or surpasses many dreams.

SHORT CONTENTS

ABOUT THE EDITORS

Marc N. Potenza, MD, PhD, is a Professor of Psychiatry, Child Study and Neuroscience at the Yale University School of Medicine where he is the Director of the Problem Gambling Clinic, the Center of Excellence in Gambling Research, the Women and Addictive Disorders Core of Women's Health Research at Yale and the Yale Research Program on Impulsivity and Impulse Control Disorders. He is an Honorary Professor in Psychological Science at Eötvös Loránd University and a Senior Research Scientist at the Connecticut Council on Problem Gambling. He is on the editorial boards of fifteen journals and has received multiple national and international awards for excellence in research and clinical care. He has consulted to multiple agencies (Substance Abuse and Mental Health Services Administration, National Institutes of Health, American Psychiatric Association and World Health Organization) on matters of addiction. He has published widely on internet use and related behaviors with addictive potential, having provided input into the DSM-5 and ICD-11.

Kyle A. Faust is a clinical psychologist working at Home Base, Massachusetts General Hospital, and Harvard Medical School. He has published numerous articles on the positive and negative applications of digital technology, and works to apply these methods in his clinical work. He has also received mentorship from Dr. James Prochaska, who developed the Transtheoretical model of behaviour change, and is working to apply this model to treatment of problematic use of digital technology.

David Faust is a Full Professor in the Department of Psychology, College of Health Science, and a Ryan Research Professor of Neuroscience, George and Ryan Institute for Neuroscience, at the University of Rhode Island; and holds an affiliate appointment in the Department of Psychiatry and Human Behavior, Alpert Medical School of Brown University. Dr. Faust has published numerous articles, books, and book chapters on such topics as assessment of digital technology use and overuse, philosophy of science, psychology and law, and neuropsychology, has lectured nationally and internationally, and has been the recipient of multiple awards and honors in his field, including awards for distinguished professional contributions.

CONTRIBUTORS

Craig A. Anderson, PhD, MS
Department of Psychology, Iowa State University

Ellen Beckjord, PhD, MPH
University of Pittsburgh Medical Center Health Plan

Morris D. Bell, PhD
Yale University School of Medicine

Manfred E. Beutel, MD
Department of Psychosomatic Medicine and Psychotherapy, University Medical Center of the Johannes Gutenberg-University Mainz, Germany

Joël Billieux, PhD
Institute of Psychology, University of Lausanne, Lausanne, Switzerland.

Jorge Blanco, MA,
Iowa State University

Matthias Brand, PhD
Cognition and Center for Behavioral Addiction Research (CeBAR), University of Duisburg-Essen, Germany; Erwin L. Hahn Institute for Magnetic Resonance Imaging, Essen, Germany

Judson Brewer, MD, PhD
Brown University School of Public Health; Warren Alpert Medical School of Brown University

Shangli Cai, PhD
Mental Health Institute of the Second Xiangya Hospital, Central South University. China; National Clinical Research Center on Mental Disorders; National Technology Institute on Mental Disorders; Hunan Key Laboratory of Psychiatry and Mental Health

Deepa R. Camenga, MD, MHS
Department of Emergency Medicine; Yale School of Medicine

Kathleen M. Carroll, PhD
Yale University School of Medicine

Sulki Chung, MSW, PhD
Department of Social Welfare, Chung-Ang University, Korea

Thomas Chung, MBChB, MHA, FFPH
Department of Health, Hong Kong SAR

Aaron Cochrane, MS
Psychology Department, University of Wisconsin - Madison; McPherson Eye Research Institute, University of Wisconsin - Madison

Nathan E. Cook, PhD
Massachusetts General Hospital and Harvard Medical School

Patrick S. R. Davidson, PhD
University of Ottawa; Bruyère Research Institute

Paul H. Delfabbro, PhD
School of Psychology, University of Adelaide, Australia

Martina de Zwaan, MD
Department of Psychosomatic Medicine and Psychotherapy, Hannover Medical School, Hannover, Germany

Emese Domahidi, PhD
Ilmenau University of Technology

Michael Dreier, PhD
Outpatient Clinic for Behavioral Addictions, Department of Psychosomatic Medicine and Psychotherapy, University Medical Center of the Johannes Gutenberg-University Mainz, Germany

David Faust, PhD
University of Rhode Island; Warren Alpert Medical School of Brown University

Kyle A. Faust, PhD
Home Base; Massachusetts General Hospital; Harvard Medical School

Christopher J. Ferguson, PhD
Stetson University

Stuart G. Ferguson, PhD
University of Tasmania

Ruth Festl, PhD
Leibniz Institute for Knowledge Media

Timothy W. Fong, MD
Professor of Psychiatry, Co-Director, UCLA Gambling Studies Program

Ariadna Forray, MD
Department of Psychiatry, Yale School of Medicine

Dawn W. Foster, PhD, MPH, MA
Indiana University; Yale University

Michael D. Franzen, PhD
AHN Behavioral Health Institute, Allegheny Health Network; Allegheny General Hospital; Temple University School of Medicine

Jonathan Zachariah Gallar, MACJ
Seattle University

Kathleen A. Garrison, PhD
Department of Psychiatry, Yale School of Medicine

Charles Gaudet, MA
University of Rhode Island; Warren Alpert Medical School of Brown University

Douglas A. Gentile, PhD
Professor of Psychology, Iowa State University

Josh D. Golt, BS
University of Alabama

Heather M. Gray, PhD
Division on Addiction, Cambridge Health Alliance; Harvard Medical School

C. Shawn Green, PhD
Department of Psychology, University of Wisconsin-Madison

Mark D. Griffiths, PhD
International Gaming Research Unit, Psychology Department, Nottingham Trent University, UK

Christopher L. Groves, PhD, MS
Department of Psychology, University of Wisconsin, Oshkosh

Wei Hao, MD, PhD
Mental Health Institute of the Second Xiangya Hospital, Central South University. China; National Clinical Research Center on Mental Disorders; National Technology Institute on Mental Disorders; Hunan Key Laboratory of Psychiatry and Mental Health

Rani A. Hoff, PhD, MPH
Department of Psychiatry, Yale University School of Medicine

Ryan Holt, PhD
Independent Scholar

Daniel Kardefelt-Winther, PhD
Department of Clinical Neuroscience, Karolinska Institute

Brian D. Kiluk, PhD
Yale University School of Medicine

Daniel L. King, PhD
College of Education, Psychology, & Social Work, Flinders University, Australia

Chih-Hung Ko, MD, PhD
Kaohsiung Medical University Hospital, Taiwan; Kaohsiung Municipal Hsiao-Kang Hospital, Taiwan; Substance and Behavior Addiction Research Center, Kaohsiung Medical University, Taiwan

Grace E. Kong, PhD
Yale University School of Medicine

Rachel Kowert, PhD
Research Director, Take *This*

Shane W. Kraus, PhD, MA, BA
University of Nevada, Las Vegas, Department of Psychology; UNLV School of Medicine

Daria J. Kuss, BA, MA, MSc, PhD
International Gaming Research Unit and Cyberpsychology Research Group, Psychology Department, Nottingham Trent University, UK

Debi A. LaPlante, PhD
Division on Addiction, Cambridge Health Alliance; Harvard Medical School

Hae Kook Lee, M.D, PhD
Department of Psychiatry, The Catholic University of Korea, Korea, Uijoengbu St. Mary's Hospital

Pietro J. Lynn, Esq
Lynn, Lynn, Blackman & Manitsky, P.C.

Dawn Delfin McDaniel, PhD
Quality for Youth

Jasmine Mena, PhD
Bucknell University

Joseph F. Meyer, PhD
VA Boston Healthcare System

James E. Mitchell, MD
University of North Dakota School of Medicine and Health Sciences

Isabelle Morris, MS
University of Tasmania

Frederick Muench, PhD
Northwell Health; The Partnership to End Addiction

Astrid Müller, MD, PhD
Department of Psychosomatic Medicine and Psychotherapy, Hannover Medical School, Hannover, Germany

Kai W. Müller, PhD
Outpatient Clinic for Behavioral Addictions, Department of Psychosomatic Medicine and Psychotherapy, University Medical Center of the Johannes Gutenberg-University Mainz, Germany

Sarah E. Nelson, PhD
Division on Addiction, Cambridge Health Alliance; Harvard Medical School

Stephanie S. O'Malley, PhD
Elizabeth Mears and House Jameson Professor, Department of Psychiatry, Yale School of Medicine

Matthew J. L. Page, PhD, ABN
AHN Behavioral Health Institute, Allegheny Health Network; Allegheny General Hospital

Halley M. Pontes, PhD, MSc
University of Tasmania, Australia; The International Cyberpsychology and Addictions Research Laboratory, University of Tasmania, Australia

Marc N. Potenza, MD, PhD
Connecticut Mental Health Center, Departments of Psychiatry, Neuroscience, and Child Study Center, Yale School of Medicine

James O. Prochaska, PhD
University of Rhode Island

Janice M. Prochaska, PhD
Prochaska Change Consultants

Sara Prot, PhD
School of Psychological, Social and Behavioural Sciences, Coventry University

Thorsten Quandt, PhD
Department of Communication, University of Münster, Germany

Sheida Rabipour, PhD
University of Ottawa; Douglas Hospital Research Centre; McGill University

Ardeshir S. Rahman, MSc
Bethink Labs; UCLA

Barbara O. Rothbaum, PhD, ABPP
Emory University School of Medicine

Hans-Jurgen Rumpf, PhD
Department of Psychiatry and Psychotherapy, University of Lübeck, Germany

Howard J. Shaffer, PhD
Morris E. Chafetz Associate Professor of Psychiatry in the Field of Behavioral Sciences, Harvard Medical School; Distinguished Faculty, Division on Addiction, The Cambridge Health Alliance

Saul Shiffman, PhD
University of Pittsburgh

Wendy K. Silverman, PhD, ABPP
Child Study Center, Yale University School of Medicine

Matthew J. Smith, PhD, MSW, MPE, LCSW
University of Michigan School of Social Work

Jasmine Turna, PhD
Department of Psychiatry and Behavioural Neurosciences, McMaster University, Canada

Federico E. Vaca, MD, MPH
Yale School of Medicine, Department of Emergency Medicine; Yale Developmental Neurocognitive Driving Simulation Research Center (DrivSim Lab)

Michael Van Ameringen, MD, FRCPC
Professor, McMaster University, Department of Psychiatry and Behavioural Neurosciences

Gerrit I. van Schalkwyk, MB, ChB
Department of Psychiatry and Human Behavior, Warren Alpert Medial School of Brown University

Susan B. Varga, MD
Dartmouth Hitchcock Medical Center

Rachel P. Vitale, BA
The Feinstein Institute for Medical Research at Northwell Health; Partnership for Drug-Free Kids

Seth W. Whiting, PhD
Central Michigan University

Klaus Wölfling, PhD
Outpatient Clinic for Behavioral Addictions, Department of Psychosomatic Medicine and Psychotherapy, University Medical Center of the Johannes Gutenberg-University Mainz, Germany

Stephanie Yarnell-Mac Grory, MD, PhD
Yale University School of Medicine, Department of Psychiatry; Warren Alpert School of Medicine at Brown University, Department of Psychiatry

Yvonne H. C. Yau, BS, MSc
McGill University

Ju-Yu Yen, MD, PhD
Kaohsiung Medical University Hospital, Taiwan; Kaohsiung Municipal Ta-Tung Hospital, Taiwan; Kaohsiung Medical University, Taiwan

Marat V. Zanov, PhD, ABPP, MBA
Madigan Army Medical Center

CONTENTS

Part Two • Impact of Internet and Technology Use: Major Conceptual Issues

Part Three • Potential Positive Impacts of Internet and Technology Use

Part Four • Potential Negative Impacts of Internet and Technology Use and Patterns of Use

Part Five • Treatment, Assessment, and Legal Considerations: Digital Technology Approaches

Part Six • Applications of Digital Technology to Promote Psychological Welfare and Health in Special Groups

Part Seven • Use of Digital Technologies to Treat Specific Disorders

Introduction to The Oxford Handbook of Digital Technologies and Mental Health

Marc N. Potenza, Kyle A. Faust, and David Faust

Over the past several decades we have witnessed revolutionary advances in digital technologies. The patterns and types of Internet use have changed rapidly, and these changes have been accompanied by tremendous opportunities for advances in human health as well as a number of potential negative consequences. In this book, we have assembled contributions from expert scholars around the world to cover topics related to digital technologies and mental health.

The aims of the edited book include providing an academically oriented and scientifically based description of how technological advances may have contributed to a wide range of mental health outcomes, covering the spectrum from problems and maladies to improved and expanded healthcare services. Considerable content is also intended to be of pragmatic value to those appraising, and considering or providing treatment to individuals engaging in possible problem use of various technologies and digital technologies. Such a book is needed given substantial changes in the availability and use of technologies (including computers, video games, smart phones, and other devices) for a broad range of activities (such as social networking, shopping, gambling, and viewing of pornography). Additionally, investigators have been studying the potential of using these devices and applications for the delivery of mental health care and various other health services. Rapid changes and expansion in the study, development, and impact of digital technology, and the absence of any comparable book focusing broadly on critical issues in the interface with health, and particularly mental health, creates a void this work is intended to help fill.

This book will cover these domains in 8 sections focusing on: 1) internet use and video-gaming in the general population, including international perspectives; 2) conceptual issues regarding the impact of Internet and digital technology use; 3) potential positive impacts of technology use and digital technology use; 4) potential negative impacts of technology use and digital technology use; 5) digital technology considerations involving treatment, assessments and legal issues; 6) applications of digital technologies to improve mental health; 7) use of digital technologies to treat specific disorders; and 8) treatment of problematic video-gaming and internet use.

In the section addressing internet use in the general population, chapters cover a range of topics. First, historical contexts are provided for internet use in general and video-gaming more specifically. Next, a chapter follows that focuses on youth and technology. Thereafter, sections cover internet use from international perspectives, including the United States, Europe, Australia, and several jurisdictions in Asia including South Korea, China, and Hong Kong. The first section concludes with a chapter addressing social networking, a behavior that has developed within the context of the internet.

The second section covering conceptual issues begins with a chapter describing debates about how best to define and classify problems relating to types and patterns of internet use. A chapter on the neurobiology, cognitive neuroscience and genetics of different forms of problematic internet use follows. The section concludes with a chapter addressing key conceptual issues in evaluating and refining measurement tools for assessing forms of problematic internet use.

The third and fourth sections address potential positive and negative impacts of digital technology usage. In the former section, the possible cognitive benefits of gaming and internet use are covered. The former section also includes a chapter devoted specifically to professional gaming, which addresses both the positive and negative aspects of this growing field. In the latter section, potential problems are reviewed in the areas of violence and videogames, shopping, gambling, sex and pornography viewing, distracted driving and cyber-bullying.

The fifth section addresses digital approaches to treatment, assessment and legal matters. Approaches afforded by digital technologies, including ecological momentary assessment, virtual reality training, and mobile applications are described. A chapter on legal and ethical considerations relating to remote treatment is also included.

In the sixth section, the application of digital technologies to address specific high-risk periods and promote mental health in specific groups is covered. This section includes chapters relating to post-partum health in women, adolescent health, risky behaviors in adults, cognitive enhancement in older adults, and cultural considerations regarding provision of mental health services via digital technologies.

In the penultimate section, digital technological approaches to treating specific psychiatric disorders are described. Chapters focus on anxiety disorders, alcohol-, tobacco- and other drug-use disorders, and gambling disorder. These chapters also describe multiple approaches including ones based on mindfulness and cognitive-behavioral therapy.

The final section addresses treatment outcomes to date with a focus on internet use more broadly and cognitive-behavioral therapy approaches to internet gaming disorder more specifically. Finally, a brief description of future directions is provided. Together, this volume addresses multiple important considerations in the rapidly changing area of the interfaces between digital technologies and mental health.

PART 1

Internet and Technology Use in the General Population

CHAPTER

1 Historical Context and Upcoming Developments in Digital Technologies

Daria J. Kuss, Daniel Kardefelt-Winther, *and* Joël Billieux

Abstract

This chapter focuses on the history of four important types of digital technology, including the Internet, digital games (all types of games played electronically), virtual reality, and smartphones (particularly smartphone apps). The authors present a varied and balanced view of different digital technologies, introducing their historical developments as well as an overview of potentially positive and negative applications of each of the technologies covered. Increased governmental support is required for research into digital technologies and those applications that have been established to have beneficial effects for users, but equal effort is also needed in developing new policy, educational, and legislative frameworks that are in tune with the needs of a digital society. Research into digital technology use and its context may enable better control of how interactions with digital technology continue to shape our behavior.

Keywords: digital technologies, Internet, digital games, virtual reality, smartphones

Introduction

This chapter focuses on the history of four important types of digital technology, including the Internet, digital games (all types of games played electronically), virtual reality, and smartphones (particularly smartphone apps). Our aim is not to be completely comprehensive because space limitations restrict us to include only a selected number of topics. However, we present a varied and well-balanced view of different digital technologies, drawing on their historical developments as well as on both the positive and negative applications of each of the technologies covered.

The Internet

History

The history of the Internet begins with the US Department of Defense's efforts to create computer networks for the purpose of military research in the 1960s and 1970s, resulting in the predecessor of the Internet, the Advanced Research Projects Agency's ARPANET (Rheingold, 1993). Following on from there, the origins of the World Wide Web as we know it today can be dated back to 1989, when Tim Berners-Lee, a scientist at the European Particle Physics Laboratory (CERN) in Geneva, Switzerland, considered efficient and expeditious ways for scientists to share information and work on collaborative projects. Accordingly, the World Wide Web was developed and contained (1) a pool of retrievable information, (2) an address system (universal resource identifiers [URIs]), (3) a network protocol (hypertext transfer protocol [HTTP]), and (4) a markup language (hypertext markup language [HTML]). URIs refer to the webpage "addresses." The HTTP transfers information, such as text, images, videos, etc., onto the screen. HTML is a computer language particularly developed for usage on web interfaces (Berners-Lee, Cailliau, Luotonen, Nielsen, & Secret, 1994). The High Performance Computing Act, signed in 1991, significantly contributed to rapid and global developments in computing technology and resulted in what is referred to as the "information superhighway," initially coined by visual artist Nam June Paik in 1974 (BBC News, 2012).

Virtual communities emerged early in the history of the Internet and have been propagated by writers such as Howard Rheingold as offering the possibility to "exchange pleasantries and argue, engage in intellectual discourse, conduct commerce, exchange knowledge, share emotional support, make plans, brainstorm, gossip, feud, fall in love, find friends and lose them, play games, flirt, create a little high art and a lot of idle talk" (Rheingold, 1993, p. 17). In essence, virtual communities offer members all the opportunities of real-life communities while being disembodied, including the psychological exploration of aspects of one's identity (Turkle, 1995). Subsequently, the development of new online technologies which allowed users to adapt and share content in an interactive and participatory fashion led to the creation of "web 2.0" (Jenkins, 2006). Web 2.0 was initially coined by DiNucci (1999) and was popularized by O'Reilly in the early 2000s (2005). Web 2.0 offers the framework for social media, allowing users to generate and share content (Kaplan & Haenlein, 2010) and led to the establishment of *collective intelligence* (indicating knowledge that is greater than the sum of its parts because it entails the possibility of sharing and interacting) (Lévy, 1997). Some have claimed that web 2.0 is now superseded by web 3.0 (Hempel, 2009) due to the growing emphasis on personalization (O'Brolchain et al., 2015).

Today, Internet use is widespread and large numbers of people have access to it both in Great Britain and worldwide (International Telecommunication Union, 2014; Internet Live Stats, 2014; Internet World Stats, 2014). Of British adults, 73% access the Internet every day (Office for National Statistics, 2013), and 74.4% of Americans have access to the Internet (File & Ryan, 2014), denoting the significance and ubiquity of this type of digital technology.

Positive Applications of Using the Internet

There are various positive applications of using the Internet, including in mental health, education, the military, communication, and global connectivity. Large-scale research including a representative sample of more than 20,000 participants from 13 different countries has indicated that, rather than contributing to loneliness among users, the Internet may have positive impacts on their social lives (Amichai-Hamburger & Hayat, 2011). The Internet has led to the establishment of a "global village" where everybody is connected to everybody else through the means of media (McLuhan, 1964).

In addition to this, the Internet allows users access to other individuals who share their interests, and this is of particular benefit to those who would otherwise have limited social contacts due to disabilities or caring responsibilities (Young, 1996). The inherent anonymity of the Internet furthermore offers the opportunity to explore different aspects of one's identity (Turkle, 1995) and may therefore have a liberating potential, given the disembodiment and consequent lack of potentially "judge-able" physical characteristics, such as age, gender, and ethnicity (Markham, 1998). The *New Yorker* cartoon of two dogs chatting to each other is a case in point, with one telling the other: "On the Internet, nobody knows you're a dog."

In terms of education, the Internet has offered many opportunities for students at various levels who can now virtually connect to each other via online campuses, thus revolutionizing learning and teaching on a global scale (Sharma & Maleyeff, 2003). It is noted however that, particularly in higher education institutions, social inclusion and actual participation (rather than access alone) need to be taken into consideration when developing modes of learning and engaging students with learning materials and with one another (David & Marc, 2003).

Furthermore, the Internet has come to be an important tool in the delivery of tailored treatment approaches, including online therapy, which is defined as "any type of professional therapeutic interaction that makes use of the Internet to connect qualified mental health professionals and their clients" (Rochlen, Zack, & Speyer, 2004, p. 270). Currently, online therapy is conducted via email or other Internet-delivered methods (Stofle, 2001), and a meta-analysis of trials indicates that it might complement or even function as an equivalent of real-life therapy (Andersson, Cuijpers, Carlbring, Riper, & Hedman, 2014; Yager, 2001). Its benefits include convenience, increased access, disinhibition, internalization, and reflection. However, a number of challenges have also been identified, and these relate to fewer modalities of communication, misreading information, time delay, skill deficiency, crisis intervention, cultural clashes, and security (Rochlen et al., 2004).

In addition to this, the Internet has supported the emergence of self-help groups for individuals suffering from various mental health conditions via accessible online support forums (Orgad, 2005). The Internet allows people with mental health problems to participate in supportive and anonymous online communities, which reduces barriers to communication about sensitive topics (Ybarra & Suman, 2006) such as physical (Leimeister, Schweizer, Leimeister, & Krcmar, 2008) and mental health (Leach, Christensen, Griffiths, Jorm, & Mackinnon, 2007). Webb et al. (2008) explored the potential dangers and risks of participation in mental health support forums and stressed the need to assess the effectiveness or potential dangers of online forums in mental health prevention and early intervention work and highlighted that there are caveats involved in using this form of mental health support. The Internet has furthermore contributed to accelerating the introduction of innovative services which benefit mental health patients. The National Healthcare System (NHS) in the United Kingdom offers an Expert Patients Programme (EPP), which is a self-management program for individuals with chronic conditions (NHS, 2015) and may make use of the propensities afforded by self-governed and self-regulated online forums.

Negative Applications of Using the Internet

Internet use may come at a price. There appear to be a number of negative consequences and repercussions that can come with using the Internet. Scholars have long warned about the potential dangers of using any form of new media, including books, the telephone, and television, which have since been disconfirmed (Eco, 1964), thus suggesting that fears associated with the Internet are similarly a passing fad (Giedd, 2012). However, it needs to be kept in mind that, unlike previous forms of media, the Internet offers a greater possibility of interactivity, which distinguishes it from earlier forms of media (Manovich, 2001).

Among others, Sherry Turkle (2011) noted how using the Internet may lead individuals to be "alone together": on the one hand, they are connected via technology, but, on the other hand, they are physically (and emotionally) disconnected. Research supports this view as it has been found that excessive Internet use can lead to loneliness (Ang, Chong, Chye, & Huan, 2012) and is associated with depression (Ceyhan & Ceyhan, 2008), insomnia (Cheung & Wong, 2011), anxiety (Dalbudak et al., 2013), and personality traits such as neuroticism and low agreeableness (Kuss, Griffiths, & Binder, 2013). Additionally, extraversion and conscientiousness appear as protective factors for Internet overuse (Kuss, van Rooij, Shorter, Griffiths, & van de Mheen, 2013).

Excessive Internet use has been shown to be associated with a number of behavioral outcomes traditionally associated with substance dependence (Kuss, Griffiths, Karila, & Billieux, 2014), namely salience, mood modification, tolerance, withdrawal, relapse, and conflict (Kuss, Shorter, van Rooij, Griffiths, & Schoenmakers, 2014), as well as neurobiological abnormalities in brain function and structure (Kuss & Griffiths, 2012c). Over the past few decades, many researchers have started to investigate the rising problem of Internet addiction, leading the American Psychiatric Association (APA) to consider including it as mental disorder in the fifth edition of the *Diagnostic and Statistical Manual for Mental Disorders* (DSM-5). This resulted in the inclusion of *Internet Gaming Disorder* in the third section of the DSM-5, which contains conditions that require further research for it to be officially accepted in the main manual (American Psychiatric Association, 2013). It appears that the Internet is too diverse a medium to warrant a comprehensive diagnosis for overuse—instead, research suggests online gaming is the most common online application used by individuals who experience addiction-like symptoms (Kuss & Griffiths, 2012b).

In addition to this, research suggests that the proliferation of Internet use may in some instances lead to cases of cyberbullying and cyberstalking as Internet use allows individuals to access information and contact others online, thus opening up possibilities for monitoring, pursuing, and harassing individuals. However, a representative European-wide study concluded that cyberbullying was not more common in countries where the Internet was more established, which suggests that cyberbullying is a new form of a long-established childhood problem rather than the consequence of digital technology (Livingstone, Haddon, Görzig, & Ólafsson, 2011). Cyberstalking is an online form of stalking perpetrated primarily via online means using emails, messaging, chats, forums, and social networking sites (Spitzberg & Hoobler, 2002). Cyberstalkers may contact their victims either directly or by proxy via their friends and family, sharing both accurate and contrived information about the victim, hacking their computer, and possibly even impersonating their victims. This can lead to severe psychological problems also associated with real-life stalking, such as posttraumatic stress disorder (PTSD), various anxiety disorders, and depression (Purcell, Pathé, & Mullen, 2004; Westrup, Fremouw, Thompson, & Lewis, 1999). Cyberstalking intersects with cyber-harrassment/cyberbullying due to the involvement of repeated engagement in behaviors that produce fear, safety concerns, and distress. Cyberstalking and cyberbullying differ in that cyberstalking typically takes place over extended time spans, relative to the shorter time spans in cyberbullying (Sheridan & Grant, 2007). Taken together, Internet use has made some behaviors more accessible and may have lowered the bar for engaging in ethically questionable behaviors due to the propensity of anonymity which may lead to online disinhibition (Suler, 2004).

Digital Games

History

Although there is considerable debate as to when the very first digital game was produced, commercial gaming arguably started with the release of the arcade version of Pong in 1972, a two-dimensional simulated tennis game created by the American company Atari (Donovan, 2010; Kent, 2001). Pong saw considerable commercial success, and, in 1975, it made it into households as an electronic device that people could connect to their televisions (Newman, 2002; Kent, 2001). This success was followed by the release of a number of well-known titles such as Taito's Space Invaders in 1978 and Namco's Pac-Man in 1980 (Kent, 2001). The popularity of these games helped establish digital gaming as a mainstream hobby. However, although the early successes of arcade games like Pong and Space Invaders paved the way for a proliferation of home gaming, first via consoles and later via computers, the arcade market ultimately fell behind and saw its profits decline rapidly from 1994 onward (Donovan, 2010).

Early computer games were typically based on simple 2D graphics or text only, which was the norm until Id Software released a new first-person shooter game called Wolfenstein 3D in 1992, followed by Doom in 1993. Doom marked a shift in the use of 3D graphics (Donovan, 2010; Lowood, 2008) and allowed for networked multiplayer gameplay. Id Software also allowed players to access Doom's source code and engine, which opened up possibilities for user-generated content. Access to the source code for major titles was unusual at the time, but enabled players to expand on the networked multiplayer mode to also allow online multiplayer gameplay (Donovan, 2010). Coinciding with increased public Internet access, this brought about a shift in gaming from being confined to a physical space to an activity also taking place online (mostly[1]) unconstrained by geographic location.

Ever since Doom, online multiplayer gameplay has remained a highly popular activity among gamers. The most popular games today tend to be multiplayer games, some of which do not even feature a single-player mode. At present, multiplayer online battle arenas (MOBA) seem to be the genre with the greatest amount of daily players, represented by games like DOTA2 and League of Legends: the latter game alone has more than 67 million people playing every month and 27 million playing every day (Riot Games, 2015). MOBAs have overtaken genres that were previously considered to be more popular, such as the massively multiplayer online role-playing game (MMORPG), typified by the game World of Warcraft, which musters around 10 million monthly players (Blizzard Entertainment, 2014).

MOBAs are also at the forefront of the rising e-Sports movement, which has turned the playing of certain computer games into a professionalized sport bearing many similarities to traditional sports and arguably boasting a greater following than some Olympic disciplines (Taylor, 2012). More than 11 million people watched live as two Korean teams battled in the finals of the 2014 League of Legends World Championships, and the prize pool for The International, the largest DOTA2 competition in 2015, has currently exceeded US$13 million, out of which 80% has been donated voluntarily by regular players. Against this background it may not come as a surprise that the video gaming industry is now reported to have exceeded the movie and music industries in terms of revenue and is expected by market analysts to reach a total revenue of US$93 billion by 2019 (PricewaterhouseCoopers, 2015).

Positive Applications

Playing digital games can be a highly creative activity. By releasing the source code for Doom, Id Software opened up a "modding" culture where the community could alter (or modify) the game as they pleased and create user-generated content. When Id Software released Quake, the successor to Doom, they also released the game engine with which the community was able to develop new, stand-alone games. An example of one such game is Team Fortress, which was created by a team of three avid Quake fans. Following major acclaim, Team Fortress was picked up by software publisher Valve and remade as a new commercial game, released in 1999 (Donovan, 2010). The release of Quake also provided players with a video recording feature so that they could share their gameplay with others. Rather than only recording gameplay however, this feature inspired a culture of movie-making in Quake, which is referred to as *machinima*; players staged scenes and played out scripts in the game and distributed their movies online (Lowood, 2008; Donovan, 2010). The popularity of user-generated content continued with the release of The Sims, a sandbox game featuring the home and life of characters controlled and directed by the player, as in a traditional dollhouse. The creators included a feature that allowed players to take photos of their characters and add a story, then publish the story on a website for others to read. Writing these stories became a means of self-expression for many players of The Sims, and, shortly after the official release of the game, more than 100,000 individual stories had been published online (Donovan, 2010).

As the sharing of user-generated content would suggest, digital games are highly social in nature and facilitate long-term friendship formation (Cole & Griffiths, 2007; Hussain & Griffiths, 2009; Kuss, 2013a). Gentile and colleagues (2009) showed in a summary of correlational, longitudinal, and experimental studies that playing pro-social games seemed to predict short-term and long-term increases in pro-social behaviors that transfer also to the non-gaming environment. Furthermore, Enevold (2012) argues based on qualitative work with children and families that playing games together has become an everyday practice in the home, increasing social interaction among family members. Importantly for people's well-being, cross-sectional and longitudinal evidence suggests that digital games may be particularly beneficial for people who are more introverted or lonely, or find it difficult to socialize face to face as these games can provide a safe environment for social interaction (Lemmens, Valkenburg, & Peter, 2011; McKenna & Bargh, 2000; McKenna, Green, & Gleason, 2002; Peter, Valkenburg, & Schouten, 2005).

In addition to fostering creativity and social interaction, there is considerable empirical evidence that playing games improves a wide range of cognitive skills (Granic, Lobel, & Engels, 2014). For example, experimental studies have showed that playing shooter/action games is associated with faster and more accurate attention allocation, higher spatial resolution in visual processing, and enhanced mental rotation abilities (Green & Bavelier, 2012). A meta-analysis concluded that improvements in spatial skills from playing shooter games are comparable to the effects of formal high-school and university-level courses aimed at enhancing the same skills and that these effects are obtained after a relatively brief period of playing, are persistent over time, and are transferrable to other contexts (Uttal et al., 2013). Additionally, longitudinal evidence showed that playing strategic video games was associated with improved problem-solving ability, which was associated with better academic grades (Adachi & Willoughby, 2013). However, this was not the case for those who played fighting or racing games, which indicates that the gaming context and motivations for playing might also influence the effects (e.g., Shen & Williams, 2011). Neuroscience evidence suggests that some of these cognitive advantages might be expressed in terms of measurable changes in neural processing and efficiency (Granic et al., 2014). In other words, adept gamers might learn to allocate attentional resources more efficiently and filter out disturbances more effectively (Bavelier, Achtman, Mani, & Focker, 2012).

In the healthcare sector, digital games have been investigated as a way to train medical professionals and patients, and they have various benefits in the context of physio- and psychotherapy (Griffiths, Kuss, & Ortiz de Gortari, 2013). Results have so far been promising and suggest that games may have some utility in improving surgical skills and health outcomes (Kato, 2010). Early studies showed that digital games could be successfully used for cognitive distraction in cancer patients during and prior to chemotherapy, resulting in decreases in reported nausea (Redd et al., 1987; Vasterling, Jenkins, Tope, & Burish, 1993). Digital games have also been used to reduce anxiety among surgery patients (Patel et al., 2006), to distract patients from pain (Hoffman et al., 2008; Sharar et al., 2007), to improve diabetes self-management behaviors (Brown et al., 1997) and to improve self-medication among cancer patients (Kato, Cole, Bradlyn, & Pollock, 2008). Research also showed that physicians who were avid gamers (play > 3 h/week) made fewer errors and performed at a faster rate in simulated laparoscopic procedures and suturing compared to non-playing counterparts (Rosser et al., 2007). Similar results have been replicated in a number of studies (e.g., Grantcharov, Bardram, Funch-Jensen, & Rosenberg, 2003; Shane, Pettitt, Morgenthal, & Smith, 2008). While these results are promising, it is as of yet unclear how to best leverage the full potential of digital games in healthcare, which opens up many avenues for future research in this area (Kato, 2010).

Negative Applications

In line with classic media and communications research (e.g., Blumler & Katz, 1974; Katz, Gurevitch, & Haas, 1973), it has been suggested that one of the main reasons for using different forms of media is to manage moods. While a number of studies have shown a causal relation between playing a preferred game and increases in positive emotion (Russoniello,

O'Brien, & Parks, 2009; Ryan, Rigby, & Przybylski, 2006), playing games to manage moods might also have a negative impact on well-being (Kardefelt-Winther, 2014a, 2014b; Kuss, Louws, & Wiers, 2012). It is possible that some people might come to depend too much on digital games to keep their negative thoughts at bay, followed by repeated excessive use and a neglect of other important things in life (Kardefelt-Winther, 2014b, 2015). This is why playing games to manage moods has been proposed as an indication of *Internet Gaming Disorder* (American Psychiatric Association, 2013) and suggests that mood management via digital games, while positive for some, might not be a suitable strategy for everyone. Excessive use of digital games has been associated with a great number of negative health outcomes (for comprehensive reviews, see Kuss and Griffiths, 2012a, 2012b, 2012c) but more research is needed to determine the direction of these associations, whether they are direct or indirect effects, and whether they persist over time (Griffiths et al., 2015).

While games are a healthy source of social interaction that foster long-term friendship formation (Cole & Griffiths, 2007; Hussain & Griffiths, 2009), a report from the Pew Internet & American Life Project (Lenhart et al., 2008) also suggests that teenagers frequently encounter anti-social behavior while gaming with others. Anti-social behavior in games typically refers to behavior that intends to ruin the experience of others either via disruptive interactions in the game world, such as scamming and cheating, or by personal insults (Lin & Sun, 2005). Although research in this area is scarce, attention is likely to increase as the player bases of multiplayer games continue to grow. For example, the producers of League of Legends saw the need to implement a player-run justice system in response to increased anti-social behavior among their players (Kou & Nardi, 2013). Research suggests that anti-social behavior in games is more frequent among skilled, younger male gamers with a decreased sense of responsibility for their in-game character (Bowman, Schultheiss, & Schumann, 2012). Such behaviors are thought to be facilitated by the anonymity that online games afford (Chen, Duh, & Ng, 2009) and may be attributed to online disinhibition (Joinson, 1998).

Finally, it needs to be mentioned that there is a persistent debate around whether violent digital games increase aggressive behavior, with a range of studies indicating support for this claim (e.g., Anderson et al., 2010). However, opponents argue that these studies suffer from severe methodological weaknesses and produce unreliable results, while pointing to additional studies showing that no video game effects on aggressive behaviors exist (e.g., Ferguson, 2007; Ferguson & Kilburn, 2010). This debate is much too broad to recount here, but, after two decades of research, the debate is still ongoing and disagreements seem to revolve around the ecological validity of different operationalization's of "aggressive behavior."

Virtual Reality

History

Virtual reality (VR) refers to any computer or multimedia environment that individuals can participate and feel present in. *Presence*, in this respect, can be defined as a "psychological state or subjective perception in which even though part of or all of an individual's current experience is generated by and/or filtered through human-made technology, part or all of the individual's perception fails to accurately acknowledge the role of the technology in the experience" (International Society for Presence Research, 2000). The idea of VR was first introduced by Sutherland in 1965, as he intended to "make that [virtual] world in the window look real, sound real, feel real, and respond realistically to the viewer's actions" (Sutherland, 1965). Accordingly, in the early 1960s, the multisensory simulator called Sensorama was created, consisting of a film that integrated different sensory experiences (namely, sound, scent, wind, and vibration); however, it lacked interactivity. Soon thereafter, the Sword of Damocles was introduced, the first VR hardware system and the first head-mounted display (HMD) allowing for head movement tracking. In 1975, the artificial reality environment Videoplace was developed, allowing users to interact with one another using image processing. In 1982, a *visually coupled airborne systems simulator* (VCASS) was created, and, using an HMD, individuals partook in flight simulations (Mazuryk & Gervautz, 1996). In the mid-1980s, the *virtual visual environment display* (VIVED) was created by the NASA Ames Research Center, consisting of a multisensory and interactive HMD interface that lets users engage with a 360-degree virtual environment (Fisher, McGreevy, Humphries, & Robinett, 1986).

At the same time, the first VR company, VPL, headed by Jaron Lanier, presented another significant development in VR technology, the DataGlove and the DataSuit, a motion-tracking system that included an HMD (the EyePhone—doesn't this sound vaguely familiar?) and RB2 (Reality Built for Two), a VR system that two individuals could use simultaneously. On June 7, 1989, VPL announced "Virtual Reality Day," a clever marketing strategy for their now personalized and computer-based RB2 system Autodesk VR CAD (computer-aided design). Lanier has been since credited with the conception of the term "virtual reality" as a materialization of "cyberspace" (Lowood, 2015). "Cyberspace" itself was coined by William Gibson in his famous science-fiction novel *Neuromancer* (Gibson, 1984), setting the framework for popular movies depicting dystopian simulated futures, such as the cult classic *The Matrix*, directed by the Wachowskis. The late 1980s and early 1990s saw a boom in the blossoming VR industry, with many VR companies founded; however, the initial explosive appeal gradually waned, leaving companies to create VR applications for lower key location-based technologies (rather than personal applications), including video games, arcades, and theme park rides that produced increasingly immersive experiences (Lowood, 2015).

In 1992, the *computer automatic virtual environment* (CAVE) Automatic Virtual Environment was introduced, topping the heretofore popular HMD displays because the CAVE allowed users to navigate an actual virtual world consisting of a cubicle that projects stereoscopic images onto its walls, thus visualizing a more immersive VR environment. Finally, *augmented reality* (AR) emerged, which uses an HMD and allows users to integrate their perception of reality with a superimposed virtual add-on consisting of graphics, data, and objects (Mazuryk & Gervautz, 1996). This development recently culminated in Google introducing Google Glass, a fashionable wearable computer based on *peripheral head-mounted technology* (PHMD) initially designed for personal use (Matthies, Haescher, Alm, & Urban, 2015). Its sale was quickly discontinued in early 2015, however, with the company continuing its work on improved versions of Google Glass with a new developer team, according to Google. However, various criticisms by users and other stakeholders appear to have contributed to the discontinuation of sales as concerns regarding lack of promised development, privacy, and safety were raised (Cellan-Jones, 2015).

More recent developments have seen the emergence of Oculus Rift, developed by Oculus VR, a VR HMD designed for immersive gaming experiences and considered "the first really professional PC-based VR headset" (Shanklin, 2015). Facebook has recently bought the Virtual Reality technology company Oculus for US$2 billion (Cellan-Jones, 2014) so that Facebook users can actively engage in creating new experiences with their Facebook friends rather than merely sharing them (Zuckerberg, 2014).

With a view to the future, recent developments have led to the suggestion that a convergence of VR and social networks (VRSN) may take place in such a way that social networks would allow users to directly interact with their friends via realistically represented avatars of themselves within the established immersive virtual environments, effectively leading to lives being lived online. This may potentially revolutionize important services, such as healthcare (O'Brolchain et al., 2015), but may also have implications for tourism and other leisure activities.

Media have been integral to human lives ever since the conception of the printing press. Already in 1964, Marshall McLuhan understood media as extensions of man, denoting the impact of media (rather than their content) on society as "the medium becomes the message" (McLuhan, 1964). Along these lines, digital technologies may not only be beneficial for purposes of social engagement, education, and mental health, but they also appear relevant from a more fundamental perspective as they become the actual means by which we experience, engage with, and reconfigure reality. Scholars claim that we move from a variety of "virtual realities" to a culture of "real virtuality," "a system in which reality itself (that is people's material/symbolic existence) is entirely captured, fully immersed in a virtual image setting, in the world of make believe, in which appearances are not just on the screen through which experience is communicated, but they become the experience" (Castells, 1996, p. 404).

Positive Applications

VR has been successfully applied in the context of mental health, and its implementations include treatment approaches for a number of mental disorders (Griffiths et al., 2013). *VR exposure therapy* (VRET) is a form of cognitive-behavioral therapy (CBT) that uses the intersection between in vivo and imaginal therapy as it takes place in virtual environments that have been designed specifically to treat various mental conditions. Different types of technology are used, including an HMD consisting of glasses and speakers worn by the individual. Alternatively, an immersive CAVE, a virtual cubicle allowing the individual to move freely via an electromagnetic tracking system, can be used. Research also indicates that 150-degree screens (semi-immersive interfaces) and common desktop computers are useful devices for delivering VRET (Tichon &

Banks, 2006). Individuals receiving this form of treatment feel present within the mediated environments, and the treatment of anxiety disorders often utilizes effective exposure to anxiety-provoking situations and stimuli (Krijn, Emmelkamp, Olafsson, & Biemond, 2004).

Positive results of applying VRET have been found for acrophobia (Krijn, Emmelkamp, Biemond, et al., 2004), claustrophobia (Botella, Banos, Villa, Perpina, & Garcia-Palacios, 2000), panic disorder with agoraphobia (Vincelli et al., 2003), fear of flying (Rothbaum, Hodges, Smith, Lee, & Price, 2000), driving phobia (Wald & Taylor, 2000), spider phobia (Garcia-Palacios, Hoffman, Carlin, Furness, & Botella, 2002), social phobia (Roy et al., 2003), and PTSD (Rothbaum, Hodges, Ready, Graap, & Alarcon, 2001; Wiederhold & Wiederhold, 2010). A meta-analysis comparing VRET with control and in vivo therapy conditions revealed VRET is efficient in treating anxiety disorders and even outperforms the golden standard of therapy—in vivo procedures—in efficacy (Powers & Emmelkamp, 2008).

Negative Applications

Alongside various positive applications of VR technologies, their rapid development may come at a price. Researchers have identified a number of concerns, including privacy and autonomy. Regarding privacy, three main concerns appear. First, *informational privacy* denotes privacy of one's personal records, thoughts, and communications from access by third parties, and online data are more vulnerable to being accessed, distributed, and misused online. Second, *physical privacy* refers to privacy of one's physical being and actions (e.g., bodily integrity) from access by third parties, and breaches are on the rise given the prevalence of recording devices, unintended revelation of physical information, and lack of anonymity. Finally, *associational privacy* relates to third-party access to one's social interactions, which are freely available through online socializing using various channels. Participation in VR environments may pose threats to each of these as a wealth of personal information accumulated using virtual technologies may become easily available (and distributable, sellable) by third parties (O'Brolchain et al., 2015).

In addition to privacy concerns, problems regarding the individual's autonomy (i.e., "self-government") may arise via threats to knowledge, freedom, and authenticity. Threats to knowledge may derive from technological filters, "cyberbalkanisation" (i.e., users having access to particular sites only), and gatekeepers (including prominent search engines but also particular governments) who may or may not make required information accessible and/or censor it (O'Brolchain et al., 2015). Various countries have limited citizens' access to the Internet, including China (Reporters Without Borders, 2012). Threats to freedom may derive from addiction to using technology (which is in line with the APA's efforts to include Internet Gaming Disorder in the updated diagnostic manual) or from governments limiting individuals' freedoms and manipulating them to behave in certain ways. Finally, threats to authenticity may entail the propagation of social conformity (i.e., peer pressures to abide by certain "norms" may be established and maintained via technology), becoming an "experience machine" that leads a virtual life rather than a real life, and shallowness due to overengagement and overreliance on technology for decision-making (O'Brolchain et al., 2015). One can claim that privacy and autonomy concerns are applicable to most modern technologies, including the Internet. However, in the context of VR environments, these dangers may become exacerbated as physical dimensions are added to the initially exclusively virtual dimension, thus adding to the threats to privacy and individual autonomy.

Mobile Phones and Smartphones

History

Mobile communication operates through the connection to a mobile network provided by a mobile phone operator, allowing access to the public telephone network. Although the first mobile phones were limited to telephony and text/picture messaging (SMS and MMS), the latest generations of mobile phones (smartphones) support a wide range of other functions, such as emailing and Internet access, short-range wireless communications (e.g., Bluetooth), gaming and gambling, business applications, social networking, photography, or geo-localization (e.g., GPS). With the continuous development of new hardware devices and mobile software and applications, mobile phones are becoming the most used technology in human history. As an example, in most Asian and European countries, there are more mobile phone subscriptions than inhabitants. As a corollary of its ubiquity, mobile phone–related research developed exponentially over the past 20 years, transcending individual research fields (e.g., ergonomics, psychology, sociology, law, business, medicine). Indeed, according to Yan and Chen (2015), approximately 4,000 peer-reviewed articles published from 1991 to 2013 investigated different types of human behaviors in using mobile phones.

The first prototype of a handheld mobile phone (which weighted around 4.5 pounds) was developed in 1973 by Motorola. Then first commercial mobile network was initiated in Japan in 1979. The next step was the creation of the Nordic Mobile Telephone, in 1981, which was simultaneously launched in several countries in Northern Europe (Finland, Norway, Denmark, and Sweden). Following these initial networks, others countries progressively launched their own cellular networks. This first generation of mobile networks (1G) was still using analog transmission. In 1990s, the second generation of mobile networks (2G) emerged, which used digital instead of analog transmission. The dissemination of this new system resulted in a rise of mobile phone use and the emergence of prepaid mobile communication. The third generation of mobile phone systems (3G) appeared in 2001, in the context of an increasing demand for greater data speeds. The high connection speeds characterizing 3G technology resulted in important changes for the industry (e.g., facilitation of Internet surfing on the mobile phone). A few years later, it had become clear that 3G networks were overwhelmed by the increased use of bandwidth-intensive applications, such as streaming media or online games. This led to the development and launching of the fourth generation of networks (4G). The 4G system, launched in 2007 in South Korea and available in Europe since 2012, is now disseminated worldwide.

Along with blossoming research regarding the influence of mobile phones on human behavior, a constantly increasing number of studies are conducted to disentangle the positive and negative consequences associated with mobile phone use.

Positive Applications

Positive outcomes were initially restricted to the optimization of communication (Geser, 2004). Initial research thus emphasized how mobile phone communication can promote communication at the individual level (e.g., via the enlargement of the number of potential communication partners), but also at the collective level (e.g., via the improvement of the efficacy of rescues services). It is however interesting to note that, from a social point of view, the mobile phone may change from the status of an instrument that promotes social exchanges to an object that interferes with face-to-face social communication (Jauréguiberry, 1998; Nickerson, Isaac, & Mak, 2008). Indeed, the use of mobile phones is today perceived as impolite or asocial in certain contexts (e.g., restaurants, libraries, theaters) and is also more frequently banned in public spaces, such as in commuting networks, and administrations.

A growing number of researchers emphasized the benefits of mobile communication in terms of health-related and behavior change interventions and applications. In particular, the efficacy of mobile phone interventions based on text message delivery to promote healthy behaviors was evidenced in different contexts, such as the self-management of diabetes, physical activity, diet, or smoking cessation (Blake, 2008; Fjeldsoe, Marshall, & Miller, 2009; Heather & Kershaw, 2010). Mobile phone–based interventions are easy to disseminate at a large scale (e.g., to reach people who would not necessarily have asked for help in a traditional face-to-face situation), can be individually tailored (e.g., adjusting to one's schedule, obligations, or objectives), and allow instant delivery, whereas they also offer the possibility to respond asynchronously. These characteristics make mobile communication a channel of choice to deliver health behavior interventions. Importantly, the last generation of mobile phone–based interventions can be supported by specific smartphone applications, which increases their potential (i.e., the intervention no longer only relies on instant messaging or emails) and makes them more ergonomic and customizable (see Heffner, Vilardaga, Mercer, Kientz, & Bricker, 2015, for an example in the context of smoking cessation). Recent research also emphasized the usefulness of smartphones to assist self-help–based psychotherapies (e.g., self-monitoring of psychopathological symptoms, psycho-education) (Shapiro et al., 2010; Watts et al., 2013). It appears, however, that such types of interventions are especially adapted to CBT and related therapies and have proved less effective in supporting other psychotherapeutic approaches, such as interpersonal therapies (Dagöö et al., 2014). However, despite mobile phone–based interventions appearing acceptable and feasible (even for severe disorders such as those of the schizophrenia spectrum), the early state of current research and the inconsistency of existing results preclude any definitive conclusions regarding their efficacy (Alvarez-Jimenez et al., 2014). Finally, it is worth noting that, as shown earlier in this chapter, it has been suggested that some cognitive functions (perceptual, attentional, and visuomotor skills) can be enhanced by the practice of video games (Green & Bavelier, 2012; Griffiths et al., 2013), which undoubtedly opens up new perspectives for mobile phone–based interventions.

Negative Applications

On the other side, the negative consequences resulting from mobile phone use have also received growing scientific attention during the past decade (see Billieux, 2012; Billieux, Maurage, Lopez-Fernandez, Kuss, & Griffiths, 2015, for reviews). Negative outcomes associated with dysfunctional mobile phone use include (but are not limited to) self-reported dependence and addiction-like symptoms (Bianchi & Phillips, 2005; Billieux, Van der Linden, & Rochat, 2008), financial problems (Billieux et al., 2008), risky driving (White, Eiser, & Harris, 2004), use in prohibited areas (Nickerson et al., 2008), sleep interference (Thomée, Harenstam, & Hagberg, 2011), or cyberbullying (Nicol & Fleming, 2010). Mobile phone use has also been related to potentially but not necessarily harmful behaviors such as *sexting* (i.e., exchanging sexually suggestive pictures or messages via mobile phones; Dir, Cyders, & Coskunpinar, 2013). Importantly, the physical health consequences of prolonged mobile phone use remain understudied, although some preliminary evidence reports increased risk of meningioma in heavy mobile phone users (Carlberg & Hardell, 2015).

Dysfunctional (or excessive) mobile phone use has generally been conceptualized as a behavioral addiction that shares many features with more established drug addictions. However, to date, the evidence supporting dysfunctional mobile phone use as an addictive disorder is scarce, and studies are lacking that identify behavioral and neurobiological similarities between mobile phone "addiction" and other types of established addictive behaviors (Billieux et al., 2015). Nonetheless, previous research emphasized that mobile phone addiction-like symptoms are frequently displayed by individuals presenting high impulsivity traits, elevated anxiety and depression, poor self-esteem, insecure attachment, or increased emotional instability (Billieux, 2012). Recently, and notwithstanding limited evidence regarding its etiology, dysfunctional mobile phone use has raised sufficient concerns among health professionals for being viewed as a potential public health problem. For example, in 2014, the World Health Organization (WHO) organized a meeting to discuss the public health implications and excessive behaviors associated with the use of information and communication technology, including mobile phones and smartphones.

Conclusion

It is clear that the rise of digital technology has had a fundamental impact on society, and it now serves an important function in everyday life. As this chapter has illustrated, it is also clear that the ways in which we engage with digital technology can have a significant impact on our health and well-being. It is less clear, however, whether these changes are ultimately positive or negative—in fact, based on the evidence reviewed here, it seems likely to be a bit of both. Despite decades of research into the positive and negative effects of digital technology on health and well-being, there are still a number of fundamental questions that remain unanswered. One such question, which was raised in this chapter, is the question of whether digital technology makes us more or less social. Are we alone together, as Sherry Turkle would suggest, or are we in fact enjoying a wider social space than ever before? While there is considerable evidence suggesting the latter, it is important also to remember that digital technologies such as the Internet have essentially reconfigured what it means to be social. This has implications for how social behaviors need to be studied, but it also highlights that it might be too soon yet to determine whether the long-term effects of digital technology are truly positive or negative. Until we are better able to understand, precisely, how society has been reconfigured by digital technology, it will be difficult to draw conclusions about the outcomes. Research has outlined the importance of understanding online and technology-assisted behaviors in the context of the individual, the respective technology, and the culture the behavior takes place in (Kuss, 2013b). Without contextualization, a comprehensive understanding of positive and negative applications of digital technology cannot be built.

Accordingly, it might be worth considering that a focus on positive and negative effects may not be the optimal way to approach research on digital technologies and their impact on behavior and well-being in the future. It might be more worthwhile to ask what changes digital technology has brought to society and from there on assess what the consequences of these changes might be without necessarily passing judgment in terms of their positive and negative effects. Therefore, contextualization of technology-supported behaviors is indispensable to carry research in the area forward. As the sections on Internet use and digital games discussed, both the act of playing games and being addicted to them might bring about changes in the brain (Kuss & Griffiths, 2012c) and cognitive functioning (Griffiths et al., 2013). However, rather than focusing on whether these changes are positive or negative, it might be more useful to investigate why they occur and what we might do to hinder or facilitate certain changes.

This chapter has discussed a number of situations where we might wish to prevent changes in behavior (such as Internet addiction) and facilitate other changes (such as improvements to cognitive ability and physicians' surgical skills; Griffiths et al., 2013). As the section on medical applications for games suggested, digital technology has the potential to contribute to better healthcare, but its full potential has yet to be discovered. Instead of focusing research on isolating the positive and negative effects of digital technology, we suggest a shift in focus onto the processes through and contexts in which such effects may occur. This may lead us toward a future where we can forestall undesirable changes in behavior by inhibiting processes involved in risk behaviors, including raising awareness of potential dangers and harm and facilitating prevention efforts on public policy and education levels.

At the same time, desirable changes should be enabled by facilitating other processes related to improved psycho-, social, and cognitive skills, as well as strengthening of digital literacies. This can possibly be accomplished through evidence-based education of the general public and increased efforts to empower parents as informed and critical technology users, which is crucial to enable children as competent users. These efforts require increased governmental support of research into the digital technologies and applications that have been established to have beneficial effects for users, as recounted in this chapter, but also into the development of new policy, educational, and legislative frameworks that are in tune with the needs of a digital society. Research into digital technology use and its context may enable better control of how the interactions with digital technology continue to shape our behavior.

Note

1. Before high-speed broadband was introduced, geographic location was still relevant because slower Internet connections produced higher latency in the commands sent to and from the game, thus giving certain players a disadvantage.

References

Adachi, P. J., & Willoughby, T. (2013). More than just fun and games: The longitudinal relationships between strategic video games, selfreported problem solving skills, and academic grades. *Journal of Youth and Adolescence, 42*, 1041–52.

Alvarez-Jimenez, A., Alcazar-Corcoles, M. A., Gonzàlez-Blanch, C., Bendall, S., McGorry, P. D., & Gleeson, J. F. (2014). Online, social media and mobile technologies for psychosis treatment: A systematic review on novel user-led interventions. *Schizophrenia Research, 156*, 96–106.

American Psychiatric Association. (2013). *Diagnostic and statistical manual of mental disorders (DSM-5)*. Arlington, VA: American Psychiatric Association.

Amichai-Hamburger, Y., & Hayat, Z. (2011). The impact of the Internet on the social lives of users: A representative sample from 13 countries. *Computers in Human Behavior, 27*, 585–89.

Anderson, C. A., Shibuya, A., Ihori, N., Swing, E. L., Bushman, B. J., Sakamoto, A., et al. (2010). Violent video game effects on aggression, empathy, and prosocial behavior in Eastern and Western countries: A meta-analytic review. *Psychological Bulletin, 136*, 151–73.

Andersson, G., Cuijpers, P., Carlbring, P., Riper, H., & Hedman, E. (2014). Guided Internet-based vs. face-to-face cognitive behavior therapy for psychiatric and somatic disorders: A systematic review and meta-analysis. *World Psychiatry, 13*, 288–95.

Ang, R. P., Chong, W. H., Chye, S., & Huan, V. S. (2012). Loneliness and generalized problematic Internet use: Parents' perceived knowledge of adolescents' online activities as a moderator. *Computers in Human Behavior, 28*, 1342–47.

Bavelier, D., Achtman, R. L., Mani, M., & Focker, J. (2012). Neural bases of selective attention in action video game players. *Vision Research, 61*, 132–43.

BBC News. (2012). Visual artist Nam June Paik predicted Internet age. http://www.bbc.co.uk/news/magazine-20649028

Berners-Lee, T., Cailliau, R., Luotonen, A., Nielsen, H. F., & Secret, A. (1994). The world-wide web. *Communications of the ACM, 37*, 907–12.

Bianchi, A., & Phillips, J. G. (2005). Psychological predictors of problem mobile phone use. *Cyberpsychology & Behavior, 8*, 39–51.

Billieux, J. (2012). Problematic mobile phone use: A literature review and a pathways model. *Current Psychiatry Reviews, 8*, 299–307.

Billieux, J., Maurage, P., Lopez-Fernandez, O., Kuss, D. J., & Griffiths, M. D. (2015). Can disordered mobile phone use be considered a behavioral addiction? An update on current evidence and a comprehensive model for future research *Current Addiction Reports, 2*, 156–62.

Billieux, J., Van der Linden, M., & Rochat, L. (2008). The role of impulsivity in actual and problematic use of the mobile phone. *Applied Cognitive Psychology, 22*, 1195–10.

Blake, H. (2008). Innovation in practice: Mobile phone technology in patient care. *British Journal of Community Nursing, 13*, 160–65.

Blizzard Entertainment. (2014). World of Warcraft surpasses 10 million subscribers as Warlords of Draenor launch begins. http://blizzard.gamespress.com/world-of-warcraft-surpasses-10-million-subscribers-as-warlords-of-drae

Blumler, J., & Katz, E. (1974). *The uses of mass communications*. Beverly Hills, CA: Sage.

Botella, C., Banos, R. M., Villa, H., Perpina, C., & Garcia-Palacios, A. (2000). Virtual reality in the treatment of claustrophobic fear: A controlled, multiple-baseline design. *Behavior Therapy, 31*(3), 583–95.

Bowman, N. D., Schultheiss, D., & Schumann, C. (2012). "I'm attached, and I'm a good guy/gal!": How character attachment influences pro- and anti-social motivations to play MMORPGs. *CyberPsychology, Behavior, and Social Networking, 15*, 169–74.

Brown, S. J., Lieberman, D. A., Germeny, B. A., Fan, Y. C., Wilson, D. M., & Pasta, D. J. (1997). Educational video game for juvenile diabetes: Results of a controlled trial. *Medical Informatics, 22*, 77–89.

Carlberg, M., & Hardell, L. (2015). Pooled analysis of Swedish case-control studies during 1997–2003 and 2007–2009 on meningioma risk associated with the use of mobile and cordless phones. *Oncology Reports, 33,* 3093–98.

Castells, M. (1996). *The rise of the network society.* Oxford: Blackwell.

Cellan-Jones, R. (2014). Facebook buys the future. BBC News. http://www.bbc.co.uk/news/technology-26746694

Cellan-Jones, R. (2015). Google Glass sales halted but firm says kit is not dead. BBC News. http://www.bbc.co.uk/news/technology-30831128

Ceyhan, A. A., & Ceyhan, E. (2008). Loneliness, depression, and computer self-efficacy as predictors of problematic internet use. *Cyberpsychology & Behavior, 11,* 699–701.

Chen, V., Duh, H., & Ng, C. (2009). Players who play to make others cry: The influence of anonymity and immersion. In *Proceedings of the International Conference on Advances in Computer Entertainment Technology* (ACE 2009), pp. 341–44.

Cheung, L. M., & Wong, W. S. (2011). The effects of insomnia and internet addiction on depression in Hong Kong Chinese adolescents: An exploratory cross-sectional analysis. *Journal of Sleep Research, 20,* 311–17.

Cole, H., & Griffiths, M. D. (2007). Social interactions in massively multiplayer online role-playing gamers. *Cyberpsychology & Behavior, 10,* 575–83.

Dagöö, J., Asplund, R. P., Bsenko, H. A., Hjerling, S., Holmberg, A., Westh, S., et al. (2014). Cognitive behavior therapy versus interpersonal psychotherapy for social anxiety disorder delivered via smartphone and computer: A randomized controlled trial. *Journal of Anxiety Disorders, 28,* 410–17.

Dalbudak, E., Evren, C., Aldemir, S., Coskun, K. S., Ugurlu, H., & Yildirim, F. G. (2013). Relationship of internet addiction severity with depression, anxiety, and alexithymia, temperament and character in university students. *Cyberpsychology, Behavior and Social Networking, 16*(4), 272–78.

David, T., & Marc, F. (2003). Widening access and participation in UK higher education. *International Journal of Educational Management, 17,* 26–36.

DiNucci, D. (1999). Fragmented future. *Print, 53,* 32.

Dir, A. L., Cyders, M. A., & Coskunpinar, A. (2013). From the bar to the bed via mobile phone: A first test of the role of problematic alcohol use, sexting, and impulsivity-related traits in sexual hookups. *Computers in Human Behavior, 29,* 1664–70.

Donovan, T. (2010). *Replay: The history of video games.* East Sussex, UK: Yellow Ant.

Eco, U. (1964). *Apocalypse postponed.* London: Flamingo.

Enevold, J. (2012). *Domesticating play, designing everyday life: The practice and performance of family gender, and gaming.* Paper presented at the Proceedings of 2012 DiGRA Nordic. Tampere: University of Tampere.

Ferguson, C., & Kilburn, J. (2010). Much ado about nothing: The misestimation and overinterpretation of violent video game effects in Eastern and Western nations: Comment on Anderson et al. (2010). *Psychological Bulletin, 136,* 174–78.

Ferguson, C. J. (2007). The good, the bad and the ugly: A meta-analytic review of positive and negative effects of violent video games. *Psychiatric Quarterly, 78,* 309–16.

File, T., & Ryan, C. (2014). *Computer and Internet use in the United States: 2013* (pp. 1–16). Washington, DC: US Department of Commerce, US Census Bureau.

Fisher, S. S., McGreevy, M., Humphries, J., & Robinett, W. (1986). *Virtual environment display system.* Paper presented at the ACM 1986 Workshop on Interactive 3D graphics. Chapel Hill, North Carolina.

Fjeldsoe, B. S., Marshall, A. L., & Miller, Y. D. (2009). Behavior change interventions delivered by mobile telephone short-message service. *American Journal of Preventive Medicine, 36,* 165–73.

Garcia-Palacios, A., Hoffman, H., Carlin, A., Furness, T. A., & Botella, C. (2002). Virtual reality in the treatment of spider phobia: A controlled study. *Behaviour Research and Therapy, 40,* 983–93.

Gentile, D. A., Anderson, C. A., Yukawa, S., Ihori, N., Saleem, M., Lim Kam Ming, et al. (2009). The effects of prosocial video games on prosocial behaviors: International evidence from correlational, longitudinal, and experimental studies. *Personality and Social Psychology Bulletin, 35,* 752–63.

Geser, H. (2004). *Toward a sociological theory of the mobile phone.* Soziologisches Institut der Universität Zürich. Zürich. http://socio.ch/mobile/t_geser1.htm

Gibson, W. (1984). *Neuromancer.* London: Voyager.

Giedd, J. N. (2012). The digital revolution and adolescent brain evolution. *Journal of Adolescent Health, 51,* 101–105.

Granic, I., Lobel, A., & Engels, R. (2014). The benefits of playing video games. *American Psychologist, 69,* 66–78.

Grantcharov, T., Bardram, L., Funch-Jensen, P., & Rosenberg, J. (2003). Impact of hand dominance, gender, and experience with computer games on performance in virtual reality laparoscopy. *Surgical Endoscopy, 17,* 1082–85.

Green, C. S., & Bavelier, D. (2012). Learning, attentional control, and action video games. *Current Biology, 22,* 197–206.

Griffiths, M. D., Kuss, D. J., & Ortiz de Gortari, A. (2013). Videogames as therapy: A review of the medical and psychological literature. In I. M. Miranda & M. M. Cruz-Cunha (Eds.), *Handbook of research on ICTs for healthcare and social services: Developments and applications* (pp. 43–68). Hershey, PA: IGI Global.

Griffiths, M. D., van Rooij, A., Kardefelt-Winther, D., Starcevic, V., Király, O., Pallesen, S., et al. (2015). Working towards an international consensus on criteria for assessing Internet Gaming Disorder: A critical commentary on Petry et al. (2014). *Addiction, 111,* 167–175.

Heather, C.-L., & Kershaw, T. (2010). Text messaging as a tool for behavior change in disease prevention and management. *Epidemiologic Reviews, 32,* 56–69.

Heffner, J. L., Vilardaga, R., Mercer, L. D., Kientz, J. A., & Bricker, J. B. (2015). Feature-level analysis of a novel smartphone application for smoking cessation. *American Journal of Drug and Alcohol Abuse, 41,* 68–73.

Hempel, J. (2009). Web 2.0 is over. Welcome to web 3.0. *Fortune, 159,* 36.

Hoffman, H. G., Patterson, D. R., Seibel, E., Soltani, M., Jewett-Leahy, L., & Sharar, S. R. (2008). Virtual reality pain control during burn wound debridement in the hydrotank. *Clinical Journal of Pain, 24,* 299–304.

Hussain, Z., & Griffiths, M. D. (2009). The attitudes, feelings, and experiences of online gamers: A qualitative analysis. *CyberPsychology & Behavior, 12,* 747–53.

International Society for Presence Research. (2000). The concept of presence: Explication statement. http://ispr.info/about-presence-2/about-presence/

International Telecommunication Union. (2014). Statistics. http://www.itu.int/en/ITU-D/Statistics/Pages/stat/default.aspx

Internet Live Stats. (2014). Internet users by country. http://www.internetlivestats.com/internet-users-by-country/

Internet World Stats. (2014). World internet usage and population statistics, 2012. http://www.internetworldstats.com/stats.htm

Jauréguiberry, F. (1998). Lieux publics, téléphone mobile et civilité. *Réseaux*, *16*, 71–84.

Jenkins, H. (2006). *Fans, gamers, and bloggers—Exploring participatory culture*. New York: New York University Press.

Joinson, A. N. (1998). Causes and effects of disinhibition on the Internet. In J. Gackenback (Ed.), *The psychology of the Internet* (pp. 43–60). New York: Academic Press.

Kaplan, A. M., & Haenlein, M. (2010). Users of the world, unite! The challenges and opportunities of social media. *Business Horizons*, *53*, 59–68.

Kardefelt-Winther, D. (2014a). A conceptual and methodological critique of internet addiction research: Towards a model of compensatory internet use. *Computers in Human Behavior*, *31*, 351–54.

Kardefelt-Winther, D. (2014b). The moderating role of psychosocial well-being on the relationship between escapism and excessive online gaming. *Computers in Human Behavior*, *38*, 68–74.

Kardefelt-Winther, D. (2015). *Excessive internet use—fascination or compulsion?*. PhD thesis. London School of Economics and Political Science, London. http://etheses.lse.ac.uk/1062/

Kato, P. M. (2010). Video games in health care: Closing the gap. *Review of General Psychology*, *14*, 113–21.

Kato, P. M., Cole, S. W., Bradlyn, A. S., & Pollock, B. H. (2008). A video game improves behavioral outcomes in adolescents and young adults with cancer: A randomized trial. *Pediatrics*, *122*, E305–17.

Katz, E., Gurevitch, M., & Haas, H. (1973). On the use of the mass media for important things. *American Sociological Review*, *38*, 164–81.

Kent, S. (2001). *The ultimate history of video games: From Pong to Pokemon and beyond—The story behind the craze that touched our lives and changed the world*. Roseville, CA: Prima.

Kou, Y., & Nardi, B. (2013). *Regulating anti-social behavior on the Internet: The example of League of Legends*. Paper presented at the iConference 2013.

Krijn, M., Emmelkamp, P. M. G., Biemond, R., de Ligny, C. D., Schuemie, M. J., & van der Mast, C. (2004). Treatment of acrophobia in virtual reality: The role of immersion and presence. *Behaviour Research and Therapy*, *42*, 229–39.

Krijn, M., Emmelkamp, P. M. G., Olafsson, R. P., & Biemond, R. (2004). Virtual reality exposure therapy of anxiety disorders: A review. *Clinical Psychology Review*, *24*(3), 259–81.

Kuss, D. J. (2013a). *For the Horde! How playing World of Warcraft reflects our participation in popular media culture*. Saarbrücken: LAP LAMBERT Academic Publishing.

Kuss, D. J. (2013b). Internet gaming addiction: Current perspectives. *Psychology Research and Behavior Management*, *6*, 125–37.

Kuss, D. J., & Griffiths, M. D. (2012a). Online gaming addiction in children and adolescents: A review of empirical research. *Journal of Behavioral Addictions*, *1*, 3–22.

Kuss, D. J., & Griffiths, M. D. (2012b). Internet gaming addiction: A systematic review of empirical research. *International Journal of Mental Health and Addiction*, *10*, 278–96.

Kuss, D. J., & Griffiths, M. D. (2012c). Internet and gaming addiction: A systematic literature review of neuroimaging studies. *Brain Sciences*, *2*, 347–74.

Kuss, D. J., Griffiths, M. D., & Binder, J. F. (2013). Internet addiction in students: Prevalence and risk factors. *Computers in Human Behavior*, *29*, 959–66.

Kuss, D. J., Griffiths, M. D., Karila, L., & Billieux, J. (2014). Internet addiction: A systematic review of epidemiological research for the last decade. *Current Pharmaceutical Design*, *20*, 4026–52.

Kuss, D. J., Louws, J., & Wiers, R. W. W. (2012). Online gaming addiction? Motives predict addictive play behavior in massively multiplayer online role-playing games. *Cyberpsychology, Behavior & Social Networking*, *15*, 480–85.

Kuss, D. J., Shorter, G. W., van Rooij, A. J., Griffiths, M. D., & Schoenmakers, T. (2014). Assessing Internet addiction using the parsimonious Internet addiction components model: A preliminary study. *International Journal of Mental Health and Addiction*, *12*, 351–66.

Kuss, D. J., van Rooij, A., Shorter, G. W., Griffiths, M. D., & van de Mheen, D. (2013). Internet addiction in adolescents: Prevalence and risk factors. *Computers in Human Behavior*, *29*, 1987–96.

Leach, L. S., Christensen, H., Griffiths, K. M., Jorm, A. F., & Mackinnon, A. J. (2007). Websites as a mode of delivering mental health information: Perceptions from the Australian public. *Social Psychiatry and Psychiatric Epidemiology*, *42*, 167–72.

Leimeister, J. M., Schweizer, K., Leimeister, S., & Krcmar, H. (2008). Do virtual communities matter for the social support of patients? Antecedents and effects of virtual relationships in online communities. *Information Technology & People*, *21*, 350–74.

Lemmens, J. S., Valkenburg, P. M., & Peter, J. (2011). Psychosocial causes and consequences of pathological gaming. *Computers in Human Behavior*, *27*, 144–52.

Lenhart, A., Kahne, J., Middaugh, E., Macgill, A., Evans, C., & Vitak, J. (2008). Teens' gaming experiences are diverse and include significant social interaction and civic engagement. http://files.eric.ed.gov/fulltext/ED525058.pdf

Lévy, P. (1997). *Collective intelligence: Mankind's emerging world in cyberspace*. Cambridge, MA: Perseus.

Lin, H., & Sun, C. (2005). *The "white-eyed" player culture: Grief play and construction of deviance in MMORPGs*. Paper presented at the DiGRA 2005 Conference: Changing Views—Worlds in Play.

Livingstone, S., Haddon, L., Görzig, A., & Ólafsson, K. (2011). *Risks and safety on the internet: The perspective of European children. Full findings*. London: LSE, London.

Lowood, H. (2008). 'Found technology: Players as innovators in the making of machinima. Digital youth, innovation, and the unexpected. In McPherson, T. (Ed.). *The John D. and Catherine T. MacArthur Foundation series on digital media and learning* (pp. 165–96). Cambridge, MA: MIT Press.

Lowood, H. E. (2015). Virtual reality. http://www.britannica.com/technology/virtual-reality/Entertainment#ref884340

Manovich, L. (2001). *The language of new media*. Cambridge, MA: MIT.

Markham, A. N. (1998). *Life online. Researching real experience in virtual space*. Walnut Creek, CA: AltaMira.

Matthies, D. J. C., Haescher, M., Alm, A., & Urban, B. (2015). *Properties of a peripheral head-mounted display (PHMD)*. Paper presented at the 17th International Conference on Human-Computer Interaction. Los Angeles, California.

Mazuryk, T., & Gervautz, M. (1996). Virtual reality: History, applications, technology and future. Citeseer. http://citeseerx.ist.psu.edu/viewdoc/summary?doi=10.1.1.42.7849

McKenna, K. Y. A., & Bargh, J. A. (2000). Plan 9 from cyberspace: The implications of the internet for personality and social psychology. *Personality and Social Psychology Review, 4*(1), 57–75.

McKenna, K. Y. A., Green, A. S., & Gleason, M. E. J. (2002). Relationship formation on the internet: What's the big attraction? *Journal of Social Issues, 58*, 9–31.

McLuhan, M. (1964). *Understanding media: The extensions of man.* New York: Routledge and Kegan Paul.

Newman, J. (2002). In search of the video gameplayer: The lives of Mario. *New Media and Society, 4*, 405–22.

NHS. (2015). The Expert Patients Programme (EPP). http://www.nhs.uk/NHSEngland/AboutNHSservices/doctors/Pages/expert-patients-programme.aspx

Nickerson, R. C., Isaac, H., & Mak, B. (2008). A multi-national study of attitudes about mobile phone use in social settings. *International Journal of Mobile Communication, 6*, 541–63.

Nicol, A., & Fleming, M. J. (2010). "i h8 u" : The influence of normative beliefs and hostile response selection in predicting adolescents' mobile phone aggression: A pilot study. *Journal of School Violence, 9*, 212–31.

O'Brolchain, F., Jacquemard, T., Monaghan, D., O'Connor, N., Novitzky, P., & Gordijn, B. (2015). The convergence of virtual reality and social networks: Threats to privacy and autonomy. *Science and Engineering Ethics, 1*, 1.

Office for National Statistics. (2013). Internet access: Households and individuals. http://www.ons.gov.uk/ons/dcp171778_322713.pdf

O'Reilly, T. (2005). What is web 2.0? Design patterns and business models for the next generation of software. http://www.oreilly.com/pub/a/web2/archive/what-is-web-20.html

Orgad, S. (2005). *Storytelling online: Talking breast cancer on the Internet.* New York: Peter Lang.

Patel, A., Schieble, T., Davidson, M., Tran, M. C. J., Schoenberg, C., Delphin, E., et al. (2006). Distraction with a hand-held video game reduces pediatric preoperative anxiety. *Pediatric Anesthesia, 16*, 1019–27.

Peter, J., Valkenburg, P. M., & Schouten, A. P. (2005). Developing a model of adolescent friendship formation on the Internet. *Cyberpsychology & Behavior, 8*, 423–30.

Powers, M. B., & Emmelkamp, P. M. G. (2008). Virtual reality exposure therapy for anxiety disorders: A meta-analysis. *Journal of Anxiety Disorders, 22*, 561–69.

PricewaterhouseCoopers. (2015). Outlook insights: An analysis of the Global entertainment and media outlook 2015–2019. http://www.pwc.com/gx/en/global-entertainment-media-outlook/assets/2015/video-games-key-insights-1-global-revenue.pdf

Purcell, R., Pathé, M., & Mullen, P. (2004). Editorial: When do repeated intrusions become stalking? *Journal of Forensic Psychiatry & Psychology, 15*, 571–83.

Redd, W. H., Jacobsen, P. B., DieTrill, M., Dermatis, H., McEvoy, M., & Holland, J. C. (1987). Cognitive-attentional distraction in the control of conditioned nausea in pediatric cancer patients receiving chemotherapy. *Journal of Consulting & Clinical Psychology, 55*, 391–95.

Reporters Without Borders. (2012). China. https://en.rsf.org/china-china-12-03-201242077.html

Rheingold, H. (1993). *The virtual community: Homesteading on the electronic frontier.* Cambridge, MA: MIT Press.

Riot Games. (2015). Key statistics for League of Legends. http://www.riotgames.com/our-games

Rochlen, A. B., Zack, J. S., & Speyer, C. (2004). Online therapy: Review of relevant definitions, debates, and current empirical support. *Journal of Clinical Psychology, 60*, 269–83.

Rosser, J., Lynch, P., Caddihy, L., Gentile, D., Klonsky, J., & Merrell, R. (2007). The impact of video games on training surgeons in the 21st century. *Archives of Surgery, 142*, 181–86.

Rothbaum, B. O., Hodges, L., Smith, S., Lee, J. H., & Price, L. (2000). A controlled study of virtual reality exposure therapy for the fear of flying. *Journal of Consulting and Clinical Psychology, 68*, 1020–26.

Rothbaum, B. O., Hodges, L. F., Ready, D., Graap, K., & Alarcon, R. D. (2001). Virtual reality exposure therapy for Vietnam veterans with posttraumatic stress disorder. *Journal of Clinical Psychiatry, 62*, 617–22.

Roy, S., Klinger, E., Legeron, P., Lauer, F., Chemin, I., & Nugues, P. (2003). Definition of a VR-based protocol to treat social phobia. *Cyberpsychology & Behavior, 6*, 411–20.

Russoniello, C. V., O'Brien, K., & Parks, J. M. (2009). EEG, HRV and psychological correlates while playing Bejeweled II: A randomized controlled study. In B. K. Wiederhold & G. Riva (Eds.), *Annual review of cybertherapy and telemedicine 2009: Advance technologies in the behavioral, social and neurosciences, Vol. 7* (pp. 189–92). Amsterdam: Interactive Media Institute and IOS Press.

Ryan, R. M., Rigby, C. S., & Przybylski, A. (2006). The motivational pull of video games: A self-determination theory approach. *Motivation and Emotion, 30*, 347–63.

Shane, M., Pettitt, B., Morgenthal, C., & Smith, C. (2008). Should surgical novices trade their retractors for joysticks? Videogame experience decreases the time needed to acquire surgical skills. *Surgical Endoscopy, 22*, 1294–97.

Shanklin, W. (2015). Extended interview: The Oculus Rift, in its' creators own words. http://www.gizmag.com/oculus-rift-interview/38002/

Shapiro, J. R., Bauer, S., Andrews, E., Pisetsky, E., Bulik-Sullivan, B., Hammer, R. M., et al. (2010). Mobile therapy: Use of text-messaging in the treatment of bulimia nervosa. *International Journal of Eating Disorders, 43*, 513–19.

Sharar, S., Carrougher, G., Nakamura, D., Hoffman, H., Blough, D., & Patterson, D. (2007). Factors influencing the efficacy of virtual reality distraction analgesia during postburn physical therapy: Preliminary results from 3 ongoing studies. *Archives of Physical Medicine and Rehabilitation, 88*, 43–49.

Sharma, P., & Maleyeff, J. (2003). Internet education: Potential problems and solutions. *International Journal of Educational Management, 17*, 19–25.

Shen, C., & Williams, D. (2011). Unpacking time online: Connecting internet and massively multiplayer online game use with psychosocial well-being. *Communication Research, 38*, 123–49.

Sheridan, L. P., & Grant, T. (2007). Is cyberstalking different? *Psychology, Crime & Law, 13*, 627–40.

Spitzberg, B. H., & Hoobler, G. (2002). Cyberstalking and the technologies of interpersonal terrorism. *New Media & Society, 4*, 71–92.

Stofle, G. S. (2001). *Choosing an online therapist.* Harrisburg, PA: White Hat Communications.

Suler, J. (2004). The online disinhibition effect. *CyberPsychology & Behavior, 7*, 321–26.

Sutherland, I. E. (1965). *The ultimate display.* Paper presented at the Information Processing: Proceedings of the IFIP Congress. New York City.

Taylor, T. L. (2012). *Raising the stakes: E-sports and the professionalization of computer gaming.* Cambridge, MA: MIT Press.

Thomée, S., Harenstam, A., & Hagberg, M. (2011). Mobile phone use and stress, sleep disturbances, and symptoms of depression among young adults-a prospective cohort study. *BMC Public Health, 11*, 66.

Tichon, J., & Banks, J. (2006). Virtual reality exposure therapy: 150-degree screen to desktop PC. *Cyberpsychology & Behavior, 9*, 480–88.

Turkle, S. (1995). *Life on the screen*. New York: Simon & Schuster.

Turkle, S. (2011). *Alone together. Why we expect more from technology and less from each other*. Philadelphia, PA: Basic Books.

Uttal, D. H., Meadow, N. G., Tipton, E., Hand, L. L., Alden, A. R., Warren, C., et al. (2013). The malleability of spatial skills: A meta-analysis of training studies. *Psychological Bulletin, 139*, 352–402.

Vasterling, J., Jenkins, R. A., Tope, D. M., & Burish, T. G. (1993). Cognitive distraction and relaxation training for the control of side effects due to cancer chemotherapy. *Journal of Behavioral Medicine, 16*, 65–80.

Vincelli, F., Anolli, L., Bouchard, S., Wiederhold, B. K., Zurloni, V., & Riva, G. (2003). Experiential cognitive therapy in the treatment of panic disorders with agoraphobia: A controlled study. *Cyberpsychology & Behavior, 6*, 321–28.

Wald, J., & Taylor, S. (2000). Efficacy of virtual reality exposure therapy to treat driving phobia: A case report. *Journal of Behavior Therapy and Experimental Psychiatry, 31*, 249–57.

Watts, S., Mackenzie, A., Thomas, C., Griskaitis, A., Mewton, L., Williams, A., et al. (2013). CBT for depression: A pilot RCT comparing mobile phone vs. computer. *BMC Psychiatry, 7*, 49.

Webb, M., Burns, J., & Collin, P. (2008). Providing online support for young people with mental health difficulties: Challenges and opportunities explored. *Early Intervention in Psychiatry, 2*, 108–13.

Westrup, D., Fremouw, W. J., Thompson, R. N., & Lewis, S. F. (1999). The psychological impact of stalking on female undergraduates. *Journal of Forensic Sciences, 44*, 554–57.

White, M. P., Eiser, J. R., & Harris, P. R. (2004). Risk perceptions of mobile phone use while driving. *Risk Analysis, 24*, 323–34.

Wiederhold, B. K., & Wiederhold, M. D. (2010). Virtual reality treatment of posttraumatic stress disorder due to motor vehicle accident. *Cyberpsychology Behavior and Social Networking, 13*, 21–27.

Yager, J. (2001). E-mail as a therapeutic adjunct in the outpatient treatment of anorexia nervosa: Illustrative case material and discussion of the issues. *International Journal of Eating Disorders, 29*, 125–38.

Yan, Z., & Chen, Q. (2015). Mobile phone behavior: An emerged discipline of research. In Z. Yan (Ed.), *Encyclopedia of Mobile Phone Behavior* (pp. 415–25). Hershey, PA: IGI Global.

Ybarra, M. L., & Suman, M. (2006). Help seeking behavior and the Internet: A national survey. *international Journal of Medical Informatics, 75*, 29–41.

Young, K. S. (1996). Addictive use of the Internet: A case that breaks the stereotype. *Psychological Reports, 79*, 899–902.

Zuckerberg, M. (2014). Facebook excited to acquire Oculus VR. Facebook. https://www.facebook.com/zuck/posts/10101319050523971

CHAPTER

2 A History and Overview of Video Game Addiction

Mark D. Griffiths *and* Halley M. Pontes

Abstract

The past decade has witnessed a significant increase in the number of empirical studies examining various aspects of problematic video game play, video game addiction, and, more recently, gaming disorder. This chapter begins with a brief past history of how research into video game addiction has developed during the past four decades in the 1980s (arcade video game addiction), 1990s (home console video game addiction), and 2000s and beyond (online video game addiction). The chapter also overviews the features of gaming addiction, its prevalence rates, demographics and gaming addiction, negative consequences of excessive video game use, Internet gaming disorder and the DSM-5, and treatment of gaming addiction. Based on the published evidence, particularly from studies conducted in the past decade, it appears that, in extreme cases, excessive gaming can have potentially damaging effects on individuals who appear to display compulsive and/or addictive behavior similar to other more traditional addictions. However, the field has been hindered by the use of inconsistent and nonstandardized criteria to assess and identify problematic and/or addictive video game use.

Keywords: excessive gaming, video game addiction, gaming addiction, gaming disorder, Internet gaming disorder, problematic gaming

According to the Entertainment Software Association (ESA, 2014), 59% of the entire American population plays video games, with an average of two gamers in each game-playing household. Additionally, among US households 68% play video games on consoles, 53% play on smartphones, and 41% play on wireless devices (ESA, 2014). During 2012, playing video games via smartphones and wireless devices increased by 22% and 37%, respectively. The average video game player is 31 years old - and about 52% of these video game players are male and 48% are female (ESA, 2014).

Given the pervasiveness of gaming across several countries and different segments of the population, the study of its associated effects on general human behavior, physical and mental health has become an important topic for dedicated research agendas from various scientific domains in addition to psychology and psychiatry (e.g., Blocher, 2015; Dreier, Wölfling, & Müller, 2013; Johnston, Boyle, MacArthur, & Manion, 2013). Taken together, findings in this developing field suggest both favorable and unfavorable effects of gaming, outcomes that could inform decisions made by healthcare professionals, parents, policymakers (Przybylski, 2014) and other stakeholders such as researchers and the video game industry (Yousafzai, Hussain, & Griffiths, 2013).

One topic that has become of increasing research interest is gaming addiction and *Internet Gaming Disorder* (IGD). The past decade has witnessed a significant increase in the number of empirical studies examining various aspects of problematic video gameplay and video game addiction (Pontes & Griffiths, 2014). This chapter begins with a brief past history of how research into video game addiction has changed over the past three decades (i.e., the 1980s, 1990s, and 2000s). The chapter addresses concerns related to video game addiction and how it made its way into the latest (fifth) edition of the *DSM* (DSM-5; American Psychiatric Association, 2013). The chapter also briefly examines features of video game addiction and examines the contemporary research literature by analyzing the prevalence of video game addiction, factors associated with video game addiction, and the treatment of video game addiction.

Gaming Addiction in the 1980s

Following the release of the first commercial video games in the early 1970s, it took until the 1980s for the first reports of video game addiction to appear in the psychological and psychiatric literature. In the early 1980s, Ross, Finestone, and Lavin reported three cases of "Space Invaders obsession" and Nilles (1982) described a similar phenomenon but called it "computer catatonia." Arguably the first reference to "video game addiction" was by Soper and Miller (1983) who, based on their observations as school counselors, claimed the disorder was like any other behavioral addiction and consisted of a compulsive behavioral involvement, a lack of interest in other activities, association mainly with other addicts, and physical and mental symptoms when attempting to stop the behavior (e.g., the shakes). Some credence was given to these claims that video game addiction existed following papers on the seemingly successful treatment of video game addiction using cognitive behavioral therapy (CBT) (Keepers, 1990; Kuczmierczyk, Walley, & Calhoun, 1987). However, all of these studies were somewhat observational, anecdotal, and/or case studies, primarily based on teenage males and all based on a particular type of video game in a particular medium (i.e., "pay-to-play" arcade video games).

Shotton (1989) carried out the first empirical study specifically on gaming addiction on a relatively small sample of 127 people (almost all teenage or young adult males) who described themselves as "hooked" on home video games for at least 5 years. Shotton's conceptualization of gaming addiction was more positive than negative, and she reported that her "addicts" were on the whole highly intelligent, motivated, and achieving people who were often misunderstood by others in society. Despite this, the main problem with the study was that no standardized measure of addiction was actually used. The only criterion for being "addicted" was the individuals own admission that they were "hooked" on computer games. Despite this major shortcoming, recent research by Widyanto, Griffiths, and Brunsden (2011) reported that a person's positive self-diagnosis to the Internet was correlated highly with more standardized measures of Internet addiction.

Gaming Addiction in the 1990s

The 1990s saw a small but significant increase of research into video game addiction, with almost all of these studies being carried out by surveying children in school settings in the United Kingdom (e.g., Brown & Robertson, 1993; Fisher, 1994; Griffiths, 1997; Griffiths & Hunt, 1995, 1998; Parsons, 1995; Phillips, Rolls, Rouse, & Griffiths, 1995). In contrast to studies from the early 1980s, these studies mainly examined non-arcade video game playing (i.e., home console games, handheld games, PC gaming). However, all of these studies were self-report surveys, relatively small in scale, and all of them assessed video game addiction using adapted versions of the Diagnostic and Statistical Manual of Mental Disorders (DSM), such as the DSM-III or the DSM-IV criteria for pathological gambling (American Psychiatric Association, 1987, 1994). Based on further analysis of the adapted DSM criteria used, these studies were later criticized as being more likely to be assessing video game preoccupation rather than video game addiction (Charlton, 2002).

Gaming Addiction in the 2000s and Beyond

The 2000s saw a substantial growth in the number of studies on video game addiction, particularly as gaming expanded into the new online medium where games could be played as part of a gaming community (i.e., massively multiplayer online role playing games [MMORPGs] such as World of Warcraft and Everquest). Approximately 60 studies were published on gaming addiction between 2000 and 2010 (Kuss & Griffiths, 2012) and a vast majority of these studies examined MMORPG addiction and were not limited to only studying adolescent males. Furthermore, many of these studies collected their data online, and a significant number of studies examined various aspects of video game addiction using non–self-report methodologies. These include studies using polysomnographic measures and visual and verbal memory tests (Dworak, Schierl, Bruns, & Struder, 2007); medical examinations including the patient's history, and physical, radiologic, intraoperative, and pathologic findings (Cultrara & Har-El, 2002); functional magnetic resonance imaging (fMRI; Han, Hwang, &

Renshaw, 2010; Hoeft, Watson, Kesler, Bettinger, & Reiss, 2008; Ko et al., 2009); electroencephalography (Thalemann, Wölfling, & Grüsser, 2007); and genotyping (Han et al., 2007). Given the methodological shortcomings of the studies published prior to 2000 and the fact that gaming has evolved substantially over the past decade, the remainder of this chapter will mainly focus on studies published in the past decade or so (i.e., post-2000 studies) with the exception of those concerning the health and medical consequences of excessive video game play.

Features of Gaming Addiction

There are a multitude of psychological perspectives on addiction, which has led to addiction being defined in many different ways. However, most models of addictive behavior refer to a persistent and uncontrollable urge to consume a substance or engage in an activity that results in significant personal harm and interpersonal conflict for the user (King, Delfabbro, & Griffiths, 2013). Thus, gaming addiction is often said to be present when individuals have completely lost control over gaming and the excessive playing behavior has had a detrimental effect on all aspects of the individuals life, compromising job and/or educational activities, interpersonal relationships, hobbies, general health, and psychological well-being (King, Delfabbro, & Griffiths, 2013). These two criteria (impaired control and harmful consequences) are regarded as fundamentally important criteria for addiction. An alternative model of addictive behavior has proposed six features or *components* of gaming addiction (Griffiths, 2005). To indicate addiction, it is thought that these criteria must be sustained for at least 3–6 months. Otherwise, they may simply indicate a temporary absorption in video games. These criteria include:

- *Salience.* This occurs when gaming becomes the most important activity in a person's life, dominating thoughts (preoccupation and cognitive distortions), emotions (cravings), and behavior (deterioration of normal behaviors). An addicted gamer is obsessed with all aspects of video games and, when not playing, will be anticipating or planning the next playing session.
- *Mood modification.* This refers to changes in a person's mood state that occur as a result of gaming. Mood change may involve a subjective feeling of euphoria as well as an increase in physiological arousal (increased heart rate, muscle tension, or shaky hands) or, alternatively, a tranquilizing feeling of calm or a numbing sensation.
- *Tolerance.* This refers to the process whereby increasing amounts of gaming are required to achieve the former mood-modifying effects. This means that players gradually increase the amount of time they spend engaged in gaming. It could be argued that addicted gamers build up their tolerance to the point that they will end a playing session only when they have become mentally or physically exhausted.
- *Withdrawal.* These are the aversive mood states and/or physical effects that occur when gaming is suddenly discontinued or reduced. Psychological withdrawal symptoms include feelings of frustration, irritability, and flattened affect. Withdrawal motivates the individual to play video games on a regular basis and to minimize periods of absence from a video game in order to alleviate these unpleasant feeling states.
- *Relapse.* This refers to the tendency for the player to make repeated reversions to earlier patterns of gaming and for even the most extreme patterns typical of the height of excessive gaming to be quickly restored after periods of abstinence or moderation. Relapse usually indicates that the individual has lost personal agency over the behavior.
- *Conflict (harm).* This refers to the negative consequences of excessive gaming. Harm includes conflicts between the addicted video game player and other people (family members and friends), other activities (job, school, social life, hobbies and interests), and from within the addict him/herself (psychological distress).

Charlton (2002) suggests that three of these features may not be reliable indicators of video game addiction. His research suggests that cognitive salience (preoccupation), euphoria (mood modification), and tolerance also indicate *high engagement,* or a type of healthy obsession, with gaming. Therefore, studies may overestimate the prevalence of problem video game play if high engagement with gaming is not properly distinguished from gaming addiction. Given these issues of reliability, many addiction specialists maintain that impaired control and harmful effects are the most appropriate criteria for identifying gaming addiction.

Prevalence of Problematic Video Game Use and Gaming Addiction

At present, it is quite difficult to estimate the prevalence of problematic gaming due to the lack of a clear definition, the application of measures without proper psychometric characteristics, and studies using different samples and different research methodologies. Large-sample studies generally report prevalence values of lower than 10%. A study conducted in the United States on a national representative sample of teenagers (Gentile, 2009), as well as on a large sample of Singaporean children (Gentile et al., 2011) both reported a problematic game use of approximately 9%. Results of another representative study in Germany showed that 3% of the male and 0.3% of the female students studied were diagnosed as dependent on video games, while another 4.7% of male and 0.5% of female students were at risk of becoming dependent (Rehbein et al., 2010). On a large Hungarian online gamer sample 3.4% of gamers belonged to the high-risk group of problematic gaming and another 15.2% to the medium-risk group (Demetrovics et al., 2012). A proportion of 4.6% of Hungarian adolescents (approximately 16 years old) belonging to a national sample were classified as high-risk users (Pápay et al., 2013) (see Table 2.1).

Demographics and Gaming Addiction

According to an online survey examining all types of online gamers (Nagygyörgy et al., 2013) ($N = 4{,}374$), the mean age was 21 years, and participants were mostly male (91%) and single (66%). Their average weekly game time varied between less than 7 hours (10%) and more than 42 hours (also 10%) with most of the gamers playing 15–27 hours weekly (35%). Furthermore, 16% of all gamers were playing either professionally (i.e., they make a living off of sponsorships and money won from tournaments) or competitively (i.e., they participate in competitions and earn money if they win). The majority of the sample (79%) had a clear gaming preference: namely, they played one single game type most of the time.

Data regarding the three main game types give a more nuanced view. The proportion of female gamers is the lowest in the case of massively multiplayer online first-person shooter (MMOFPS) games (1–2%) (Jansz & Tanis, 2007; Nagygyörgy et al., 2013) and the highest between MMORPG users (15–30%) (Cole & Griffiths, 2007; Nagygyörgy et al., 2013; Yee, 2006a). MMOFPS users are the youngest (18–19.8 years) (Jansz & Tanis, 2007; Nagygyörgy, et al., 2013), while both massively multiplayer online real-time strategy (MMORTS) (22 years) (Nagygyörgy et al., 2013) and MMORPG players (21–27 years) (Nagygyörgy et al., 2013; Yee, 2006a) are significantly older. Among the three main groups, MMORPG gamers spend the most time playing (Nagygyörgy et al., 2013). Since MMORPGs are the most researched games (most likely because they allow players to interact to form friendships, create communities, and work together to accomplish a variety of goals [Barnett & Coulson, 2010]), there is additional information regarding such players that is still unknown in the case of other game types. For instance, half of MMORPG players work full time, 22.2% are students, and 14.8% are homemakers (89.9% of whom were female). Furthermore, 36% of the gamers are married and 22% of them have children (Yee, 2006a, 2006b). Overall, the demographic composition of MMORPG users is quite varied and probably more diverse than the composition of MMORTS and MMOFPS users (although this needs to be empirically established).

From a substantive perspective, there are some generalizations that can be made with regard to the demographic characteristics of gamers and problem gamers. The literature to date suggests that adolescent males and young male adults appear to be at greater risk of experiencing problematic video game play. However, the course and severity of these problems is not well known (King, Delfabbro, & Griffiths, 2012) and the finding that this group is more at risk may be a consequence of sampling bias and the fact that this group plays video games more frequently than do other sociodemographic groups. It has also been suggested that university students may be vulnerable to developing problematic video gaming. Reasons for this include their flexible tuition and study hours, ready access to high-speed broadband on a 24/7 basis, and multiple stressors associated with adjusting to new social obligations and/or living out-of-home for the first time (King, Delfabbro et al., 2012; Young, 1998a).

Negative Consequences of Excessive Video Game Use

Irrespective of whether problematic video game play can be classed as an addiction, there is now a relatively large number of studies all indicating that excessive video game play can lead to a wide variety of negative psychosocial consequences for a minority of affected individuals. These include sacrificing work, education, hobbies, socializing, time with partner/family, and sleep (Batthyány, Müller, Benker, & Wölfling, 2009; Griffiths, Davies, & Chappell, 2004; King & Delfabbro, 2009; Liu & Peng, 2009; Peng & Liu, 2010; Peters & Malesky, 2008; Rehbein et al., 2010; Yee 2006a, 2006b), increased stress (Batthyány et al., 2009), an absence of real-life relationships (Allison, von Wahlde, Shockley, & Gabbard, 2006), lower

Table 2.1 Prevalence of problematic online gaming involving large samples

Author(s) (reference)	Location	Research subjects (mean age (M), standard deviation (SD))	Method	Measure	Criteria of problematic use	Life-prevalence value
Yee (2006)	USA, Canada	3,166 persons, MMORPG gamers	Online survey	Direct question ("Do you consider yourself addicted to MMORPGs?" yes/no question)	Yes to the direct question	50%
Grüsser, Thalemann, and Griffiths (2007)	Germany	7,069 gamers (M: 21,1 years, SD: 6,4)	Online survey	6 criteria of key symptoms of a dependence syndrome as outlined in WHO's ICD-10	3 or more criteria fulfilled	11,9%
Gentile (2009)	USA	1,178 persons (adolescents aged 8 – 18 years)	Nationally representative online survey	Pathological Video-Game Use	6 or more yes answers	8,5%
Porter et al. (2010)	USA, Canada, Europe, Australia, New Zeeland, Asia, Central and South America	1,945 persons, gamers older than 14 years	Online survey	Video Game Use Questionnaire, (VGUQ), 10 criteria: 3 (preoccupation), 7 (adverse consequences), yes/no answers	2 or more criteria (preoccupation) + 3 or more criteria (adverse consequences)	8%
Van Rooij et al. (2011)	Netherlands	4,559 persons (M: 14.4 years, SD: 1.2) (T1) and 3740 persons (M: 14.3 years SD: 1.0) (T2)	Paper-and-pencil survey	Compulsive Internet Use Scale (CIUS) + weekly hours online gaming	Latent profile analysis	1,6% (T1), 1,5% (T2) ~ 1,5%
Gentile et al. (2011)	Singapore	3,034 persons elementary and secondary school students	2 years longitudinal study paper-and-pencil survey	Pathological Video-Game Use	5 or more yes answer	7,6% – 9,9%
Lemmens, Valkenburg, and Peters (2011)	Netherlands	543 adolescent gamers (M: 13.9 years, SD: 1.4)	Longitudinal paper-and-pencil survey	Game Addiction Scale (GAS)	Score of 3 or higher	6% (T1), 4% (T2)
Rehbein et al. (2010)	Germany	15,168 ninth graders (15.3 years, SD: 0.69)	Nationally representative survey	Video Game Dependency Scale (KFN-CSAS-II)	Score higher than 42 dependent players; score between 35 and 41: players at risk	dependent: boys 3%, girls 0,3%; at risk: boys 4,7%, girls 0,5%

Thomas and Martin (2010)	Australia	2,031 persons (705 university students, 1,326 secondary and college students)	Paper-and-pencil survey	Adaptation of YDQ (Young's Diagnostic Questionnaire) to computer games	Score of 5 or higher	5%
Jeong and Kim (2011)	South Korea	600 persons (12-18 years)	Nationally representative paper-and-pencil survey	Young's internet Addiction Test (IAT) modified by replacing the word "Internet" with "gaming"	Score above 80	2,2%
Demetrovics et al. (2012)	Hungary	3,415 persons, online gamers (M: 21 years, SD: 5,9)	Online survey	Problematic Online Gaming Questionnaire (POGQ)	Latent profile analysis	high risk problematic online gamers: 3,4%; medium risk of problematic use: 15,2%
Pápay et al. (2013)	Hungary	5,045 students from secondary general and secondary vocational schools (M: 16.4 years, SD: 0.9)	Nationally representative survey	Problematic Online Gaming Questionnaire Short Form (POGQ-SF)	Latent profile analysis	4.6%
Strittmatter et al. (2015)	Estonia, Germany, Italy, Romania, Spain, and Sweden	8,807 European adolescents (M: 15 years, SD: 1.3)	Nationally representative survey	Adaptation of YDQ (Young's Diagnostic Questionnaire) to computer games	Score of 5 or higher	3.1%
Baggio et al. (2015)	Switzerland	5,663 young adults aged between 17, 14, and 20 years	Nationally representative survey	GAS	Responding "sometimes" or more on all 7 items	2.3%
Brunborg et al. (2015)	Norway	10,081 individuals from the general population (M: 35 years, SD: 13.76)	Nationally representative survey	GAS	Responding "sometimes" or more on all 7 items	0.7%
Müller et al. (2015)	Germany, Greece, Iceland, Netherlands, Poland, Romania, and Spain	12,938 European adolescents aged between (M: 15.8 years, SD: 0.7)	Nationally representative survey	Assessment of Internet and Computer game Addiction-Scale (AICA-S)	Score above 13.5	1.6%
Henchoz et al. (2016)	Switzerland	5,990 young adults (M: 19.95, SD: 1.2)	Nationally representative survey	GAS	Scores of 3 or more on at least any four of the seven criteria	2.2%

(continued)

Table 2.1 Continued

Author(s) (reference)	Location	Research subjects (mean age (M), standard deviation (SD))	Method	Measure	Criteria of problematic use	Life-prevalence value
Lemmens et al. (2016)	Netherlands	2,442 individuals from the general population with ages between 13 to 14 years	Nationally representative survey	The Internet Gaming Disorder Scale (IGDS)	Endorsing at least 5 criteria	5.8%
Pontes et al. (2016)	Slovenia	1,071 adolescents	Nationally representative survey	Internet Gaming Disorder Scale – Short-Form (IGDS9-SF)	Endorsing at least 5 criteria	2.5%
Ustinavičienė et al. (2016)	Lithuania	1,806 young adolescents aged between 13 to 18 years	Nationally representative survey	Adaptation of YDQ (Young's Diagnostic Questionnaire) to computer games	Score of 5 or higher	9.3%
Yu et al. (2016)	South Korea	2,024 young adolescents aged between 13 to 15 years (M: 15.5, SD: 0.50)	Nationally representative survey	DSM-5 criteria for IGD	Endorsing at least 5 criteria	5.9%
Carras et al. (2017)	Netherlands	9,773 adolescents (M: 14.1 years)	Nationally representative survey	Video Game Addiction Test (VAT)	Latent class analysis	1.3%
Park et al. (2017)	South Korea	7,650 adults	Nationally representative survey	DSM-5 criteria for IGD	Endorsing at least 5 criteria	4%
Rosenkranz et al. (2017)	Germany	5,667 adolescents aged between 12 to 19 years (M: 15.44, SD: 1.73)	Nationally representative survey	AICA-S	Score above 13.5	3.6%
Wartberg et al. (2017)	Germany	1,531 adolescents and young adults (M: 18.86 years, SD: 4.06)	Nationally representative survey	IGDS	Endorsing at least 5 criteria	5.7%

psychosocial well-being and loneliness (Lemmens, Valkenburg, & Peter, 2011), poorer social skills (Griffiths, 2010; Zamani, Kheradmand, Cheshmi, Abedi, & Hedayati, 2010), decreased academic achievement (Chiu, Lee, & Huang, 2004; Jeong & Kim, 2011; Rehbein et al., 2010; Skoric, Teo, & Neo, 2009), increased inattention (Batthyány et al., 2009; Chan & Rabinowitz, 2006), aggressive/oppositional behavior and hostility (Chan & Rabinowitz, 2006; Chiu et al., 2004), maladaptive coping (Batthyány et al., 2009; Hussain & Griffiths, 2009a, 2009b), decreased verbal memory performance (Dworak et al., 2007), maladaptive cognitions (Peng & Liu, 2010), and suicidal ideation (Rehbein et al., 2010).

In addition to the reported negative psychosocial consequences, there are also many reported health and medical consequences that may result from excessive video game playing. These include epileptic seizures (Chuang, 2006; Graf, Chatrian, Glass, & Knauss, 1994; Harding & Jeavons, 1994; Maeda et al., 1990; Millett, Fish, & Thompson, 1997; Quirk et al., 1995); auditory hallucinations (Ortiz de Gortari & Griffiths, 2014a; Spence, 1993); visual hallucinations (Ortiz de Gortari & Griffiths, 2014b); enuresis (Schink, 1991); encopresis (Corkery, 1990); obesity (Deheger, Rolland-Cachera, & Fontvielle, 1997; Johnson & Hackett, 1997; Shimai, Yamada, Masuda, & Tada, 1993; Vandewater, Shim, & Caplovitz, 2004); wrist pain (McCowan, 1981); neck pain (Miller, 1991); elbow pain (Miller, 1991); tenosynovitis—also called "nintendinitis" (Brasington, 1990; Casanova & Casanova, 1991; Reinstein, 1983; Siegal, 1991); blisters, calluses, sore tendons, and numbness of fingers (Loftus & Loftus, 1983); hand-arm vibration syndrome (Cleary, McKendrick, & Sills, 2002); sleep abnormalities (Allison et al., 2006; Dworak et al., 2007); psychosomatic challenges (Batthyány et al., 2009); and repetitive strain injuries (Mirman & Bonian, 1992).

Taken together, this relatively long list of potential psychosocial and medical negative consequences indicates that excessive gaming is an issue irrespective of whether it is an addiction. It also suggests that more extensive recognition is needed of the wide range of potential negative and life-limiting consequences of excessive video play.

Factors Associated with Problematic Video Game Use and Video Game Addiction

A number of studies have examined the role of different personality factors, comorbidity factors, and biological factors and their association with gaming addiction. In relation to personality traits, gaming addiction has been shown to have association with neuroticism (Mehroof & Griffiths, 2010; Peters & Malesky, 2008), aggression and hostility (Caplan, Williams, & Yee, 2009; Chiu et al., 2004; Kim, Namkoong, Ku, & Kim, 2008; Mehroof & Griffiths, 2010), avoidant and schizoid interpersonal tendencies (Allison et al., 2006), loneliness and introversion (Caplan et al., 2009), social inhibition (Porter, Starcevic, Berle, & Fenech, 2010), boredom inclination (Chiu et al., 2004), sensation-seeking (Chiu et al., 2004; Mehroof & Griffiths, 2010), diminished agreeableness (Peters & Malesky, 2008), diminished self-control and narcissistic personality traits (Kim et al., 2008), low self-esteem (Ko, Yen, Chen, Chen, & Yen, 2005), state and trait anxiety (Mehroof & Griffiths, 2010), and low emotional intelligence (Parker et al., 2008). It is hard to assess the etiological significance of these associations with gaming addiction as they may not be unique to the disorder. Further research is therefore needed.

Research has also shown gaming addiction to be associated with a variety of comorbid disorders. This includes attention deficit hyperactivity disorder (Allison et al., 2006; Batthyány et al., 2009; Chan & Rabinowitz, 2006; Han et al., 2009) and symptoms of generalized anxiety disorder, panic disorder, depression, social phobia (Allison et al., 2006), school phobia (Batthyány et al., 2009), and various psychosomatic symptoms (Batthyány et al., 2009).

Through use of fMRI, biological research has shown that gaming addicts show similar neural processes and increased activity in brain areas associated with substance-related addictions and other behavioral addictions, such as pathological gambling (significant activation in the left occipital lobe, parahippocampal gyrus, dorsolateral prefrontal cortex, nucleus accumbens, right orbitofrontal cortex, bilateral anterior cingulate, medial frontal cortex, and the caudate nucleus (Han et al., 2010; Hoeft et al., 2008; Ko et al., 2009). It has also been reported that gaming addicts (like substance addicts) have a higher prevalence of two specific polymorphisms of the dopaminergic system (i.e., Taq1A1 allele of the dopamine D_2 receptor and the Val158Met in the catecholamine-o-methyltransferase receptor) (Han et al., 2007).

Internet Gaming Disorder and the DSM-5

Prior to the publication of the DSM-5 (American Psychiatric Association, 2013), there had been some debate as to whether "Internet addiction" should be introduced into the text as a separate disorder (Block, 2008; Petry & O'Brien, 2013). Alongside this, there was debate as to whether those researching the online addiction field should be researching generalized Internet use and/or the potentially addictive activities that can be engaged on the Internet (e.g., gambling, video gaming, sex, shopping, etc.) (Griffiths, 2000; Griffiths, King, & Demetrovics, 2014). Following these debates, the Substance Use Disorder Work Group (SUDWG) recommended that the DSM-5 include a subtype of problematic Internet use (i.e., Internet gaming disorder [IGD]) in Section 3 ("Emerging Measures and Models") as an area that needed future research before being included in future editions of the DSM (Petry & O'Brien, 2013). According to Petry and O'Brien (2013), IGD will not be included as a separate mental disorder until the (1) defining features of IGD have been identified, (2) reliability and validity of specific IGD criteria have been obtained cross-culturally, (3) prevalence rates have been determined in representative epidemiological samples across the world, and (4) etiology and associated biological features have been evaluated.

One of the key reasons that IGD was not included in the main text of the DSM-5 was that the SUDWG concluded that no standard diagnostic criteria were used to assess gaming addiction across these many studies (Griffiths et al., 2014). A review of instruments assessing problematic, pathological, and/or addictive gaming by King and colleagues (2013) reported that 18 different screening instruments had been developed and that these had been used in 63 quantitative studies comprising 58,415 participants. This comprehensive review identified both strengths and weaknesses of these instruments. The main strengths of the instrumentation included (1) the brevity and ease of scoring; (2) excellent psychometric properties, such as convergent validity and internal consistency; and (3) robust data that will aid the development of standardized norms for adolescent populations. However, the main weaknesses identified in the instrumentation included (1) core addiction indicators being inconsistent across studies, (2) a general lack of any temporal dimension, (3) inconsistent cutoff scores relating to clinical status, (4) poor and/or inadequate interrater reliability and predictive validity; and (5) inconsistency and/or dimensionality. It has also been noted by a number of authors that the criteria for IGD assessment tools are theoretically based on a variety of different potentially problematic activities including substance use disorders, pathological gambling, and/or other behavioral addiction criteria (King et al., 2013; Petry & O'Brien, 2013). There are also issues surrounding the settings in which diagnostic screens are used, as those used in clinical practice settings may require a different emphasis than those used in epidemiological, experimental, and neurobiological research settings (King et al., 2013; Koronczai et al., 2011).

A recent review by Pápay and colleagues (2014) argued that some researchers consider video games as the starting point for examining the characteristics of IGD, while others consider the Internet as the main platform that unites different addictive Internet activities, including online games. Recent studies (Demetrovics et al., 2012; Kim & Kim, 2010) have made an effort to integrate both approaches. Consequently, IGD can either be viewed as a specific type of video game addiction, as a variant of Internet addiction, or as an independent diagnosis (Griffiths et al., 2014).

Griffiths (2005) has argued that although all addictions have particular and idiosyncratic characteristics, they share more commonalities than differences (i.e., salience, mood modification, tolerance, withdrawal symptoms, conflict, and relapse) and likely reflect a common etiology of addictive behavior. Consequently, online game addiction is viewed as a specific type of video game addiction. Similarly, Porter and colleagues (2010) do not differentiate between problematic video game use and problematic online game use. They conceptualized problematic video game use as excessive use of one or more video games resulting in a preoccupation with and a loss of control over playing video games and their various negative psychosocial and/or physical consequences. However, unlike Griffiths (2005), their criteria for problematic video game use does not include other features usually associated with dependence or addiction (e.g., tolerance, physical symptoms of withdrawal) as they say there is no clear evidence that problematic gaming is associated with such phenomena. Researchers such as Young (1998b) view online gaming addiction as a subtype of Internet addiction, as they believe the Internet itself provides situation-specific characteristics that facilitate gaming becoming problematic and/or addictive.

Kim and Kim's (2010) Problematic Online Game Use (POGU) model takes a more integrative approach and claims that neither of the approaches just outlined adequately capture the unique features of online games such as MMORPGs. They argue that the Internet is just one channel where people may access the content they want (e.g., gambling, shopping, sex, etc.) and that such users may become addicted to the particular content rather than to the channel itself. This is analogous to the argument by Griffiths (2000) that there is a fundamental difference between addiction *to* the Internet and addictions *on* the Internet. MMORPGs also differ from single-player video games as there are social and/or role-playing dimensions that allow interaction with other gamers.

The POGU model resulted in five underlying dimensions of addictive gameplay (i.e., euphoria, health problems, conflict, failure of self-control, and preference of virtual relationships). Demetrovics and colleagues (2012) also support the integrative approach and stress the need to include all types of online games in addiction models in order to make comparisons between genres and gamer populations possible (such as those who play online real-time strategy (RTS) games and online first-person shooter (FPS) games in addition to the widely researched MMORPG players). Their model comprises six dimensions (i.e., preoccupation, overuse, immersion, social isolation, interpersonal conflicts, and withdrawal).

Irrespective of approach or model, the components and dimensions that comprise online gaming addiction just outlined are very similar to the IGD criteria in Section 3 of the DSM-5. For instance, Griffiths's (2005) six addiction components directly map onto the nine proposed criteria for IGD (of which five or more need to be endorsed and result in clinically significant impairment). More specifically: (1) preoccupation with Internet games (salience); (2) withdrawal symptoms when Internet gaming is taken away (withdrawal); (3) the need to spend increasing amounts of time engaged in Internet gaming (tolerance), (4) unsuccessful attempts to control participation in Internet gaming (relapse/loss of control); (5) loss of interest in hobbies and entertainment as a result of, and with the exception of, Internet gaming (conflict); (6) continued excessive use of Internet games despite knowledge of psychosocial problems (conflict); (7) deception of family members, therapists, or others regarding the amount of Internet gaming (conflict); (8) use of the Internet gaming to escape or relieve a negative mood (mood modification); and (9) loss of a significant relationship, job, or educational or career opportunity because of participation in Internet games (conflict).

Treatment of Gaming Addiction

Clinical interventions and treatment for problematic and/or addictive gaming vary considerably in the literature, with most of the very few published studies employing some type of CBT, pharmacotherapy, and/or self-devised psychological interventions (Griffiths & Meredith, 2009; Han et al., 2009, 2010; King, Delfabbro, & Griffiths, 2010, 2012). Han et al. (2010) presented some successful case studies regarding pharmacotherapeutic treatment. After a 6-week (Han et al., 2010) and a 12-week (Han & Renshaw, 2012) period of bupropion sustained-release treatment, problematic gamers showed significant improvement, evident in both decreased problem behavior and decreased depression scores. The researchers' pharmacological choice had been driven by the similarities in neurological activity of different behavioral addictions (Han et al., 2010; Ko et al., 2009; Kuss & Griffiths, 2012).

Currently, the evidence base on the treatment of problematic and/or addictive gaming is limited. Furthermore, the lack of consistent approaches to treating problematic video game playing and video game addiction makes it difficult to produce any definitive conclusions as to the efficacy of treatment, although at this stage CBT (as with the treatment efficacy of other addictions) appears to show good preliminary support (King et al., 2012). There remains a need for controlled, comparative studies of psychological and pharmacological treatments, administered individually and in combination with each other, to determine the optimal treatment approach.

The lack of comparative treatment studies might suggest that there is a general lack of demand for psychological services for problematic video game play and/or video game addiction (King et al., 2010). However, this may not necessarily be the case. For instance, Woog (2004) surveyed a random sample of 5,000 US mental health professionals. Although only 229 participants completed the questionnaire, two-thirds had treated someone with excessive computer use problems in the year prior to the survey. Woog also reported that problematic gaming was most common among 11- to 17-year-old clients. However, this may not be truly representative as this age group may be more likely to present in therapy. Anecdotal evidence suggests that 11- to 17-year-old clients are typically forced by concerned parents to attend treatment. Adult gaming addicts may not seek treatment or may seek treatment at a later stage for other psychological problems (e.g., depression) that develop after experiencing the severe negative consequences of gaming.

In South East Asia there appears to be significant demand for treatment for online-related problems, including gaming addiction. The South Korean government has reportedly established a network of more than 140 counseling centers for treatment of online addiction (Kim, 2008). In Western countries, gaming addiction clinics have also started to emerge in places such as Holland and the United Kingdom (Griffiths & Meredith, 2009; King, Delfabbro, Griffiths, & Gradisar, 2011). There are also treatment groups that are modeled on 12-step self-help treatment (e.g., Online Gamers Anonymous) (Griffiths & Meredith, 2009). However, little detail is known about the treatment protocols or their efficacy.

Conclusion

Based on the published empirical studies, and particularly those published over the past decade, it appears that, in extreme cases, excessive gaming can have potentially damaging effects on individuals who appear to display compulsive and/or addictive behavior similar to other more traditional addictions. However, the field has been hindered by the use of inconsistent and nonstandardized criteria to assess and identify problematic and/or addictive video game use. Furthermore, most studies' recruitment methods have serious sampling biases, with an overreliance on self-selected samples.

Despite these shortcomings, there are several noticeable trends that can be drawn from this review of problematic video game play and gaming addiction.

- There has been a significant increase in empirical research decade by decade since the early 1980s.
- There has been a noticeable (and arguably strategic) shift in researching the mode of video game play. In the 1980s, research mainly concerned "pay-to-play" arcade video games. In the 1990s, research mainly concerned stand-alone (offline) video games played at home on consoles, PCs or handheld devices. In the 2000s, research mainly concerned online massively multiplayer video games.
- There has been a noticeable shift in how data are collected. Up until the early 2000s, data about video game behavior were typically collected face to face, whereas contemporary studies collect data online, strategically targeting online forums where gamers are known to (virtually) congregate. These samples are typically self-selecting and (by default) unrepresentative of the general population. Therefore, generalization is almost always one of the methodological shortcomings of this data collection approach.
- Survey study sample sizes have generally increased. In the 1980s and 1990s, sample sizes were typically in the low hundreds. In the 2000s, sample sizes in the thousands—even if unrepresentative—are not uncommon.
- There has been a diversification in the way data are collected, including experiments, physiological investigations, secondary analysis of existing data (such as data collected from online forums), and behavioral tracking studies.
- There has been increased research on adult (i.e., non-child and non-adolescent) samples, reflecting the fact that the demographics of gaming have changed.
- There has been increasing sophistication in relation to issues concerning assessment and measurement of problematic video game play and video game addiction. In the past few years, instruments have been developed that have more robust psychometric properties in terms of reliability and validity. However, there are still some concerns as many of the most widely used screening instruments were adapted from adult screens and much of the video game literature has examined children and adolescents. King et al. (2012) assert that to enable future advances in the development and testing of interventions for video game–related problems, there must be some consensus among clinicians and researchers as to the precise classification of these problems.

The fact that IGD was included in Section 3 of the DSM-5 appears to have been well received by researchers and clinicians in the gaming addiction field (and by those individuals who have sought treatment for such disorders and had their experiences psychiatrically validated). However, for IGD to be included in the section on "Substance-Related and Addictive Disorders" along with "Gambling Disorder," the gaming addiction field must unite and start using the same assessment measures so that comparisons can be made across different demographic groups and different cultures. For epidemiological purposes, Koronczai and colleagues

(2011) assert that the most appropriate measures in assessing problematic online use (including Internet gaming) should meet six requirements. Such an instrument should have (1) brevity (to make surveys as short as possible and help overcome question fatigue), (2) comprehensiveness (to examine all core aspects of problematic gaming as possible), (3) reliability and validity across age groups (e.g., adolescents vs. adults), (4) reliability and validity across data collection methods (e.g., online, face-to-face interview, paper-and-pencil), (5) cross-cultural reliability and validity, and (6) clinical validation. It was also noted that an ideal assessment instrument should serve as the basis for defining adequate cutoff scores in terms of both specificity and sensitivity.

Clearly, there exist a number of gaps in our current understanding of problematic video game play and gaming addiction. King, Delfabbro, and Griffiths (2013) note a need for epidemiological research to determine the incidence and prevalence of clinically significant problems associated with video game play in the broader population. There are too few clinical studies that describe the unique features and symptoms of problematic video game play and/or video game addiction. Most of the studies tend to examine problematic video play from the perspective of the individual. However, there is a small body of research suggesting that the characteristics of the video games themselves may have a role in the acquisition, development, and maintenance of video game addiction. These studies have investigated the role of structural characteristics of video games in maintaining problem playing behavior (King et al., 2011; Westwood & Griffiths, 2010; Wood, Griffiths, Chappell, & Davies, 2004), but there is little empirical research that examines why some individuals may be protected from developing excessive playing habits or whether some individuals simply mature out of their problem playing behavior.

Another growing concern is the recent explosion of online and mobile gaming although, as yet, little research has been done. There are also strong links between online gaming, gambling, non-gambling fantasy games, role-playing games, board games, and card games. These may be an additional cause for concern as youth migrate from free gaming sites to online gambling sites. It should also be noted that video game playing does not occur in a vacuum, but is one behavior engaged in alongside many others. To date, very few studies have been used to examine links between video games and other risk behaviors (e.g., gambling, drug and alcohol use, seatbelt use, poor school performance, conduct problems, truancy, delinquency, violence and sexual activity).

Acknowledgments

Some of the material in this chapter was previously published in the following previous works:

Griffiths, M. D., Kuss, D. J., & King, D. L. (2012). Video game addiction: Past, present and future. *Current Psychiatry Reviews, 8*(4), 308–18. doi:10.2174/157340012803520414

Griffiths, M. D. (2015). Online games, addiction and overuse of. In *The International Encyclopedia of Digital Communication and Society*. Chichester: John Wiley & Sons, Inc.

King, D. L., Delfabbro, P. H., & Griffiths, M. D. (2013). Chapter 82 - Video Game Addiction. In P. M. Miller (Ed.), *Principles of Addiction* (pp. 819–25). San Diego: Academic Press.

References

Allison, S. E., von Wahlde, L., Shockley, T., & Gabbard, G. O. (2006). The development of the self in the era of the Internet and role-playing fantasy games. *American Journal of Psychiatry, 163*, 381–85.

American Psychiatric Association. (1987). *Diagnostic and Statistical Manual for Mental Disorders* (3rd ed.). Washington, DC: Author.

American Psychiatric Association. (1994). *Diagnostic and Statistical Manual for Mental Disorders* (4th ed.). Washington, DC: Author.

American Psychiatric Association. (2013). *Diagnostic and Statistical Manual of Mental Disorders—Text Revision* (5th ed.). Washington, DC: Author.

Barnett, J., & Coulson, M. (2010). Virtually real: A psychological perspective on massively multiplayer online games. *Review of General Psychology, 4*, 167–79.

Batthyány, D., Müller, K. W., Benker, F., & Wölfling, K. (2009). Computer game playing: Clinical characteristics of dependence and abuse among adolescents. *Wiener Klinsche Wochenschrift, 121*(15–16), 502–09.

Blocher, J. M. (2015). Gaming. In R. Papa (Ed.), *Media Rich Instruction* (pp. 219–34). Champaign, IL: Springer International Publishing.

Block, J. J. (2008). Issues for DSM-V: Internet addiction [Editorial]. *American Journal of Psychiatry, 165*, 306.

Brasington, R. (1990). Nintendinitis. *New England Journal of Medicine, 322*, 1473–74.

Brown, R. I. F., & Robertson, S. (1993). Home computer and video game addictions in relation to adolescent gambling: Conceptual and developmental aspects. In W. R. Eadington & J. A. Cornelius (Eds.), *Gambling behavior and problem gambling* (pp. 451–71). Reno: University of Nevada Press.

Caplan, S. E., Williams, D., & Yee, N. (2009). Problematic internet use and psychosocial well-being among MMO players. *Computers in Human Behavior, 25*, 1312–19.

Casanova, J., & Casanova, J. (1991). Nintendinitis. *Journal of Hand Surgery, 16*, 181.

Chan, P. A., & Rabinowitz, T. (2006). A cross-sectional analysis of video games and attention deficit hyperactivity disorder symptoms in adolescents. *Annals of General Psychiatry, 5*(1), 16–26.

Charlton, J. P. (2002). A factor-analytic investigation of computer 'addiction' and engagement. *British Journal of Psychology, 93*, 329–44.

Chiu, S. I., Lee, J. Z., & Huang, D. H. (2004). Video game addiction in children and teenagers in Taiwan. *CyberPsychology and Behavior, 7*, 571–81.

Chuang, Y. C. (2006). Massively multiplayer online role-playing game-induced seizures: A neglected health problem in Internet addiction. *CyberPsychology and Behavior, 9*, 451–56.

Cleary, A. G., Mckendrick, H., & Sills, J. A. (2002). Hand-arm vibration syndrome may be associated with prolonged use of vibrating computer games. *British Medical Journal, 324*, 301.

Cole, H. & Griffiths, M. D. (2007). Social interactions in Massively Multiplayer Online Role-Playing gamers. *CyberPsychology and Behavior, 10*, 575–583.

Corkery, J. C. (1990). Nintendo power. *American Journal of Diseases in Children, 144*, 959.

Cultrara, A., & Har-El, G. (2002). Hyperactivity-induced suprahyoid muscular hypertrophy secondary to excessive video game play: A case report. *Journal of Oral and Maxillofacial Surgery, 60*, 326–27.

Deheger, M., Rolland-Cachera, M. F., & Fontvielle, A. M. (1997). Physical activity and body composition in 10-year-old French children: Linkages with nutritional intake? *International Journal of Obesity, 21*, 372–79.

Demetrovics, Z., Urbán, R., Nagygyörgy, K., Farkas, J., Griffiths, M. D., Pápay, O., . . . Oláh, A. (2012). The development of the Problematic Online Gaming Questionnaire (POGQ). *Plos One, 7*(5), e36417.

Dreier, M., Wölfling, K., & Müller, K. W. (2013). Psychological research and a sociological perspective on problematic and addictive computer game use in adolescents. In A. Tsitsika, M. Janikian, D. E. Greydanus, H. A. Omar, & J. Merrick (Eds.), *Internet addiction: A public health concern in adolescence* (pp. 87–110). New York: Nova Science Publishers.

Dworak, M., Schierl, T., Bruns, T., & Struder, H. K. (2007). Impact of singular excessive computer game and television exposure on sleep patterns and memory performance of school-aged children. *Pediatrics, 120*, 978–85.

Entertainment Software Association. (2014). *Essential facts about the computer and video game industry.* Washington, DC: Entertainment Software Association. www.theesa.com/facts/pdfs/esa_ef_2013.pdf

Fisher, S. E. (1994). Identifying video game addiction in children and adolescents. *Addictive Behaviors, 19*, 545–53.

Gentile, D. A. (2009). Pathological video-game use among youth ages 8 to 18: A national study. *Psychological Science, 20*(5), 594–602.

Gentile, D. A., Choo, H., Liau, A., Sim, T., Li, D. D., Fung, D., & Khoo, A. (2011). Pathological video game use among youths: A two-year longitudinal study. *Pediatrics, 127*(2), 319–29.

Graf, W. D., Chatrian, G. E., Glass, S. T., & Knauss, T. A. (1994). Video-game related seizures: A report on 10 patients and a review of the literature. *Pediatrics, 3*, 551–56.

Griffiths, M. D. (1997). Computer game playing in early adolescence. *Youth and Society, 29*, 223–37.

Griffiths, M. D. (2000). Internet addiction—Time to be taken seriously? *Addiction Research, 8*, 413–18.

Griffiths, M. D. (2005). A 'components' model of addiction within a biopsychosocial framework. *Journal of Substance Use, 10*, 191–97.

Griffiths, M. D. (2010). Computer game playing and social skills: A pilot study. *Aloma: Revista de Psicologia, Ciències de l'Educació i de l'Esport, 27*, 301–10.

Griffiths, M. D., Davies, M. N. O., & Chappell, D. (2004). Demographic factors and playing variables in online computer gaming. *CyberPsychology and Behavior, 7*, 479–87.

Griffiths, M. D., & Hunt, N. (1995). Computer game playing in adolescence: Prevalence and demographic indicators. *Journal of Community and Applied Social Psychology, 5*, 189–93.

Griffiths, M. D., & Hunt, N. (1998). Dependence on computer games by adolescents. *Psychological Reports, 82*, 475–80.

Griffiths, M. D., King, D. L., & Demetrovics, Z. (2014). DSM-5 Internet gaming disorder needs a unified approach to assessment. *Neuropsychiatry, 4*(1), 1–4.

Griffiths, M. D., & Meredith, A. (2009). Videogame addiction and treatment. *Journal of Contemporary Psychotherapy, 39*(4), 47–53.

Grüsser, S. M., Thalemann, R., & Griffiths, M. D. (2007). Excessive computer game playing: Evidence for addiction and aggression? *CyberPsychology and Behavior, 10*, 290–92.

Han, D. H., Hwang, J. W., & Renshaw, P. F. (2010). Bupropion sustained release treatment decreases craving for video games and cue-induced brain activity in patients with Internet video game addiction. *Experimental and Clinical Psychopharmacology, 18*, 297–304.

Han, D. H., Lee, Y. S., Na, C., Ahn, J. Y., Chung, U. S., Daniels, M. A., . . . Renshaw, P. F. (2009). The effect of methylphenidate on Internet video game play in children with attention-deficit/hyperactivity disorder. *Comprehensive Psychiatry, 50*, 251–56.

Han, D. H., Lee, Y. S., Yang, K. C., Kim, E. Y., Lyoo, I. K., & Renshaw, P. F. (2007). Dopamine genes and reward dependence in adolescents with excessive internet video game play. *Journal of Addiction Medicine, 1*, 133–38.

Han, D. H., & Renshaw, P. F. (2012). Bupropion in the treatment of problematic online game play in patients with major depressive disorder. *Journal of Psychopharmacology, 26*, 689–696.

Harding, G. F. A., & Jeavons, P. M. (1994). *Photosensitive epilepsy.* London: Mac Keith Press.

Hoeft, F., Watson, C. L., Kesler, S. R., Bettinger, K. E., & Reiss, A. L. (2008). Gender differences in the mesocorticolimbic system during computer game-play. *Journal of Psychiatric Research, 42*, 253–58.

Hussain, Z., & Griffiths, M. D. (2009a). The attitudes, feelings, and experiences of online gamers: A qualitative analysis. *CyberPsychology and Behavior, 12*, 747–53.

Hussain, Z., & Griffiths, M. D. (2009b). Excessive use of massively-multi-player online role-playing games: A pilot study. *International Journal of Mental Health and Addiction, 7*, 563–71.

Jansz, J., & Tanis, M. (2007). Appeal of playing online first person shooter games. *CyberPsychology & Behavior, 10*(1), 133–136.

Jeong, E. J., & Kim, D. W. (2011). Social activities, self-efficacy, game attitudes, and game addiction. *Cyberpsychology, Behavior & Social Networking, 14*, 213–21.

Johnson, B., & Hackett, A. F. (1997). Eating habits of 11–14-year-old schoolchildren living in less affluent areas of Liverpool, UK. *Journal of Human Nutrition and Dietetics, 10*, 135–44.

Johnston, B., Boyle, L., MacArthur, E., & Manion, B. F. (2013). The role of technology and digital gaming in nurse education. *Nursing Standard, 27*(28), 35–38.

Keepers, G. A. (1990). Pathological preoccupation with video games. *Journal of the American Academy of Child and Adolescent Psychiatry, 29*, 49–50.

Kim, E. J., Namkoong, K., Ku, T., & Kim, S. J. (2008). The relationship between online game addiction and aggression, self-control, and narcissistic personality traits. *European Psychiatry, 23*, 212–18.

Kim, J. (2008). The effect of a R/T group counselling program on the Internet addiction level and self-esteem of Internet addiction university students. *International Journal of Reality Therapy, 17*, 4–12.

Kim, M. G., & Kim, J. (2010). Cross-validation of reliability, convergent and discriminant validity for the problematic online game use scale. *Computers in Human Behavior, 26*, 389–98.

King, D. L., & Delfabbro, P. (2009). Understanding and assisting excessive players of video games: A community psychology perspective. *The Australian Community Psychologist, 21*(1), 62–74.

King, D. L., Delfabbro, P. H., & Griffiths, M. D. (2010). Cognitive behavioural therapy for problematic video game players: Conceptual considerations and practice issues. *Journal of CyberTherapy and Rehabilitation, 3*, 261–73.

King, D. L., Delfabbro, P. H., & Griffiths, M. D. (2011). The role of structural characteristics in problematic video game play: An empirical study. *International Journal of Mental Health and Addiction, 9*, 320–33.

King, D. L., Delfabbro, P. H., & Griffiths, M. D. (2012). Clinical interventions for technology-based problems: Excessive Internet and video game use. *Journal of Cognitive Psychotherapy, 26*, 43–56.

King, D. L., Delfabbro, P. H., & Griffiths, M. D. (2013). Video game addiction. In P. Miller (Ed.), *Principles of addiction: Comprehensive addictive behaviors and disorders.* (Vol. 1, pp. 819–25). San Diego: Academic Press.

King, D. L., Delfabbro, P. H., Griffiths, M. D., & Gradisar, M. (2011). Assessing clinical trials of Internet addiction treatment: A systematic review and CONSORT evaluation. *Clinical Psychology Review, 31*, 1110–16.

King, D. L., Haagsma, M. C., Delfabbro, P. H., Gradisar, M. S., & Griffiths, M. D. (2013). Toward a consensus definition of pathological video-gaming: A systematic review of psychometric assessment tools. *Clinical Psychology Review, 33*, 331–42.

Ko, C. H., Liu, G. C., Hsiao, S. M., Yen, J. Y., Yang, M. J., Lin, W. C., et al. (2009). Brain activities associated with gaming urge of online gaming addiction. Journal of Psychiatric Research, 43, 739–47.

Ko, C. H., Yen, J. Y., Chen, C. C., Chen, S. H., & Yen, C. F. (2005). Gender differences and related factors affecting online gaming addiction among Taiwanese adolescents. *Journal of Nervous and Mental Disease, 193*, 273–77.

Koronczai, B., Urban, R., Kokonyei, G., Paksi, B., Papp, K., Kun, B., . . . Demetrovics, Z. (2011). Confirmation of the three-factor model of problematic internet use on off-line adolescent and adult samples. *Cyberpsychology, Behavior and Social Networking, 14*, 657–64.

Kuczmierczyk, A. R., Walley, P. B., & Calhoun, K. S. (1987). Relaxation training, in vivo exposure and response-prevention in the treatment of compulsive video-game playing. *Scandinavian Journal of Behaviour Therapy, 16*, 185–90.

Kuss, D. J., & Griffiths, M. D. (2012). Online gaming addiction: A systematic review. *International Journal of Mental Health and Addiction, 10*, 278–96.

Lemmens, J. S., Valkenburg, P. M., & Peter, J. (2011). Psychosocial causes and consequences of pathological gaming. *Computers in Human Behavior, 27*, 144–52.

Liu, M., & Peng, W. (2009). Cognitive and psychological predictors of the negative outcomes associated with playing MMOGs (massively multiplayer online games). *Computers in Human Behavior, 25*, 1306–11.

Loftus, G. A., & Loftus, E. F. (1983). *Mind at play: The psychology of video games.* New York: Basic Books.

Maeda, Y., Kurokawa, T., Sakamoto, K., Kitamoto, I., Kohji, U., & Tashima, S. (1990). Electroclinical study of video-game epilepsy. *Developmental Medicine and Child Neurology, 32*, 493–500.

McCowan, T. C. (1981). Space Invaders wrist. *New England Journal of Medicine, 304*, 1368.

Mehroof, M., & Griffiths, M. D. (2010). Online gaming addiction: The role of sensation seeking, self-control, neuroticism, aggression, state anxiety, and trait anxiety. *CyberPsychology and Behavior, 13*, 313–16.

Miller, D. L. G. (1991). Nintendo neck. *Canadian Medical Association Journal, 145*, 1202.

Millett, C. J., Fish, D. R., & Thompson, P. J. (1997). A survey of epilepsy-patient perceptions of video-game material/electronic screens and other factors as seizure precipitants. *Seizure, 6*, 457–59.

Mirman, M. J., & Bonian, V. G. (1992). "Mouse elbow": A new repetitive stress injury. *Journal of the American Osteopath Association, 92*, 701.

Nagygyörgy, K., Urbán, R., Farkas, J., Griffiths, M. D., Zilahy, D., Kökönyei, G., . . . & Harmath, E. (2013). Typology and sociodemographic characteristics of massively multiplayer online game players. *International Journal of Human-Computer Interaction, 29*(3), 192–200.

Nilles, J. M. (1982). *Exploring the world of the personal computer.* Englewood Cliffs, NJ: Prentice Hall.

Ortiz de Gortari, A. B., & Griffiths, M. D. (2014a). Auditory experiences in Game Transfer Phenomena: An empirical self-report study. *International Journal of Cyber Behavior, Psychology and Learning, 4*(1), 59–75.

Ortiz de Gortari, A. B., & Griffiths, M. D. (2014b). Altered visual perception in Game Transfer Phenomena: An empirical self-report study. *International Journal of Human-Computer Interaction, 30*, 95–105.

Pápay, O., Nagygyörgy, K., Griffiths, M. D., & Demetrovics, Z. (2014). Problematic online gaming. In K. Rosenberg & L. Feder (Eds.), *Behavioral addictions: Criteria, evidence and treatment* (pp. 61–95). New York: Elsevier.

Pápay, O., Urbán, R., Griffiths, M. D., Nagygyörgy, K., Farkas, J., Elekes, Z., . . . Demetrovics, Z. (2013). Psychometric properties of the Problematic Online Gaming Questionnaire Short-Form (POGQ-SF) and prevalence of problematic online gaming in a national sample of adolescents. *Cyberpsychology, Behavior and Social Networking, 16*, 340–48.

Parker, J. D. A., Taylor, R. N., Eastabrook, J. M., Schell, S. L., & Wood, L. M. (2008). Problem gambling in adolescence: Relationships with internet misuse, gaming abuse and emotional intelligence. *Personality and Individual Differences, 45*(2), 174–80.

Parsons, K. (1995, April). Educational places or terminal cases: Young people and the attraction of computer games. Paper presented at the British Sociological Association Annual Conference, University of Leicester.

Peng, W., & Liu, M. (2010). Online gaming dependency: A preliminary study in China. *Cyberpsychology, Behavior and Social Networking, 13*, 329–33.

Peters, C. S., & Malesky, L. A. (2008). Problematic usage among highly-engaged players of massively multiplayer online role-playing games. *CyberPsychology and Behavior, 11*, 480–83.

Petry, N. M., & O'Brien, C. P. (2013). Internet gaming disorder and the DSM-5. *Addiction, 108*, 1186–87.

Phillips, C. A., Rolls, S., Rouse, A., & Griffiths, M. D. (1995). Home video game playing in schoolchildren: A study of incidence and pattern of play. *Journal of Adolescence, 18*, 687–91.

Pontes, H., & Griffiths, M. D. (2014). The assessment of internet gaming disorder in clinical research. *Clinical Research and Regulatory Affairs, 31*(2–4), 35–48.

Porter, G., Starcevic, V., Berle, D., & Fenech, P. (2010). Recognizing problem video game use. *The Australian and New Zealand Journal of Psychiatry, 44*(2), 120–28.

Przybylski, A. K. (2014). Electronic gaming and psychosocial adjustment. *Pediatrics, 134*(3), e716–e722.

Quirk, J. A., Fish, D. R., Smith, S. J. M., Sander, J. W., Shorvon, S. D., & Allen, P. J. (1995). First seizures associated with playing electronic screen games: A community based study in Great Britain. *Annals of Neurology, 37*, 110–24.

Rehbein, F., Kleimann, M., & Mossle, T. (2010). Prevalence and risk factors of video game dependency in adolescence: Results of a German nationwide survey. *CyberPsychology, Behavior and Social Networking, 13*, 269–77.

Reinstein, L. (1983). De Quervain's stenosing tenosynovitis in a video games player. *Archives of Physical and Medical Rehabilitation, 64*, 434–35.

Schink, J. C. (1991). Nintendo enuresis. *American Journal of Diseases in Children, 145*, 1094.

Shimai, S., Yamada, F., Masuda, K., & Tada, M. (1993). TV game play and obesity in Japanese school children. *Perceptual and Motor Skills, 76*, 1121–22.

Shotton, M. (1989). *Computer addiction? A study of computer dependency*. London: Taylor and Francis.

Siegal, I. M. (1991). Nintendonitis. *Orthopedics, 14*, 745.

Skoric, M. M., Teo, L. L. C., & Neo, R. L. (2009). Children and video games: Addiction, engagement, and scholastic achievement. *CyberPsychology and Behavior, 12*, 567–72.

Soper, W. B., & Miller, M. J. (1983). Junk time junkies: An emerging addiction among students. *School Counsellor, 31*, 40–43.

Spence, S. A. (1993). Nintendo hallucinations: A new phenomenological entity. *Irish Journal of Psychological Medicine, 10*, 98–99.

Thalemann, R., Wölfling, K., & Grüsser, S. M. (2007). Specific cue reactivity on computer game-related cues in excessive gamers. *Behavioral Neuroscience, 12*, 614–18.

Thomas, N. J., & Martin, F. H. (2010). Video-arcade game, computer game and Internet activities of Australian students: Participation habits and prevalence of addiction. *Australian Journal of Psychology, 62*, 59–66.

Vandewater, E. A., Shim, M., & Caplovitz, A. G. (2004). Linking obesity ad activity level with children's television and game use. *Journal of Adolescence, 27*, 71–85.

Van Rooij, A. J., Schoenmakers, T. M., Vermulst, A. A., Van den Eijnden, R. J., & Van de Mheen, D. (2011). Online video game addiction: Identification of addicted adolescent gamers. *Addiction, 106*(1), 205–12.

Westwood, D., & Griffiths, M. D. (2010). The role of structural characteristics in video game play motivation: A Q-Methodology study. *Cyberpsychology, Behavior and Social Networking, 13*, 581–85.

Widyanto, L., Griffiths, M. D., & Brunsden, V. (2011). A psychometric comparison of the Internet Addiction Test, the Internet Related Problem Scale, and self-diagnosis. *Cyberpsychology, Behavior, and Social Networking, 14*, 141–49.

Wood, R. T. A., Griffiths, M. D., Chappell, D., & Davies, M. N. O. (2004). The structural characteristics of video games: A psycho-structural analysis. *CyberPsychology and Behavior, 7*, 1–10.

Woog, K. (2004). A survey of mental health professionals' clinical exposure to problematic computer use. Unpublished study. http://www.wooglabs.com/

Yee, N. (2006a). The demographics, motivations and derived experiences of users of massively-multiuser online graphical environments. *PRESENCE: Teleoperators and Virtual Environments, 15*, 309–29.

Yee, N. (2006b). The psychology of MMORPGs: Emotional investment, motivations, relationship formation, and problematic usage. In R. Schroeder & A. Axelsson (Eds.), *Avatars at work and play: Collaboration and interaction in shared virtual environments* (pp. 187–207). London: Springer.

Young, K. (1998a). *Caught in the net*. Chichester, UK: Wiley.

Young, K. S. (1998b). Internet addiction: The emergence of a new clinical disorder. *Cyberpsychology and Behavior, 1*, 237–44.

Yousafzai, S., Hussain, Z., & Griffiths, M. D. (2013). Social responsibility in online videogaming: What should the videogame industry do? *Addiction Research & Theory, 22*(3), 181–85.

Zamani, E., Kheradmand, A., Cheshmi, M., Abedi, A., & Hedayati, N. (2010). Comparing the social skills of students addicted to computer games with normal students. *Journal of Addiction and Health, 2*, 59–69.

CHAPTER

3 Youth and Technology

A Developmental Perspective on Internet Use

Gerrit I. van Schalkwyk, Joshua D. Golt, *and* Wendy K. Silverman

Abstract

Use of the Internet for interpersonal communication has dramatically altered the lives of youth. Awareness of the unique properties of this style of communication has given rise to both concern and optimism about its developmental consequences. Current findings suggest that the Internet may act to supplement offline relationships and offer some utility to socially anxious youth, with relatively limited evidence for adverse effects on psychological well-being. However, there continue to be concerns about how Internet-mediated communication may affect certain vulnerable groups. In addition, although this technology may provide a new platform for sharing of information, current data points to negative consequences for overall academic performance. Further study is indicated given the complexity of this area.

Keywords: Internet-mediated communication, peer relationships, psychological well-being, academic performance, social media

Introduction

Technology is increasingly dominant in the lives of children and adolescents (Subrahmanyam & Greenfield, 2008). Whereas early developments like television and video games provided compelling new media for entertainment, the Internet has become a pervasive platform for engaging in an extremely broad range of activities—from online shopping to sexual engagement. The use of the Internet for interpersonal communication is widespread, with multiple studies in developed countries reporting high rates of use: 84% in the Netherlands (Valkenburg & Peter, 2007b) and 73% in the United States (Lenhart, Purcell, Smith, & Zickuhr, 2010). Facebook remains the most popular social networking site and is used by 71% of adult Internet users in the United States (Duggan, Ellison, Lampe, Lenhart, & Madden, 2015). The pace at which Internet-mediated communication (IMC) has become a dominant form of communication for adolescents is dramatic.

This trend has not gone unnoticed by the popular news media or the academic community, with the creation of multiple new journals dedicated to the study of IMC and other Internet-related issues (e.g., *Cyberpsychology; Behavior and Social Networking*; *Journal of Computer Mediated Communication*). Concerns about the potential risks of IMC, as well as optimism about its unique potential utilities, predate the development of Facebook and have been the subject of systematic study since about 1998 (Kraut et al., 1998). Much of the interest relates to developmental considerations, including the potential consequences on the social and academic development of youth (Subrahmanyam, Greenfield, Kraut, & Gross, 2001). Attention has further been drawn to the consequences of IMC on psychological well-being (Shaw & Gant, 2002). The discourse in each of these areas highlights both specific concerns (such as cyberbullying and the development of depression) and sources of optimism (such as the potential for IMC to help socially anxious individuals).

After almost two decades of research, the literature now includes multiple theories and a growing body of empirical data. Early patterns have been identified in existing data, such as the increasingly substantiated finding that IMC serves to enhance communication with existing friends (e.g., Valkenburg & Peter, 2009). It is also recognized however that further progress in understanding will necessitate more specific inquiry, as the consequences of IMC may vary across contexts (Mitchell, Lebow, Uribe, Grathouse, & Shoger, 2011).

In this chapter, we summarize some of the most salient literature regarding Internet use and its developmental consequences in children and adolescents (broadly referred to as "youth" when considered together). To this end, we draw attention to the available empirical data and theoretical ideas which continue to influence research in this field.

Chapter Overview and Conceptual Issues

It has been noted that, given the diversity and ubiquity of the Internet, it is important to frame inquiry into its effects in specific terms (Mitchell et al., 2011). Otherwise, the "Internet" cannot reasonably be investigated for its capacity to have "negative" developmental consequence—this would be akin to attempting to describe the developmental consequences of talking to others. Equally important, in summarizing the literature for this chapter, we sought to define our focus in a way that would facilitate analysis of key ideas and findings. In the process of establishing this focus, we have chosen not to summarize the literature regarding video game use, which is covered elsewhere in this book. Although video game use has been viewed as a discrete construct and handled as such in meta-analysis (Anderson & Bushman, 2001), multiple dimensions to video gaming experiences have been described (Kolo & Baur, 2004). Online video gaming has, in some instances, given prominence to cooperative play and, in some instances, parallel virtual lives, with their own social dynamics (Kolo & Baur, 2004). This shift is an example of the capacity of how the Internet may facilitate social connectedness—albeit one that is qualitatively distinct from connections based on face-to-face interactions. It is this phenomenon on which we focus in this chapter, under the broad label of IMC.

IMC remains a broad concept, encompassing a number of distinct types of communicative activity. Perhaps the earliest example of IMC was simple, one-to-one communication using email or messaging services. This continues to be a highly prevalent form of IMC and is often incorporated into other more complex platforms (e.g., private chat functions on web forums). Platforms such as Facebook create the potential for a range of interactions, including private messaging, broadcasting (whereby content is posted to be viewed by a broad audience), and the monitoring of content made available by others (Lenhart & Madden, 2007).

In considering the consequences of IMC, it thus becomes important to consider what in particular is under study. Whereas it is understandably common that people may ask the question, "Is it good for my kids?," the most accurate response is that this may vary greatly depending on specific developmental outcomes. On one hand, there is research highlighting the value of electronic messaging for enhancing peer relationships (Valkenburg & Peter, 2007b). On the other hand, other research highlights ways in which features of IMC may lead to increased stress, such as the ability of users of social networking sites such as Facebook to monitor posts by friends. In a survey of 425 undergraduate students engaging in this type of monitoring, this activity was associated with a belief that one is less happy than one's peers (Chou & Edge, 2012). It would therefore seem that whereas one type of IMC may have social benefits, another application of the technology might lead to stress.

In this chapter, we focus on three categories of developmental outcomes as they relate to IMC use: social, psychological, and academic development. In addressing social development, we review literature related to the potential consequences of IMC on the development of adolescents' relationships. We focus on peer relationships specifically as they have been most heavily researched by investigators (Subrahmanyam & Greenfield, 2008).

In discussing psychological well-being, we summarize the literature on the relation between use of IMC and factors like self-esteem in youth, as well as possible associations with psychiatric illness. Regarding the latter, we also highlight interesting descriptions of how IMC may be of particular use to certain psychiatric populations. Regarding academic development, we discuss emerging understanding of how IMC may influence this process in youth, again drawing attention to both relevant concerns (such as possible effects on writing ability) and areas of optimism (such as enhanced access to information).

We begin the chapter with a general discussion of some of the features of IMC that distinguishes it from other forms of communication, and we substantiate the importance of it being a specific focus of research. We make limited reference to the construct of cyberbullying, which, although trans-theoretically applicable to a number of topics in this chapter, is the focus of another chapter in this volume.

Features of Internet-Mediated Communication

Although there is little dispute that communication over the Internet is distinct from face-to-face interaction, it is worth considering what these distinctions are. These distinctions relate to specific hypotheses about how IMC may be experienced by youth—and in turn, how it may be developmentally consequential. It has been suggested that, owing to IMC's properties, it is likely to constitute a less stressful form of interaction for some individuals (Baker & Oswald, 2010). For example, the decreased reliance on nonverbal cues and increased capacity for control of the interaction may be significant factors which facilitate online self-disclosure (Schouten, Valkenburg, & Peter, 2007).

In a qualitative study of 20 adolescents (aged 13–18 years) with psychiatric illness, participants highlighted how the capacity to formulate responses slowly and deliberately when using IMC reduced the overall stress of the social interaction, particularly when sharing sensitive content. Participants also highlighted the unique value of being able to broadcast messages to a broad but selective audience (their Facebook "friends"), such that anyone who was available could respond to them (van Schalkwyk et al 2015). The potentially greater anonymity of certain types of IMC may further serve to reduce stress as individuals may feel there are fewer consequences in sharing and requesting information. Current popular platforms (like Facebook) are less anonymous, however, and do not offer this advantage. Taken together, these features of IMC have given rise to ideas about how it may be an especially useful communicative platform for socially anxious individuals (Baker & Oswald, 2010). Recent empirical work in youth with autism spectrum disorder (ASD) has identified an association between social media use and friendship quality, although this relationship is absent in youth with higher levels of social anxiety (van Schalkwyk et al., 2017).

Other unique features of IMC may be considered as disadvantages. In the course of IMC, content is often restricted to text, and much of the additional social message may be lost, with increased potential for misunderstanding (Byron, 2008). Relatedly, it has been suggested that interpersonal relationships that develop over the Internet likely constitute weaker bonds than those that include a face-to-face component (Cummings, Butler, & Kraut, 2002), although the empirical findings in this regard are mixed (discussed further later). In addition, the 24/7 nature of IMC appears to be a significant feature, facilitating a major increase in the connectedness of adolescents to their peer group. This may serve as a source of anxiety for vulnerable youth (van Schalkwyk et al., 2015) as it may exacerbate pressure for constant engagement (Turkle, 2008). Constant engagement may also place individuals at increased risk for cyberbullying (Campbell, Spears, Slee, Butler, & Kift, 2012; see other chapters in this volume).

Awareness of the specific ways in which IMC differs from face-to-face communication has led to the development of hypotheses about how IMC may influence the development of relationships, psychological well-being, and academic performance of adolescents. We discuss these further next.

Internet-Mediated Communication and Peer Relationships

It has been suggested that understanding the social consequences of IMC may be organized around two lines of inquiry (Cummings et al., 2002). First, there are questions about how IMC may influence the pattern of individuals' social engagement and whether it is likely to supplement existing online relationships or serve to displace offline social activities. Second, there is a question of how IMC may influence the quality of relationships and how online relationships compare in quality to offline relationships.

Internet-Mediated Communication and Social Engagement

Early empirical work exploring the social consequences of Internet use led to the description of the "Internet paradox" (Kraut et al., 1998). Kraut et al. examined the effects of having Internet access in a sample of 169 people (all 10 years of age and older, with three times as many adults as teenagers) in 73 households. Kraut et al. noted that despite the fact that the Internet was a "social technology," its use was associated with decreased communication among family members and smaller social circles. These effects were not sustained in the sample after a 3-year follow-up, but the initial description nevertheless gave prominence to the *displacement hypothesis*. This hypothesis suggests that engagement on the Internet may have negative social consequences by acting to "displace" other, more enriching activities, such as spending time with friends or family (Kraut et al., 2002).

By contrast, another prominent hypothesis in the literature is the *increase hypothesis*. Early evidence for this hypothesis came from a large-scale Internet-based survey conducted on the National Geographic Society Website in 1998, in which participants reported using IMC to "supplement" offline communication, increasing the overall time spent in contact with others (Wellman, Haase, Witte, & Hampton, 2001). Also referred to as the *stimulating hypothesis*, further support for this hypothesis came from a subsequent survey of 1,210 Dutch teenagers (Valkenburg & Peter, 2007a). Results of a mediation analysis showed that instant messaging use led to increased time spent with existing friends and improved peer relationships.

Attempts to further confirm the validity of the preceding hypotheses have led to more specific research efforts aimed at answering questions about which types of individuals are likely to experience benefit from using the Internet and social networking sites in particular (Caplan, 2007; Mitchell et al., 2011; Sheeks & Birchmeier, 2007; Valkenburg & Peter, 2009). This line of research has led to at least two additional hypotheses (Lee, 2009). First, the *rich-get-richer hypothesis* suggests that online communication is of greatest value to individuals who are non-lonely and have strong social skills. These individuals use the Internet as yet another way to maintain and build these established connections—a model initially supported by a follow-up study by Kraut et al. (2002). The *social-compensation hypothesis*, a contrasting idea to the rich-get-richer hypothesis, suggests that, owing to particular qualities of online communication that may make it less anxiety-provoking than face-to-face communication, it may be especially helpful to those with social anxiety (McKenna & Bargh, 2000).

Although frequently framed as opposing, recent work has emphasized that each hypothesis may have explanatory power in different contexts. For example, Valkenburg and Peter (2007b) conducted a large cross-sectional survey (N = 794) that included the goal of evaluating the contrasting rich-get-richer and social-compensation hypotheses. Results suggested that whereas socially anxious respondents communicated less often with peers than did non–socially anxious respondents (consistent with the rich-get-richer hypothesis), socially anxious respondents considered the Internet more valuable for the purposes of intimate self-disclosure. A subsequent longitudinal study conducted with grade 9 secondary school students examined the linkages between IMC and friendship quality over 4 years (Desjarlais & Willoughby, 2010). The authors reported a main effect of computer use and friendship quality in girls (supporting both hypotheses), but found that, in boys, this effect was moderated by social anxiety (supporting the social-compensation hypothesis).

Internet-Mediated Communication and Quality of Relationships

An additional area of focus relates to the quality of interactions and resultant relationships formed online. Multiple different perspectives have been proposed. The *hyperpersonal perspective* emphasizes how computer-mediated communication may provide a mechanism for a type of interaction that is in some ways even richer than face-to-face interactions (Walther, 1996). The hyperpersonal perspective highlights how computer-mediated communication may lead to an individual's "greater allocation of cognitive resources" to the process of crafting and editing social responses, leading to enhanced capacity for "impression development" and, resultantly, improved relationship intimacy (Walther, 2007).

Although it had been suggested that IMC leads primarily to the development of "weak ties" (Kraut et al., 1998) (i.e., relationships that are useful for information exchange, rather than emotional support), empirical work suggests that, over time, interpersonal relationships developed. Oher work exploring national survey data reported a high prevalence of 'close' relationships that intersected with offline peer groups in a sample of teenagers (Wolak, Mithcell and Finkelor, 2002). Taken together, this literature challenges early ideas about online relationships being of lower quality.

Implications

What are the developmental implications of these findings with respect to peer relationships? Clearly, the capacity exists for IMC to provide an additional platform for relationships to develop. This may act to further enrich the social development of those individuals who previously had large social networks. In addition, IMC may serve as an important lifeline for individuals who experience significant difficulties with face-to-face interactions, for whom the Internet may facilitate relationship-building self-disclosures.

Further research is needed to better understand ways in which vulnerable subgroups may be socially disadvantaged as a result of IMC's 24/7 nature. The importance of strong peer relationships on social development is well-described (Greenberg, Siegel, & Leitch, 1983). Although emerging data suggest intimate relationships are possible through online interactions, it remains unclear whether online relationships fulfill all the requirements to be developmentally formative.

Internet-Mediated Communication and Psychological Well-Being

Research examining the association between IMC and psychological well-being has focused on a range of related outcomes, perhaps most commonly, symptoms of depression, feelings of loneliness, self-esteem, and perceived social support (Huang, 2010; Shaw & Gant, 2002; van den Eijnden, Meerkerk, Vermulst, Spijkerman, & Engels, 2008; Weiser, 2001). Several studies have also examined the relation between IMC and social anxiety (Bonetti, Campbell, & Gilmore, 2010; Gross, Juvonen, & Gable, 2002). Frequently, these outcomes are combined within individual studies to represent the summative construct of psychological well-being. As such, this section will discuss findings related to these outcomes in parallel.

In addition to enhancing our understanding of the interaction between IMC and social relationships, Kraut et al. (1998) found Internet use led to increased symptoms of depression and perceived decreases in social support. This finding was more prominent in teenage participants relative to adult participants. In the absence of a comparison control sample, further research is needed, especially since reduced social support may be a normative teenage experience (Gross et al., 2002).

More than 40 studies have been conducted aimed at understanding the relations between Internet use and psychological well-being since the initial work of Kraut (Kraut et al., 1998). Multiple studies have found the absence of significant statistical associations between Internet use and psychological well-being (Gross, 2004; Gross et al., 2002; Wästlund, Norlander, & Archer, 2001), although a recent study in adults did find an association with depression (Lin et al., 2016). Among studies of youth, one study is noteworthy in its use of an experimental design to determine whether engagement in structured online communication may lead to improvements in psychological well-being (Shaw & Gant, 2002). University students in an introductory psychology course were administered a pre-test in which self-ratings of loneliness, self-esteem, and perceived social support were obtained. Subsequently, participants engaged in five structured, anonymous chat sessions, being paired with other participants within same-gender dyads. These chat sessions were structured in that specific questions were supplied by the investigators, but participants were allowed to discuss these questions for as long as they wanted. Measures were readministered midway (after completion of two sessions) and again upon study conclusion, at which point four sessions had occurred. Findings indicated significant decreases in participants' self-ratings of depressive symptoms and loneliness, along with significant increases in self-esteem and social support. The authors presented their results as a source of optimism, but acknowledged their experimental paradigm did not necessarily mirror a "typical" online experience, given its scripted nature.

Huang (2010) synthesized the literature on this topic and conducted a meta-analysis of 43 studies, representing a total of 21,258 participants. Huang's overall finding was that a small negative association (−0.0504 using a fixed-effects model and.0385 for the random-effects model) between high use of the Internet and negative psychological well-being. The author highlighted that the magnitude of the effect size was small but similar to effect sizes noted in other meta-analyses of correlations between Internet use and psychological well-being indicators. The effects of all variables examined as potential moderators, including type of Internet use and participant well-being, age, and gender, were not significant. Huang (2010) urged caution, though, in interpreting the absence of significant moderator effects as not all the studies reported data on these variables, thus leading to reduced statistical power although the specifics of the "missingness" (e.g., which variables and how much) was not indicated.

Multiple studies have examined associations between use of social-network sites and psychiatric illness—in particular, major depressive disorder. Pantic et al. (2012) conducted a cross-sectional study focusing on depressive symptoms as rated by the Beck Depression Inventory in a sample of 160 high school students. Results indicated a significant, positive association between depression scores and reported time spent on social networking sites. By contrast, a subsequent study using the Patient Health Questionnaire 9 in a sample of 190 individuals (average age = 18.9 years) found a lack of an association between self-ratings of depression and social networking site usage (Jelenchick, Eickhoff, & Moreno, 2013). These inconsistent findings led Pantic (2014) to conclude that further longitudinal work is needed before it is possible to draw inferences between depression and time spent on social networking sites (Pantic, 2014).

There has also been interest in the potential utility of IMC for mental health treatment. In a study examining the Facebook disclosures of 200 college students, it was found that 25% of the participants included posted symptoms consistent with DSM criteria for depression, with the authors highlighting the potential for Facebook to aid in the identification of at-risk students (Moreno et al., 2011). In a qualitative study, adolescents with psychiatric illness (mostly major depressive disorder) expressed interest in communicating with mental health providers using IMC. The participants suggested that the Internet may represent a less anxiety-provoking form of communication, could facilitate more continued access to support, and could allow providers to monitor their patients' ongoing mental states (van Rensburg, Klingensmith, McLaughlin, Qayyum, & van Schalkwyk, 2015). However, participants also emphasized the importance of providers being able to respond within a brief period of time (such as a few minutes). The challenge of patients attempting to use IMC for more urgent communication has previously been described (Stubbe, 2012).

In summary, there is currently no convincing empirical evidence of a significant relation between use of IMC and negative outcomes on psychological well-being. In the absence of such evidence, it is nevertheless appropriate that youth be supported with difficulties they may experience in the course of engaging IMC. Future research efforts should aim to more precisely clarify which individuals may be at risk for negative impacts on their psychological well-being. In addition, the potential for IMC to enhance access and engagement with psychiatric care may be a fruitful avenue for continued investigation.

Internet-Mediated Communication and Academic Development

Concern and optimism about the academic consequences of Internet use stem from a broad range of ideas. One significant area of concern is Internet addiction and how this may distract youth from focusing on school tasks to the detriment of their academic performance (Kubey, Lavin, & Barrows, 2001). The topic of Internet addiction is discussed elsewhere in this book. In this section, we reference briefly its relation with academic performance. In addition, we highlight ways in which IMC has been found to enhance aspects of academic development.

The results of a survey completed by 572 students at a large public university found a positive correlation between heavy recreational Internet use (such as chat rooms) and poor academic performance (Kubey et al., 2001). More recent studies have focused on Facebook use in particular. A study of both undergraduate and graduate students at an unnamed university in the Midwestern United States ($N = 219$) found Facebook users had significantly lower grade point averages than non-users, and they also reported spending significantly fewer hours studying (Kirschner & Karpinski, 2010). However, two other studies in similar samples found no statistically significant associations between use of social networking sites and academic performance (Kolek & Saunders, 2008; Pasek, More, & Hargittai, 2009).

These findings may be explained by the hypothesis that the academic impact of Internet use, and IMC use in particular, may depend on the purposes for which the technology is being used (Bliuc, Ellis, Goodyear, & Piggott, 2010). A large study of college students ($N = 1{,}839$) replicated prior findings of a negative association between Facebook use and grade point average (GPA) (Junco, 2012). However, when looking at specific activities on Facebook, "status updates" and "chatting," which the authors broadly group under "socializing," was negatively associated with a higher GPA, whereas checking on friends and sharing links, which the authors group under "collecting and sharing information," was positively associated with a higher GPA. The authors describe potential ways that faculty members, for example, could capitalize on such a finding by creating Facebook groups for specific courses. This recommendation echoes other reports in the literature on how Facebook may be used as an educational tool through the development of education "micro-communities," among other mechanisms (Bosch, 2009).

Taken together, these findings highlight the potential risks of IMC on academic performance insofar as this may represent a time-consuming activity that has been linked to reduced time spent on academic work. However, this is not a universal finding, and more recent work provides evidence of ways in which IMC may lead to improved academic performance through facilitation of information gathering and sharing.

Conclusion

The use of the Internet for communication and social engagement represents a significant change in the lives of youths. Understanding the developmental consequences of this change is a considerable challenge given the wide range of potential influences and outcomes. Recognition of the ways in which IMC differs from other forms of communication has informed further efforts to clarify its specific effects. However, to date, existing data have only begun to answer the growing lists of questions about ways in which IMC may affect the peer relationships, psychological well-being, and academic performance of youths.

Regarding peer relationships, there are data suggesting that IMC may act to supplement and enhance offline relationships. Other areas of potential benefit (such as IMC being of potentially unique value in vulnerable populations) and risk (such as IMC acting as a source of anxiety) remain areas of interest that require further investigation. In terms of psychological well-being, although current empirical work has failed to show consistent, statistically significant impacts of IMC use in this regard, further work is needed to clarify whether specific individuals may be at greater risk, even if effects are not clearly detectable in samples drawn from the general population. The potential for IMC to displace academic activities has been shown in several large studies, with potentially significant consequences on academic performance.

Encouragingly, there appears to be increasing interest in conducting research into the effects of IMC. Future research efforts may benefit from focused approaches looking at specific types of IMC in different populations and with specific, hypothesis-driven outcomes in mind. In addition, research looking at vulnerable populations in particular should be prioritized. The potential advantages of IMC in these populations should be acknowledged although a better understanding of the difficulties youth may encounter is perhaps more urgent. Such an understanding could equip parents and clinicians to better protect these individuals from suffering negative developmental consequences.

References

Anderson, C. A., & Bushman, B. J. (2001). Effects of violent video games on aggressive behavior, aggressive cognition, aggressive affect, physiological arousal, and prosocial behavior: A meta-analytic review of the scientific literature. *Psychological Science, 12*, 353–59. doi:10.1111/1467-9280.00366

Baker, L. R., & Oswald, D. L. (2010). Shyness and online social networking services. *Journal of Social and Personal Relationships, 27*(7), 873–89. doi:10.1177/0265407510375261

Bliuc, A. M., Ellis, R., Goodyear, P., & Piggott, L. (2010). Learning through face-to-face and online discussions: Associations between students' conceptions, approaches and academic performance in political science. *British Journal of Educational Technology, 41*, 512–24. doi:10.1111/j.1467–8535.2009.00966.x

Bonetti, L., Campbell, M. A., & Gilmore, L. (2010). The relationship of loneliness and social anxiety with children's and adolescents' online communication. *Cyberpsychology, Behavior and Social Networking, 13*, 279–85. doi:10.1089/cyber.2009.0215

Bosch, T. E. (2009). Using online social networking for teaching and learning: Facebook use at the University of Cape Town. *Communication, 35*, 185–200. doi:10.1080/02500160903250648

Byron, K. (2008). Carrying too heavy a load? The communication and miscommunication of emotion by email. *Academy of Management Review, 33*, 309–27. doi:10.5465/AMR.2008.31193163

Campbell, M., Spears, B., Slee, P., Butler, D., & Kift, S. (2012). Victims' perceptions of traditional and cyberbullying, and the psychosocial correlates of their victimisation. *Emotional and Behavioural Difficulties, 17*(3–4), 389–401. doi:10.1080/13632752.2012.704316

Caplan, S. E. (2007). Relations among loneliness, social anxiety, and problematic Internet use. *Cyberpsychology & Behavior: The Impact of the Internet, Multimedia and Virtual Reality on Behavior and Society, 10*(2), 234–42. doi:10.1089/cpb.2006.9963

Chan, D. K.-S., & Cheng, G. H.-L. (2004). A Comparison of Offline and Online friendship qualities at different stages of relationship development. *Journal of Social and Personal Relationships, 21*(3), 305–320. doi:10.1177/0265407504042834

Chou, H.-T. G., & Edge, N. (2012). "They are happier and having better lives than I am": The impact of using Facebook on perceptions of others' lives. *Cyberpsychology, Behavior and Social Networking, 15*(2), 117–21. doi:10.1089/cyber.2011.0324

Cummings, J. N., Butler, B., & Kraut, R. (2002). The quality of online social relationships. *Communications of the ACM, 45*(7), 103–108. doi:10.1145/514236.514242

Desjarlais, M., & Willoughby, T. (2010). A longitudinal study of the relation between adolescent boys and girls' computer use with friends and friendship quality: Support for the social compensation or the rich-get-richer hypothesis? *Computers in Human Behavior, 26*(5), 896–05. doi:10.1016/j.chb.2010.02.004

Duggan, M., Ellison, N. B., Lampe, C., Lenhart, A., & Madden, M. (2015). Demographics of key social networking platforms. Pew Research Center. https://www.pewresearch.org/internet/2015/01/09/demographics-of-key-social-networking-platforms-2/

Greenberg, M. T., Siegel, J. M., & Leitch, C. J. (1983). The nature and importance of attachment relationships to parents and peers during adolescence. *Journal of Youth and Adolescence, 12*(5), 373–86. doi:10.1007/BF02088721

Gross, E. F. (2004). Adolescent internet use: What we expect, what teens report. *Journal of Applied Developmental Psychology, 25*, 633–49. doi:10.1016/j.appdev.2004.09.005

Gross, E. F., Juvonen, J., & Gable, S. L. (2002). Internet use and well-being in adolescence. *Journal of Social Issues, 58*(1), 75–90. doi:10.1111/1540–4560.00249

Huang, C. (2010). Internet use and psychological well-being: A meta-analysis. *Cyberpsychology, Behavior and Social Networking, 13*(3), 241–49. doi:10.1089/cyber.2009.0217

Jelenchick, L. A., Eickhoff, J. C., & Moreno, M. A. (2013). Facebook depression? Social networking site use and depression in older adolescents. *Journal of Adolescent Health, 52*, 128–30. doi:10.1016/j.jadohealth.2012.05.008

Junco, R. (2012). Too much face and not enough books: The relationship between multiple indices of Facebook use and academic performance. *Computers in Human Behavior, 28*, 187–98. doi:10.1016/j.chb.2011.08.026

Kirschner, P. A., & Karpinski, A. C. (2010). Facebook and academic performance. *Computers in Human Behavior, 26*, 1237–45. doi:10.1016/j.chb.2010.03.024

Kolek, E. A., & Saunders, D. (2008). Online disclosure: An empirical examination of undergraduate Facebook profiles. *Journal of Student Affairs Research and Practice, 45*(1), 1–25. doi:10.2202/1949–6605.1905

Kolo, C., & Baur, T. (2004). Living a virtual life: Social dynamics of online gaming. *Game Studies, 4*(1). http://www.gamestudies.org/0401/kolo/

Kraut, R., Kiesler, S., Boneva, B., Cummings, J., Helgeson, V., & Crawford, A. (2002). Internet paradox revisited. *Journal of Social Issues, 58*, 49–74. doi:10.1111/1540–4560.00248

Kraut, R., Patterson, M., Lundmark, V., Kiesler, S., Mukopadhyay, T., & Scherlis, W. (1998). Internet paradox. A social technology that reduces social involvement and psychological well-being? *The American Psychologist, 53*, 1017–31. doi:10.1037/0003-066X.53.9.1017

Kubey, R. W., Lavin, M. J., & Barrows, J. R. (2001). Internet use and collegiate academic performance decrements: Early findings. *Journal of Communication, 51*, 366–82. doi:10.1093/joc/51.2.366

Lee, S. J. (2009). Online communication and adolescent social ties: Who benefits more from internet use? *Journal of Computer-Mediated Communication, 14*, 509–31. doi:10.1111/j.1083–6101.2009.01451.x

Lenhart, A., & Madden, M. (2007). Social networking websites and teens: An overview. http://htlab.psy.unipd.it/uploads/Pdf/lectures/technology_for_young/Social Networking Websites and Teens text.pdf

Lenhart, A., Purcell, K., Smith, A., & Zickuhr, K. (2010). Social media & mobile internet use among teens and young adults. *Pew Internet & American Life Project, 01.* http://eric.ed.gov/?id=ED525056

Lin, L. Y, Sidani, J. E., Shensa, A., Radovic, A., Miller, E., Colditz, J. B., . . . Primack, B. A. (2016). Association between social media use and depression among US young adults. *Depression and Anxiety, 33*(4), 323–31. doi:10.1002/da.22466

McKenna, K. Y. A., & Bargh, J. A. (2000). Plan 9 From Cyberspace: The implications of the internet for personality and social psychology. *Personality and Social Psychology Review, 4*(1), 57–75. doi:10.1207/S15327957PSPR0401_6

Mitchell, M. E., Lebow, J. R., Uribe, R., Grathouse, H., & Shoger, W. (2011). Internet use, happiness, social support and introversion: A more fine grained analysis of person variables and internet activity. *Computers in Human Behavior, 27*(5), 1857–61. doi:10.1016/j.chb.2011.04.008

Moreno, M. A., Jelenchick, L. A., Egan, K. G., Cox, E., Young, H., Gannon, K. E., & Becker, T. (2011). Feeling bad on Facebook: Depression disclosures by college students on a social networking site. *Depression and Anxiety, 28*, 447–55. doi:10.1002/da.20805

Pantic, I. (2014). Online social networking and mental health. *Cyberpsychology, Behavior, and Social Networking, 17*(10), 652–57. doi:10.1089/cyber.2014.0070

Pantic, I., Damjanovic, A., Todorovic, J., Topalovic, D., Bojovic-Jovic, D., Ristic, S., & Pantic, S. (2012). Association between online social networking and depression in high school students: Behavioral physiology viewpoint. *Psychiatria Danubina, 24*, 90–93.

Pasek, J., More, E., & Hargittai, E. (2009). Facebook and academic performance: Reconciling a media sensation with data. *First Monday, 14(5)*. doi:10.5210/fm.v14i5.2498

Schouten, A. P., Valkenburg, P. M., & Peter, J. (2007). Precursors and underlying processes of adolescents' online self-disclosure: Developing and testing an "internet-attribute-perception" model. *Media Psychology, 10*(2), 292–315. doi:10.1080/15213260701375686

Shaw, L. H., & Gant, L. M. (2002). In defense of the internet: The relationship between Internet communication and depression, loneliness, self-esteem, and perceived social support. *Cyberpsychology & Behavior: The Impact of the Internet, Multimedia and Virtual Reality on Behavior and Society, 5*(2), 157–71. doi:10.1089/109493102753770552

Sheeks, M. S., & Birchmeier, Z. P. (2007). Shyness, sociability, and the use of computer-mediated communication in relationship development. *Cyberpsychology & Behavior: The Impact of the Internet, Multimedia and Virtual Reality on Behavior and Society, 10*(1), 64–70. doi:10.1089/cpb.2006.9991

Stubbe, D. (2012). Communication commentary: Communicating with the internet generation: Challenges and opportunities. *Focus, 10*(3):323–26.

Subrahmanyam, K., & Greenfield, P. (2008). Online communication and adolescent relationships. *The Future of Children, 18*(1), 119–46. http://www.ncbi.nlm.nih.gov/pubmed/21338008

Subrahmanyam, K., Greenfield, P., Kraut, R., & Gross, E. (2001). The impact of computer use on children's and adolescents' development. *Journal of Applied Developmental Psychology, 22*, 7–30. doi:10.1016/S0193-3973(00)00063–0

Turkle, S. (2008). Always-on/always-on you: The tethered self. In J. Katz (Ed.), *Handbook of mobile communication studies* (pp. 121–38). Cambridge, MA: MIT Press.

Valkenburg, P. M., & Peter, J. (2007a). Online communication and adolescent well-being: Testing the stimulation versus the displacement hypothesis. *Journal of Computer-Mediated Communication, 12*, 1169–82. doi:10.1111/j.1083–6101.2007.00368.x

Valkenburg, P. M., & Peter, J. (2007b). Preadolescents' and adolescents' online communication and their closeness to friends. *Developmental Psychology, 43*(2), 267–77. doi:10.1037/0012–1649.43.2.267

Valkenburg, P. M., & Peter, J. (2009). Social Consequences of the Internet for adolescents: A decade of research. *Current Directions in Psychological Science, 18*(1), 1–5. doi:10.1111/j.1467–8721.2009.01595.x

van den Eijnden, R. J. J. M., Meerkerk, G.-J., Vermulst, A. A., Spijkerman, R., & Engels, R. C. M. E. (2008). Online communication, compulsive Internet use, and psychosocial well-being among adolescents: A longitudinal study. *Developmental Psychology, 44*(3), 655–65. doi:10.1037/0012–1649.44.3.655

van Rensburg, S. H., Klingensmith, K., McLaughlin, P., Qayyum, Z., & van Schalkwyk, G. I. (2015). Patient-provider communication over social media: Perspectives of adolescents with psychiatric illness. *Health Expectations, 19*(1), 112–120. doi:10.1111/hex.12334

van Schalkwyk, G. I., Klingensmith, K., McLaughlin, P & Qayyum, Z. (2015). The use of social networking sites by adolescents with psychiatric illnesses: A qualitative study. *Scandinavian Journal of Child and Adolescent Psychiatry and Psychology, 3*(2).

van Schalkwyk, G. I., Marin, C. E., Ortiz, M., Rolison, M., Qayyum, Z., McPartland, J. C., . . . Silverman, W. K. (2017). Social media use, friendship quality, and the moderating role of anxiety in adolescents with Autism Spectrum Disorder. *Journal of Autism and Developmental Disorders, 47*(9), 2805–13. doi:10.1007/s10803-017-3201-6

Walther, J. B. (1996). Computer-mediated communication: Impersonal, interpersonal, and hyperpersonal interaction. *Communication Research, 23*(1), 3–43. doi:10.1177/009365096023001001

Walther, J. B. (2007). Selective self-presentation in computer-mediated communication: Hyperpersonal dimensions of technology, language, and cognition. *Computers in Human Behavior, 23*, 2538–57. doi:10.1016/j.chb.2006.05.002

Wästlund, E., Norlander, T., & Archer, T. (2001). Internet blues revisited: Replication and extension of an Internet paradox study. *Cyberpsychology & Behavior : The Impact of the Internet, Multimedia and Virtual Reality on Behavior and Society, 4*, 385–91. doi:10.1089/109493101300210295

Weiser, E. B. (2001). The functions of internet use and their social and psychological consequences. *Cyberpsychology & Behavior: The Impact of the Internet, Multimedia and Virtual Reality on Behavior and Society, 4*(6), 723–43. doi:10.1089/109493101753376678

Wellman, B., Haase, A. Q., Witte, J., & Hampton, K. (2001). Does the Internet increase, decrease, or supplement social capital? Social networks, participation, and community commitment. *American Behavioral Scientist, 45*(3), 436–455. doi:10.1177/00027640121957286

Wolak, J., Mitchell, K. J., & Finkelhor, D. (2002). Close online relationships in a national sample of adolescents. *ADOLESCENCE, 37*, 441–456.

CHAPTER

4

Epidemiology of Technology Use and Mental Health in the United States

Seth W. Whiting *and* Rani A. Hoff

Abstract

Advancements in technologies and their mass-scale adoption throughout the United States create rapid changes in how people interact with the environment and each other and how they live and work. As technologies become commonplace in society through increased availability and affordability, several problems may emerge, including disparate use among groups, which creates divides in attainment of the beneficial aspects of a technology's use and coinciding mental health issues. This chapter briefly overviews new technologies and associated emerging applications in information communication technologies, social media networks, video games and massively multiplayer online role-playing games, and online gambling, then examines the prevalence of use among the general population and its subgroups and further discusses potential links between mental health issues associated with each technology and implications of overuse.

Keywords: information communication, digital divide, epidemiology, online gambling, Internet, social media, smart devices, video games

Technology shapes the way we work, interact, gather information, learn, spend leisure time, and live. Consider news media, for example. Newspapers and other print sources were once the quickest and most common means of learning about recent events and getting a weather report. This same information later became more widely available with quicker notice via radio and television. Since the development of the Internet in a more connected world, news of virtually any form is available at a moment's notice on a personal computer or mobile device. Of the three-fourths of Americans who consume news media every day, almost as many people get news from a cell phone as they do from newspapers and magazines (56% vs. 61%, respectively), and about 13% of adults prefer social media, such as Facebook, as their primary source of news (Media Insight Project, 2014).

Few innovations in recent history have affected daily living as much as computers and the Internet. Modern processing speeds and momentary access to information of almost any kind were once fictional imaginations, but are now commonplace. In the 1990s, 56k dial-up Internet services frequently required users to endure a series of what may be considered iconic, albeit discordant, noises and a delay of several minutes prior to access. Through advances in technology, the Internet is often available on an almost instantaneous basis, and even minor delays in access or downloading speed might be a cause for annoyance. Everything from health information, to correspondence, personal files, shopping, and geolocation and navigation are possible from a home computer or on a smart wireless device that fits inside one's pocket.

Similarly, social interactions have been evolving with advances in technology. Great changes in the way interactions took place were observed as technology allowed for radio transmission and telephone calls, and modern connectivity and online software have again greatly altered the way people interact and share information. Social media networks have emerged on the Internet as increasingly popular sources of social behavior. Websites such as Facebook, Twitter, and YouTube allow anyone with an Internet connection to create a profile, share information about themselves, create a circle of "friends," keep up with distant relationships, and share photos, videos, audio, and other rich media among groups of people all over the world. For many, a great proportion of life is taking place through social media because experiences may be shared as they happen.

Along with social media, video games offer an increasingly interactive experience and, in some cases, may be used as a form of a second life or identity. As processing and graphical capabilities of computers, video game consoles, and mobile devices have increased, video games have become increasingly realistic, interactive, and immersive. Two-dimensional pixilated games with very limited commands have evolved into three-dimensional online virtual communities where players can trade goods and services, hold social status among live peers, and create factions or guilds for competitive or cooperative play. The potential to create and live a virtual life has been actualized, and growing numbers of users are spending more time interacting in these virtual worlds than in real-life communities.

Next, as technology is changing the way we interact socially and access information, other leisure activities are evolving in kind. Casino gambling already ranks among the most popular leisure activities in the United States (Ghezzi, Lyons, & Dixon, 2000), and increasingly real and available virtual casinos are in operation, with further development in several states around the country. With these virtual casinos, gamblers can now place a bet online against a sponsoring casino establishment within the state, such that a wager is only a few clicks away.

As the Internet becomes faster and more accessible, virtual social networks become more interactive, virtual worlds in video games increasingly simulate real life, gambling opportunities become increasingly accessible and available, and technology allows for more generalized accessibility, anonymity, convenience, and momentary gratification, the widespread use of these technologies might engender mental health issues. Furthermore, differences in use among groups might signal a divide by which some are more likely at risk for distress or are at a disadvantage due to limited access to beneficial technologies. In the sections that follow, patterns of technology use among various populations and subgroups are examined and the potential for relationships with mental health disorders are discussed.

Information and Communication Technologies

Background and Use

Emerging as early as the 1940s, computers were cumbersome machines designed and produced with the intent to solve complex mathematical equations and analyze data (Gustafson, 2000). Now much more flexible in function, computers can be used to write, save work, transmit massive amounts of data, record video and audio, play games, and do many other tasks. Similarly, the Internet has transformed the functional utility of computers and allows one access to a global network of millions of computer devices. Rapid dissemination of Internet technology began in the mid-1990s with the release of the Netscape browser and subsequent commercialization of online content (Mowery & Simcoe, 2002). With the Internet, users are connected to practically endless data, global communication is momentarily feasible, and many daily life activities, from buying groceries to setting an appointment for a haircut, are possible. As computers shrink in size and wireless technologies develop, Internet access is increasingly available through smart devices and the "Internet of Things." That is, rather than a standard desktop or laptop computer, the Internet may be accessed through a multitude of mobile devices such as cell phones that can be used to send and receive email, download software, navigate travel routes, transmit files, and listen to music, to name a few activities. Other devices will be equipped with Internet technology such as home thermostats and advanced medical devices, with estimates of "things" connected to the Internet approximating 26 billion units by 2020 (Gartner, Inc., 2013a). In this way, information and communication technologies (ICTs) are an established part of modern life and an ongoing source of development.

As computers have become reduced in price over the years to levels that most individuals in the United States can afford, this technology has gained widespread use. As a part of the American Community Survey program, the US Census Bureau reported results from a national-scale sample of approximately 3.5 million households in regard to Internet and technology use (File & Ryan, 2014). This report provided several key facts related to ICT use among Americans. First, ownership of a desktop or laptop computer is now the rule rather than the exception. As early as 1984, only 8% of households reported home computer use, and this figure has regularly increased to 79% in 2013. All age groups reported similar rates of computer ownership (except those aged 65 and older) ranging from 82% to 86%, with the senior group lagging behind at an approximate 62%. In comparison to age, race and ethnicity categories tend to be more divisive on this measure. Asian and white individuals reported the greatest frequencies, with 90% and 81% computer ownership, respectively. Hispanic (70%) and black (66%) individuals reported less frequent computer ownership. Similarly, a gap of close to 9% has been observed between metropolitan (79%) and nonmetropolitan (71%) citizens. A stepwise increase in computer use was observed as a function of income level, with households earning less than $25,000 per year representing a significant deficit (54%) and households earning more than $150,000 representing almost universal (97%) computer ownership. Educational divisions have replicated this stepwise pattern, with rates ranging from 47% in those with less than a high school education to 94% in those with bachelor's degrees or greater.

As might be expected, similar trends in Internet use were observed in the same report. From 1997 to 2013, home Internet use increased from 18% to 74% as high-speed Internet services permeated throughout the country. Again, those aged 65 or older represent a deficit in Internet subscription at 58%, while all other age groups report approximately 20% higher use. About three-fourths of the metropolitan population has an Internet subscription, with the nonmetropolitan population lagging behind with rates of almost 65%. Internet use increases with education and income, with large disparities between households with less than $25,000 annual income or less than high school education and those earning excesses of $150,000 or bachelor's degrees (File & Ryan, 2014). Finally, divided by ethnicity, disparities in household Internet use appear to be shrinking. In 2000, roughly half as many black and Hispanic households reported Internet use as white and Asian households. As of 2013, differences remained apparent yet less pronounced with about 75% of black, 80% of Hispanic, 85% of white, and 93% of Asian households accessing the Internet (File, 2013).

Next, smartphones have increased in popularity and were used by approximately half of those 15 and older as of 2011 (File, 2013). Trends in smartphone use resembled those of general Internet and computer use. First, as age increases, the rate of smartphone ownership diminishes. Slightly more than two out of every three people aged 15–25 years and 25–34 years own a smartphone, while use decreases in those 35–44 years (59%), again in those 45–54 years (45%), and drops again significantly in those older than 54 (23%). For educational divides, rates decreased in turn with education: those with a bachelor's degree or more education demonstrated the greatest rate of smartphone use at 59% with each lower educational subdivision including fewer and fewer. Differing from computer and Internet trends, all races and ethnicities reported approximately 50% adoption. In addition, researchers noted a similar approximate one out of two rate in both male and female genders (File, 2013).

Last, handheld computers and other mobile devices have risen in popularity and are worth mention. When these devices, such as iPads and wireless tablet personal computers, were included (with smartphones) in the survey, the US Census Bureau (File & Ryan, 2014) observed trends similar to general smartphone ownership but found that all wireless devices were used by 64% of the population older than 15 years and that more than 5% of households used handheld computers or smart devices in place of a laptop or computer. Research more specifically targeting rates of ownership of different types of devices suggests that approximately 19% of Americans own an e-book (e.g., Kindle or Nook) and the same amount own a tablet device, with both demonstrating an increasing trend. For general cell phones and Mp3 or portable music players, stable trends of ownership were observed at 88% and 44%, respectively (Zickuhr & Smith, 2012).

Mental Health Concerns

As use of the Internet and smart devices likely continues to grow, special attention should be paid to coinciding mental health issues. One issue garnering attention in ICT is the controversy of Internet addiction. Despite the lack of status as a formally recognized disorder, some research in problematic Internet use is suggestive of significant risk and similar patterns to other addictions, but more extensive research is required (see Pies, 2009). Several measurement tools have been developed to assess Internet addiction, and studies have been conducted throughout the world, with a large proportion taking place outside of the United States. Based on criteria generated from impulse-control and substance-use disorders as well as clinical experiences, Ko, Yen, Chen, Chen, and Yen (2005) found that approximately 20% of adolescents in schools in Taiwan (22% males and 14% of females) exhibited

Internet addiction. Using the Internet Addiction Test, in older teens and adults in the United Kingdom, Morrison and Gore (2010) found a prevalence rate of 1.2%, with greater rates observed in men, and, of more than 17,000 US citizens, an approximate 6% of online respondents scored in the range of Internet addiction (Greenfield, 1999). Overall, estimates of general Internet addiction rates range from 1.5% to 8.2% across the United States and Europe (see Weinstein & Lejoyeux, 2010, for a review), with data suggesting that teens and males may be more susceptible to problematic Internet use.

With Internet addiction, substantial comorbid psychiatric disorders and related negative conditions have been identified. In a preliminary analysis involving only 20 participants with problematic Internet use, all participants had one or more lifetime psychiatric diagnosis beyond Internet addiction, most frequently bipolar disorder and phobias (Shapira, Goldsmith, Keck, Khosla, & McElroy, 2000). Further research has found that those with more severe Internet use frequently reported symptoms such as disruptions in academic efforts, relationships, finances, and occupations similar to presumably related addiction phenomena (Young, 1998), and such features may be particularly prevalent when ICT use has negatively affected sleeping habits and waking-time tiredness (Punamäki, Wallenius, Nygård, Saarni, & Rimpelä, 2007). One of the more frequently pervasive comorbid conditions is depression, as several observations of increased rates have been noted in the literature (e.g., Morrison & Gore, 2010; Young & Rodgers, 1998), and such a phenomenon has been observed across age groups, but may be most common in younger men (Morrison & Gore, 2010). Similar to depression, cross-sectional studies conducted in countries around the world have revealed significant associations between attention deficit hyperactivity disorder (ADHD), social anxiety disorder, increased presence of general psychiatric symptoms in children and adults, substance use disorders in adults and teens, and obsessive compulsive disorder and increased hostility in adolescents and teens (See Ko, Yen, Yen, Chen, & Chen, 2012, for a review). Overall, these conditions may be quite common in those with Internet addiction. In the 20 participants studied by Shapira et al. (2000), all reported at least one Axis-I diagnosis in his or her life. In an additional 15 participants screened by Bernadi and Pallanti (2009), depression was observed in 5 (34%), sleep disturbance in 2 (13%), ADHD in 3 (20%), mood fluctuation in 1 (7%), and anxiety in 2 participants (13%).

Despite some of these observed links with negative mental health issues, some researchers suggest that computers and the Internet have positive, protective effects on mental health. Wellman et al. (1996) argued that computer networks function to link people together and that significant social communities, support, and personal relationships may be achieved through online interaction. To support this assertion, for example, Shaw and Gant (2002) found that participants improved on measures of loneliness, depression, self-esteem, and perceived social support following arranged online chat sessions with another person. Such information suggests that how and why ICT is used may have implications for mental health outcomes.

Social Media Platforms

Background and Use

Social media has emerged as a significant pastime across the US population. As the availability of Internet access and general computer use increases, activity on the Internet is becoming more interactive, both in terms of sharing information and ideas with other people and of active social interaction. Many commercial websites or programs have been developed on the Internet for the primary purpose of social interaction, and the popularity of such content prompts constant development and introduction of new networks and websites with social aims. *Social media*, or Internet-based applications where content is continuously generated and modified by its community of users, includes a wide array of applications ranging from collaborative projects such as Wikipedia to virtual social worlds where users can exist as a representative avatar and live a virtual life among other users (Kaplan & Haenlein, 2010). Altogether, online social media outlets are those interactive websites or online programs that possess the following characteristics in some degree: other users are available, content is shared, communication between users occurs, personal information is divulged, users form communities, users relate to each other, and the reputation of social standing and content is portrayed (Kietzmann, Kermkens, McCarthy, & Silvestre, 2011).

Across the range of social media, the most popular tend to fall within categories of social networking sites and content communities. The former are distinguished by the inclusion of personal information profiles, exchanges with other users granting access to each other's personal profiles, and interuser messaging and content sharing. Social networking sites include Facebook and LinkedIn, among others. Content communities share the same social presence and media richness as the aforementioned social networking sites but typically involve less disclosure of personal information (Kaplan & Haenlein, 2010). Such communities include networks such as YouTube and Pinterest, where relatively little personal information is divulged in a user's profile but the sharing of video and images is commonplace.

Membership in social networking sites and content communities appears to be the rule rather than the exception. In a telephone-based survey administered to 1,445 Internet users of adult age (18 years or older), approximately 71% of respondents indicated that they used Facebook in 2013, the most popular of these websites. Other popular social networking and content sharing sites register many millions of users but at a reduced rate in comparison to Facebook. Within the same survey, 22% of adults on the Internet are LinkedIn users, 21% use Pinterest, 18% use Twitter, and 17% use Instagram. In total, approximately 73% of online adults reported use of at least one social networking site, 42% of whom reported membership with more than one (Duggan & Smith, 2013). Furthermore, engagement with all of these social media outlets has increased among adults with Internet access every year since 2005, suggesting that these data may continue on an upward trend in coming years (Brenner & Smith, 2013).

Also demonstrating a yearly increase in use of social networking websites, a 2009 nationally representative sample of 800 American teenagers aged 12–17 years found that 73% of American teenagers used social media. Broken down further, 82% of those aged 14–17 years reported use of social media, and online teens aged 12–13 years only used these social networking sites at a rate of 55%, with the lower proportion likely attributable to age restrictions of these sites (e.g., Facebook requires that users be at least 13 years old), though the age limits may not be consistently imposed (Lenhart, Purcell, Smith, & Zickur, 2010). By 2012, overall teenage use of social networking sites has increased to 81%, including 94% using Facebook, 26% using Twitter, 11% using Instagram, and 7% using Youtube and MySpace (Madden et al., 2013).

Although frequently represented less in terms of online activity, older adults continue to represent a significant proportion of social media users. Out of a national sample of 1,526 adults aged 65 years or older, 27% used social networking websites. Because a lesser proportion of this demographic group tends to use the Internet, it must be noted that 46% of those who do go online use social media. Similar to other age groups, older adults show a general increasing trend of social media use over recent years (Smith, 2014).

In terms of other demographic characteristics, several differences in social media use have been noted. From a survey of 1,802 internet users, women (71%) were found to use social media at a significantly greater proportion than men (62%). No statistical differences were observed with respect to race and ethnicity, as 65% of white, 68% of black, and 72% of Hispanic respondents reported using social media. Similarly, education and income levels were not significant predictors as 65–69% of college graduates, those with some college experience, and those who completed high school or less reported social media use, as did 66–72% of respondents across all income ranges, indicating little variability among categories. A final difference was noted in geography as 70% of those in urban areas used social media, a greater rate than those in rural areas, of which only 61% reported the same (Duggan & Brenner, 2013).

Mental Health Concerns

As noted previously, about three out of every four online adults and just as many teens use a social media website. With prevalent use of social media, any problems coinciding with such use are likely widespread. Issues may arise, for example, through overuse, where increasing amounts of time are allocated to social networking at the expense of other opportunities, and increased engagement appears linked to loneliness (Burke, Marlow, & Lento, 2010). Approximately 40% of adults on Facebook reported multiple sessions per day. Similar trends have been observed for Instagram and Twitter users: 35 and 29% of users log in to these services more than once per day, respectively (Duggan & Smith, 2013). Such behavior may be more extreme with teens as an estimated 51% are engaged with social media services at least once a day, and nearly one out of four teens (22%) check social networking sites 10 or more times per day. Engagement in content communities with streaming video occurs 10 or more times per day in 13% of teens (Common Sense Media, 2009). Overall, self-report estimates suggest that 20%, or one out of every five teens, may show signs of being addicted to social networking (Common Sense Media, 2012).

Relatedly, the pervasiveness of engagement in risky behavior on social media appears both common and generally underestimated by parents. In terms of risky online behavior, about 4 out of 10 teens (39%) have posted something on a social media website that they have later regretted, about 2 of 10 have illegally downloaded or shared files (23%), and approximately 1 out of 10 teens has sent or posted naked or semi-naked images or videos of themselves (13%). Of these risky online behaviors, about half of the parents know what their teens are doing, as 20% of parents report that their teens have made a regretful post, 10% know their children are engaged in illegal file downloading and sharing, and only 2% of parents are aware that their teens are sharing illicit pictures or videos of themselves (Common Sense Media, 2009).

Beyond overly frequent use and risky behavior, social media use may have implications for mental health. To start, depressive symptoms following extended use of social media have been termed "Facebook Depression" (see O'Keeffe & Clarke-Pearson, 2011). Behavioral indicators of depression have been observed on social media, and an overall decrease in activity, increased negative affect, high self-attentional focus, and increases in frequency of expression of religious thoughts and relational focus during interactions on Twitter have been found to predict onset of depression. Here, roughly 36% of users in the sample scored positive for this disorder (De Choudhury, Gamon, Counts, & Horvitz, 2013). Similarly, Moreno et al. (2011) screened public Facebook profiles of college students and found that 25% displayed at least some depressive symptoms and 2.5% of profiles met the criteria for a major depressive episode. Though a majority report positive experiences with social networking websites, a survey of teens found that approximately 5% reported increased feelings of depression resulting from social media use (Common Sense Media, 2012). In a similar sample of high school students, time spent on social networking websites and depression demonstrated a significant, positive relationship (Pantic et al., 2012).

Gaming

Background and Use

With advances in computing and technology, computer games have evolved from text-based or two-dimensional format to three-dimensional worlds including live interactions with numerous other players and increasingly realistic visual aesthetics. Furthermore, whereas arcade video games may have been most popular in past decades, video game consoles are available for the home, and smartphones and handheld systems offer numerous video games available to download on demand and/or take anywhere. In total, the video game industry has demonstrated a consistently increasing growth trend, to where this market has increased to total more than $90 billion per year (Gartner, Inc., 2013b).

As might be expected with a large and growing market, video games have become an almost universal leisure activity. Video games are produced across many genres for broad appeal, ranging from sports simulation to fantasy role play. In addition, each game involves varying levels of motivational factors of achievement, social interaction, and immersion in the experience offered (Yee, 2006), and various combinations of these factors may hold appeal to different groups of gamers. For instance, for those who prefer greater depth in the experience, some online multiplayer games may function to serve as a "third place" beyond the workplace (or school setting) and home where the player can regularly interact with an extended community of diverse individuals and choose an alternate identity (Steinkuehler & Williams, 2006); for lighter, more casual players, games to simply pass time are widely available on mobile phones.

Due to a vast array of genre possibilities and varying motivational factors, typifying a gamer stereotype may be difficult as use is commonplace across the population, especially in teens and children. In a survey regarding technology use, 80% of teens aged 12–17 reported owning a video game console, such as those in the Microsoft Xbox or Sony PlayStation series, including 89% of males and 70% of females in this age range. Along with consoles, approximately 51% of teens reported ownership of a portable gaming device such as a Sony PSP or Nintendo Gameboy, including 56% of males and 47% of females. After the teen years, video game ownership generally declines across age groups: 59% of young adults aged 18–29 years, 51% of adults aged 30–49 years, 20% of adults 50–64 years, and 4% of adults 65 years or older reported owning a video game console, for a total of 37% of all adults. Portable gaming devices are less popular among adults, with ownership ranging from 30% (30–49 years) to only 1% of adults 65 years or older, for a total rate of 18%. Gender differences were also observed within this sample as more adult men owned a console (39% compared to 34%) and slightly more women owned a portable gaming device (20% compared to 16%). Beyond the age and gender differences noted here, no further differences were observed among income, ethnicity, or education divides (Lenhart et al., 2010; see also Jackson et al., 2008). Additional estimates support these values regarding widespread use and suggest that 40% of adults and upward of 83% of teens play video games on a regular basis (Williams, Yee, & Caplan, 2008).

Although consoles and even handheld gaming devices are now capable of accessing the Internet and gaming networks, much online gaming, such as massively multiplayer online role-playing games (MMORPGs) must be set apart from more casual online game play. MMORPGs are characterized by an immersive world in which a player creates an avatar to represent himself or herself, and live play consists of interactions between many players simultaneously (Steinkeuhler & Williams, 2006); these must be given particular attention for several reasons. First, online games may be more immersive than most as these games frequently allow players to develop their own unique identities and essentially create a 3D visual representation of themselves (Brian & Wiemer-Hastings, 2005) or a closer approximation to their ideal selves (Bessiére, Seay, & Kiesler, 2007). Players of MMORPGs are often observed to engage in online "social realism" such that players save and collect resources to purchase in-game items, participate via trading and bartering within the confines of a virtual economy, form relationships with social status, and worry about crimes (Kolbert, 2001). Second, MMORPGs are among the most popular games. As of 2006, the online gaming community consisted of 11–12 million registered users, and the numbers have since increased to an approximate 18–19 million (Van Geel, 2013). Third, such games may be more addictive than classic-type console games, such that some players have referred to them as "heroinware" (Brian & Wiemer-Hastings, 2005).

Several attempts to describe the demographics of MMO players have been conducted through interactions with online communities. In a survey provided across two fan websites associated with the game Everquest (a non-ending fantasy MMORPG), Griffiths, Davies, and Chappell (2003) found that a majority of players (60–74%) were older than 19 years of age and 84–86% registered as male. The sample was academically diverse as 42% of the sample had earned an undergraduate diploma or greater, and another 14% were currently registered in college courses. In a similar survey across three Everquest fan sites, 81% of respondents were male, a majority of the sample (59%) was between 18 and 30 years old, slightly more than half (55%) of respondents were unmarried, and 29% reported having earned an undergraduate degree or were working toward earning a higher degree (Griffiths, Davies, & Chappell, 2004). The demographic evaluations of these studies are supported by additional Internet-based surveys by Brian and Wiemer-Hastings (2005) who found that 88% of MMORPG players were male and 37% reported student status. Williams and colleagues (2008) noted Everquest 2 players predominantly consisted of white (88%) males (81%), with 39% aged between 18 and 29 years and another 37% of whom are 30–39 years. Billieux et al. (2012) reported a World of Warcraft (a similar MMORPG) sample consisted of 87% males with a mean age of 26 years. In sum, video games have emerged as a commonplace activity across teens and adults, and while males tend toward video game play more than do females, other demographic factors are often not predictive of use. MMORPG players often do not fit the stereotype of middle school-aged males, but are diverse in educational background and consist mostly of young-adult, white, male users.

Mental Health

With the prevalent use of video games across many demographic categories, several mental health issues have been suggested. Directly related to the amount of use, *Internet gaming disorder* (IGD) has been proposed as a diagnosis in its own right. Gamers have reported compulsive play, conflicts with gaming and other interests or job duties, significant distress, and withdrawal symptoms from reduced gaming, but more clinical research is required before consideration for formal inclusion in the *Diagnostic and Statistical Manual of Mental Disorders* (DSM) (Hiller, 2013). Supporting evidence for excessive gaming and potential for addiction has been collected across several samples. For excessive play, as suggested previously, gamers who play online games may be at greater risk for addiction due to frequently observed extended play times and increased engagement. In general population teens (a higher risk group of gamers), estimates of daily use of online gaming sites approximate 30%, and 12% of teens log in to online gaming sites more than 10 times per day (Common Sense Media, 2009). In sum, based on a nationally representative sample of American youth aged 8–18 years, approximately 8% exhibited pathological gaming (Gentile, 2009).

Addiction characteristics may be more prevalent in those who play certain types of games. Brian and Wiemer-Hastings (2005) noted further disparities in play duration between MMORPG and non-MMORPG players. While almost half of non-MMORPG gamers play less than 2 hours per week, only 6% of MMORPG players reported similar play durations. In contrast, 45% of MMORPG gamers played at least 21 hours per week (including 11% with more than 40 hours) while only 6% of non-MMORPG gamers played that long. Griffiths and colleagues noted similar findings with Everquest players, as between 48% (2004) and 66% (2003) spent more than 21 hours per week gaming online. Time allocation to other MMORPGs, such as World of Warcraft, is within a similar range, with players reporting an average of 25.17 hours per week playing (Billieux et al., 2013). In addition to excessive time duration, Williams et al. (2008) noted that MMORPG gamers, on average, replace other hobbies or pastimes such as television viewing with playing games online. More significant substitutions have been noted as 26% of MMORPG gamers have stated that they have sacrificed other hobbies, 18% have sacrificed sleep, 10% have sacrificed work or school, and many have forgone opportunities to socialize with their friends (10%), partner/significant other (5%), and family (5%). Overall, a greater prevalence of video game addiction has been observed in MMORPG players, as a large sample of online gamers found a pathological gaming rate of 12% (Grüsser, Thalemann, & Griffiths, 2007).

Along with potential addiction, another related topic garnering attention is a possible linkage between video game play and aggression. Many video games contain some measure of violence, which may range from cartoon fights or explosions to realistic-looking battle experiences and graphic large-scale wars in a first-person perspective. These games remain popular as approximately half of players reported that their favorite game genre was either fantasy violence or human violence (Funk, 1993), so further discussion is warranted.

Relationships and causality between video games and violent and aggressive behavior remain a source for debate. In a meta-analysis of related studies, Anderson (2004) found frequent links between exposure to violent video games and aggressive behavior, cognition, and physiological arousal. As these types of studies, including those reviewed by Anderson, often demonstrate relationships between aggression and video game exposure generally judged to be weak by scientific convention, the practical significance of the findings is frequently questioned (General Assembly of the Commonwealth of Pennsylvania, Joint State Government Commission [JSGC], 2008). Furthermore, the definition of aggression often varies from study to study (Kutner & Olson, 2008), and directionality of a possible relationship has not been definitively determined. That is, whether video games may cause aggression, aggression attracts a person to violent video games, or whether some other variable, such as masculinity, is responsible for both aggression and interest in violent games has yet to be determined precisely (Ferguson et al., 2008). Furthermore, other analyses of the literature have failed to support conclusions that violence and engagement with violent video games are significantly linked (Ferguson, 2007). Overall, conclusive evidence of causality and practical effects are still required to settle the issue.

Beyond addiction and implications of aggressive behavior, research has found multiple links between mental health conditions and video game activity. To start, pathological gaming has been linked to attention problems. Gentile (2009) found that children and teens scoring as pathological gamers more frequently reported trouble paying attention in school and qualified for ADHD at more than twice the rate of nonpathological gamers. Similarly, a significant relationship was discovered between playing video games for more than 1 hour per day and inattention and ADHD both for players of console video games and Internet video games (Chan & Rabinowitz, 2006).

Across a 2-year longitudinal study, Gentile and colleagues (2011) identified several additional mental health factors related to gaming. A total of 3,034 students in grades 3, 4, 7, and 8 were surveyed three times across a period of 2 years. When comparing survey responses of those classified as having pathological gaming and those not, analyses found differences in ADHD symptoms, anxiety, social phobia, and depression, all of which were significantly higher in the former group. Similarly, impulsivity acted as a significant predictor of the development of pathological gaming. Investigations into the relationships of mental health and MMORPG play have yielded similar results, including indications of greater depression (Desai, Krishnan-Sarin, Cavallo, & Potenza, 2010; Mentzoni et al., 2011; Williams et al., 2008), anxiety (Mentzoni et al., 2011), cigarette smoking (Desai et al., 2010), and substance abuse (Williams et al., 2008). In addition to the previously discussed concerns, lower life satisfaction (Mentzoni et al., 2011), Internet addiction (Chan & Rabinowitz, 2006), worse health and sleep quality (Smyth, 2007), lower school performance (Chan & Rabinowitz, 2006; Jackson et al., 2008; Smyth, 2007), and serious fights (Desai et al., 2010) have been noted in greater frequencies among individuals with varying levels of problem-gaming severities.

Technology and Gambling

Background and Use

Gambling consistently ranks as a top leisure activity within the United States, with yearly revenues of more than $35 billion from commercial casinos alone (American Gaming Association [AGA], 2013). Gambling is now legal in some form in 48 out of 50 states, excluding only Utah and Hawaii (AGA, 2014). Prevalence estimates of pathological gambling frequently range from 0.4% to 2%, including a past-year rate of approximately 1% (Petry & Blanco, 2013), indicating a problem of social concern.

Legalized gambling opportunities have emerged on the Internet such that one can place wagers against a casino or other poker players from a home computer, smartphone, or tablet with access to the Internet. Online poker is fully legal within the borders of Nevada (Nevada Gaming Commission, 2014), whereas Delaware and New Jersey have passed laws legalizing not only poker, but also roulette, blackjack, slot machines, and other classic and modern simulated forms of casino gambling (New Jersey Division of Gaming Enforcement, n.d.; Delaware Gaming Competitiveness Act of 2012). Furthermore, websites not explicitly approved for gambling take in billions of dollars per year, and very few people have been prosecuted for gambling online; other types of "convenience" gambling might include wagers on horse racing, which may often be placed legally from a remote, out-of-state location (Rose, 2006). Because of advancing technology and policy development, online gambling provides greater accessibility, convenience, interactivity, anonymity, and disinhibition and represents an increasing source for further gambling activity (Griffiths, 1999, 2003).

Although research in online gambling may be difficult due to the anonymity and limited legality of online wagering, a number of samples have been collected to investigate characteristics associated with Internet gambling. Similar to some other forms of gambling, Internet gambling is predominantly done by males, with gender composition estimates ranging from 56% (Wood & Williams, 2007) to 85% (Griffiths & Barnes, 2008). Differences in ethnic composition have been noted. In a sample of 389 university healthcare patients, 16% reported a non-Caucasian ethnicity, but these participants represented 36% of the group who reported having gambled money on the Internet, and non-Caucasian status was identified as a significant predictor of problem and pathological gambling (Ladd & Petry, 2002). In another sample across North America, similar patterns were evident: excluding the "other" category, groups of participants in all non-European ancestries consisted of greater proportions of problem and pathological gamblers than did those with European ancestry (Wood & Williams, 2007). Next, analyses have suggested that Internet gambling occurs across a range of ages, incomes, and education levels, with online gambling present across all groups (Ladd & Petry, 2002; Wood & Williams, 2007). College students may represent a particularly problematic group as approximately one-fourth have gambled on the Internet and about 6% have done so on a weekly basis (Petry & Weinstock, 2007). Additionally, anonymity and accessibility of Internet gambling may allow for increased access among underage populations. For example, out of 4,523 students sampled from public high schools, 2,006 reported past-year gambling, 20.5% of whom had gambled on the Internet (Potenza et al., 2011).

Mental Health Concerns

General gambling behavior has been frequently linked to a variety of mental health disorders and concerns (e.g., Black & Moyer, 1998; Petry, 2004), and although gambling online is similar in many ways to gambling within a casino, additional mental health concerns have been noted. In scores on the General Health Questionnaire, those who gambled online infrequently and frequently scored significantly higher, indicating relatively poorer mental health than those who have never done so regardless of pathological-gambling status (Petry & Weinstock, 2007). Next, substance use may be common while gambling online, and illicit substance use may be more likely due to the privacy afforded by the Internet. In a general sample of Internet gamblers, almost one-half reported drinking alcohol while gambling online, one-third reported using tobacco, about 9% reported using marijuana while gambling, and almost 4% reported using other illicit drugs during play (McBride & Derevensky, 2009). For adolescents, for whom casino gambling is illegal, Potenza et al. (2011) established links between gambling online and several negative conditions, including increased odds of substance abuse and poorer academic performance.

As gambling opportunities expand, rates of pathological gambling are of particular interest. Research has found on several occasions that pathological gamblers may be drawn to Internet gambling. In a group of college students who have gambled on the Internet, more than 60% were pathological gamblers (Petry & Weinstock, 2007). Similar patterns were evident in adolescents as almost 60% of Internet gamblers endorsed at least one of the DSM criteria for pathological gambling (Potenza et al., 2011). Adult samples demonstrated similar findings, with estimates of problem and pathological gambling ranging from 23% (McBride & Derevensky, 2009) to 74% (Ladd & Petry, 2002).

Conclusion and Future Directions

Because of the utility of the Internet, computer systems, and modern technology as a whole, differential access to such systems may be disadvantageous for the unconnected. Whereas the term "Digital Divide" formerly referred to differences in access to ICT, with the high rates of adoption and widespread accessibility the term may now also refer to differences in the type and intensity of use (Jackson et al., 2008). Several large-scale research efforts noted previously have found groups more slowly adopting the discussed technologies, thus representing significant gaps. Also, due to mental health issues related to overuse, overuse of ICT warrants further attention.

Information and Communication Technologies

Because ICT use is largely ubiquitous among the general population, specifying a typical computer, Internet, or smart device user is difficult. However, with respect to less computer use, several demographic factors likely predict a divide. Older adults stand out with respect to age, black and Hispanic households with respect to race and ethnicity, and non-metropolitan citizens with respect to urban/rural designations. These patterns are mostly shared in terms of both Internet and smartphone usage.

Despite differences in general use of these technologies, research suggests that divides among racial/ethnic groups may be closing. Trends in online access suggest that divides in ICT are decreasing among racial/ethnic groups, and adoption of smartphone technology among racial/ethnic groups (File, 2013; File & Ryan, 2014) suggests that they may serve as a functional replacement for computers.

For those aged 65 years or older, research suggests that those with limited access to ICT may be self-excluders. For example, Zickuhr and Smith (2012) noted that half of non-Internet users do not go online because it isn't relevant to them. Other studies suggest that self-exclusion is not the case. Ennis, Rose, Denis, Pandit, and Wykes (2012) found that older individuals reported reduced levels of familiarity and confidence as the main reasons for abstinence. Furthermore, Smith (2014) found that difficulties learning to use ICT served as an additional barrier. Overall, rates of older adults using ICT have demonstrated steady increases, but a gap remains between older adults and younger age groups (Smith, 2014).

Relatively consistent disparities in ICT adoption have been noted among those in rural areas, even when effects of income level are removed (US Department of Commerce, 1999). However, as more wireless Internet coverage is offered throughout the country, Farrell and McKinnon (2003) suggested that use of emerging technologies may pose as an acceptable and feasible means for rural populations to access mental health services. Such disparities may be overcome, again, through the implementation of mobile devices. That is, as cell phone towers and wireless hotspots permeate, mobile technologies may allow those in more remote locations access to resources otherwise not available.

Overall, although adoption of ICT is steadily growing, several divides persist. Further attention must be given to monitoring such group differences and examining barriers to adoption. Once the barriers are firmly identified, increased efforts can be placed toward addressing and overcoming any obstacles to eliminate divides and to ensure that all individuals have equal opportunity to contact the advantages offered by connectivity. Because smartphones and other mobile devices are now capable of performing a wide variety of functions, further research in this area would be fruitful.

Last, because of the high frequency of comorbid mental health problems, much investigation into ICT is required. Though not officially designated as a disorder in its own right, Internet addiction may represent a future problem of social concern. Smartphone use may be habit-forming (Oulasvirta, Rattenbury, Ma, & Raita, 2012), and almost continuous, immediate reinforcement is available from Internet use, suggesting that overuse may become increasingly common. However, whether the Internet is "good" or "bad" for mental health appears to depend on how it is used. In this way, future research on Internet addiction may wish to further clarify the characteristics of use that result in each type of outcome.

Social Media Platforms

The spectrum of social media has increased in popularity due to widespread acceptance, but several predictive factors have been noted. Women tend to engage with social media more frequently than do men, older teens more than younger teens, and urban more than rural populations. Less so do seniors engage with social media, and no differences in race or ethnicity, education, or income have been observed. Again, because social media is a frequent source for maintaining relationships, obtaining news, promoting political interactions, and furthering social interactions, identifying barriers to use may be beneficial for older-adult and rural populations that appear to lag behind.

Furthermore, much research is warranted in the relationships between social media use and mental health. For instance, "Facebook depression" is a phenomenon warranting further examination. Because social media is quite popular and frequently used throughout the day, investigations into how, why, and whether social media may lead to deterioration in mental health should be explored so that ill effects may be better understood and prevented. Though arguably less frequently examined, scientists should also investigate positive or desirable effects of social media use so that websites may be designed in a way that promotes increased well-being. Similar to other aspects of Internet use, improvement and impairment are likely a function of how social media is used. Comparisons in functioning between high social media users and those who have never before used social media might suggest additional positive or negative effects of frequent use, and further examination into how healthy users and unhealthy users interact with social media differently may yield information toward mechanisms relating to mental health considerations. Several studies have begun to examine the utility of scanning behavior on Twitter (De Choudhury et al., 2013) and Facebook (Moreno et al., 2011) to detect potential depressive episodes. It may be beneficial to determine how to best implement systems using such information so that depression and other mental health concerns do not go untreated.

Finally, the extent to which virtual social interaction is replacing live, real-world interaction is a source for ongoing consideration. As a significant proportion of teens log in to social networking sites or content communities more than 10 times per day, the impact of such behaviors may be particularly important to determine. For example, with extensive interaction on social networking websites, it may be possible that some people may be more likely to partake in real-life experiences for the sole function of sharing pictures or videos of the activity on the Internet. Thus, an audience and attention may always be available for both seemingly positive and negative behaviors. Understanding the relationship between social networking and overt behavior may reveal potential avenues for mental health treatment or prevention of risky behavior that is common on the Internet and in the lives of teens and others.

Gaming

Considering gaming consoles such as Xbox and PlayStation, video game use is largely ubiquitous across younger age groups regardless of ethnicity, income, and level of education and is especially common for male teens. MMORPG games, which may harbor greater potential for the development of mental health problems, are played predominantly by adult, white males who are otherwise diverse in background.

Pathological gaming, or IGD, affects a significant proportion of the population and has been found to co-occur with anxiety disorders, depression, attentional problems, substance abuse, social phobia, and heightened impulsivity. Although IGD has not yet been designated as an official diagnosis, the observed rates of compulsive play and frequent comorbidity with other mental health disorders warrant ongoing investigation in this area. First, many of the studies noted here and throughout the literature on this topic were conducted in Asian countries (see Hiller, 2013). Because many video games and systems are designed and manufactured in those areas, differences may emerge between pathological gaming and mental health disorders between these countries and the United States. Thus, further research more applicable to US and worldwide populations is important in considering IGD as a formal diagnosis, including the validation of a standard tool used for measurement across many regions of study. Second, a proportion of the data suggesting increased addiction and behavioral problems associated with online gaming comes from convenience samples (e.g., participants recruited from gaming websites who may be more immersed in gaming culture and may not be perfectly representative of the whole) such that rates of problem gaming might be overestimated. The existing data are valuable in that they suggest a problem of social significance and a need for further evaluation in this area of study. Because of the problems observed in these populations and the observation that millions of Americans register to play these games, more expansive efforts are necessary. Third, debate continues on the relationship between exposure to video games and overt aggressive and violent behavior. Evidence exists both supporting and failing to support relationships between aggressive behavior and video game play (see General Assembly of the Commonwealth of Pennsylvania, 2008, for a review). Scientists should strive toward more highly controlled, precise studies identifying practical effects of playing violent video games and evidence of causal, directional relationships to better inform the public and policy development. Last, online games, especially MMORPGs, have been related to addictive tendencies more so than console play, and special attention should be given to these outlets moving forward.

Technology and Gambling

In sum, gambling online is legal in several states, with more likely to follow. Online gambling has been linked to being male and having a non-Caucasian ethnic background. Also, this activity has been linked with problem/pathological gambling and poor psychiatric health, including major depressive, anxiety, and substance use disorders.

In light of the mental health issues noted within the research in this area, several concerns are noteworthy. To begin, one should consider the extent to which online gambling is particularly problematic for individuals with existing gambling problems. Rates of problem and pathological gambling in states where online gambling has been legalized should be monitored to inform policy development in other states. This could further serve as a prompt for treatment development and dissemination, which may already be a concern in the gambling community (Petry & Blanco, 2013). In contrast, relatively large percentages of casino earnings are returned to the government via gaming taxes in a manner that online gambling may provide several benefits to the state. Cost-benefit analyses considering tax and revenue benefits, increases in job availability, rates of pathological gambling, economic effects concerning gamblers and communities, and treatment quality and availability may be important considerations moving forward.

Online gambling is currently not an "all-or-nothing" case. Nevada has legalized online poker, and more recently other states, including Delaware and New Jersey, offer a much wider variety of online casino gambling. Comparisons between economic and health changes among Internet gamblers in these states could provide information relevant to potential risks associated with various types of online gambling. Similarly, differences among Internet gambling and live gambling should be studied further in terms of operative effects on gambling behavior. For example, gathering money and traveling to a casino involves a response cost, while turning on a tablet PC removes much effort and motivational barriers. The anonymity of online gambling may also have an effect on the frequency that individuals with gambling problems seek treatment. Substance abuse that may be restricted in public may occur at increased likelihood while gambling in private settings, and gambling while decision-making skills are impaired may result. Overall, online gambling offers many potential benefits and leisure opportunities, but ongoing investigation into who is gambling, mental health associations, changes in the prevalence of disordered gambling, and the relationship of costs and benefits should be carefully monitored in future investigations.

References

American Gaming Association (AGA). (2013). *2013 State of the states: The AGA survey of casino entertainment.* http://www.americangaming.org/sites/default/files/uploads/docs/aga_sos2013_fnl.pdf

American Gaming Association (AGA). (2014). *Fact sheets: Type of gaming by state.* http://www.americangaming.org/industry-resources/research/fact-sheets/states-gaming

Anderson, C. A. (2004). An update on the effects of playing violent video games. *Journal of Adolescence, 27,* 113–22. doi:10.1016/j.adolescence.2003.10.009

Bernardi, S., & Pallanti, S. (2009). Internet addiction: A descriptive clinical study focusing on comorbidities and dissociative symptoms. *Comprehensive Psychiatry, 50,* 510–16. doi:10.1016/j.comppsych.2008.11.011

Bessiére, K., Seay, A. F., & Kiesler, S. (2007). The ideal elf: Identity exploration in World of Warcraft. *CyberPsychology & Behavior, 10,* 530–35. doi:10.1089/cpb.2007.9994

Billieux, J., Van der Linden, M., Achab, S., Khazaal, Y., Paraskecopoulos, L., Zullino, D., & Thorens, G. (2013). Why do you play World of Warcraft? An in-depth exploration of self-reported motivations to play online and in-game behaviours in the virtual world of Azeroth. *Computers in Human Behavior, 29,* 103–109. doi:10.1016/j.chb.2012.07.021

Black, D. W., & Moyer, T. (1998). Clinical features and psychiatric comorbidity of subjects with pathological gambling behavior. *Psychiatric Services, 49*, 1434–39. doi: 10.1176/ps.49.11.1434

Brenner, J., & Smith, A. (2013). 72% of online adults are social networking site users. *Pew Research Center's Internet and American Life Project.* http://www.pewinternet.org/files/old-media//Files/Reports/2013/PIP_Social_networking_sites_update_PDF.pdf

Brian, D., & Wiemer-Hastings, P. (2005). Addiction to the internet and online gaming. *CyberPsychology and Behavior, 8*, 110–13. doi:10.1089/cpb.2005.8.110.

Burke, M., Marlow, C., & Lento, T. (2010). Social network activity and social well-being. In *Proceedings of the SIGCHI Conference on Human Factors in Computing Systems* (pp. 1909–12). New York: ACM.

Chan, P. A., & Rabinowitz, T. (2006). A cross-sectional analysis of video games and attention deficit hyperactivity disorder symptoms in adolescents. *Annals of General Psychiatry, 5*, 16–26. doi:10.1186/1744-859X-5-16

Common Sense Media. (2009). Is technology networking changing childhood? A national poll. https://www.commonsensemedia.org/sites/default/files/uploads/pdfs/social_networking_poll_summary_results.pdf

Common Sense Media. (2012). Social media, social life: How teens view their digital lives. https://www.commonsensemedia.org/research/social-media-social-life-how-teens-view-their-digital-lives

De Choudhury, M., Gamon, M., Counts, S., & Horvitz, E. (2013). Predicting depression in social media. *Proceedings of the 7th International AAAI Conference on Weblogs and Social Media (ICWSM).*

Delaware Gaming Competitiveness Act of 2012, Dela. Stat. § 78–285. (2012). http://legis.delaware.gov/lis/lis146.nsf/vwlegislation/16D3B2FBA90AE777852579F90058959E

Desai, R. A., Krishnan-Sarin, S., Cavallo, D., & Potenza, M. N. (2010). Video-gaming among high school students: Health correlates, gender differences, and problematic gaming. *Pediatrics, 126*, e1414–24. doi: 10.1542/peds.2009–2706

Duggan, M., & Brenner, J. (2013). The demographics of social media users – 2012. *Pew Research Center's Internet and American Life Project.* http://www.pewinternet.org/files/old-edia//Files/Reports/2013/PIP_SocialMediaUsers.pdf

Duggan, M., & Smith, A. (2013). Social media update 2013. *Pew Research Center's Internet and American Life Project.* http://pewinternet.org/Reports/2013/Social-Media-Update.aspx

Ennis, L., Rose, D., Denis, M., Pandit, N., & Wykes, T. (2012). Can't surf, won't surf: The digital divide in mental health. *Journal of Mental Health, 21*, 395–203. doi: 10.3109/09638237.2012.689437

Farrell, S. P., & McKinnon, C. R. (2003). Technology and rural mental health. *Archives of Psychiatric Nursing, 27*, 20–26. doi:10.1053/apnu.2003.4

Ferguson, C. J. (2007). The good, the bad and the ugly: A meta-analytic review of positive and negative effects about violent video games. *The Psychiatric Quarterly, 78*, 309–16. doi:10.1007/s11126-007-9056-9

Ferguson, C. J., Rueda, S. M., Cruz, A. M., Ferguson, D. E., Fritz, S., & Smith, S. M. (2008). Violent video games and aggression: Causal relationship or byproduct of family violence and intrinsic violence motivation. *Criminal Justice and Behavior, 35*, 311–32. doi:10.1177/0093854807311719

File, T. (2013). Computer and Internet use in the United States: Population characteristics (Report No. P20-569). US Census Bureau. http://www.census.gov/prod/2013pubs/p20-569.pdf

File, T., & Ryan, C. (2014). Computer and Internet use in the United States: 2013 (Report No. ACS-28). US Census Bureau. http://www.census.gov/content/dam/Census/library/publications/2014/acs/acs-28.pdf

Funk, J. B. (1993). Reevaluating the impact of video games. *Clinical Pediatrics, 32*, 86–90. doi:10.1177/000992289303200205

Gartner, Inc. (2013a). Gartner says the Internet of Things installed base will grow to 26 billion units by 2020 [Press Release]. http://www.gartner.com/newsroom/id/2636073

Gartner, Inc. (2013b). Gartner says worldwide video game market to total $93 billion in 2013 [Press Release]. http://www.gartner.com/newsroom/id/2614915

General Assembly of the Commonwealth of Pennsylvania, Joint State Government Commission. (2008). *The Report of the Task Force on Violent Interactive Video Games.* http://jsg.legis.state.pa.us

Gentile, D. (2009). Pathological video-game use among youth ages 8 to 18: A national study. *Psychological Science, 20*, 594–02. doi:10.1111/j.1467–9280.2009.02340.x

Gentile, D. A., Choo, H., Liau, A., Sim, T., Li, D., Fung, D., & Khoo, A. (2011). Pathological video game use among youths: A two-year longitudinal study. *Pediatrics, 127*, 319–29. doi:10.1542/peds.2010–1353

Ghezzi, P., Lyons, C., & Dixon, M. R. (2000). Gambling from a socioeconomic perspective. In W. K. Bickel & R. E. Vuchinich (Eds.), *Reframing health behavior change with behavioral economics* (pp. 315–341). New York: Erlbaum.

Greenfield, D. N. (1999). Psychological characteristics of compulsive Internet use: A preliminary analysis. *CyberPsychology & Behavior, 2*, 403–12. doi:10.1089/cpb.1999.2.403

Griffiths, M. (1999). Gambling technologies: Prospects for problem gambling. *Journal of Gambling Studies, 15*, 265–83. doi:10.1023/a:1023053630588

Griffiths, M. (2003). Internet gambling: Issues, concerns, and recommendations. *CyberPsychology & Behavior, 6*, 557–68. doi: 10.1089/109493103322725333

Griffiths, M., & Barnes, A. (2008). Internet gambling: An online empirical study among student gamblers. *International Journal of Mental Health and Addiction, 6*, 194–204. doi:10.1007/s11469-007-9083-7

Griffiths, M. D., Davies, M. N. O., & Chappell, D. (2003). Breaking the stereotype: The case of online gaming. *CyberPsychology & Behavior, 6*, 81–91. doi:10.1089/109493103321167992

Griffiths, M. D., Davies, M. N. O., & Chappell, D. (2004). Demographic factors and playing variables in online computer gaming. *CyberPsychology & Behavior, 7*, 479–87. doi:10.1089/cpb.2004.7.479

Grüsser, S. M., Thalemann, R., & Griffiths, M. D. (2007). Excessive computer game playing, Evidence for addiction and aggression? *CyberPsychology & Behavior, 10*, 290–92. doi:10.1089/cpb.2006.9956

Gustafson, J. (2000). Reconstruction of the Atanasoff-Berry computer. In R. Rojas & U. Hashagen (Eds.), *The first computers: History and architectures* (pp. 91–106). Cambridge, MA: MIT Press.

Hiller, A. (2013). *Internet gaming disorder fact sheet.* http://www.dsm5.org/Documents/Internet%20Gaming%20Disorder%20Fact%20Sheet.pdf

Jackson, L. A., Zhao, Y., Kolenic, A., Fitzgerald, H., Harold, R., & Von Eye, A. (2008). Race, gender, and information technology use: The new digital divide. *CyberPsychology & Behavior, 11*, 437–42. doi:10.1089/cpb.2007.0157

Kaplan, A. M., & Haenlein, M. (2010). Users of the world, unite! The challenges and opportunities of social media. *Business Horizons, 53,* 59–68. doi:10.1016/j.bushor.2009.09.003

Kietzmann, J. H., Hermkens, K., McCarthy, I. P., & Silvestre, B. S. (2011). Social media? Get serious! Understanding the functional building blocks of social media. *Business Horizons, 54,* 241–51. doi:10.1016/j.bushor.2011.01.005

Ko, C.-H., Yen, J.-Y., Chen, C.-C., Chen, S.-H., & Yen, C.-F. (2005). Proposed diagnostic criteria of internet addiction for adolescents. *Journal of Nervous and Mental Disease, 193,* 728–33. doi:10.1097/01.nmd.0000185891.13719.54

Ko, C.-H., Yen, J.-Y., Yen, C.-F., Chen, C.-S., & Chen, C.-C. (2012). The association between Internet addiction and psychiatric disorder: A review of the literature. *European Psychiatry, 27,* 1–8. doi:10.1016/j.eurpsy.2010.04.011

Kolbert, E. (2001). Pimps and dragons: How an online world survived a social breakdown. *The New Yorker, 77,* 88.

Kutner, L., & Olson, C. K. (2008). *Grand theft childhood: The surprising truth about violent video games and what parents can do.* New York: Simon and Schuster.

Ladd, G. T., & Petry, N. M. (2002). Disordered gambling among university-based medical and dental patients: A focus on internet gambling. *Psychology of Addictive Behaviors, 16,* 76–97. doi:10.1037//0893-164X.16.1.76

Lenhart, A., Purcell, K., Smith, A., & Zickuhr, K. (2010). Social media and mobile internet use among teens and young adults. *Pew Research Center's Internet and American Life Project.* http://www.pewinternet.org/Reports/2010/Social-Media-and-Young-Adults.aspx

Madden, M., Lenhard, A., Cortesi, S., Gasser, U., Duggan, M., Smith, A., & Beaton, M. (2013). Teens, social media, and privacy. *Pew Research Center's Internet and American Life Project.* http://www.pewinternet.org/files/2013/05/PIP_TeensSocialMediaandPrivacy_PDF.pdf

McBride, J., & Derevensky, J. (2009). Internet gambling behavior in a sample of online gamblers. *International Journal of Mental Health and Addiction, 7,* 149–67. doi:10.1007/s11469-008-9169-x

Media Insight Project. (2014). The Personal News Cycle. http://www.apnorc.org/PDFs/Media%20Insight/News%20Cycle/The_Personal_News_Cycle_Final.pdf

Mentzoni, R. A., Brunborg, G. S., Molde, H., Myrseth, H., Skouverøe, K. J., Hetland, J., & Pallesen, S. (2011). Problematic video game use: Estimated prevalence and associations with mental and physical health. *Cyberpsychology, Behavior, and Social Networking, 14,* 591–96. doi:10.1089/cyber.2010.0260

Moreno, M. A., Jelenchick, L. A., Egan, K. G., Cox, E., Young, H., Gannong, K. E., & Becker, T. (2011). Feeling bad on Facebook: Depression disclosures by college students on a social networking site. *Depression and Anxiety, 28,* 447–55. doi:10.1002/da.20805

Morrison, C. M., & Gore, H. (2010). The relationship between excessive internet use and depression: A questionnaire-based study of 1,319 young people and adults. *Psychopathology, 43,* 121–26. doi:10.1159/000277001

Mowery, D. C., & Simcoe, T. (2002). Is the Internet a US invention? An economic and technological history of computer networking. *Research Policy, 31,* 1369–87. doi:10.1016/s0048-7333(02)00069–0

Nevada Gaming Commission. (2014). Online gaming: Nevada Gaming Commission approved and licensed operators of interactive gaming. http://gaming.nv.gov/index.aspx?page=265

New Jersey Division of Gaming Enforcement. (n.d.). *Internet gaming.* http://www.nj.gov/oag/ge/internetgaming.html

O'Keefe, G. S., & Clarke-Pearson, K. (2011). The impact of social media on children, adolescents, and families. *Pediatrics, 127,* 800–804. doi:10.1542/peds.2011–0054

Oulasvirta, A., Rattenbury, T., Ma, L., & Raita, E. (2012). Habits make smartphone use more pervasive. *Personal and Ubiquitous Computing, 16,* 105–14. doi:10.1007/s00779-011-0412-2

Pantic, I., Damjanovic, A., Todorovic, J., Topalovic, D., Bojovic-Jovic, D., Ristic, S., & Pantic, S. (2012). Association between online social networking and depression in high school students: Behavioral physiology viewpoint. *Psychiatria Danubina, 24,* 90–93.

Petry, N. M. (2004). *Pathological gambling: Etiology, comorbidity, and treatments.* Washington, DC: American Psychological Association.

Petry, N. M., & Blanco, C. (2013). National gambling experiences in the US: Will history repeat itself? *Addiction, 108,* 1032–37. doi:10.1111/j.1360–0443.2012.03894.x

Petry, N. M., & Weinstock, J. (2007). Internet gambling is common in college students and associated with poor mental health. *The American Journal on Addictions, 16,* 325–30. doi:10.1080/10550490701525673

Pies, R. (2009). Should DSM-V designate 'Internet addiction' a mental disorder? *Psychiatry, 6,* 31–37.

Potenza, M. N., Wareham, J. D., Steinberg, M. A., Rugle, L., Cavallo, D. A., Skrishnan-Sarin, S., & Desaid, R. A. (2011). Correlates of at-risk/problem internet gambling in adolescents. *Journal of the American Academy of Child & Adolescent Psychiatry, 50,* 150–59. doi:10.1016/j.jaac.2010.11.006

Punamäki, R., Wallenius, M., Nygård, C., Saarni, L., & Rimpelä, A. (2007). Use of information and communication technology (ICT) and perceived health in adolescence. The role of sleeping habits and waking-time tiredness. *Journal of Adolescence, 30,* 569–85. doi:10.1016/j.adolescence.2006.07.004

Rose, I. N. (2006). Gambling and the Law: An introduction to the law of internet gambling. *UNLV Gaming Research & Review Journal, 10,* 1–14. doi:10.1089/glr.2006.10.537

Shapira, N. A., Goldsmith, T. D., Keck, P. E., Khosla, U. M., & McElroy, S. L. (2000). Psychiatric features of individuals with problematic internet use. *Journal of Affective Disorders, 57,* 267–72. doi:10.1016/s0165-0327(99)00107-x

Shaw, L. H., & Gant, L. M. (2002). In defense of the Internet: The relationship between internet communication and depression, loneliness, self-esteem, and perceived social support. *CyberPsychology & Behavior, 2,* 157–71. doi:10.1089/109493102753770552

Smith, A. (2014). Older adults and technology use. *Pew Research Center's Internet and American Life Project.* http://www.pewinternet.org/2014/04/03/older-adults-and-technology-use/

Smyth, J. M. (2007). Beyond self-selection in video game play: An experimental examination of the consequences of massively multiplayer online role-playing game play. *CyberPsychology & Behavior, 10,* 717–21. doi:10.1089/cpb.2007.9963

Steinkuehler, C., & Williams, D. (2006). Where everybody knows your (screen) name: Online games as 'third places.' *Journal of Computer-Mediated Communication, 11,* 885–909. doi:10.1111/j.1083–6101.2006.00300.x

United States Department of Commerce. (1999). *Falling through the net: Defining the digital divide.* Washington, DC: Author.

Van Geel, I. (2013). *Total active subscriptions.* http://users.telenet.be/mmodata/Charts/TotalSubs.png

Weinstein, A., & Lejoyeux, M. (2010). Internet addiction or excessive internet use. *The American Journal of Drug and Alcohol Abuse, 36,* 277–83. doi:10.3109/00952990.2010.491880

Wellman, B., Salaff, J., Dimitrova, D., Garton, L., Gulia, M., & Haythornthwaite, C. (1996). Computer networks as social networks: Collaborative work, telework, and virtual community. *Annual Review of Sociology, 22,* 213–38. doi:10.1146/annurev.soc.22.1.213

Williams, D., Yee, N., & Caplan, S. E. (2008). Who plays, how much, and why? Debunking the stereotypical gamer profile. *Journal of Computer-Mediated Communication, 13,* 993–1018. doi:10.1111/j.1083-6101.2008.00428.x

Wood, R. T., & Williams, R. J. (2007). Problem gambling on the internet: Implications for internet gambling policy in North America. *New Media & Society, 9,* 520–42. doi:10.1177/1461444807076987

Yee, N. (2006). Motivations for play in online games. *CyberPsychology & Behavior, 9,* 772–75. doi:10.1089/cpb.2006.9.772

Young, K. S. (1998). Internet addiction: The emergence of a new clinical disorder. *CyberPsychology & Behavior, 1,* 237–44. doi:10.1089/cpb.1998.1.237

Young, K. S., & Rodgers, R. C. (1998). The relationship between depression and Internet addiction. *CyberPsychology & Behavior, 1,* 25–28. doi:10.1089/cpb.1998.1.25

Zickuhr, K., & Smith, A. (2012). Digital differences. *Pew Research Center's Internet and American Life Project.* http://www.pewinternet.org/files/old-media/Files/Reports/2012/PIP_Digital_differences_041312.pdf

CHAPTER

5

General Population-Based Studies of Problematic Internet Use

Data from Europe

Hans-Jürgen Rumpf

Abstract

In Europe, 16 studies based on general population samples show a wide range of prevalence estimations ranging from 0.2% to 11.8% for Internet addiction and from 2.8% to 25.1% for at-risk use. Differences are due to assessment instruments, age groups, regions under study, and whether surveys focus on Internet gaming alone or on broader use of different Internet applications. The disorders are associated with male gender, younger age, mental health problems, and unfavorable social conditions. Prevalence estimations in most of the European studies show that relevant proportions of the population suffer from problematic Internet use, particularly in young age groups. Effective prevention and early intervention and treatment are necessary to face this new disorder. Future studies would benefit from generally accepted criteria and assessment tools for problematic Internet use.

Keywords: Internet gaming disorder, Internet addiction, prevalence, risk factors, general population, Europe

The Need for Population-Based Studies

Quite a number of prevalence estimations on Internet addiction (IA) or problematic use of the Internet (PUI) have been published. Some of these studies are restricted to problems associated with online and computer games, which is described as Internet gaming disorder (IGD) in the fifth edition of the *Diagnostic and Statistical Manual of Mental Disorders* (DSM-5; American Psychiatric Association, 2013; Petry, Blanco, et al., 2014; Petry, Rehbein, et al., 2014). The term IGD is used here for studies restricted to gaming and for conditions like addiction, dependence, or compulsive use. However, IGD does not imply that the DSM-5 criteria were applied.

Most prevalence studies are based on convenience samples recruited via online surveys or consisting of subgroups with elevated prevalence rates, such as students. Such approaches are likely to result in biased data and tend to overestimate true prevalence. Moreover, most such studies are not representative (Byun et al., 2009) and, therefore, lack generalizability. As a result, inferences about predictors, comorbidities, or other associations with IA, PUI, or IGD may well also be biased.

Another methodological concern is that no generally accepted approach exists for defining IA or PUI. As a result, studies are based on a number of different concepts and definitions, which is likely one reason for varying prevalence rates. Some studies have published data on more severe conditions like addiction or dependence, whereas other studies have focused on compulsive use or milder forms like problematic use.

Moreover, a plethora of assessment instruments have been used, each with different types of thresholds and cutoff points (Kuss, Griffiths, Karila, & Billieux, 2014; Lortie & Guitton, 2013). Most of these instruments have to be regarded as screening questionnaires and have not been thoroughly tested with respect to validity and reliability. In general, screening instruments can lead to significant and considerable over- or underestimations of true prevalence. The accuracy of prevalence estimations based on screening instruments depends on the number of false-positive and false-negative results according to the specificity and sensitivity of the questionnaire as well as the true prevalence in the population under study. In particular, disorders with low prevalence are widely overestimated the more the specificity of an instrument falls short of optimal.

Pragmatic concerns contribute to these difficulties. General population studies are quite expensive, which is a key reason for the small amount of existing data gathered through such an approach. The first general population study on the prevalence of IA was conducted in the United States and found a rather low prevalence of 0.3–0.7% depending on different diagnostic algorithms (Aboujaoude, Koran, Gamel, Large, & Serpe, 2006). This chapter focuses on general population studies conducted in Europe, published in the English language, and appearing in peer-reviewed journals.

Data from Adolescent Samples

In general, adolescent samples are recruited in schools. Strictly speaking, these approaches cannot be considered general population studies, but they cover a subsample fairly well, particularly when they are large and conducted nationwide. For that reason, they are included here. Nevertheless, bias has to be considered due to absenteeism or students leaving school early (especially in older age groups). We found six nationwide studies that estimated IGD or IA in adolescent samples and three cross-national studies on IGD or IA. One study on IGD was considered, despite being an online survey, due to its representative approach. Other studies were not included because the samples could not be considered nationwide or representative (e.g., Van Rooij, Schoenmakers, Vermulst, Van den Eijnden, & Van de Mheen, 2011). One study recruited adolescents only if one caregiver agreed to take part as well and was excluded due to doubtful representativeness (Wartberg, Kriston, Kammerl, Petersen, & Thomasius, 2015).

Gaming

In a European study (Müller et al., 2015), 12,983 students (10th grade) aged 14–17 years completed the Assessment of Internet and Computer Game Addiction—Gaming Module (AICA-S-Gaming; Wölfling, Müller, & Beutel, 2011). This study used a stratified random probability sample from seven countries across Europe, which included Germany, Greece, Iceland, the Netherlands, Poland, Romania, and Spain. The lowest prevalence could be found in Spain (0.6%) and the Netherlands (1.0) whereas estimates were highest in Poland (2.0) and Greece (2.5). IGD was associated with psychopathology—in particular, aggressive and rule-breaking behavior—as well as social problems.

Two nationwide studies estimated the occurrence of IGD in schools, one based on a German sample (Rehbein, Kleimann, & Mössle, 2010) and another originating in Hungary (Papay et al., 2013). The German study included 15,168 participants recruited in schools, drawn from a larger sample of 44,610 students from schools in 61 randomly selected regions in Germany. In this representative sample of ninth-graders, every third was asked to complete the 14-item Video Game Dependency Scale (KFN-CSAS-II; Rehbein & Borchers, 2009), which yields a total score ranging from 14 to 56. A total of 10,402 individuals responded to at least 13 items and were included in the prevalence estimation. The authors used cut-points of 35 and 42 on the Video Game Dependency Scale to identify risk for developing IGD and the presence of IGD, respectively. Across the total sample, 2.8% were identified as being at risk and 1.7% as having IGD (Rehbein & Borchers, 2009). The respective figures were 4.7% and 3.0% for boys and 0.5% and 0.3% for girls, thereby showing a preponderance of game-related problems in male participants. IGD was associated with decreased school achievement, increased truancy, reduced sleep time, reduced leisure activities, and increased suicidal ideation.

The Hungarian study (Papay et al., 2013) collected data using the European School Survey Project on Alcohol and Other Drugs (ESPAD). The sample on IGD covered grades 9 and 10 in secondary general and secondary vocational schools. Among the 5,045 participants, 2,774 had played online games in the past month and filled in an abbreviated 12-item version of the 18-item Problematic Online Gaming Questionnaire (POGQ; Demetrovics et al., 2012). The authors used a two-step approach in analyzing their data. First, a confirmatory factor analysis revealed that the six dimensions yielded an appropriate fit. Second, a latent profile analysis based on the six dimensions was applied and resulted in a three-class solution: no risk for problematic use of online games, low risk for problematic use, and high risk for problematic use. Based on these classes the prevalence was estimated to be 4.6% for the high risk group and 13.3% for the low risk group. Belonging to the high-risk class was associated with being male, playing for more than 5 hours a day, having a lower grade point average, having lower self-esteem, and having a higher depression score.

A German study recruited 1,531 participants aged 12–25 in an online survey (Wartberg, Kriston, & Thomasius, 2017). In contrast to other online studies, an extensive pool of addresses was used for a multistage random procedure, and data were analyzed using weights to qualify representative findings. The 9-item Internet Gaming Disorder Scale (IGDS; Lemmens, Valkenburg, & Gentile, 2015) was used to assess IGD according to DSM-5 with a threshold of 5 points. The estimated prevalence was 5.7% and markedly higher than in other German samples (Muller et al., 2015; Rehbein et al., 2010; Rehbein, Kliem, Baier, Mossle, & Petry, 2015).

Another study was conducted in Slovenia and recruited schoolchildren based on a random probability selection of all eight graders with a final samples size of 1,071 students aged 12–16 (Pontes, Macur, & Griffiths, 2016). The Internet Gaming Disorder Scale—Short Form (IGDS9-SF) was used as screening instrument (Pontes & Griffiths, 2015). Participants were classified as having IGD if they answered with "very often" to at least 5 of the 9 items tapping the DSM-5 criteria. Using this threshold resulted in a prevalence estimate of 2.5%.

Internet Use in General

A European study with adolescents provided a broader focus by covering not only gaming but other forms of Internet addiction as well (Durkee et al., 2012). This project was conducted in 10 European countries (Austria, Estonia, France, Germany, Hungary, Ireland, Italy, Romania, Slovenia, and Spain) and in Israel, with a total of 11,956 participants and a mean age of 14.9 years. Students from 178 randomly selected schools were recruited within the framework of the Saving and Empowering Young Lives in Europe (SEYLE) trial (Wasserman et al., 2010). IA was assessed using the 8-item Young Diagnostic Questionnaire (YDQ; Young, 1998b) and differentiated between maladaptive users (3–4 points) and pathological users (≥5 points). Overall, 4.4% (5.2% of males and 3.8% of females) were classified as IA (pathological use) and 13.5% (12.4% of males and 14.3% of females) as PUI (maladaptive use).

Prevalence rates varied between countries: The highest prevalence rates for IA were observed in Israel with 11.8% and Slovenia with 5.8%, with the lowest rates found in Hungary with 1.6% and Italy with 1.2%. IA and PIU was related to not living with a biological parent, low parental involvement, and parental unemployment. Another study conducted a second assessment in five of the countries (Estonia, Germany, Italy, Romania, and Spain; $n = 5{,}939$) 2 years later ($n = 9{,}758$) and revealed an increase of prevalence estimations in all countries except Germany (Kaess et al., 2016). In the second assessment, prevalence for PUI was 17.6, ranging between 12.2% (Italy) and 25.1% (Estonia); and prevalence for IA was 6.9%, ranging between 4.4% (Italy) and 11.5% (Estonia).

In a study from Greece, 5,590 students aged 12–18 were recruited in middle and high schools using a multistage stratified random sampling technique (Tsimtsiou et al., 2017). Participants completed a Greek version of the Internet Addiction Test (IAT; Young, 1998a). This 20-item questionnaire was used with a threshold of 50 or higher indicating moderate IA and 80 or higher indicating severe IA. Among all participants, 9.6% were classified as exhibiting PUI and 0.5% as exhibiting IA when applying the preceding thresholds.

Another study in schoolchildren was conducted in Lithuania (Ustinaviciene et al., 2016). A multilevel sampling method (country, school, and class) was used to recruit 1,806 participants aged 13–18 years. Based on an 8-item version of Young's Diagnostic Questionnaire (Young, 1998b), 10.6% of males and 7.7% of females were identified as having IA when using a cutoff score of 5 or more.

Data from Samples Including Adults

In total, seven European general population studies have been conducted with adult participants. Of these, three focused on IGD and four on IA.

Gaming

A nationwide study recruited participants aged 15–40 from the Norwegian National Registry to estimate the prevalence of IGD (Mentzoni et al., 2011). Among the 2,500 individuals sampled, 816 (34.0%) responded to a questionnaire via post or website. The authors weighted the data according to the Norwegian demographic structure. Among the respondents, 56.3% reported using video games on a regular basis. IGD was assessed using the Gaming Addiction Scale for Adolescents (GAS; Lemmens, Valkenburg, & Peter, 2009), a seven-item questionnaire covering the dimensions of salience, tolerance, mood modification, withdrawal, relapse, conflict, and problems. Following Lemmens et al.'s guidelines, "video game addiction" was classified as responding at least with "sometimes" to all seven items. Based on this criterion, 0.6% of the sample was classified as having IGD. Problematic use was defined as responding at least with "sometimes" to four or more items (but less than all seven items), resulting in a prevalence of 4.1%. For both groups, young age and male gender were strong predictors (Mentzoni et al., 2011). A relationship was found between problematic use of video games and lower life satisfaction, as well as with elevated levels of anxiety and depression.

In the Netherlands, Haagsma and colleagues (Haagsma, Pieterse, & Peters, 2012) used a national panel to conduct an online survey. Using a stratified random sampling procedure, 3,200 subscribers were invited to participate and 902 (aged 14–81) took part. No differences were found between responders and nonresponders with respect to sociodemographic factors. This study used the GAS (Lemmens et al., 2009), again using responding at least with "sometimes" to all seven items to identify IGD. In the total sample, 1.3% fulfilled the preceding criterion suggesting IGD. Consistent with other studies on gaming, prevalence was higher in males and in younger age groups. The results of this study have to be regarded with caution because the sample is based on an online survey. Nevertheless, it was included here because a representative sample was pursued with respect to sociodemographic variables. However, a selection bias with an overestimation of prevalence estimates due to only including online participants cannot be ruled out.

Another study focusing on IGD in the general population comes from Germany and consists of 4,382 participants aged 14–90 (Festl, Scharkow, & Quandt, 2012). In a representative telephone survey (response rate 55%), 50,000 participants were asked about their gaming behavior, with 12,578 indicating at least occasional game use. This pool of affirmative responders was used to draw a stratified random sample of 3,500 who played multiplayer games at least occasionally and 1,000 who played only single-player titles. The response rate for this part of the survey was 79.6%; 118 participants were excluded due to missing data. The sample was subdivided into 580 adolescents between 14 and 18 years, 1,866 younger adults between 19 and 39 years, and 1,936 adults aged 40 years and older. Again, as in the two preceding studies, the GAS (Lemmens et al., 2009) was used to distinguish between nonproblematic use, problematic use, and dependence. For dependence, a low prevalence rate (0.2%) was obtained for the total sample (Festl et al., 2012). In contrast to other studies, this proportion was the same across all age groups. The prevalence of problematic use was 3.7% across the total sample. Here, however, rates varied with age, with the highest prevalence obtained in the 14–18 age group (7.6%), followed by the 19–39 group (3.3%) and the 40 and older group (3.0%). High GAS scores were associated with higher aggression, lower sociability, lower self-efficacy, lower satisfaction with life, and higher gaming intensity.

Internet Use in General

In a Norwegian study, stratified probability sampling was used to estimate the prevalence of IA as part of a national postal gambling survey that included individuals from 16 to 74 years of age (Bakken, Wenzel, Gotestam, Johansson, & Oren, 2009). The sample of 10,000 drawn from the population database of Norway resulted in 9,638 valid addresses and in turn generated a 35.3% response rate (3,399 respondents). The authors used the YDQ (Young, 1998b) to tap IA, setting 5 yes-answers among the 8 YDQ-items as the threshold for IA. Responding affirmatively to 3–4 criteria was considered indicative of PUI. Looking at the entire sample, 1% was classified as having IA and 5.2% as being at risk (PUI). Rates for both IA and PUI were higher for males (1.4%/6.4%) than for females (0.7%/4.1%). In addition, and as in most other studies, prevalence for both IA and PUI was higher in younger age groups. The authors performed a logistic regression analysis to look for predictors associated with IA or PUI. Besides young age and male gender, university-level education and an unsatisfactory financial situation were identified as risk factors. Higher YDQ scores were associated with self-reported mental health problems such as sleeping disorder or depression.

A study from Germany implemented a random-route procedure that produced a total of 2,512 participants ranging from 14 to 94 years of age (Müller, Glaesmer, Brähler, Wölfling, & Beutel, 2013). Participants were interviewed at their homes and filled in questionnaires. The final response rate was 54.9%, and the resulting sample could be considered representative of the German general population. IA was defined by using the Assessment of Internet and Computer Game Addiction (AICA-S), which is a 14-item questionnaire based on a scale measuring Computer Game Addiction (CSV-S; Wölfling et al., 2011). Based on the distribution of scores and comparisons with clinical judgments, a cut-point of 7 was used. This criterion yielded a prevalence of 2.1% across the sample for IA (Müller et al., 2013). The authors compared "regular" and "addicted" users on a variety of measures and found male gender, being unmarried, unemployment, being a student, and low income as risk factors.

Another general population study from Germany (Rumpf et al., 2014) followed a different approach by applying a statistical, data-driven concept to estimate the prevalence of IA and PUI. This approach, latent profile or latent class analysis (LCA), was comparable to the method used by Papay et al. (2013) and in a study originating in the Netherlands (Van Rooij et al., 2011). LCA has the advantage of not depending on cutoffs. Assessment instruments used in other research on problematic Internet use often suffer from insufficient validation or formal support for selected classification thresholds. In contrast, LCA is a statistical method that identifies groups of respondents based on similarity of response patterns and a specific probability of belonging to a latent class of respondents.

The sample for the present study was drawn from a large representative general population study on Pathological Gambling and Epidemiology (PAGE; Meyer et al., 2015), which included landline telephone (n = 14,022) and cell phone numbers (n = 1,001) in participants aged 14–64. Participants who reported using the Internet for private purposes at least 1 hour on a typical weekday or at least 1 hour a day at the weekend (n = 8,130) completed the 14-item Compulsive Internet Use Scale (CIUS; Meerkerk, Van Den Eijnden, Vermulst, & Garretsen, 2009). The CIUS covers core criteria of problematic Internet use: salience, withdrawal, loss of control, conflict, and coping with unpleasant mood. A six-classes model showed good fit with two of the groups likely to represent IA and PUI. Based on these groups, prevalence was estimated to be 1.0% for IA in the entire sample (N = 15.023), with higher proportions observed in younger age groups (e.g., 4% in participants 14–16 years of age). There were no significant gender differences. The prevalence rates for PUI were 4.6% in the entire sample and 15.4% in the youngest age group (14–16 years). Unemployment and migration background were related to IA. Among those with IA, males reported games as their main Internet activity more often than did females, with females reporting social network use more often than males.

In Slovenia, the prevalence of problematic Internet use was estimated in the general population aged 18 years or older (Macur, Kiraly, Maraz, Nagygyorgy, & Demetrovics, 2016). From the Central Registry of Slovenia and using a stratified sampling method, a total of 6,029 participants were recruited. The assessment was administered via computer-assisted personal interviewing and computer-assisted web interviewing. A weighting procedure was used to account for nonresponse bias. The Problematic Internet Use Questionnaire Short-Form (PIUQ-SF) was selected for assessment, which is an abbreviated version (6 items; PIUQ-SF-6) of the original 18-item PIUQ (Demetrovics, Szeredi, & Rozsa, 2008). Scores on this measure range from 6 to 30, and, based on a latent profile analysis, 15 points or higher was used as a cutoff. The results showed that 3.1% of the sample had problematic Internet use, with higher prevalence for males (3.6%) compared to females (2.6%). The strongest risk factors for problematic Internet use were young age, high educational status, and student status. Other risk factors were being unemployed or unable to work.

Conclusion

Studies on prevalence rates are summarized in Table 5.1. Estimates range from 0.2% to 11.8% for IA and from 2.8% to 17.0% for PUI. In general, prevalence estimates are higher in adolescents and in studies focusing on the broader construct or proposed class of IA compared to IGD. Furthermore, across the studies, groups exhibiting at-risk use are between 1.6 and 6.8 times larger than the IA/IGD groups, with the exception of Festl et al.'s (2012) and Tsimtsiou et al.'s (2017) results showing a considerably higher ratio (18.5:1.0 and 19.2:1.0, respectively). The European cross-national study clearly shows marked variation in prevalence rates for IA and PUI across countries, with respective ranges of 1.2–11.8% and 8.8–17.0% (Durkee et al., 2012). Much of the variation across other studies is likely due to the use of different instruments for assessing IA or IGD. Three studies used a different approach by applying LPA or LCA (which are basically the same), however, the studies are difficult to compare because one focused on IGD (Papay et al., 2013) and two on IA (Macur et al., 2016; Rumpf et al., 2014). Furthermore, two studies used latent classes or latent profiles directly for prevalence estimation whereas the third used the latent profile to find a cutoff for the screening tool and then used this cutoff for prevalence estimation (Macur et al., 2016). Overall, factors found to be associated with IA or IGD are quite similar, with most studies showing associations with male gender, young age, mental health problems, and unfavorable or stressful social conditions (e.g., negative financial circumstances, unemployment, or migration background). However, gender differences may change with the increased availability and use of

Table 5.1 General population studies from Europe

Authors	Sample size (age)	Assessment	Country	Problematic or at-risk use of the Internet or games (%)	Internet addiction or Internet gaming disorder (%)
Adolescents: Gaming					
Müller et al. (2015)	12,983 (14–17)	AICA-S-gaming	7 European countries	–	0.6–2.5
Rehbein et al. (2010)	15,168 (mean: 15.3)	KFN-CSAS-II	Germany	2.8	1.7
Papay et al. (2013)	5,045 (mean: 16.4)	LPA based on POGQ	Hungary	13.3	4.6
Wartberg et al. (2017)	1,531 (12–25)	IGDS	Germany	–	5.7
Pontes et al. (2016)	1,071 (12–16)	IGDS9-SF	Slovenia	–	2.5
Adolescents: Internet use in general					
Durkee et al. (2012)	11,956 (mean: 14.9)	YDQ	11 European countries	13.5 (8.8–17.0)	4.4 (1.2–11.8)
Kaess et al.	5,839 first study (mean: 14.8) 9,758 second study (mean: 15.3)	YDQ	European countries	17.6 (12.2–25.1	6.9 (4.4–11.5)
Tsimtsiou et al. (2017)	5,590 (12–18)	IAT	Greece	9,6	0,5
Ustinaviciene (2016)	1,806 (13–18)	YDQ	Lithuania	–	Males: 10.6 Females: 7.7
All age groups: Gaming					
Mentzoni et al. (2011)	816 (15–40)	GAS	Norway	4.1	0.6
Haagsma et al. (2012)	902 (14–81)	GAS	Netherlands	–	1.3
Festl et al. (2012)	4,382 (14–90)	GAS	Germany	3.7	0.2
All age groups: Internet use in general					
Bakken et al. (2009)	3,399 (16–74)	YDQ	Norway	5.2	1.0
Müller et al. (2013)	2,512 (14–94)	AICA-S	Germany	–	2.1
Rumpf et al. (2014)	15,023/8,103 (14–64)	LCA based on CIUS	Germany	4.6	1.0
Macur et al. (2016)	6,029 (≥18)	PIUQ-SF-6	Slovenia	3.1	–

AICA-S, Assessment of Internet and Computer Game Addiction; AICA-S-Gaming, Assessment of Internet and Computer Game Addiction–Gaming Module; CIUS, Compulsive Internet Use Scale; GAS, Gaming Addiction Scale; IGDS, Internet Gaming Disorder Scale; IGDS9-SF, Internet Gaming Disorder Scale–Short Form; KFN-CSAS-II, German acronym for the Video Game Dependency Scale; LCA, latent class analysis; LPA, latent profile analysis; PIUQ-6, Problematic Internet Use Questionnaire Short-Form; POGQ, Problematic Online Gaming Questionnaire; YDQ, Young Diagnostic Questionnaire.

social networks. Although data are rare (Andreassen & Pallesen, 2014; Kuss & Griffiths, 2011), more recent studies show that women tend to develop problematic use of social networks more often than men (Rehbein & Mössle, 2013; Rumpf et al., 2014). As shown earlier, one large general population study found no overall gender differences with respect to IA, but males reported Internet gaming significantly more often as a main activity and females social networking (Rumpf et al., 2014).

Of note, one European study found an increase of IA in adolescents in four out of five countries (Kaess et al., 2016). Nevertheless, more data are definitely needed to clarify trends with respect to the prevalence of PUI, IA, or IGD.

To conclude, prevalence estimations in most of the European studies generally show that substantial numbers of individuals suffer from PUI, IA, and IGD, particularly in young age groups. Therefore, we need to be prepared to provide effective prevention, early intervention, and treatment. However, the data that are available thus far are compromised by varying approaches used to define IA/IGD or at-risk Internet use. Therefore, comparison of data is difficult due to the different methods used (c.f. Mihara & Higuchi, 2017). In the 16 studies that were reviewed in this chapter, 10 different assessment instruments had been used, with a tendency to use instruments developed by the same group of researchers who conducted the prevalence study. For future research, generally accepted criteria are a worthwhile goal, with the suggested criteria in DSM-5 (Petry & O'Brien, 2013; Petry, Rehbein, et al., 2014) and ICD-11 (Saunders et al., 2017) potentially serving as good starting points. Furthermore, generally accepted and sound assessment tools are needed to make comparisons between different studies.

References

Aboujaoude, E., Koran, L. M., Gamel, N., Large, M. D., & Serpe, R. T. (2006). Potential markers for problematic Internet use: A telephone survey of 2,513 adults. *CNS Spectrums, 11*(10), 750–55.

American Psychiatric Association. (2013). *Diagnostic and statistical manual of mental disorders* (5th ed.). Washington, DC: American Psychiatric Association. https://doi.org/10.1176/appi.books.9780890425596

Andreassen, C. S., & Pallesen, S. (2014). Social network site addiction—an overview. *Current Pharmaceutical Design, 20*(25), 4053–61.

Bakken, I. J., Wenzel, H. G., Gotestam, K. G., Johansson, A., & Oren, A. (2009). Internet addiction among Norwegian adults: A stratified probability sample study. *Scandinavian Journal of Psychology, 50*(2), 121–27. doi:10.1111/j.1467-9450.2008.00685.x

Byun, S., Ruffini, C., Mills, J. E., Douglas, A. C., Niang, M., Stepchenkova, S., . . . Blanton, M. (2009). Internet addiction: Metasynthesis of 1996–2006 quantitative research. *Cyberpsychology and Behavior, 12*(2), 203–07. doi:10.1089/cpb.2008.0102

Demetrovics, Z., Szeredi, B., & Rozsa, S. (2008). The three-factor model of Internet addiction: The development of the Problematic Internet Use Questionnaire. *Behavior Research Methods, 40*(2), 563–74.

Demetrovics, Z., Urban, R., Nagygyoergy, K., Farkas, J., Griffiths, M. D., Papay, O., . . . Olah, A. (2012). The Development of the Problematic Online Gaming Questionnaire (POGQ). *PLoS One, 7*(5). e36417 doi:10.1371/journal.pone.0036417

Durkee, T., Kaess, M., Carli, V., Parzer, P., Wasserman, C., Floderus, B., . . . Wasserman, D. (2012). Prevalence of pathological internet use among adolescents in Europe: Demographic and social factors. *Addiction, 107*(12), 2210–22. doi:10.1111/j.1360-0443.2012.03946.x

Festl, R., Scharkow, M., & Quandt, T. (2012). Problematic computer game use among adolescents, younger and older adults. *Addiction, 108*(3), 592–99. doi:10.1111/add.12016

Haagsma, M. C., Pieterse, M. E., & Peters, O. (2012). The prevalence of problematic video gamers in the Netherlands. *Cyberpsychology, Behavior and Social Networking, 15*(3), 162–68. doi:10.1089/cyber.2011.0248

Kaess, M., Parzer, P., Brunner, R., Koenig, J., Durkee, T., Carli, V., . . . Wasserman, D. (2016). Pathological Internet use is on the rise among European adolescents. *Journal of Adolescent Health, 59*(2), 236–39. doi:10.1016/j.jadohealth.2016.04.009

Kuss, D. J., & Griffiths, M. D. (2011). Online social networking and addiction: A review of the psychological literature. *International Journal of Environmental Research and Public Health, 8*(9), 3528–52. doi:10.3390/ijerph8093528

Kuss, D. J., Griffiths, M. D., Karila, L., & Billieux, J. (2014). Internet addiction: A systematic review of epidemiological research for the last decade. *Current Pharmaceutical Design, 20*(25), 4026–52.

Lemmens, J. S., Valkenburg, P. M., & Gentile, D. A. (2015). The Internet Gaming Disorder Scale. *Psychol Assess, 27*(2), 567–82. doi:10.1037/pas0000062

Lemmens, J. S., Valkenburg, P. M., & Peter, J. (2009). Development and validation of a game addiction scale for adolescents. *Media Psychology, 12*(1), 77–95. doi:10.1080/15213260802669458

Lortie, C. L., & Guitton, M. J. (2013). Internet addiction assessment tools: Dimensional structure and methodological status. *Addiction, 108*(7), 1207–16. doi:10.1111/add.12202

Macur, M., Kiraly, O., Maraz, A., Nagygyorgy, K., & Demetrovics, Z. (2016). Prevalence of problematic internet use in Slovenia. *Zdr Varst, 55*(3), 202–11. doi:10.1515/sjph-2016-0026

Meerkerk, G. J., Van Den Eijnden, R., Vermulst, A. A., & Garretsen, H. F. L. (2009). The Compulsive Internet Use Scale (CIUS): Some psychometric properties. *Cyberpsychology & Behavior, 12*(1), 1–6. doi:10.1089/cpb.2008.0181

Mentzoni, R. A., Brunborg, G. S., Molde, H., Myrseth, H., Skouveroe, K. J. M., Hetland, J., & Pallesen, S. (2011). Problematic video game use: Estimated prevalence and associations with mental and physical health. *Cyberpsychology Behavior and Social Networking, 14*(10), 591–96. doi:10.1089/cyber.2010.0260

Meyer, C., Bischof, A., Westram, A., Jeske, C., deBrito, S., Glorius, S., . . . Rumpf, H. J. (2015). The Pathological Gambling and Epidemiology (PAGE) study program: Design and fieldwork. *International Journal of Methods in Psychiatric Research*, 24(1), 11–31. https://doi.org/10.1002/mpr.1458

Mihara, S., & Higuchi, S. (2017). Cross-sectional and longitudinal epidemiological studies of Internet gaming disorder: A systematic review of the literature. *Psychiatry Clinical Neurosciences*, *71*(7), 425–44. doi:10.1111/pcn.12532

Müller, K. W., Glaesmer, H., Brähler, E., Wölfling, K., & Beutel, M. E. (2013). Prevalence of internet addiction in the general population: Results from a German population-based survey. *Behaviour & Information Technology*, 33(7), 757-66; *http://dx.doi.org/10.1080/0144929X.2013.810778.*

Müller, K. W., Janikian, M., Dreier, M., Wolfling, K., Beutel, M. E., Tzavara, C., . . . Tsitsika, A. (2015). Regular gaming behavior and internet gaming disorder in European adolescents: Results from a cross-national representative survey of prevalence, predictors, and psychopathological correlates. *European Child and Adolescent Psychiatry*, *24*(5), 565–74. doi:10.1007/s00787-014-0611-2

Papay, O., Urban, R., Griffiths, M. D., Nagygyorgy, K., Farkas, J., Kokonyei, G., . . . Demetrovics, Z. (2013). Psychometric properties of the problematic online gaming questionnaire short-form and prevalence of problematic online gaming in a national sample of adolescents. *Cyberpsychology, Behavior, and Social Networking*, *16*(5), 340–48. doi:10.1089/cyber.2012.0484

Petry, N. M., Blanco, C., Auriacombe, M., Borges, G., Bucholz, K., Crowley, T. J., . . . O'Brien, C. (2014). An overview of and rationale for changes proposed for pathological gambling in DSM-5. *Journal of Gambling Studies*, *14*, 493–02. doi:10.1007/s10899-013-9370-0

Petry, N. M., & O'Brien, C. P. (2013). Internet gaming disorder and the DSM-5. *Addiction*, *108*(7), 1186–87. doi:10.1111/add.12162

Petry, N. M., Rehbein, F., Gentile, D. A., Lemmens, J. S., Rumpf, H. J., Mossle, T., . . . O'Brien, C. P. (2014). An international consensus for assessing internet gaming disorder using the new DSM-5 approach. *Addiction, 109(9), 1399-406.* doi:10.1111/add.12457

Pontes, H. M., & Griffiths, M. D. (2015). Measuring DSM-5 internet gaming disorder: Development and validation of a short psychometric scale. *Computers in Human Behavior*, *45*, 137–43. doi:10.1016/j.chb.2014.12.006

Pontes, H. M., Macur, M., & Griffiths, M. D. (2016). Internet Gaming Disorder Among Slovenian Primary Schoolchildren: Findings from a nationally representative sample of adolescents. *Journal of Behavioral Addictions*, *5*(2), 304–10. doi:10.1556/2006.5.2016.042

Rehbein, F., & Borchers, M. (2009). Süchtig nach virtuellen welten? Exzessives Computerspielen und Computerspielabhängigkeit in der Jugend [Addicted to virtual worlds? Excessive videogaming and video game addiction in adolescents]. *Kinderärztliche Praxis, 80(3), 42-49*, 42–49.

Rehbein, F., Kliem, S., Baier, D., Mossle, T., & Petry, N. M. (2015). Prevalence of internet gaming disorder in German adolescents: Diagnostic contribution of the nine DSM-5 criteria in a state-wide representative sample. *Addiction*, *110*(5), 842–51. doi:10.1111/add.12849

Rehbein, F., Kleimann, M., & Mössle, T. (2010). Prevalence and risk factors of video game dependency in adolescence: Results of a German nationwide survey. *Cyberpsychology Behavior and Social Networking*, *13*(3), 269–77. doi:10.1089/cyber.2009.0227

Rehbein, F., & Mössle, T. (2013). Video game and Internet addiction: Is there a need for differentiation? *Sucht*, *59*, 129–42.

Rumpf, H. J., Vermulst, A. A., Bischof, A., Kastirke, N., Gürtler, N., Bischof, G., . . . Meyer, C. (2014). Occurrence of internet addiction in a general population sample: A latent class analysis. *European Addiction Research*, *20*, 159–66.

Saunders, J. B., Hao, W., Long, J., King, D. L., Mann, K., Fauth-Bühler, M., . . . Poznyak, V. (2017). Gaming disorder: Its delineation as an important condition for diagnosis, management and prevention. *Journal of Behavioral Addictions*, *6*, 271–79. doi:10.1556/2006.6.2017.039

Tsimtsiou, Z., Haidich, A. B., Drontsos, A., Dantsi, F., Sekeri, Z., Drosos, E., . . . Arvanitidou, M. (2017). Pathological Internet use, cyberbullying and mobile phone use in adolescence: A school-based study in Greece. *International Journal of Adolescent Medicine and Health, 30(6), 20160115.* doi:10.1515/ijamh-2016–0115

Ustinaviciene, R., Skemiene, L., Luksiene, D., Radisauskas, R., Kaliniene, G., & Vasilavicius, P. (2016). Problematic computer game use as expression of Internet addiction and its association with self-rated health in the Lithuanian adolescent population. *Medicina (Kaunas)*, *52*(3), 199–04. doi:10.1016/j.medici.2016.04.002

Van Rooij, A. J., Schoenmakers, T. M., Vermulst, A. A., Van den Eijnden, R. J., & Van de Mheen, D. (2011). Online video game addiction: Identification of addicted adolescent gamers. *Addiction*, *106*, 205–12. doi:10.1111/j.1360–0443.2010.03104.x

Wartberg, L., Kriston, L., Kammerl, R., Petersen, K. U., & Thomasius, R. (2015). Prevalence of pathological Internet use in a representative German sample of adolescents: Results of a latent profile analysis. *Psychopathology*, *48*(1), 25–30. doi:10.1159/000365095

Wartberg, L., Kriston, L., & Thomasius, R. (2017). The prevalence and psychosocial correlates of Internet Gaming Disorder. *Dtsch Arztebl Int*, *114*(25), 419–24. doi:10.3238/arztebl.2017.0419

Wasserman, D., Carli, V., Wasserman, C., Apter, A., Balazs, J., Bobes, J., . . . Hoven, C. W. (2010). Saving and empowering young lives in Europe (SEYLE): A randomized controlled trial. *BMC Public Health, 10*, 192. doi:1471-2458-10-192 [pii] 10.1186/1471-2458-10-192

Wölfling, K., Müller, K. W., & Beutel, M. (2011). [Reliability and validity of the Scale for the Assessment of Pathological Computer-Gaming (CSV-S)]. *Psychotherapie, Psychosomatik, Medizinische Psychologie*, *61*(5), 216–24. doi:10.1055/s-0030–1263145

Young, K. S. (1998a). *Caught in the net: How to recognize the signs of internet addiction—and a winning strategy for recovery.* New York: Wiley. ISBN:978-0-471-19159-9

Young, K. S. (1998b). Internet addiction: The emergence of a new clinical disorder. *Cyberpsychology and Behavior*, *1*(5), 237–44. doi:10.1089/cpb.1999.2.381

CHAPTER

6

The Natural History of Problematic Internet Use and Gaming

Recent Findings, Challenges, and Future Directions

Daniel L. King *and* Paul H. Delfabbro

Abstract

Internet use and gaming technologies may, under certain conditions, be associated with clinically significant harm across multiple domains of functioning. However, relatively little is known about the natural history of these problems, including their etiology, symptom trajectory, and risk factors. The aim of this chapter is to summarize and discuss some of the literature on the natural course of Internet-related disorders, with a focus on gaming disorder, and to highlight potentially useful areas for further investigation. The chapter is organized into two main sections which provide summaries of qualitative and quantitative research. It is shown that qualitative evidence is relatively limited in scope. Case reports suggest that problematic Internet and gaming behaviors can have a rapid onset that often arises in the context of busy and unfulfilled lives, particularly among individuals with preexisting psychological issues (e.g., depression, anxiety). The quantitative evidence is more developed and growing. Most studies have focused on adolescence. Studies suggest that social factors such as family life and parent–child relationships play a strong role in the development of persistent behaviors (e.g., gaming to escape from parental conflict). Preexisting poorer social skills, attention issues, and neurotic personality type are risk factors. Overall, the evidence suggests that many individuals, representing a diverse range of social background and psychological vulnerabilities, report long-term problems with Internet and gaming activities. Future research is needed to gain better understanding of these problems to assist affected individuals and their families.

Keywords: gaming disorder, longitudinal, qualitative, risk factor, profile, Internet

Introduction

There is mounting evidence that Internet use and gaming technologies may, under certain conditions, be associated with clinically significant harm across multiple domains of functioning (King, Delfabbro, & Griffiths, 2013; Sim et al., 2012). Research evidence has so far guided the development of some preliminary taxonomies and clinical descriptions of Internet-related problems to support further empirical inquiry, particularly in relation to online video games (e.g., Internet gaming disorder [IGD] in the fifth edition of the *Diagnostic and Statistical Manual of Mental Disorders* [DSM-5]). However, as noted by several reviews over the past decade (King, Haagsma, Delfabbro, Gradisar, & Griffiths, 2013, 2014; Lam, 2014), considerably less is known about the natural history of Internet-related problems, including their etiology, symptom trajectory, and risk factors. Put simply: How and when do these difficulties begin, how do they tend to progress, how long do they last, and what other factors might play a role?

These questions remain difficult to answer despite the growing international level of interest and resources directed toward understanding them. Current gaps in knowledge may be attributed to several factors, including (1) the relative infancy of the field of study, (2) inconsistencies in conceptualization and measurement across research studies, (3) the reliance on cross-sectional designs based on self-report and (4) a lack of clinical research with follow-up observation. Recently, however, there have been a number of research studies that employ designs more capable of examining the longitudinal course of Internet-related disorders. According to Lam (2014), for example, there have been 24 published papers that detail the prospective longitudinal study of Internet-related disorders. Although this evidence base remains small, a review of these findings may be useful for identifying points of consensus and debate and for informing future research agendas. Therefore, the aim of this chapter is to summarize and discuss some of the recent literature on the natural course of Internet-related disorders and to highlight potentially useful areas for further investigation. Given that the scope of Internet activities is quite broad, encompassing social media, digital games, and web browsing among other activities unique to the Internet, this chapter focuses mostly on online gaming because this activity has arguably received the most attention for its association with excessive and problematic behavior. At the same time, this chapter will discuss a number of under-researched topics of a methodological and conceptual nature that will be broadly applicable to many other Internet-related activities.

Qualitative Research

Overview

Detailed case reports of Internet-related disorders are unusually rare in the area of technology-based behavior. In the area of problematic video gaming, for example, there have been approximately only a dozen qualitative studies published in the past decade, representing fewer than 120 people with recognized Internet gaming problems. This figure stands in sharp contrast to the many thousands of individuals surveyed in cross-sectional online surveys. The extent to which published papers are able to provide a detailed account of the natural history of problems varies across this body of work, with some papers focused on examining current symptoms and associated harm and/or difficulties. However, there are some well-documented cases of problematic Internet users that include descriptions of the nature and history of the problem.

Early Qualitative Research

A notable case study by Shotton (1989) is one of the first psychological studies of excessive computer use. Shotton conducted interviews with 106 individuals who reported being "dependent" on their computers. "Dependents" were described as highly intelligent and congenial, but their fascination with computer technology was often misunderstood and judged negatively by those around them. They were drawn to computers because they offered a safe retreat from an uncertain world. Some users were reported to value time spent on their computer above all other life activities, including work and interpersonal relationships. Shotton speculated that many "dependents" had not received adequate parental warmth during childhood and therefore began using computers to fulfill unmet attachment needs. She theorized that, over time, these users had developed a stable preference for technology-based rewards and therefore avoided participation in other life activities. While dependency was the primary focus of the research, Shotton also argued that computer technology was appealing for other reasons. "Dependents" used computers extensively in their adult lives in many contexts. Some worked in vocations that involved computers, such as programming, whereas others merely used computers at home each night for recreational purposes. "Dependents" were primarily motivated to increase their knowledge of computers and to develop a mastery over the intellectual challenges posed by computers. Although these intrinsic goals reportedly gave "dependents" a great deal of personal fulfillment, Shotton also found that high levels of computer use were not always beneficial. Some users developed minor strain injuries or muscle pains. Despite this, home computer use did not appear to have a substantially negative impact on the quality of spousal relationships. In fact, spouses reported to be understanding and supportive of their partners' computer activities. It was concluded that the potential for harm resulting from dependency was often outweighed by the many positive aspects of computer use.

Anecdotal evidence on Internet-related disorders has accumulated in the two decades since Shotton's study. There have been many described cases of lonely teenage males with social skill deficits using a reliance on technology to compensate. However, several recent qualitative studies have highlighted the fact that Internet-related disorders can also present in older populations, for both genders, married or in a long-term relationship, and across the spectrum of socioeconomic advantage (Griffiths, 2000; Lee, 2011; Tsai & Lin, 2003). In this way, the multiple demographic profiles observed in qualitative research are not in line with the stereotype that is commonly perpetuated in popular media. The paucity of detailed case reports or qualitative studies as compared to quantitative method-based studies may reflect a number of factors. These include (1) the difficulty in recruiting people who experience problems with technology and who are willing to admit that a problem exists, (2) the relative lack of academic interest in qualitative studies given the perceived difficulty in publishing such work, or (3) an assumption that qualitative studies are unlikely to contribute as meaningfully to knowledge in the area to the same extent as quantitative work.

Recent Reports on Adults and Adolescents

The extant qualitative research has proved valuable in providing useful insights into the natural history of problematic behaviors, particular in relation to gaming. Several studies (e.g., Griffiths, 2000, 2010; Lee, 2011; Tsai & Lin, 2003) have documented that problems can often develop rather quickly (i.e., within a 3-month period) from initial use of certain video games, particularly in the case of massively multiplayer online role-playing games (MMORPGs) such as World of Warcraft that typically require a considerable time investment as compared to other video games. Often a sudden increase in use, which may lead to excessive use, is described as being preceded by a longer term familiarity with or exposure to gaming and/or multiple previous episodes of binge-style gaming at a younger age. Additionally, while gaming can start at a very young age (e.g., 4 years old), it is not often detected by parents or others as being problematic or causing interference (i.e., harmful) usually until the individual reaches middle adolescence, when schooling responsibilities become more demanding (e.g., more difficult and requiring nightly homework) and less compatible with frequent gaming activity. Resistance to parental boundaries and limit-setting may occur at this stage, with problematic cases often involving parents becoming fatigued and/or overwhelmed by the emotional reactivity (i.e., sadness, anger) of the child. Ultimately, many parents of problem gamers relent to the young person's demands for persistent and uninterrupted gaming activity.

In the case of adult gamers, two somewhat different cases are described in qualitative studies. The first may be generally characterized as the psychologically normal, "busy" adult gamer with multiple life commitments that become disrupted due to (usually suddenly) increased gaming activity. Increased gaming appears to cause particular interference for individuals with competing demands in both full-time employment and family life (marriage, children). It is noted that certain high levels of gaming (e.g., consistently playing 4–6 hours per night and 12 hours per day on the weekend) may initially cause only minor consequences, such as decreased sleep producing lethargic mood and irritability. However, a problematic habit may then form quickly as the individual becomes more preoccupied with the game and with planning the next time they will play. Such a trajectory usually evolves into a schedule of gaming that notably includes only rare (if any) non-gaming days, with limited efforts to control or reduce gaming in the early stages. Some accounts suggest that emerging problematic adult gamers will deceive partners and/or employers (e.g., faking illness) in order to spend more time gaming without interruption by other responsibilities. For example, Griffiths (2000) describes the case of an unemployed problematic gamer who created the pretence that he was actively (but continually unsuccessfully) searching for a new job by leaving his résumé and formal interview clothes in sight of his living partner so he could instead play an online game during the day without her knowledge.

The second type of adult problem gamer appears to be the more psychologically vulnerable gamer who is often socially isolated and who then becomes, or has long been, immersed in gaming both as a way of coping with life difficulties and as means of empowerment (King & Delfabbro, 2009, 2014). It is notable that the feeling of self-empowerment associated with attaining status and achievements in the gaming environment often contrasts with the reverse situation in real life. Such situations may lead to a further abrogation of real-life responsibilities and a further elevation of the cyberworld for the maintenance of self-worth. Such individuals often may not necessarily need to engage in secrecy or deception related to gaming given that there are so few significant others in the person's life to necessitate this tactic. For example, in one such case known to the authors, a 40-year-old man with a 20-year history of problem gaming had become long-term unemployed (following an earlier career in video game testing) and then socially isolated from friends and family. This individual spent all available time in his small apartment engaged in gaming, with very few attempts made to control or reduce his gaming. Following a crisis that involved an attempted suicide triggered by feeling worthless about spending so much time gaming, as well as overwhelming disgust in the poor sanitary condition of his living space, this individual sought counseling to address his gaming and other related problems.

Other qualitative accounts have eschewed the addiction conceptualization when discussing Internet-related problems. This is illustrated, for example, in a paper by Allison and colleagues (Allison, von Wahlde, Shockley, & Gabbard, 2006) who describe the case of an 18-year-old man who presented to an outpatient multidisciplinary clinic for evaluation of his obsession with gaming. The individual had a life-long history of school refusal and various anxiety issues and often engaged in excessive gaming as a means of escape and coping. This gaming behavior was reported as being relatively stable over the period of adolescence, with multiple failed attempts to reduce or abstain from gaming to attend to school or job responsibilities. In the case of this individual, severe gaming-related problems manifested rapidly in conjunction with the deterioration of his psychological well-being, and these combined problems continued over a number of years. Alison et al.'s (2006) paper is notable in that they refrained from conceptualizing the individual's problems primarily from an addiction standpoint. Instead, they emphasized that the adverse consequences of the gaming were comparable to other known addictive behaviors, but they were content to avoid relying on conventional processes (e.g., withdrawal) in their explanation. They observed that that the gaming activity allowed the user to "express aspects of himself that served a compensatory function psychologically" while also enabling him to avoid "intimacy with peers and the expansion of his identity in the outside world" (Alison et al., 2006; p. 384). In this sense, the conventional addiction model was not the only means of explaining the development and progression of the problematic gaming habit, with developmental concerns being important to understanding the problem.

Summary

The available qualitative evidence is relatively limited in scope. However, it may be concluded on preliminary reports that problem Internet and gaming behaviors can have a rapid onset from normal levels of use. This has been described in some cases as following the "big discovery" of a particularly novel, challenging and, socially integrated type of video game. The MMORPG is particularly salient in this respect, as it is often described as catering to many players' motivations to game, including their desire to be part of a larger community and to immerse themselves in an activity that rewards mastery and persistence. Existing longitudinal evidence suggests that problematic gaming can occur over a long period of time (i.e., in excess of 6–12 months). However, it is not clear why some individuals may "age out" or otherwise naturally recover or significantly reduce their gaming. One notable aspect of the qualitative reports is the minimal ambivalence or "internal conflict" reported by problem gamers and the limited motivation to reduce gaming over time. This is particularly evident for adolescents, who may not report a desire to reduce their gaming but instead view the stress and conflict from concerned parents or teachers as the principal source of their problems. Similarly, adolescents' entry into therapy or treatment facilities is often nonvoluntary.

Qualitative data on problematic Internet-related disorders hold a lot of potential to understanding the core psychopathology, as well as to guiding many new empirical efforts toward measurement, diagnosis, and, ultimately, treatment. A review of the available studies on problematic gaming indicates that there has been a predominant focus on the phenomenological experience of gaming use and associated negative consequences. However, fewer attempts have been made to document the progression of normal healthy Internet and gaming use to more problematic types of behavior. One of the key issues is determining the role of preexisting issues (e.g., social anxiety, developmental issues, life stressors) in affecting the development of problematic gaming, particularly in the case of adult gamers with complex life histories. Nevertheless, it is apparent in many cases of problem gamers that there may be preexisting deficits, as in the area of social skills, as well as anxiety and depression. Many problem gamers appear to be more socially confident and assertive in online gaming settings. For example, they may demonstrate conversational skills (e.g., flowing conversation, persuasion, constructive feedback, appropriate humor, etc.) that may be rarely used in other social settings.

Quantitative Research

Overview

One of the primary objectives of prospective longitudinal studies is to follow a cohort of users over an extended period of time in order to study long-term patterns of behavior (Yu & Shek, 2013). This may include testing the assumption that certain behaviors may be prone to fluctuate over time or an opposing view that behavior may be relatively stable. To date, there have been several prospective longitudinal studies of Internet-related disorders (e.g., Haagsma, King, Pieterse, & Peters, 2013; Sun et al., 2012; Yang et al., 2014; Yen et al., 2012) that have attempted to identify the most salient risk and outcome factors of problematic Internet use. This section will attempt to summarize some of the most recent work conducted internationally in populations that include both adolescents and adults, including a discussion of the relative strengths and weaknesses of this literature base.

Recent Reports on Adults and Adolescents

Several major prospective longitudinal studies of problematic Internet use and gaming have been conducted in the past few years. This is particularly evident in the Eastern context, where such issues are considered a priority for research by local health authorities and governmental bodies. One task of longitudinal research has been to identify specific risk factors that might predict the incidence of problematic electronic media use. Such risk factors often include certain demographic factors (e.g., male gender, age) and media use, psychological and mental health variables, and personality factors. For example, a study by Ko et al. (2007) examined 517 students from three junior high schools in southern Taiwan. The researchers examined gender, personality, mental health, self-esteem, family function, life satisfaction, and Internet activities as predictors of Internet addiction. The results indicated that the 1-year incidence and remission rates for Internet addiction were 7.5% and 49.5%, respectively. Low self-esteem, low family function, and online (vs. offline) game playing were predictive of the emergence of Internet addiction. Poorer social competence predicted remission of Internet addiction, demonstrating that difficulties in managing socially in the real world may contribute to "relapse" or returning to the safety of the online world.

One of the first (and also largest) longitudinal studies of youth gamers was reported by Gentile et al. (2011), who conducted a 2-year follow-up study involving 3,034 school students in Singapore. Their analysis showed that increased amounts of gaming, lower social competence, and greater impulsivity seemed to act as risk factors for becoming pathological gamers, whereas depression, anxiety, social phobias, and lower school performance seemed to act as outcomes of pathological gaming. An additional finding was that the majority (84%) of youths who were initially identified as pathological gamers were still pathological gamers 2 years later. On this basis, the study supported the notion that problematic video gaming behavior was persistent or stable over time in many cases.

However, the evidence does not appear to be wholly supportive of the notion that problematic gaming tends to be a stable behavioral pattern. A study by Scharkow, Festl, and Quandt (2014) examined a total of 112 adolescents aged between 14 and 18 years over a period of 2 years. Their total sample also included 363 adults aged between 19 and 39 years and 427 adults aged 40 years and older. The authors assessed problematic video gaming using an addiction-based checklist known as the Game Addiction Scale (GAS). They observed generally low GAS scores which were very stable in yearly intervals. However, only nine participants consistently exhibited symptoms of problematic game use across all waves, while no respondent could be classified consistently as being addicted according to the GAS criteria. Changes in problematic gaming were not related consistently to changes in psychosocial well-being, although some cross-lagged effects were statistically significant in younger and older adult groups. Within a 2-year time-frame, problematic use of computer games was observed to be a less stable behavior than reported in other studies and not related systematically to negative changes in the gamers' lives. A similar finding was reported by King, Delfabbro, et al. (2013) who found that problem gaming symptoms generally declined among both normal and problematic gamers over an 18-month period.

Researchers often acknowledge the importance of studying adolescent behavior in relation to the family context. Several longitudinal studies have therefore explored the role of parenting in influencing problematic media use, including parental strategies targeted at limiting media use as well as the quality of parent–child relationships. A study by Ko et al. (2015) investigated a total of 2,293 adolescents assessing Internet addiction status, family function, and family factors with a 1-year follow-up. Their analysis showed that parent–child conflict predicted the incidence of Internet addiction after 12 months and that the next most important factors were that the young person did not live with his or her mother or was permitted to use the Internet for more than 2 hours per day by parents or caregivers. A similar study was reported by Choo, Sim, Liau, Gentile, and Khoo (2015), who surveyed 2,974 secondary students in Singapore over a 2-year period. The authors examined the main effects of parent–child closeness and parental restriction of child video gaming on children and adolescents' pathological video gaming symptoms. Their results showed that poor parent–child bonding increased risk of problematic gaming and that restrictive rules and regulations set by parents on the child's video gaming behaviors were not effective in reducing the pathological symptoms. These findings together are also consistent with van den Eijnden et al.'s (2010) study of 510 Dutch adolescents. They found that good parent–child communication regarding Internet use was protective against the development of compulsive digital media use.

A number of research projects have focused on identifying risk factors for problematic Internet use and gaming. One of the objectives of such research is to identify variables that are significantly likely to precede the development of problematic behavior. Family and social factors are often considered in such studies as being relatively impactful on the trajectory toward problem behavior. For example, a 5-year, two-wave longitudinal study conducted by Rehbein and Baier (2013) examined the development of problematic gaming in 406 students from Grades 4 to 9. Their findings suggested that 15-year-old video game addicts had already exhibited a number of specific risk factors at the age of 10. Students from single-parent families seemed to be particularly at risk, as were students with low school well-being and weaker social integration in the classroom.

Several individual psychological factors have been strongly implicated in the development and maintenance of gaming-related problems. One common hypothesis is that prolonged gaming may affect some cognitive capabilities of users, such as memory, concentration, and attention. For example, a study by Ferguson and Ceranoglu (2014) tracked the development of attention problems and occurrence of pathological gaming in 144 adolescents during a 1-year prospective analysis. Attention problems tended to precede pathological gaming behaviors; however, gaming did not precede attention issues. The authors argued that gaming problems may be symptomatic of attention problems, rather than being a distinct problem in their own right.

Social competence and social skills have also been implicated in problem gaming, perhaps owing to observations in case studies that many heavy gamers may choose to avoid social interaction in the real world. A study by Lemmens, Valkenburg, and Peter (2011) involved a two-wave panel study of 851 Dutch adolescents, including 543 gamers. Their analyses indicated that social competence, self-esteem, and loneliness were significant predictors of pathological gaming at 6-month follow-up. The authors stated that lower psychosocial well-being could be considered an antecedent of pathological gaming among adolescent gamers. Furthermore, it was suggested that loneliness may be a consequence of pathological gaming, on the basis that excessive gaming displaced real-world social interaction and therefore existing relationships deteriorated.

Relatively fewer longitudinal studies have been conducted in adult populations. It is notable that many studies involve the administration of clinical measures (i.e., psychometric tests for mental disorders) to general population or university samples. A study by Dong, Lu, Zhou, and Zhao (2011), for example, examined 59 university students using the Symptom CheckList-90 prior to and after becoming addicted to the Internet. The authors reported that participants who developed problematic Internet use issues tended to score in the abnormal range on the obsessive-compulsive dimension at baseline. At follow-up, addicted participants reported significantly higher scores of depression, anxiety, hostility, interpersonal sensitivity, and psychoticism, suggesting that these may be outcomes of Internet addiction. A similar 2-year longitudinal study by Dong, Wang, Yang, and Zhou (2013) examined the role of personality factors in determining Internet addiction status in 868 university students. Their results indicated that students addicted to the Internet demonstrated higher neuroticism and psychoticism. A subgroup of 49 individuals (all male) classified as "addicted" at baseline were found to be addicted at follow-up.

Summary

This brief review of the quantitative research has shown that there increasing efforts are being made to systematically measure and track problematic Internet and gaming behaviors over time. A notable methodological strength is that follow-up periods of 2 years are often employed, but very few studies conduct interim observations that are sensitive to changes that may occur within this time interval. Particular attention has been paid to understanding the development of gaming problems in adolescence. Consistent findings suggest that social factors such as family life and parent–child relationships play a strong role in the development of patterns of gaming behavior, indicating that gaming becomes an avenue to escape from parental conflict. To date, there have been several studies documenting a variety of risk factors, with convergent evidence on the role of preexisting poorer social skills as a precursor for the development of problematic gaming. Individual factors such as neurotic personality traits, poor attention, and poor mental health have been identified in empirical studies. Less is known about adult problem gamers, and there are particular limitations to the evidence base relying on nongeneral populations rather than sampling from clinical populations. Given these mixed results, there does not appear to be a consensus regarding the stability and course of problematic gaming, but there are a large number of cases that demonstrate symptoms over and beyond a 2-year period.

Limitations and Methodological Improvements

The preceding analysis has revealed several areas of improvement for research on the natural history of Internet-related disorders. Primarily, there is a strong need for theory building to develop testable assumptions about etiological mechanisms underlying problematic Internet-related behaviors. Theoretical frameworks designed for specific Internet-related behaviors (e.g., social media use, video gaming, etc.) may be particularly useful given the known differences in usage patterns and user profiles across such activities. Another important issue is improving consistency in research designs across research teams and regions to ensure comparability and synthesis of research findings. This is especially pertinent to the issue of measurement or instrumentation (i.e., consistency in the use of survey tools), but also in relation to other design characteristics such as population and recruitment processes, as well as frequency and duration of follow-up measures. Similarly, as noted by Lam (2014), many longitudinal studies do not meet all quality standards of design or reporting, and therefore there is a need for general improvement in study quality. However, such improvements and innovations in research design may arguably require more funding and resources than are currently available in particular regions.

Another issue is the reliance on self-report measurement, a criticism often raised in this area (King, Haagsma, et al., 2013). There do not appear to be any studies that involve naturalistic observation of gaming. It seems possible to use more sophisticated approaches than basic paper or online surveys to gather self-report data to improve recall or accuracy. Personal diaries or apps on mobile devices can be used more dynamically in relevant situations to record usage and/or other psychometric information. Another possibility is the use of behavioral tracking data that are gathered by the Internet application itself (e.g., an online video game or social media application), given this information is likely to be the most reliable source of data. However, one major obstacle is that access to such information may be blocked or made unavailable without the permission of the IP owner. Industry collaboration may be one potential avenue for research to circumvent this problem. For example, an academic study of problematic gaming in collaboration with a major MMO company could provide anonymized user account information and facilitate additional survey procedures. However, there are significant concerns about potential conflicts of interest associated with academic collaboration with a commercial entity. The lack of collaboration may suggest that, within the gaming industry, there is a lack of interest in or receptiveness to research on the negative aspects of gaming, or a perception of research as having limited financial or other (e.g., social responsibility) value. One explanation may be that the industry views parents as having the primary social responsibility for addressing excessive gaming in adolescents.

Another observation of the field of Internet-related disorders is that it encompasses a very broad range of activities and functions related to digital online technologies. Many of these activities and devices are rapidly evolving, becoming more structurally complex and socially connected and adopting or evolving new functionalities. They are also often situated within a changing social/cultural context that may normalize certain aspects of their use (e.g., the widespread adoption of digital tablet technology in junior schools). For these reasons, there is a need to carefully delineate between certain types of activities, even within known types or classes of activities (e.g., social media use). In the case of video gaming, for example, it may be necessary to track progression across different types of games (e.g., playing offline role-playing games to playing online massively multiplayer style games). Just as a football player may not refer to him- or herself as a "sportsperson," many video gamers may be more likely to identify themselves as players of specific games (e.g., FIFA, World of Warcraft, or League of Legends) than as simply a "gamer." Recognizing these more micro-level aspects of an activity may lead to accurate and useful longitudinal observations. Specific user/player actions in certain activities (e.g., spending real money in an MMO, having a higher number of followers on a social media site) may be predictive of increasing prioritization of technology use or of developing excessive use of the activity. In short, moving beyond simple classification of activities, such as "gaming," may yield more useful observations of patterns of use.

Knowledge Gaps and Future Directions

A review of the quantitative evidence on the natural history of problematic Internet and gaming has highlighted several potential gaps in knowledge. First, there is a need to better understand the course and stability of problematic gaming behavior. This requires prospective research designs that include more frequent measurement intervals or waves of data collection in order to maximize sensitivity to user changes. The reliance on normal populations (e.g., university samples, online convenience samples) has arguably hindered the investigation of different clinical presentations. For example, based on the qualitative research base, it is possible that some problematic gamer types may be more likely to report specific clusters of symptoms. For example, some gamers may be more likely to lie or act furtively (i.e., those who conceal their gaming from a partner or employer vs. those without partners or other commitments) or experience withdrawal symptoms (i.e., those who experience difficulty in balancing their gaming vs. those who almost exclusively spend their time gaming). Another interesting avenue of research would be to follow individuals who have received treatment for problem gaming to identify differences in those who do or do not return to gaming activities, including problematic levels of use. With respect to adolescent research, it is notable that parental limiting and monitoring of electronic media has only a minimal relationship to the development and maintenance of problematic gaming. Understanding why parental strategies are relatively ineffectual may be a useful line of inquiry given its utility to public health and parenting help forums.

There are many promising avenues for future qualitative research studies. Qualitative studies are particularly important for their role in helping to shape conceptualization and in therefore influencing clinical concepts applied to Internet-related activities. For example, further qualitative work may be influential to the wording and inclusion of criteria for the psychiatric diagnosis of IGD in the DSM-5. Additional promising avenues include the investigation of comorbidity factors in problem Internet users and how these factors directly influence the onset, development, and relapse of problem behavior. Qualitative data may inform basic knowledge of the user relationship to certain technologies (e.g., different types of gaming activities) and how this relationship may be problematic. With respect to the addiction model, there is only a limited understanding of the concepts of withdrawal and tolerance as they relate to gaming and other activities. For example, do problem gamers develop a need to play longer, or more often, or to achieve certain goals or have certain experiences? Another needed qualitative research agenda concerns the experiences of problematic technology users who recovered spontaneously (i.e., without formal treatment) and how these experiences may differ from those engaged in therapy. The phenomenon of "binge" gaming (or other Internet activity) that often occurs in periods of stress or life adjustment for many users may also develop our understanding of the appeal and associated motivations of the activity.

Other important considerations for future research relate to novelty of study scope and design. First, there is a need to include more adults in longitudinal studies of Internet-related disorders, given the overreliance on adolescent samples. In the case of gaming, for example, the average age of video gamers in Australia (and many other regions) is purportedly greater than 30 years (Brand, Borchard, & Holmes, 2009). Therefore, expanding the age range in studies focused on Internet-related problems is likely to ensure greater representativeness of those who experience problems and to develop a better understanding of the user base in general. Additionally, it is likely that older (i.e., adult) users may report different types of problems (e.g., interference with marriage or similar long-term relationship, social isolation, job productivity) and associated risk factors (e.g., low job satisfaction, financial difficulties, physical health complaints, such as injury or chronic pain) as compared to younger samples.

In studies of adolescents, it may be helpful to explore and gather more information related to cognitive and social development. Understanding how symptom profiles differ demographically and by Internet activity may also provide useful clinical insights. Another avenue for future research is to consider nonpathological aspects of digital technology use alongside the study of addictive/harmful behaviors. Unlike many substance-based disorders (e.g., heroin, cocaine, and so on), digital technology use itself is not considered inherently harmful, and many millions of people use the technology on a daily basis without any negative impact. Furthermore, research has shown that many individuals who experience Internet-related problems may do so in a transient way, including those who "recover" without any formal intervention (King, Delfabbro et al., 2013). There is limited understanding of the possible reasons that some people may recover naturally from an Internet-based disorder. Research on protective factors, as well as on healthy or adaptive Internet use, may provide some useful insights while also serving to contextualize research findings related to risks and harms related to Internet use.

Conclusion

Internet use and other related disorders are preliminary conditions in need of further clinical research to validate their proposed set of clinical features and descriptions. This chapter has highlighted some of the important quantitative and qualitative studies that may inform our current understanding of the natural course of Internet-related disorders. The study of such disorders represents a major challenge given the diverse range of available online activities as well as their rapidly changing nature and functionality. There is undoubtedly a need for greater international consistency in how researchers conceptualize such disorders, as well as greater collaborative efforts and funding to more efficiently and productively study these disorders. The emerging knowledge base suggests that there are numerous individuals, representing a diverse range of social background and psychological vulnerabilities, who report long-term problems with Internet us and gaming. This chapter suggests multiple avenues, including new possibilities as well as refinements, to guide further research on such individuals. Ultimately, it is hoped that this may guide the development of appropriate and effective measures to assist individuals whose lives have been negatively affected by problematic gaming habits.

References

Allison, S. E., von Wahlde, L., Shockley, T., & Gabbard, G. O. (2006). The development of the self in the era of the Internet and role-playing fantasy games. *American Journal of Psychiatry, 163*, 381–85.

Brand, J. E., Borchard, J., & Holmes, K. (2009). *Interactive Australia 2009*. Gold Coast, Australia: Bond University Press.

Choo, H., Sim, T., Liau, A. K. F., Gentile, D. A., & Khoo, A. (2015). Parental influences on pathological symptoms of video-gaming among children and adolescents: A prospective study. *Journal of Child and Family Studies, 24*, 1429–41.

Dong, G., Lu, Q., Zhou, H., & Zhao, X. (2011). Precursor or sequela: Pathological disorders in people with Internet addiction disorder. *PLoS ONE, 6*, e14703.

Dong, G., Wang, J., Yang, X., & Zhou, H. (2013). Risk personality traits of Internet addiction: A longitudinal study of Internet-addicted Chinese university students. *Asia-Pacific Psychiatry, 5*, 316–21.

Ferguson, C. J., & Ceranoglu, T. A. (2014). Attention problems and pathological gaming: Resolving the 'chicken and egg' in a prospective analysis. *Psychiatric Quarterly, 85*, 103–10.

Gentile, D. A., Choo, H., Liau, A., Sim, T., Li, D., Fung, D., & Khoo, A. (2011). Pathological video game use among youths: A two-year longitudinal study. *Pediatrics, 127*(2), e319–29.

Griffiths, M. D. (2000). Does Internet and computer "addiction" exist? Some case study evidence. *Cyberpsychology and Behavior, 3*, 211–18.

Griffiths, M. D. (2010). The role of context in online gaming excess and addiction: Some case study evidence. *International Journal of Mental Health and Addiction, 8*, 119–25.

Haagsma, M. C., King, D. L., Pieterse, M. E., & Peters, O. (2013). Assessing problematic video gaming using the theory of planned behavior: A longitudinal study of Dutch young people. *International Journal of Mental Health and Addiction, 11*, 172–85.

King, D. L., & Delfabbro, P. H. (2009). Understanding and assisting excessive players of video games: A community psychology perspective. *Australian Community Psychologist, 21*, 62–74.

King, D. L., & Delfabbro, P. H. (2014). The cognitive psychology of Internet gaming disorder. *Clinical Psychology Review, 34*, 298–308.

King, D. L., Delfabbro, P. H., & Griffiths, M. D. (2013). Trajectories of problem video gaming among adult regular gamers: An 18-month longitudinal study. *Cyberpsychology, Behavior, and Social Networking, 16*, 72–76.

King, D. L., Haagsma, M. C., Delfabbro, P. H., Gradisar, M., & Griffiths, M. D. (2013). Toward a consensus definition of pathological video-gaming: A systematic review of psychometric assessment tools. *Clinical Psychology Review, 33*, 331–42.

Ko, C.-H., Wang, P.-W., Liu, T.-L., Yen, C.-F., Chen, C.-S., & Yen, J.-Y. (2015). Bidirectional associations between family factors and Internet addiction among adolescents in a prospective investigation. *Psychiatry and Clinical Neurosciences, 69*, 192–300.

Ko, C.-H., Yen, J. Y., Yen, C. F., Lin, H. C., & Yang, M. J. (2007). Factors predictive for incidence and remission of Internet addiction in young adolescents: A prospective study. *Cyberpsychology and Behavior, 10*, 545–51.

Lam, L. T. (2014). Risk factors of Internet addiction and the health effect of Internet addiction on adolescents: A systematic review of longitudinal and prospective studies. *Current Psychiatry Reports, 16*, 508.

Lee, E. J. (2011). A case study of Internet Game Addiction. *Journal of Addictions Nursing, 22*, 208–13.

Lemmens, J. S., Valkenburg, P. M., & Peter, J. (2011). Psychosocial causes and consequences of pathological gaming. *Computers in Human Behavior, 27*, 144–52.

Rehbein, F., & Baier, D. (2013). Family-, media-, and school-related risk factors of video game addiction: A 5-year longitudinal study. *Journal of Media Psychology, 25*, 118–28.

Scharkow, M., Festl, R., & Quandt, T. (2014). Longitudinal patterns of problematic computer game use among adolescents and adults: A 2-year panel study. *Addiction, 109*, 1910–17.

Shotton, M. A. (1989). *Computer addiction? A study of computer dependency*. Basingstoke, UK: Taylor and Francis.

Sim, T., Gentile, D. A., Bricolo, F., Serpelloni, G., & Gulamoydeen, F. (2012). A conceptual review of research on the pathological use of computers, video games, and the Internet. *International Journal of Mental Health and Addiction, 10*(5), 748–769.

Sun, P., Johnson, C. A., Palmer, P., Arpawong, T. E., Unger, J. B., Xie, B., . . . Sussman, S. (2012). Concurrent and predictive relationships between compulsive Internet use and substance use: Findings from vocational high school students in China and the USA. *International Journal of Environmental Research and Public Health, 9*, 660–73.

Tsai, C.-C., & Lin, S. S. J. (2003). Internet addiction of adolescents in Taiwan: An interview study. *Cyberpsychology and Behavior, 6*, 649–52.

van den Eijnden, R. J. J. M., Spijkerman, R., Vermulst, A. A., van Rooij, T. J., & Engels, R. C. M. E. (2010). Compulsive Internet use among adolescents: Bidirectional parent-child relationships. *Journal of Abnormal Child Psychology, 38*(1), 77–89.

Yang, S. J., Stewart, R., Lee, J. Y., Kim, J. M., Kim, S. W., Shin, I. S., & Yoon, J. S. (2014). Prevalence and correlates of problematic Internet experiences and computer-using time: A two-year longitudinal study in Korean school children. *Psychiatry Investigation, 11*, 24–31.

Yen, J.-Y., Yen, C.-F., Chen, C.-S., Chang, Y.-H., Yeh, Y.-C., & Ko, C.-H. (2012). The bidirectional interactions between addiction, behaviour approach and behaviour inhibition systems among adolescents in a prospective study. *Psychiatry Research, 200*, 588–92.

Yu, L., & Shek, D. T. L. (2013). Internet addiction in Hong Kong adolescents: A three-year longitudinal study. *Journal of Pediatric and Adolescent Gynecology, 26*, S10–17.

CHAPTER 7

Research Findings and Clinical Perspectives on Asian Media Technology Use, Mental Health Networking, and Other Social Aspects of Technology Use

Past, Present, and Future Considerations

Chih-Hung Ko *and* Ju-Yu Yen

Abstract

Digital technologies are powerful tools for connecting individuals to each other and the world. Although concerns about the effects of mass media in varying forms (e.g., television and movies) on violence have been raised for decades, causal relationships between long-standing and more recently developed technologies and mental health considerations often remain obscure. Furthermore, variations and use of digital technologies and the Internet have expanded rapidly in recent years in Asia areas, as in Western society, and are increasingly impacting peoples' lives. This review covers research on potential positive and negative effects of digital technologies, with an emphasis on Asian children and adolescents. The authors focus on problem Internet use or addiction, risky behaviors, and mental health problems related to excessive use of digital technologies, which appear to have a sizeable impact on children and adolescents, particularly in Asia. They also review how digital technologies may benefit child and adolescent mental health. As scientific knowledge in this field lags far behind the evolution of digital technologies, expansion and advancement in research is essential to address such issues as prevention and the design of effective treatment strategies.

Keywords: media, Asia, communication, violence, addiction, sex, media education

The Evolution of Electronic Media

Today, we live in an environment full of digital technological tools for media, communication, and the exchange of information. In recent decades, media technologies have developed rapidly, consequently changing methods of communication. Information written on paper progressed to analog images displayed on television and was then transformed to three-dimensional images shown on high-definition television. Information could previously be delivered by telephone line or cable. Now, large volumes of information can be delivered with remarkable speed by optic fiber or wirelessly via Wi-Fi or the fourth generation of mobile telecommunications technology (4G). This all but eliminates the limitation of location when receiving information. Previously, we were able to read information in a book, hear a voice on the telephone, or watch a movie in a theater. Now, we can do all of this in real time using a smartphone or mobile tablet. Previously, we interacted with each other face to face or could talk with a person on the telephone. Now, we can interact with many people at the same time through the Internet using a computer, smartphone, or tablet. Previously, we played games when meeting together. Now, we play together using a computer, smartphone, or tablet, even when living in different countries (Nielsen, 2012a). The development of the Internet and smartphones has changed our way of life.

Electronic Media Technological Product Use in Asia

According to Nielsen (2014), media consumption among the young (18–34 years of age) has grown by 4% annually for all groups combined, with varying rates among subgroups, such as 2% among Hispanic individuals, 8% among black individuals, and 10%

among Asian individuals. Hence, rates of increase have been high, especially among Asian groups. The development of digital technologies, particularly smartphones and tablets, has contributed to increased media consumption. Aside from Apple (which had about 40% of the market in 2013), Asian industries such as HTC of Taiwan, LG, Samsung of Korea, and Sony of Japan, share the market worldwide (Nielsen, 2013).

The rapid increase in use among Asian groups is also reflected in the Nielsen Global Online Survey from 2010 (Nielsen, 2012b), which showed individual Asian countries to be among the top three in online and mobile video usage. Furthermore, the percentage of people making purchasing decisions according to social media information is particularly high in Asian countries (Nielsen, 2012b). The shifting of geopolitical and economic power from West to East and from developed to developing countries (Barns, 2014) has allowed individuals to access information, goods, and services within and beyond any sovereign border and resulted in globalization of media technology use. Thus, media technology is as available and popular in Asian areas as in Western societies, and understanding its effects on mental health, particularly in children and adolescents, is a pressing concern.

The Electronic Media and Mental Health

Considerable research indicates that child and adolescent development is significantly shaped by exposure to mass media, social media, and games (Kappos, 2007). These forms of technology have all evolved rapidly in the past two decades. The interactive screen has been introduced into glasses and watches, such as Google Glass and the iWatch. Kappos (2007) claimed that society has performed a vast and uncontrolled experiment on our children, exposing them as infants and toddlers to home environments that are saturated with electronic media. Previous studies have demonstrated a general pattern of childhood peaks in gray matter followed by adolescent declines, functional and structural increases in connectivity and integrative processing, and a change in the balance between limbic/subcortical and frontal lobe functions extending well into young adulthood (Giedd, 2008). This research suggests that the brains of children and adolescents are in a vulnerable stage of development (Scherf, Behrmann, & Dahl, 2012). Thus it is essential to understand the consequences of massive exposure to electronic media in such groups. However, research knowledge lags considerably behind the development of media. Furthermore, intervention to prevent negative consequences cannot wait for the results of definitive and ongoing studies within changing digital environments. Thus, a review of the research performed to date is warranted to provide important insights into the effects of media on children and adolescents and to assist in developing practical interventions.

The Electronic Media and Mental Health in the Past

One of the most important issues concerning the potential impact of media on adolescents' mental health is its influence on violent behavior. Scenes of violence include the portrayal of violence as a normal solution to problems, heroes who inflict pain and injury, callousness toward victims, aggressive attitudes, and taking pleasure in pain or humiliation (Spitzer, 2005). As television is extremely popular and is readily available to adolescents in modern society, the effect of its violent content on adolescent behavior has been investigated across decades (Frydman, 1999). In consideration of such research, the Committee on Education of the American Academy of Pediatrics described possible negative health effects of television viewing on children and adolescents, such as violent aggressive behavior, substance use, sexual activity, obesity, poor body image, and decreased academic performance (Committee on Public Education, 2001). They provided recommendations for television watching, including monitoring and regulating children's exposure to television, promoting media education for children, and initiating legislation and rules to protect children from inappropriate television content.

Video games became extremely popular once they could be played conveniently through televisions in the home. Violent content, such as fighting, punishing others, or killing enemies, is common in video games and may provoke violent thoughts and feelings and physiological arousal, at least in the short term (Anderson & Bushman, 2001). Repeated exposure to violence in games may also contribute to aggressive beliefs, hostility, violent schema, and aggressive behavioral patterns in the long term (Funk, 2005). Therefore, the violent content of games may alter and channel emotional, cognitive, and behavioral tendencies in aggressive directions (Carnagey & Anderson, 2005). As gaming typically involves not only passive viewing but also behavioral decision-making in simulated environments, the mechanisms contributing to violence are likely complex. *Cognitive neo-association theory, social learning theory, social cognition theory, excitation transfer theory,* and *social interaction theory* have all attempted to explain the mechanisms by which media may influence violence (Anderson & Bushman, 2002; Browne & Hamilton-Giachritsis, 2005).

Browne and Hamilton-Giachritsis (2005) used a multifactor approach to characterize the impact of media violence on children and adolescents. Their model incorporates personal effects (e.g., temperament, moral attitudes, and empathy for others), environmental effects (e.g., exposure to violence, culture, and socioeconomic level), and media effects (e.g., the type of media, exposure duration). Based on this multifactorial approach, the *general aggression model*, integrating the preceding theories, claims that a violent media effect is established though interaction between cognitive, affective, and physiological responses to violent media. It then contributes to aggressive decisions and violent behavior (Anderson & Bushman, 2002). Going by this model, the evidence supports the hypotheses that violent video games have an associated aggressive affect, and this may result in physiological arousal, aggressive cognition, and aggressive behavior among children and adolescents (Gentile & Stone, 2005). Furthermore, the effects of violent media content have been demonstrated in both Western and Eastern societies, with no observed differences (Anderson et al., 2010). This outcome suggests that media violence could be a global problem.

However, there is continuing debate regarding such matters as the best methodologies and models to use when studying or characterizing the impact of media on violence, the generalizability of findings from one or another set of studies, and, more broadly, the extent to which media violence affects children and adolescents (Browne & Hamilton-Giachritsis, 2005). Some investigators view studies linking media and violence as inconclusive and causal relationships as open to debate (Ferguson, 2007; Ferguson & Kilburn, 2009). A compelling argument was made for a bidirectional interaction between media violence and aggressive behavior in a previous review (Anderson & Bushman, 2002; Gentile & Stone, 2005). Furthermore, the form of media that delivers the violent content may also contribute to its impact on aggressive behavior (Gentile & Stone, 2005), and, as technology has rapidly developed, the method in which violent content is delivered has changed considerably in recent years. Studies investigating the effects of violent content in newly developed media on behavior should be updated as soon as possible.

The Electronic Media and Mental Health at Present

The Internet has been used in academia since the 1980s, with use becoming increasingly widespread during the 1990s. The commercialization of the international network resulted in its popularization in the 1990s and incorporation into virtually every aspect of modern human life. Currently, more than 2 billion people worldwide are connected to the Internet (Khan et al., 2014). The Internet is one of the most widely accessible media in the world, with characteristics that differ from those of previous media. Furthermore, more and more equipment, such as computers, notebooks, televisions, telephones, tablets, glasses, and watches can be connected to the Internet and are commonly used by children and adolescents.

The new interactive media are characterized by extensive connectivity, personalization, peer-to-peer networking, engagement, immersion, and content creation. These characteristics may create powerful attractions for youth (Montgomery & Chester, 2009). Youth users not only watch content from media, but they also participate in interactive activities. In contrast to playing classic video games, the use of new interactive media usually involves interaction with an object represented by other real people, not by a machine or artificial intelligence. This also provides individuals with the opportunity to make contact with strangers all over the world without age limitations. Owing to freedom in media use, children and adolescents can search for information with very few restrictions. It has become difficult for parents to monitor their children's interactions in these newly interactive media. Last, as youth income or access to funds has increased in recent years, this population has become a valuable target for the commercial market (Montgomery & Chester, 2009). Increasingly more Internet technologies and activities are being designed to attract children and adolescents. Thus, new interactive media technology can have a strong influence, both positive and negative, on individuals' mental health, particularly among adolescents and children.

In the past 10 years, Asian countries have developed rapidly, contributing greatly to global economic development (Barns, 2014). Interactive media through the Internet is well developed and popular in many developing countries in Asia. On the one hand, problems with the use of new media technologies has also been noted and researched in Asia. On the other hand, the new interactive media have also been utilized to improve education, provide services, and deliver preventive interventions in public mental health (Brown & Witherspoon, 2002; O'Keeffe & Clarke-Pearson, 2011). Gaining an understanding of the positive and negative impact of new interactive media on mental health is important in order to enhance the former and reduce the latter.

The Negative Effects of New Interactive Media Technology in Asia

Addiction to New Interactive Media

The Internet has rapidly developed and is widely distributed in Asia and elsewhere. (It provides an information highway without time limitations to more than 90% of youth in Canada [Norris, 2007].) Diminished control over Internet use among adolescents resulting in negative consequence has been termed *Internet addiction* (IA; Young, 1998). In Asia, IA had been researched since 2001 in Taiwan (Bai, Lin, & Chen, 2001; Chou, 2001). Diagnostic criteria for IA have been developed in Taiwan (Ko et al., 2005a; Ko et al., 2009b) and China (Tao et al., 2010) for application in clinical practice and research. The *Diagnostic and Statistical Manual of Mental Disorders* (DSM-5; American Psychiatric Association, 2013) included diagnostic criteria for Internet gaming disorder (IGD) in Section III, the location for possible conditions warranting additional research. These criteria focus on online gaming (American Psychiatric Association, 2013).

The Chen Internet Addiction Scale (Ko et al., 2005b) in Taiwan and Young's Internet Addiction Test (Widyanto & McMurran, 2004) are arguably the most popular scales for assessing the severity and prevalence of IA in Asia. Prevalence rates have been reported to be 15.1% in Turkey (Sasmaz et al., 2014), 0.7% in India (Goel, Subramanyam, & Kamath, 2013), 15.3% in Taiwan (Lin et al., 2011; Tsai et al., 2009), 18% in Hong Kong (Mak et al., 2014), and 10.7% in Korea (Park, Kim, & Cho, 2008) based on epidemiological studies using questionnaires. These results suggest that IA is highly prevalent in Asia, although it should be noted that study outcomes may vary considerably based on the diagnostic criteria and assessment methodology used (Petry, Rehbein, Ko, & O'Brien, 2015).

Owing to the development of Internet technologies, online games allow individuals to engage both socially and competitively with individuals across the globe (Latham, Patston, & Tippett., 2013). Massive multiplayer online role-playing games (MMORPGs) have a high level of complexity and involve an extensive social interaction (Granic, Lobel, & Engels, 2014). MMORPGs provide an electronic virtual setting in which users may immerse themselves in a designed virtual environment and interact with each other or with non-player characters that appear as real as those in the natural world (Yee, 2006). High levels of pleasure may be experienced during online gaming, creating a significant risk among participants for poorly controlled use (van Rooij et al., 2010). Given its potential serious impact on mental health, diminished control over online gaming was termed IGD (American Psychiatric Association, 2013). The validity of the DSM-5 IGD criteria has been evaluated among young adults in Taiwan, with the results supporting the specified cutoff point (Ko et al., 2014a).

IGD was reported to result in adolescent depression, anxiety, social phobias, and poorer academic performance in a prospective study (Gentile et al., 2011). Neurocognitive study has demonstrated impaired inhibition of proactive interference and a positive implicit response to gaming cues among subjects with IGD in Taiwan (Ko et al., 2014b; Yen et al., 2011a). Brain imaging studies have demonstrated impaired risk evaluation (Lin et al., 2014), a potential role for D_2-like dopamine receptors in the striatum (Tian et al., 2014), impaired prefrontal impulse inhibition (Ding et al., 2014), and alterations in functional connectivity and white matter integrity (Ding et al., 2013; Dong, DeVito, Huang, & Du, 2012a; Dong, Huang, & Du, 2012b) among subjects with IGD in China. In a Taiwanese study, cue-induced online gaming craving was found to provoke brain activation paralleling changes found in substance use disorders (Ko et al., 2013a; Ko et al., 2013b) and to impair brain inhibitory functions. These Asian studies all indicated that cognitive function is impaired among subjects with IGD in a manner resembling those with substance use disorders. However, the cross-sectional design of these studies could not confirm whether the brain alterations contribute to or result from IGD. In contrast, other research also suggests that gaming may improve certain cognitive functions, such as spatial skills (Granic et al., 2014). Thus, how or whether addiction to online gaming may alter brain development merits further study.

Aside from online gaming, addictions to cybersex (Lam, 2014), social media such as Facebook (Hormes, Kearns, & Timko, 2014), shopping (Duroy, Gorse, & Lejoyeux, 2014), and gambling (Gainsbury, Suhonen, & Saastamoinen, 2014) have been noted in recent years. However, evidence and research are limited. Some studies on these topics have been performed in Asia (Duroy et al., 2014; Shin et al., 2014; Wong & So, 2014). As these behaviors are addictive, demonstration of the role of the Internet or interactive media in the mechanism of these addictive behaviors is necessary before identifying these behaviors as media-associated. Furthermore, smartphone addiction has also been evaluated in Asia (Takao, 2014; Wang et al., 2014; Yen et al., 2009). Although definitions of these behaviors are not well developed, their presentations appear similar. Defining these addictive behaviors according to the equipment (e.g., phone, pad, or tablet), the technology (e.g., the Internet), or the activity (e.g., gaming or sexual behavior) is still under debate. Studies have also indicated that the interactions between media technology and people are complex, and more comprehensive theories are necessary to understand them.

Media Technology Use and Mental Health Problems

Technology usage may improve skills and generate social benefits, but there is also the potential for harm, as may be observed with sexting, cyberbullying, privacy violations, and IA, all of which may affect health (O'Keeffe, 2012). Asian research has focused considerable attention on co-occurring conditions associated with IA (Ko, Yen, Yen, Chen, & Chen, 2012). Possible relationships have been uncovered between heavy Internet use and mental health problems. A variety of Asian studies have demonstrated associations between IA and depression, social anxiety, and attention deficit hyperactivity disorder (ADHD) (Ha et al., 2007; Sasmaz et al., 2014; Yen et al., 2008). As ADHD typically develops early in childhood, the association suggests that adolescents with ADHD are vulnerable to developing IA, as per the results of a prospective study (Ko, Yen, Chen, Yeh, & Yen, 2009a).

Although an association between IA and depressive disorder was demonstrated in an interview study (Ko, Yen, Chen, Chen, & Yen, 2008), a causal relationship could not be investigated in the cross-sectional study. Prospective research has demonstrated that depression and anxiety predict IA in adolescents (Cho, Sung, Shin, Lim, & Shin, 2013; Ko et al., 2009a). Two prospective studies demonstrated that level of depression increased when adolescents became addicted to the Internet or online gaming (Gentile et al., 2011; Ko et al., 2009a). These results could suggest that heavy Internet use or online gaming contributes to mental health problems in adolescents. However, given the methodological limitations of these studies, it is difficult to confirm whether depression emerges before or after the onset of IA. Again, it might be reasonable to conclude that a bidirectional interaction exists between mental health problems and heavy Internet or online gaming use.

In contrast to the body of literature showing an association between IA and various psychiatric symptoms or disorders (Ko et al., 2006; Ko et al., 2012; Lin, Ko, & Wu, 2011; Tsai et al., 2009), research suggesting that Internet use may increase capacities to cope with stress or mental health problems has also been reported. For example, subjects with social anxiety have been found to exhibit decreased anxiety after going online (Yen et al., 2012). This could be a method of finding support from the Internet to cope with stress or mood problems in the short term (Deatherage, Servaty-Seib, & Aksoz, 2014). However, whether persistent heavy Internet use truly benefits long-term well-being has not been investigated in depth. The comorbidity of IA suggests that comorbid psychiatric disorders should be evaluated when treating subjects with IA. However, as social support may be gained from using Internet interactive media (Wang & Wang, 2013), comorbid psychiatric disorders, such as depression, may require treatment prior to aggressive intervention to decrease Internet use.

Associations Between Internet Use and Risky Behavior

Another important issue is the association between Internet use and risky behavior, such as substance exposure, sexual behaviors, and aggressive behaviors. IA has been reported to be associated with substance exposure and substance use disorders (Ko et al., 2006; Sung, Lee, Noh, Park, & Ahn, 2013; Yen et al., 2008). Furthermore, Internet advertising is a new way to promote the marketing of substances such as tobacco (Hrywna, Delnevo, & Lewis, 2007). Asian individuals have been found to be more likely to make purchasing decisions according to information obtained from interactive media versus other sources (Nielsen, 2012b). Whether advertising of alcohol, cigarettes, or illicit substances on the Internet is more available than advertising in the real world and contributes to risks of substance use in children and adolescents should be evaluated in Asia and other areas of the world.

Research into sexual behavior online is relatively limited and addresses both potential negative and positive influences. For example, adolescents may be exposed to Internet pornography and may form relationships with strangers online that can pose serious threats to their welfare (Tseng, Wang, Wang, & Chou, 2012). The Internet was also found to be associated with sexual intercourse among adolescents (Kim, 2012; Sung et al., 2013). In contrast, the Internet can be an unmatched communications platform for sex-related information and education (Tseng et al., 2012). It can be argued that digital media have become the leading sex educator for children and teenagers, as sexual education may be inadequate in many countries (Strasburger, 2012). Websites have been used to provide sexual education in Australia (Mak, Bastian, Grace, Aquilina, & Sweeting, 2012). However, given current gaps in the scientific knowledge base, more research is necessary to gain an understanding of the effects of Internet use, particularly social interactive media, on children's and adolescents' sexual health.

IA has been reported to be associated with hostility (Yen, Ko, Yen, Wu, & Yang, 2007) and aggressive behaviors (Ko, Yen, Liu, Huang, & Yen, 2009c) in Taiwan and Iran (Khoshakhlagh & Faramarzi, 2012). However, one study demonstrated that only subjects with IA exhibited increased hostility after going online and that others instead exhibited decreased hostility (Yen, Yen, Wu, Huang, & Ko, 2011b). On the other hand, hostility may increase when adolescents become addicted to the Internet and decrease when they remit (Ko et al., 2014c). This situation suggests that personal factors may contribute to the effects of Internet use on aggressive behaviors, as per the general model theory. Furthermore, IA has been reported to be associated with self-injurious behaviors (Lam, Peng, Mai, & Jing, 2009), including suicide (Lin et al., 2014). As aggressive behavior toward others or oneself, such as suicide pacts, are highly risky, more research is needed to better understand the role of interactive media in these kinds of behavior.

Aside from aggressive behavior toward oneself or others, exposure to aggressive experiences online is another important mental health issue. Cyberbullying involves hurting someone else by using information and communication technologies (Nixon, 2014), and it can be a serious mental health event for adolescents (Donnerstein, 2012). Victims of cyberbullying have been reported to exhibit increased depression, anxiety, loneliness, suicidal behavior, and somatic symptoms (Nixon, 2014). Cyberbullying was found to be associated with child death based on secondary order data analysis (Fu, Chan, & Ip, 2014).

In comparison to traditional bullying, cyberbullying reaches a virtually unlimited audience, with fewer limitations on space and time. It may also be more difficult to supervise and prevent. Perpetrators of cyberbullying do not see the faces of their targets and subsequently may not understand the full consequences of their actions, thereby decreasing important feelings of personal accountability. This has been referred to as the *online disinhibition effect* (Suler, 2004). Aside from the effects of media technologies, environmental factors (e.g., school environments) and personal factors (e.g., body image) may also contribute to the risk of cyberbullying (Landstedt & Persson, 2014). Heavy online gaming has also been reported to be associated with cyberbullying (Lam, Cheng, & Liu, 2013).

Cyberbullying and/or cybervictimization has been reported to be associated with risky Internet behavior, depression, anxiety, loneliness, and poor mental health in Taiwan (Chang et al., 2013; Yen et al., 2014) and Korea (Choi et al., 2014; Stewart, Drescher, Maack, Ebesutani, & Young, 2014). These studies in Asia also support the negative consequences of cyberbullying. A cross-culture study demonstrated that East Asian adolescents were less likely to engage in cyberbullying than European-descent participants. In addition, East Asian adolescents were more likely to be motivated to engage in cyberaggression for proactive reasons than reactive reasons, particularly among males (Shapka & Law, 2013). Considering the potentially significant harmful impact that cyberbullying may have on children's and adolescents' mental health, the emergence of such aggressive behavior deserves considerable further study and intervention in Asia and elsewhere.

Using Media Technology to Promote Mental Health or Treat Psychiatric Disorders

To maintain a balanced perspective, it is important to consider potential benefits of interactive media, such as allowing children and adolescents to stay connected with friends and family, which may contribute to their socialization. Furthermore, the Internet may enhance learning opportunities by creating unprecedented access to information and providing opportunities to ask questions and exchange information with peers (O'Keeffe & Clarke-Pearson, 2011). Through the Internet, newly developing media may provide interactive platforms to promote valuable educational and interventional programs for children and adolescents. Children and adolescents may access health information, such as mental health resources or sexual education, via the Internet (O'Keeffe & Clarke-Pearson, 2011). Thus, interactive social media may benefit mental health when used constructively.

Research indicates that using the Internet to communicate with friends and family is associated with a decline in depression (Bessiere, Pressman, Kiesler, & Kraut, 2010). Social online interaction has been found to provide support to individuals with mental health problems in Taiwan (Hou & Lu, 2013; Wang & Wang, 2013) and Korea (Oh & Lee, 2012). The Internet has also been utilized to survey psychological disorders in Korea (Son, Song, Kim, & Paick, 2010), Japan, and Taiwan (Aritake et al., 2015; Wei, Chen, Huang, & Bai, 2012). Furthermore, educational efforts utilizing online media have been implemented to reduce the stigma associated with mental health in Korea (Seo & Kim, 2010). Cognitive-behavioral psychotherapy for psychiatric disorders has been delivered via the Internet in Australia (Dear et al., 2013) and China (Choi et al., 2012). However, the real-world interactions normally associated with these programs were not present. In addition, digital media may be used to target other activities that have negative effects: on children and adolescents, such as inappropriate sexual behavior; on society, such as crimes or suicides; or worldwide, such as terrorism. Whether these educational programs, resources, and interventions delivered through new interactive media really benefit children and adolescents more than traditional media, and the balance between positive and negative influences, deserves further evaluation.

The Electronic Media and Mental Health in the Future

By 2020, 50 billion devices are expected to be connected to the Internet (Khan et al., 2014). Media technology will be an essential part of daily life for most people. Provision of healthy ways to use these new interactive media technologies is more practical than preventing people from exposure to these technologies. Based on the preceding review, the negative mental health consequences associated with media technology may include (1) poor control over use, resulting in negative consequences; (2) exposure to risky situations or materials, such as violent content or inappropriate sexual content; (3) inappropriate advertising of substances or illegal materials; and (4) inappropriate interaction through media, such cyberbullying, unselected cybersex, privacy violations, online illegal or problematic gambling, or suicide pacts. Considerable additional research is needed on the nature of these behaviors and development of adequate and practical education, preventive strategies, and intervention programs. Furthermore, how to control use, prevent risky content, and limit risky behavior are essential issues to address in media education programs provided to users, teachers, and parents.

Media Education

The most practical and essential means to promote the benefits of media and prevent negative consequences is media education. The ministry of education in Taiwan has provided systemic media education for teachers, parents, children, and adolescents (https://eteacher.edu.tw/). The website addresses IA, cyberbullying, online friendships, "netiquette," online safety, online gaming, and legal problems online. A teacher version, parental version, and student version are provided. Basic rules related to Internet use by children and adolescents are outlined; for example, computers should be in the living room or a study area and not in children's and adolescents' bedrooms.

However, the evolution of media technology is so rapid it is extremely challenging to keep pace, particularly in Asia. Media education programs should be updated as soon as possible. How to regulate media use in a reasonable way is extremely important for parents. For example, 13 years is a common minimum age for using social media (O'Keeffe & Clarke-Pearson, 2011). However, many parents provide a tablet and smartphone to children for learning or playing. Given the convenience and scope of new interactive media, it could be used as an available tool to educate or inspire children. However, the nearly unlimited information that may be accessed and the various activities users may undertake may harm children, adolescents, and some adults. More research is needed to investigate both the benefits and negative consequences of media technology and associated factors. It is also necessary to develop reasonable regulatory guides and policies to balance risks and benefits for younger users.

Research on Mental Health Problems *Related to Media Technology Use in the Future*

POOR CONTROL OVER USE: POTENTIAL NEGATIVE CONSEQUENCES

As many media technologies have arguably become essential to daily life, duration of use, by itself, does not equate with problem use. Rather, repeated evidence of poor control over use, which in turn results in significant negative consequences, arguably serves as a key identifier of problematic media technology use. Although IGD is a primary focus of IA at present, the activities to which one may become addicted vary across these new and different media technologies. The development of Internet technologies (e.g., 4G, 3D simulation, or artificial intelligence) may contribute to reward experiences for Internet users in differing ways. Tablets, watches, glasses, or various smartphones may provide various ways in which to develop an addiction. Aside from research into individual media, gaining an understanding of the unique and shared nature of these methods that may contribute to an addictive potential is also important.

The smartphone is popular worldwide and useful in daily life. Furthermore, 64% of mobile phone time is used on applications (Nielsen, 2012a). It is not only a communication tool, but also a multiple-function media. Because it is a new form of media equipment, research specific to its excessive use, benefits, or negative consequences is relatively limited. Research focusing on its positive and negative effects on mental health and the possible mechanism of poorly controlled use is necessary to develop guidelines for healthy patterns of use.

Finally, as more children and adolescents are exposed to these media technologies at earlier ages, it is also important to understand whether or the extent to which excessive exposure and massive interaction with these technologies may alter brain development. Furthermore, for some who are addicted to media technologies, such as various individuals with IGD, real-life experiences may be replaced in substantial or large part by media. The potential impact on this alteration on brain development should also be studied. How to effectively promote healthy activities in the real world, such as exercise, travel, or summer camps for children and adolescents, could well be an important area to pursue for preventing excessive media technology use.

The Effect of Media on Aggressive Behavior

According to the preceding reviews (Browne & Hamilton-Giachritsis, 2005; Escobar-Chaves & Anderson, 2008; Ferguson, 2007), exposure to violent content in the real world or in the media may increase the risk of aggressive behaviors. More research is necessary to understand whether and how new media technology may contribute to aggressive behavior. The characteristics of these media technologies, such as 3D simulation, real-time interaction, and active participation, differ from traditional media and should be evaluated in future research. Furthermore, personal factors, such as hostility cognition or impulsivity, should be considered when interpreting the potential impact of media on aggressive behavior.

In addition, aggressive behavior online, particularly cyberbullying, is another important issue related to media violence. Gaining a better understanding of the needs and motivations that may lead individuals to bully others via the Internet or other media could provide insights that help prevent risky behavior online. The development of media technology to prevent this kind of aggressive behavior and to provide resources to victims is also needed.

The Association Between Media Technology Use and Mental Health

As noted, research suggests that the association between mental health problems and excessive media is often bidirectional (Ko et al., 2012, 2014c, 2014d). Furthermore, both positive and negative effects of media use have been documented and postulated (Pantic, 2014). Moreover, levels and types of negative consequences from excessive online gaming will likely vary in relation to the individual characteristics of users. The factors that contribute to the bidirectional effect should be evaluated in the future. The media has also become a popular method by which to deliver educational or informational content, particularly health information (Fahy, Hardikar, Fox, & Mackay, 2014). Aside from understanding the negative effects of media use, professionals should also understand the benefits of using media to deliver information, educational programs, or interventions to individuals. Systematic reviews that clarify and describe how best to use newly developed media to provide better mental health information or services could promote the benefits of media to public health.

Conclusion

Previous studies on media violence have suggested a bidirectional effect between media violent content and individual aggressive behavior. The associations between excessive media technology use, such as online gaming, and mental health problems are significant not only in Asia, but also in Western societies. The impact of media technology on mental health is thus a global problem. However, media technology also provides adolescents and children with new ways to explore the world. Information, education, and interventions may be delivered through this method. The positive or negative effects of new media technologies may depend on the content delivered and the methods of use. An updated media education program should be developed as soon as possible to provide healthy and constructive ways to use new media. Ongoing research is also needed to address newly emerging problems, such as cybersex addiction, cyberbullying, and smartphone addiction.

References

American Psychiatric Association. (2013). *Diagnostic and statistical manual of mental disorders* (5th ed.). Washington, DC: Author.

Anderson, C. A., & Bushman, B. J. (2001). Effects of violent video games on aggressive behavior, aggressive cognition, aggressive affect, physiological arousal, and prosocial behavior: A meta-analytic review of the scientific literature. *Psychological Science, 12*(5), 353–59.

Anderson, C. A., & Bushman, B. J. (2002). Human aggression. *Annual Review of Psychology, 53*, 27–51.

Anderson, C. A., Shibuya, A., Ihori, N., Swing, E. L., Bushman, B. J., Sakamoto, A., . . . Saleem, M. (2010). Violent video game effects on aggression, empathy, and prosocial behavior in eastern and western countries: A meta-analytic review. *Psychological Bulletin, 136*(2), 151–73.

Aritake, S., Asaoka, S., Kagimura, T., Shimura, A., Futenma, K., Komada, Y., Yuichi, I. (2015). Internet-based survey of factors associated with subjective feeling of insomnia, depression, and low health-related quality of life among Japanese adults with sleep difficulty. *International Journal of Behavioral Medicine, 22*(2), 233-8.

Bai, Y. M., Lin, C. C., & Chen, J. Y. (2001). Internet addiction disorder among clients of a virtual clinic. *Psychiatric Services, 52*(10), 1397.

Barns, M. (2014). Uncommon sense: Global trends that will affect us all. http://www.nielsen.com/us/en/insights/news/2014/uncommon-sense-global-trends-that-will-affect-us-all.html

Bessiere, K., Pressman, S., Kiesler, S., & Kraut, R. (2010). Effects of internet use on health and depression: A longitudinal study. *Journal of Medical Internet Research, 12*(1), e6.

Brown, J. D., & Witherspoon, E. M. (2002). The mass media and American adolescents' health. *The Journal of Adolescent Health, 31*(6 Suppl), 153–70.

Browne, K. D., & Hamilton-Giachritsis, C. (2005). The influence of violent media on children and adolescents: A public-health approach. *Lancet, 365*(9460), 702–10.

Carnagey, N. L., & Anderson, C. A. (2005). The effects of reward and punishment in violent video games on aggressive affect, cognition, and behavior. *Psychological Science, 16*(11), 882–89.

Chang, F. C., Lee, C. M., Chiu, C. H., Hsi, W. Y., Huang, T. F., & Pan, Y. C. (2013). Relationships among cyberbullying, school bullying, and mental health in Taiwanese adolescents. *The Journal of School Health, 83*(6), 454–62.

Cho, S. M., Sung, M. J., Shin, K. M., Lim, K. Y., & Shin, Y. M. (2013). Does psychopathology in childhood predict internet addiction in male adolescents? *Child Psychiatry and Human Development, 44*(4), 549–55.

Choi, I., Zou, J., Titov, N., Dear, B. F., Li, S., Johnston, L., . . . Hunt, C. (2012). Culturally attuned Internet treatment for depression amongst Chinese Australians: A randomised controlled trial. *Journal of Affective Disorders, 136*(3), 459–68.

Choi, J. S., Park, S. M., Roh, M. S., Lee, J. Y., Park, C. B., Hwang, J. Y., Jung, H. Y. (2014). Dysfunctional inhibitory control and impulsivity in Internet addiction. *Psychiatry Research, 215*(2), 424–28.

Chou, C. (2001). Internet heavy use and addiction among Taiwanese college students: An online interview study. *Cyberpsychology and Behavior, 4*(5), 573–85.

Committee on Public Education. (2001). Children, adolescents, and television. *Pediatrics, 107*(2), 423–26.

Dear, B. F., Zou, J., Titov, N., Lorian, C., Johnston, L., Spence, J., . . . Knight, R. G. (2013). Internet-delivered cognitive behavioural therapy for depression: A feasibility open trial for older adults. *The Australian and New Zealand Journal of Psychiatry, 47*(2), 169–76.

Deatherage, S., Servaty-Seib, H. L., & Aksoz, I. (2014). Stress, coping, and internet use of college students. *Journal of American College Health, 62*(1), 40–46.

Ding, W. N., Sun, J. H., Sun, Y. W., Chen, X., Zhou, Y., Zhuang, Z. G., et al. (2014). Trait impulsivity and impaired prefrontal impulse inhibition function in adolescents with internet gaming addiction revealed by a Go/No-Go fMRI study. *Behavioral and Brain Functions* 10: 20.

Ding, W. N., Sun, J. H., Sun, Y. W., Zhou, Y., Li, L., Xu, J. R., . . . Du, Y. S. (2013). Altered default network resting-state functional connectivity in adolescents with Internet gaming addiction. *PLoS One, 8*(3), e59902.

Dong, G., DeVito, E., Huang, J., & Du, X. (2012a). Diffusion tensor imaging reveals thalamus and posterior cingulate cortex abnormalities in internet gaming addicts. *Journal of Psychiatric Research, 46*(9), 1212–16.

Dong, G., Huang, J., & Du, X. (2012b). Alterations in regional homogeneity of resting-state brain activity in internet gaming addicts. *Behavioral and Brain Functions, 8*, 41.

Donnerstein, E. (2012). Internet bullying. *Pediatric Clinics of North America, 59*(3), 623–33.

Duroy, D., Gorse, P., & Lejoyeux, M. (2014). Characteristics of online compulsive buying in Parisian students. *Addictive Behaviors, 39*(12), 1827–30.

Escobar-Chaves, S. L., & Anderson, C. A. (2008). Media and risky behaviors. *The Future of Children, 18*(1), 147–80.

Fahy, E., Hardikar, R., Fox, A., & Mackay, S. (2014). Quality of patient health information on the Internet: Reviewing a complex and evolving landscape. *The Australasian Medical Journal, 7*(1), 24–28.

Ferguson, C. J. (2007). The good, the bad and the ugly: A meta-analytic review of positive and negative effects of violent video games. *The Psychiatric Quarterly, 78*(4), 309–16.

Ferguson, C. J., & Kilburn, J. (2009). The public health risks of media violence: A meta-analytic review. *The Journal of Pediatrics, 154*(5), 759–63.

Frydman, M. (1999). Television, aggressiveness and violence. *International Journal of Adolescent Medicine and Health, 11*(3–4), 335–344.

Fu, K. W., Chan, C. H., & Ip, P. (2014). Exploring the relationship between cyberbullying and unnatural child death: An ecological study of twenty-four European countries. *BMC Pediatrics, 14*(1), 195.

Funk, J. B. (2005). Children's exposure to violent video games and desensitization to violence. *Child and Adolescent Psychiatric Clinics of North America, 14*(3), 387–404.

Gainsbury, S. M., Suhonen, N., & Saastamoinen, J. (2014). Chasing losses in online poker and casino games: Characteristics and game play of Internet gamblers at risk of disordered gambling. *Psychiatry Research, 217*(3), 220–25.

Gentile, D. A., Choo, H., Liau, A., Sim, T., Li, D., Fung, D., & Khoo, A. (2011). Pathological video game use among youths: A two-year longitudinal study. *Pediatrics, 127*(2), e319–29.

Gentile, D. A., & Stone, W. (2005). Violent video game effects on children and adolescents. A review of the literature. *Minerva Pediatrica, 57*(6), 337–58.

Giedd, J. N. (2008). The teen brain: Insights from neuroimaging. *The Journal of Adolescent Health, 42*(4), 335–43.

Goel, D., Subramanyam, A., & Kamath, R. (2013). A study on the prevalence of internet addiction and its association with psychopathology in Indian adolescents. *Indian Journal of Psychiatry, 55*(2), 140–43.

Granic, I., Lobel, A., & Engels, R. C. (2014). The benefits of playing video games. *The American Psychologist, 69*(1), 66–78.

Ha, J. H., Kim, S. Y., Bae, S. C., Bae, S., Kim, H., Sim, M., . . . Cho, S. C. (2007). Depression and Internet addiction in adolescents. *Psychopathology, 40*(6), 424–30.

Hormes, J. M., Kearns, B., & Timko, C. A. (2014). Craving Facebook? Behavioral addiction to online social networking and its association with emotion regulation deficits. *Addiction, 109*(12), 2079–88.

Hou, C. N., & Lu, H. Y. (2013). Online networks as a venue for social support: A qualitative study of married bisexual men in Taiwan. *Journal of Homosexuality, 60*(9), 1280–96.

Hrywna, M., Delnevo, C. D., & Lewis, M. J. (2007). Adult recall of tobacco advertising on the Internet. *Nicotine and Tobacco Research, 9*(11), 1103–107.

Kappos, A. D. (2007). The impact of electronic media on mental and somatic children's health. *International Journal of Hygiene and Environmental Health, 210*(1), 555–62.

Khan, N., Yaqoob, I., Hashem, I. A., Inayat, Z., Mahmoud Ali, W. K., Alam, M., . . . Gani, A. (2014). Big data: Survey, technologies, opportunities, and challenges. *The Scientific World Journal, 2014*, 712826.

Khoshakhlagh, H., & Faramarzi, S. (2012). The relationship of emotional intelligence and mental disorders with internet addiction in internet users university students. *Addiction and Health, 4*(3–4), 133–41.

Kim, J. Y. (2012). The nonlinear association between Internet using time for non-educational purposes and adolescent health. *Journal of Preventive Medicine and Public Health, 45*(1), 37–46.

Ko, C. H., Liu, G. C., Yen, J. Y., Chen, C. Y., Yen, C. F., & Chen, C. S. (2013a). Brain correlates of craving for online gaming under cue exposure in subjects with Internet gaming addiction and in remitted subjects. *Addiction Biology, 18*(3), 559–69.

Ko, C. H., Liu, G. C., Yen, J. Y., Yen, C. F., Chen, C. S., & Lin, W. C. (2013b). The brain activations for both cue-induced gaming urge and smoking craving among subjects comorbid with Internet gaming addiction and nicotine dependence. *Journal of Psychiatric Research, 47*(4), 486–93.

Ko, C. H., Liu, T. L., Wang, P. W., Chen, C. S., Yen, C. F., & Yen, J. Y. (2014c). The exacerbation of depression, hostility, and social anxiety in the course of Internet addiction among adolescents: A prospective study. *Comprehensive Psychiatry, 55*(6), 1377–84.

Ko, C. H., Wang, P. W., Liu, T. L., Yen, C. F., Chen, C. S., & Yen, J. Y. (2014d). Bidirectional associations between family factors and Internet addiction among adolescents in a prospective investigation. *Psychiatry and Clinical Neurosciences, 69*(4), 192–200.

Ko, C. H., Wang, P. W., Liu, T. L., Yen, C. F., Chen, C. S., & Yen, J. Y. (2014b). The inhibition of proactive interference among adults with Internet gaming disorder. *Asia-Pacific Psychiatry, 7*(2), 143–52.

Ko, C. H., Yen, J. Y., Chen, C. C., Chen, S. H., Wu, K., & Yen, C. F. (2006). Tridimensional personality of adolescents with internet addiction and substance use experience. *Canadian Journal of Psychiatry, 51*(14), 887–94.

Ko, C. H., Yen, J. Y., Chen, C. C., Chen, S. H., & Yen, C. F. (2005a). Proposed diagnostic criteria of Internet addiction for adolescents. *The Journal of Nervous and Mental Disease, 193*(11), 728–33.

Ko, C. H., Yen, J. Y., Chen, C. S., Chen, C. C., & Yen, C. F. (2008). Psychiatric comorbidity of internet addiction in college students: An interview study. *CNS Spectrums, 13*(2), 147–53.

Ko, C. H., Yen, J. Y., Chen, C. S., Yeh, Y. C., & Yen, C. F. (2009a). Predictive values of psychiatric symptoms for internet addiction in adolescents: A 2-year prospective study. *Archives of Pediatrics and Adolescent Medicine, 163*(10), 937–43.

Ko, C. H., Yen, J. Y., Chen, S. H., Wang, P. W., Chen, C. S., & Yen, C. F. (2014a). Evaluation of the diagnostic criteria of Internet gaming disorder in the DSM-5 among young adults in Taiwan. *Journal of Psychiatric Research, 53*: 103–10.

Ko, C. H., Yen, J. Y., Chen, S. H., Yang, M. J., Lin, H. C., & Yen, C. F. (2009b). Proposed diagnostic criteria and the screening and diagnosing tool of Internet addiction in college students. *Comprehensive Psychiatry, 50*(4), 378–84.

Ko, C. H., Yen, J. Y., Liu, S. C., Huang, C. F., & Yen, C. F. (2009c). The associations between aggressive behaviors and internet addiction and online activities in adolescents. *The Journal of Adolescent Health, 44*(6), 598–605.

Ko, C. H., Yen, J. Y., Yen, C. F., Chen, C. C., Yen, C. N., & Chen, S. H. (2005b). Screening for Internet addiction: An empirical study on cut-off points for the Chen Internet Addiction Scale. *The Kaohsiung Journal of Medical Science, 21*(12), 545–51.

Ko, C. H., Yen, J. Y., Yen, C. F., Chen, C. S., & Chen, C. C. (2012). The association between Internet addiction and psychiatric disorder: A review of the literature. *European Psychiatry, 27*(1), 1–8.

Lam, L. T. (2014). Internet gaming addiction, problematic use of the internet, and sleep problems: A systematic review. *Current Psychiatry Reports, 16*(4), 444.

Lam, L. T., Cheng, Z., & Liu, X. (2013). Violent online games exposure and cyberbullying/victimization among adolescents. *Cyberpsychology, Behavior and Social Networking, 16*(3), 159–65.

Lam, L. T., Peng, Z., Mai, J., & Jing, J. (2009). The association between internet addiction and self-injurious behaviour among adolescents. *Injury Prevention, 15*(6), 403–408.

Landstedt, E., & Persson, S. (2014). Bullying, cyberbullying, and mental health in young people. *Scandinavian Journal of Public Health, 42*(4), 393–99.

Latham, A. J., Patston, L. L., & Tippett, L. J. (2013). The virtual brain: 30 years of video-game play and cognitive abilities. *Frontiers in Psychology, 4*: 629.

Lin, I. H., Ko, C. H., Chang, Y. P., Liu, T. L., Wang, P. W., Lin, H. C., . . . Yen, C. F. (2014). The association between suicidality and Internet addiction and activities in Taiwanese adolescents. *Comprehensive Psychiatry, 55*(3), 504–10.

Lin, M. P., Ko, H. C., & Wu, J. Y. (2011). Prevalence and psychosocial risk factors associated with internet addiction in a nationally representative sample of college students in Taiwan. *Cyberpsychology, Behavior and Social Networking, 14*(12), 741–46.

Mak, D. B., Bastian, L., Grace, J., Aquilina, H., & Sweeting, J. (2012). Evaluation of a sexual health and blood-borne virus health education website for youth. *Health Promotion Journal of Australia,* 23(3), 194–200.

Mak, K. K., Lai, C. M., Ko, C. H., Chou, C., Kim, D. I., Watanabe, H., & Ho, R. C. M. (2014). Psychometric properties of the revised Chen Internet Addiction Scale (CIAS-R) in Chinese adolescents. *Journal of Abnormal Child Psychology, 42*(7), 1237–45.

Montgomery, K. C., & Chester, J. (2009). Interactive food and beverage marketing: Targeting adolescents in the digital age. *Journal of Adolescent Health, 45*(3 Suppl), S18–29.

Nielsen. (2012a). The digital revolution: A look through the marketer's lens. http://www.slideshare.net/emeguedes/the-digital-revolution-a-look-throu-gh-the-marketers-lens

Nielsen. (2012b). Turing digital: The Asian media landscape. http://www.nielsen.com/us/en/insights/reports/2012/turning-digital—the-asian-media-landscape.html

Nielsen. (2013). Who's winning the US smartphone market? http://www.nielsen.com/us/en/insights/news/2013/whos-winning-the-u-s-smartphone-market-.html

Nielsen. (2014). The digital consumer. http://www.nielsen.com/content/dam/corporate/us/en/reports-downloads/2014%20 Reports/the-digital-consumer-report-feb-2014.pdf

Nixon, C. L. (2014). Current perspectives: The impact of cyberbullying on adolescent health. *Adolescent Health, Medicine and Therapeutics, 5,* 143–58.

Norris, M. L. (2007). HEADSS up: Adolescents and the Internet. *Pediatrics & Child Health, 12,* 211–16.

Oh, H. J., & Lee, B. (2012). The effect of computer-mediated social support in online communities on patient empowerment and doctor-patient communication. *Health Communication, 27*(1), 30–41.

O'Keeffe, G. S. (2012). Overview: New media. *Pediatric Clinics of North America, 59*(3), 589–600.

O'Keeffe, G. S., & Clarke-Pearson, K. (2011). The impact of social media on children, adolescents, and families. *Pediatrics, 127*(4), 800–804.

Pantic, I. (2014). Online social networking and mental health. *Cyberpsychology, Behavior and Social Networking, 17*(10), 652–57.

Park, S. K., Kim, J. Y., & Cho, C. B. (2008). Prevalence of Internet addiction and correlations with family factors among South Korean adolescents. *Adolescence, 43*(172), 895–909.

Petry, N. M., Rehbein, F., Ko, C. H., & O'Brien, C. P. (2015). Internet gaming disorder in the DSM-5. *Current Psychiatry Reports, 17*(9), 72.

Sasmaz, T., Oner, S., Kurt, A. O., Yapici, G., Yazici, A. E., Bugdayci, R., & Şiş, M. (2014). Prevalence and risk factors of Internet addiction in high school students. *European Journal of Public Health, 24*(1), 15–20.

Scherf, K. S., Behrmann, M., & Dahl, R. E. (2012). Facing changes and changing faces in adolescence: A new model for investigating adolescent-specific interactions between pubertal, brain and behavioral development. *Developmental Cognitive Neuroscience, 2*(2), 199–219.

Seo, M., & Kim, H. L. (2010). Effectiveness of an education program to reduce negative attitudes toward persons with mental illness using online media. *Asian Nursing Research, 4*(2), 90–101.

Shapka, J. D., & Law, D. M. (2013). Does one size fit all? Ethnic differences in parenting behaviors and motivations for adolescent engagement in cyberbullying. *Journal of Youth and Adolescence, 42*(5), 723–38.

Shin, Y. C., Choi, S. W., Ha, J., Mok, J. Y., Lim, S. W., Choi, J. S., & Kim, D. J. (2014). Age of pathological gambling onset: Clinical and treatment-related features. *Journal of Addiction Medicine, 8*(3), 205–10.

Son, H., Song, S. H., Kim, S. W., & Paick, J. S. (2010). Self-reported premature ejaculation prevalence and characteristics in Korean young males: Community-based data from an internet survey. *Journal of Andrology, 31*(6), 540–46.

Spitzer, M. (2005). Influence of violent media on children and adolescents. *Lancet, 365*(9468), 1387–88.

Stewart, R. W., Drescher, C. F., Maack, D. J., Ebesutani, C., & Young, J. (2014). The development and psychometric investigation of the Cyberbullying Scale. *Journal of Interpersonal Violence, 29*(12), 2218–38.

Strasburger, V. C. (2012). Adolescents, sex, and the media. *Adolescent Medicine: State of the Art Reviews, 23*(1), 15–33.

Suler, J. (2004). The online disinhibition effect. *Cyberpsychology and Behavior, 7*(3), 321–26.

Sung, J., Lee, J., Noh, H. M., Park, Y. S., & Ahn, E. J. (2013). Associations between the Risk of Internet Addiction and Problem Behaviors among Korean adolescents. *Korean Journal of Family Medicine, 34*(2), 115–22.

Takao, M. (2014). Problematic mobile phone use and big-five personality domains. *Indian Journal of Community Medicine, 39*(2), 111–13.

Tao, R., Huang, X., Wang, J., Zhang, H., Zhang, Y., & Li, M. (2010). Proposed diagnostic criteria for internet addiction. *Addiction, 105*(3), 556–64.

Tian, M., Chen, Q., Zhang, Y., Du, F., Hou, H., Chao, F., & Zhang, H. (2014). PET imaging reveals brain functional changes in internet gaming disorder. *European Journal of Nuclear Medicine and Molecular Imaging, 41*(7), 1388–97.

Tsai, H. F., Cheng, S. H., Yeh, T. L., Shih, C. C., Chen, K. C., Yang, Y. C., & Yang, Y. K. (2009). The risk factors of Internet addiction: A survey of university freshmen. *Psychiatry Research, 167*(3), 294–99.

Tseng, Y. H., Wang, R. H., Wang, H. H., & Chou, F. H. (2012). [Internet use and adolescents' sexual health]. *Hu Li Za Zhi, 59*(6), 86–91.

van Rooij, A. J., Schoenmakers, T. M., van de Eijnden, R. J., & van de Mheen, D. (2010). Compulsive Internet use: The role of online gaming and other internet applications. *The Journal of Adolescent Health, 47*(1), 51–57.

Wang, E. S., & Wang, M. C. (2013). Social support and social interaction ties on internet addiction: Integrating online and offline contexts. *Cyberpsychology, Behavior and Social Networking, 16*(11), 843–49.

Wang, P. W., Liu, T. L., Ko, C. H., Lin, H. C., Huang, M. F., Yeh, Y. C., & Yen, C. F. (2014). Association between problematic cellular phone use and suicide: The moderating effect of family function and depression. *Comprehensive Psychiatry, 55*(2), 342–48.

Wei, H. T., Chen, M. H., Huang, P. C., & Bai, Y. M. (2012). The association between online gaming, social phobia, and depression: An internet survey. *BMC Psychiatry, 12*: 92.

Widyanto, L., & McMurran, M. (2004). The psychometric properties of the internet addiction test. *Cyberpsychology and Behavior, 7*(4), 443–50.

Wong, I. L., & So, E. M. (2014). Internet gambling among high school students in Hong Kong. *Journal of Gambling Studies, 30*(3), 565–76.

Yee, N. (2006). The demographics, motivations, and derived experiences of users of massively multi-user online graphical environments. *Presence, 15*(3), 21.

Yen, C. F., Chou, W. J., Liu, T. L., Ko, C. H., Yang, P., & Hu, H. F. (2014). Cyberbullying among male adolescents with attention-deficit/hyperactivity disorder: Prevalence, correlates, and association with poor mental health status. *Research in Developmental Disabilities, 35*(12) 3543–53.

Yen, C. F., Tang, T. C., Yen, J. Y., Lin, H. C., Huang, C. F., Liu, S. C., Ko, C. H. (2009). Symptoms of problematic cellular phone use, functional impairment and its association with depression among adolescents in Southern Taiwan. *Journal of Adolescence, 32*(4), 863–73.

Yen, J. Y., Ko, C. H., Yen, C. F., Chen, S. H., Chung, W. L., & Chen, C. C. (2008). Psychiatric symptoms in adolescents with Internet addiction: Comparison with substance use. *Psychiatry and Clinical Neurosciences, 62*(1), 9–16.

Yen, J. Y., Ko, C. H., Yen, C. F., Wu, H. Y., & Yang, M. J. (2007). The comorbid psychiatric symptoms of Internet addiction: Attention deficit and hyperactivity disorder (ADHD), depression, social phobia, and hostility. *The Journal of Adolescent Health, 41*(1) 93–98.

Yen, J. Y., Yen, C. F., Chen, C. S., Tang, T. C., Huang, T. H., & Ko, C. H. (2011a). Cue-induced positive motivational implicit response in young adults with Internet gaming addiction. *Psychiatry Research, 190*(2–3), 282–86.

Yen, J. Y., Yen, C. F., Chen, C. S., Wang, P. W., Chang, Y. H., & Ko, C. H. (2012). Social anxiety in online and real-life interaction and their associated factors. *Cyberpsychology, Behavior and Social Networking, 15*(1), 7–12.

Yen, J. Y., Yen, C. F., Wu, H. Y., Huang, C. J., & Ko, C. H. (2011b). Hostility in the real world and online: The effect of internet addiction, depression, and online activity. *Cyberpsychology, Behavior and Social Networking, 14*(11), 649–55.

Young, K. S. (1998). Internet addiction: The emergence of a new clinical disorder. *Cyberpsychology, Behavior and Social Networking, 1*, 237–44.

CHAPTER

8

Conceptualization of Internet Addiction Based on the Public Health Perspective

Hae Kook Lee *and* Sulki Chung

Abstract

With rapidly growing Internet and smartphone use in daily life, Internet use disorder (IUD) is gaining increased recognition, along with an associated rise in scientific evidence and public health concerns about its adverse cognitive, developmental, psychosocial, and physical consequences. Problematic use of the Internet and other technologies is directly related to social, cultural, and economic environments; examining the social and environmental factors within the public health framework is important in understanding IUD and developing intervention strategies. The authors present a conceptual model of IUD based on the public health model and the continuum model of addictive disorders and positing that health problems result from interactions among the agent mediating the disorder, those experiencing the disorder, and the social and environmental context in which the disorder occurs. Addictive online media components and predisposing biological, cognitive, psychological, and environmental factors increase risk for developing IUD, so prevention and intervention should not only target individual vulnerabilities, but also media-related risk and the environment to better address the complex phenomena of IUD. Intervention approaches to IUD must be tailored along a continuum of severity ranging from social to problematic use, and across a spectrum of intervention strategies ranging from primary to tertiary approaches. Multidisciplinary efforts are needed that combine various areas of expertise including prevention, treatment, education, and consumer protection to develop effective strategies for reducing harmful Internet use and promoting healthy digital media and device use.

Keywords: Internet use disorder, public health perspective, conceptual model, prevention, intervention strategies

Introduction

Since the introduction of the concept of Internet addiction (IA) in the late 1990s, the basis for defining Internet use disorders as a primary disease has been accumulated by many researchers to date. The issues of defining the problem as a disease and presenting accurate diagnosis criteria for the problem are still under debate (Kuss, Griffiths, Karila, & Billieux, 2014). However, consistent results have been reported regarding the consequences caused by excessive use of Internet activities like online gaming and social networking. These consequences include mental, behavioral, and physical health problems which point to the consensus that excessive Internet use is a public health problem (Hong Kong Department of Health, 2014; Smahel, Wright, & Cernikova, 2015).

These problems related to the use of the Internet are sufficient to be discussed as a matter of public health in a few aspects. First, the problems associated with Internet use have been widely reported in children and youth. Second, the adverse effects occur according to the amount and pattern of Internet use. Third, related problems are experienced on the family and community levels as well as on the individual level.

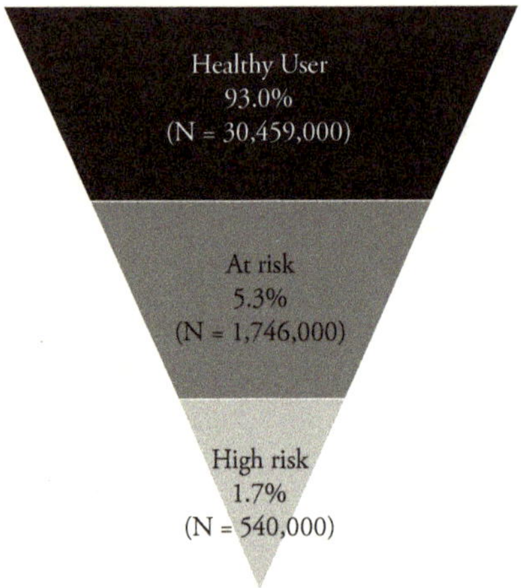

Figure 8.1 Continuum of problem spectrum (total population: aged 5–54, *N* = 32,745,000).

Problems associated with excessive Internet use are directly related to the social, cultural, and economic environments featured by the development and dissemination of new technologies. Therefore, understanding the social and environmental factors within a public health framework is important in understanding the problems associated with excessive Internet use and developing intervention strategies for reducing these problems.

IA is a problem that occurs in the process of consuming attractive digital contents by utilizing the Internet as a tool. This can be understood in a similar context as an alcohol addiction which develops in the course of purchasing and using alcohol that is legally available. As such, the public health model of alcoholism, which is composed of three factors (including host, agent, and the environment) can also be applied to excessive (or addictive) Internet use. This differs from the medical model, which explains a disease mainly based on individual vulnerability.

This chapter attempts to (1) examine the characteristics of addiction from the public health model, (2) restructure various risk factors presented by the existing literature in the public health model framework, and (3) suggest a comprehensive intervention model for reducing the problems of IA based on the comprehensive public health approach. In addition, we describe a Korean system of intervention efforts for IA problems in the public sector during the past decade.

The term "IA" is used as an umbrella concept which includes various kinds of addiction related to excessive use of Internet activities like online games, social network services, etc.

Spectrum Framework for Internet Addiction Problems

IA has similar clinical characteristics to an alcohol use disorder or a gambling disorder, and the diagnostic criteria has been applied by borrowing these similar characteristics (Young & Rogers, 1998). Therefore, the severity of symptoms and related behavioral problems can increase according to the amount and pattern of Internet use.

Internet users were classified into three categories of high-risk, potential-risk, and general user groups by the Korean IA scale (K-scale), which has been used in South Korea to assess the severity of the Internet use problems (National Information Society Agency of Korea, 2014). In other words, people using the Internet can be grouped into regular users, users at the initial stage of the addiction process, and an addicted group experiencing clear addiction symptoms with various impairments in a wide range of areas. Similar to substance addiction, IA should also be understood as a problem on a continuum. Thus, screening and the application of treatment programs should be made based on this understanding.

Many studies reported that the more severe the addiction, the worse the extent of the problems experienced (Shek, Sun, & Yu, 2013). In this context, IA from the public health perspective can be defined as a problem on a continuous spectrum rather than as a dichotomous disease. Figure 8.1 shows the continuum of the problem spectrum based on the Korean National Survey (National Information Society Agency of Korea, 2014).

Consequences Related to Excessive Internet Use

Excessive Internet use has been reported to be related to abnormality in mental health, physical health, daily functioning, and role performance. These categories can also be separated into physical health and psychosocial health.

The e-report published by the Hong Kong Department of Health and Human Services reviewed 14 problems consisting of seven physical health and seven mental health problems associated with excessive use of digital media. They then published precautions on health hazards associated with digital media use, as well as instructions on safe use (Hong Kong Department of Health, 2014). The physical health problems included health status related to physical strength and obesity, vision, musculoskeletal problems, hearing ability, injuries and accidents, infection,

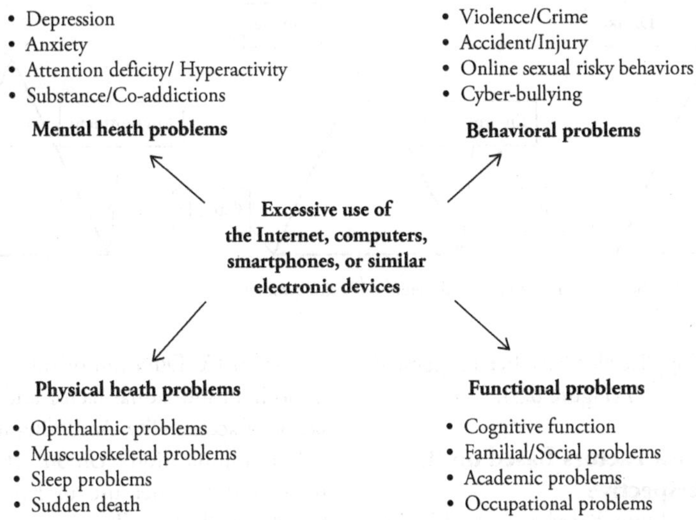

Figure 8.2 Consequences related to the excessive Internet use.

and high-frequency electromagnetism. The psychosocial health problems included addiction, cybercrime, cognitive development and learning, social development, sleep deprivation, risky sexual behaviors, and aggressive behaviors (Ahibom et al., 2008; Andersen, Fallentin, Thomsen, & Mikkelsen, 2011; Noll, Shenk, Barnes, & Haralson, 2013; Porter, 2012; Rosenfield, 2011; Tokunage, 2010).

We suggest that problems associated with Internet use can be divided into four areas, including mental health problems, behavioral safety/accidents, physical health problems, and malfunctioning. In regards to mental health problems, depression, suicidal ideation, impulsiveness, attention deficit hyperactivity disorder (ADHD), smoking, and drinking are all increased in association with IA (Choi et al., 2013; Ha et al., 2006; Han et al., 2011). In the physical health area, eye disease, musculoskeletal disorders, sleep problems, and sudden death are reported to be related to excessive Internet use (Andersen et al., 2011; Rosenfield, 2011). In the behavioral safety/accidents area, increases in aggression and violence, accidents, cyberbullying, and risky sexual behaviors are reported (Baumgartner, Sumter, Peter, & Valkenburg, 2012; Katzer, Fetchenhauer, & Belschak, 2009). In the malfunctioning problems area, learning, intellectual abilities, and family functioning are reported to all be decreased (Lee et al., 2010; Park et al., 2011) (Figure 8.2).

Public Health Model of Internet Addiction

The public health model is based on the premise that health problems occur from the interactions among three factors: the agent to mediate the disease (Agent), those who experience the disease (Host), and the social and environmental context in which the disease occurs (Environment). Based on the public health model, it is similarly presented that alcohol problems occur from interactions among alcohol as the "agent," a person as the "host," and social and cultural contexts in which alcohol is consumed (Center for Substance Abuse Prevention, 1993).

The public health model has been applied similarly to gambling disorder, a type of behavioral addiction. Korn and Shaffer (1999) defined gambling problems as problems on a spectrum rather than a simple dichotomous segmentation of disease. In addition, they applied the public health model to gambling problems, thereby conceptualizing gambling problems in three factors: gambling persons as the "host," various forms of gambling as the "agent," and social/cultural environments in which the gambling takes place.

For IA, depression and impulsiveness are considered individual risks, while high accessibility to Internet cafes and high-speed Internet connections are considered environmental risks. Both risks have been reported to be associated with IA (Stewart & Choi, 2003; Young & Rogers, 1998). In addition, as "agent" properties, games have been reported to exhibit positive reinforcing effects on the compensation circuit in the brain, similarly to the impacts of alcohol or gambling (Yuan, Qin, Liu, & Tian, 2011; Ko, Yen, Yen, Chen, & Chen, 2012). Considering the complex interactions between "host" and "agent,"

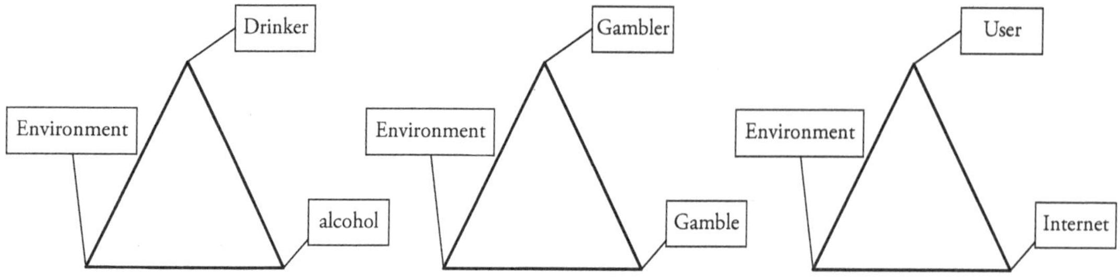

Figure 8.3 Comparison for the public health view of different addiction problem.

typologies for gaming disorder have been suggested (Lee, Lee, & Choo, 2017) (Figure 8.3).

Classifying the Risk Factors Based on the Public Health Perspective

Jacobs applied to gambling disorder the health promotion intervention model based on the ecological model proposed by McLeroy, Bibeau, Steckler, and Glanz (1988). He emphasized that gambling problems can be solved through comprehensive intervention strategies to resolve risk factors in a variety of aspects and levels (Jacobs, 1986).

Furthermore, Messerlian, Derevensky, and Gupta (2005) classified the risk factors affecting gambling behavior into five categories, of which intrapersonal and interpersonal factors correspond to "host" factors, while institutional, community, and public policy correspond to "environmental" factors. In a meta-analysis, Koo & Kwon (2014) presented the risk factors of IA as intrapersonal and interpersonal factors. As presented in Table 8.1, gambling disorder and IA share common risk factors with regard to intrapersonal and interpersonal factors.

"Agent" factors inherent in alcohol or gambling have been presented through numerous neurobiological studies (Crockford, Goodyear, Edwards, Quickfall, & el-Guebaly, 2005; Myrick et al., 2004; Potenza et al., 2003). Similar to alcohol and gambling, results show that online Internet games consistently stimulate the reward circuit among gaming addicts (Han, Kim, Lee, Min, & Renshaw, 2010; Ko et al., 2009). In addition, because the risk of addiction differs depending on the characteristics of the "agent" (i.e., type of alcohol or type of gambling), pornographic or gambling components of the Internet have been reported to increase the risk of IA (Lee, 2010; Kim, Lee, & Shin, 2008). Environmental factors such as accessibility, sociocultural awareness, and attitudes toward usage may also exert significant effects on IA. Duration of Internet use can be seen as both an individual factor and an environmental factor of accessibility. According to the International Telecommunication Union (ITU) report, the household Internet use in Korea was as high as 84.8%, with broadband penetration rate being one of the highest in the world (International Telecommunications Union, 2014). This high accessibility to high-speed Internet connection acts as an environmental risk factor and may contribute to IA risk among Korean adolescents.

Understanding the Public Health Perspective Based on the Analysis of Korean Nationwide Data

We analyzed Korean nationwide data to examine the public health model of IA. A Survey on the Internet Addiction Status was conducted by the Ministry of Science, ICT, and Future Planning and the National Information Society Agency (Kim, Lee, Chung, & Lee, 2015). This survey has been extended to a larger subject pool and its contents improved since the first survey in 2004; it has been conducted annually for 10 years (as of 2014). In order to test the public health perspective, a hierarchical linear regression model was constructed. In this model, IA scores (K-scale) were used as the dependent variable. The independent variables were entered in four blocks: host variables, agent variables, accessibilities variables, and environmental variables, following the public health model. Among the youth aged 10–19 years, male gender, lower income, online PC games (positive correlation), video games (negative correlation), adult content, longer Internet use time, and being offspring of immigrants were found to be risk factors of IA. While there were some variations in risk factors between adolescents and adults, risk factors were found in each of the four areas in the public health perspective (see Table 8.2).

Table 8.1 Risk factors for Internet addiction (IA) based on the public health model

Levels	Factors	Examples (gambling)	Example (Internet)
Host			Depression/anxiety[1]
Intrapersonal	Emotion/mood Knowledge Attitude Temperament Character Stress coping	Male Risk-taking propensity Low self-esteem Poor coping skills Impulsivity, sensation seeking Anxiety, depression	Attention problems[1] Impulsivity Novelty seeking[1] Negative stress coping[1]
Interpersonal	Relational ability Parent–child relationship Family functioning	Family history of gambling Parental or peer attitudes Family connectedness	Social anxiety[1] Unspecified[1] Negative parenting attitude[1] Family conflict/discord[1]
Environment			School policy[2]
Institutional	Social institution with formal/ informal rules or Policies	School policy/programs Industry policies and enforcement	
Community	Relationships and Network	Social norms Media Community resources Availability and accessibility factors	Social support[3]
Public policy	National system, policies and laws that regulate	Federal and provincial policies on age restrictions, enforcement, advertising, and legislations	Number of PC cafes[4] Block program to harmful websites[5] Time of use[6]
Agent	Contents		Games,[6] pornography[7]

[1] Koo & Kwon (2014);
[2] Kim et al. (2001);
[3] Park & Choi (2011);
[4] Lee & Kim (2009);
[5] Kim & Cha (2012);
[6] Kim et al. (2008);
[7] Lee (2010)

Table 8.2 Risk factors for Internet addiction (IA) based on the public health perspective

	Adolescents	Adults
Data	"A Survey on Current Internet Addiction Status," which was conducted by the Ministry of Science, ICT, and Future Planning and the National Information Society Agency	
Analysis	Hierarchical linear regression	
Age	10–19 years	20–49 years
Number of subject	2,526	8,768
Risk factors	**Host** Gender (male), lower income **Agent** Online PC game (positive correlation), video game (negative correlation) **Accessibility** Longer Internet use time **Environment** Dual-income households	**Host** Younger age, Lower income **Agent** Mobile messenger, online PC game, pornography **Accessibility** Longer Internet use time **Environment** Multicultural family

Intervention Framework Based on Public Health Model

We classified the risk factors of IA into agent, host, and environment factors. Through empirical analysis of Korean data, we found that these three risk factors can be identified in these categories. Therefore, interventions for IA problems should focus on strategies to reduce these risk factors in a public health model. The risk factor of the "agent" is the addictive nature of the content itself. Evidence can be found in functional magnetic resonance imaging (fMRI) studies that showed similar compensation circuit activation among online game addicts and alcoholics (Han et al., 2011). In addition, studies showed that adult content or online games increase the risk of IA (Kim et al., 2008; Lee, 2010). Therefore, policies to control accessibility to provocative adult content, online games, and gambling content are needed for the "agent" factor. These policies should include appropriate age regulation to access content, as well as posting warning signs.

Despite controversy in causality, one's psychological vulnerability and coexisting psychopathology may be a risk factor for addiction (Lee, Lee, & Choo, 2017; Rehbein, Kleimann, & Mößle, 2010). Therefore, intervention strategies should include a mental health promotion approach to vulnerable populations, early identification and intervention at the earliest stage for the risk group, development and dissemination of appropriate prevention and treatment programs, and building an infrastructure for the intervention.

High accessibility to Internet use (i.e., Internet cafés, personal/tablet computers in bedrooms), aggressive marketing of the Internet and gaming industry, and permissive social cultures are all potential risk factors. Campaigns to increase public awareness of the negative consequences of IA, regulations on excessive industry marketing, and systematic approaches for access restriction (i.e., shut down, cooling off, and fatigue system policies) may be possible strategies (see Table 8.3).

Constructing a Comprehensive Intervention System Based on the Public Health Model

A comprehensive intervention system can be constructed by integrating the public health model deploying intervention strategies suited to the risk factors and the continuous care model deploying a stepwise intervention strategy (the primary, secondary, and tertiary stages) based on severity of Internet use. Such a model has been applied to alcohol and gambling problems (Institute of Medicine, 1990; Skinner, 1990).

Prevention education in combination with public health promotion campaigns proposed in gambling addiction can be proposed as a primary intervention targeting the general population (Messerlian et al., 2005). Examples include slowing media exposure for children and restricting the

Table 8.3 Risk-specific intervention strategy based on the public health perspective

	Risk	Intervention
Agent	Adictiveness Sexual content Gambling Special online games	Content review rating board Regulation of content rating Warning label for age of consent
Host	Psychological vulnerability Low self esteem Poor coping skills Comorbid mental illness Parenting problems	Mental health promotion program Preventive education Early identification & intervention programs Establishment of prevention & treatment service system
Environment	Permissive culture Aggressive marketing Poor alternative sources Internet cafes	Social movement or campaign Counter-advertisement Regulation of marketing Accessibility control regulation (Shut down policy[a], Cooling off policy[b], Fatigue system policy[c])

[a] *Shut down policy*: Policy forces online game provider to shut down their service for teenagers under 16 years old from midnight to 6 AM (South Korea).

[b] *Cooling off system policy*: Policy sets up a restriction on the amount of total playing time for specific age groups.

[c] *Fatigue system policy*: Policy forces player to gain no reward points in a game after 5 hours of play (China).

exposure time to 2 hours, which was proposed by the US Institute of Children and Adolescents, and developing a guideline for using digital media similar to the guidelines developed by the Hong Kong Department of Health (Hong Kong Department of Health, 2014; Strasburger et al., 2013).

Secondary interventions would implement screening and intensive prevention programs using screening tools. Evidence-based prevention education programs can also be utilized (Ellickson & Bell, 1990; Rosenberg, McKeon, & Dinero, 1999). Educating individuals who are most likely to encounter others with IA problems and help them cope with their addiction is another form of secondary intervention. The American Academy of Pediatrics has advised teachers or pediatricians to ask children about Internet use and to check for possible problems (Strasburger et al., 2013).

Tertiary interventions involve constructing an infrastructure to employ evidence-based treatment programs (Young, 1999), fostering addiction experts, and constructing a community-based aftercare system for relapse prevention.

In addition, institutional interventions can be proposed to control the supply of the Internet. These interventions include the shutdown system, the fatigue system, and the cooling off system, which regulates Internet connection based on time of the day, age, and amount of usage time.

A Snapshot of Korean Government Response to Internet Addiction

In response to the IA problem, Korea established the Third Internet Addiction Prevention & Resolution Comprehensive Plan in 2016, led by the Ministry of Science, ICT, and Future Planning in cooperation with the Ministry of Culture, Sports, and Tourism (governing game contents); the Department of Education; the Ministry of Gender Equality and Family; and the Ministry of Health and Welfare (governing youth protection services). The Third Comprehensive Plan is still in progress. Despite a large investment of around $10 million, the plan has limitations in that it is implemented under the leadership of the ministry in charge of managing the information technology industry and gaming industry. Another limitation is that similar types of prevention counseling programs are being implemented by different ministries, creating possible overlap and confusion (Lee et al., 2013). Table 8.4 shows the detail of the intervention from different agencies.

The Ministry of Science, ICT, and Future Planning has been providing education and group counseling for prevention in conjunction with local primary and middle schools and has placed Internet Addiction Response Centers in 16 metropolitan cities. The Ministry of Education has been conducting a screening protocol utilizing the K-scale on all 4th, 7th, and 10th grade students. Students identified as either risk or high risk are provided prevention counseling services.

The Ministry of Culture, Sports, and Tourism supports IA counselors in the 45 Education District Offices. Stationed at the Education Office, they provide prevention training and counseling for children and youths exhibiting IA problems. In addition, the Ministry of Culture, Sports, and Tourism has been operating Excessive Gaming Healing Centers through the Game Culture Foundation. Furthermore, one of these centers is providing treatment through a department of child and adolescent psychiatry at a university medical center.

The Ministry of Gender Equality and Family holds the most active stance on addiction problems, but their budget is limited. The Ministry operates the Rescue School, a short-term residential treatment program, which was introduced by international media. In 2014, the Ministry established a facility to operate camps year-round for more stable operation.

In addition, the Ministry of Health and Welfare provides IA-related services through community-based Addiction Management Centers and social service institutions. Addiction Management Centers, having mostly focused on services for alcohol problems, began to expand their services to include behavioral addictions in 2014. However, most of the centers have trouble providing viable services due to the small number of staff (usually around three, except for some pilot areas). Although social service institutions have higher accessibility, they have limitation in controlling service quality.

Conclusion

With the advance of digital technology and widespread use of digital media, problems related to the excessive or inappropriate use of the Internet have also increased. The public health model of addiction could be useful when it is applied to the excessive use of Internet activities. Integrative and comprehensive intervention approaches are needed to target the risk factors identified in the public health model. Moreover, primary, secondary, and tertiary intervention services should be provided according to the severity of the addiction problems.

The digital media industry has produced many conveniences in our life, and a large party of interest

Table 8.4 Intervention services provided by government agency in Korea

Division	Institution in charge	Main activities
Ministry of Science, ICT and Future Planning (MSIP)	Under the "Framework Act on National Informatization," the MSIP plans and carries out the necessary actions for prevention of and recovery from Internet addiction (IA).	
	Internet Addiction Center	• Prevention education, counseling, investigation & research, professional training • 16 centers (as of 2015) • Budget: $9,740,000 (in 2015) • Counseling: appx. 12,000 people (12 sessions in 2012)
Ministry of Culture, Sports and Tourism (MCST)	Budget (in 2013)	$182,215 (Screening & counseling: $637,755; Prevention education: $728,862; Investigation & promotion: $455,540)
	Wee Center (Ministry of Education)	• Support counselors to 45 *Wee centers*, provide preventive services and other PR activities. • Counseling: appx. 670 people (12 sessions in 2012)
	Counseling/ Therapy centers for game addiction	• Individual counseling and therapy (inpatient/ outpatient therapy) • Three centers (as of 2015) • Budget: $706,086 (in 2012)
Ministry of Gender Equality and Family (MOGEF)	Based on the "Juvenile Protection Act," the MOGEF provides education and counseling to those suffering from IA according to their levels of risk. They operate a boarding institute for recovery called the "RESCUE School" and also hold family cure camps for juveniles.	
	Budget (2015 plan)	• $4,479,775
	Counseling & Resource Center for Youth	• 208 centers • Counseling provision: 8,772 people (in 2012)
	Boarding institute for recovery (RESCUE School)	• 12-day Lodging Camp • Middle and high school students • 25 participants per program (22 programs in 2013) • Budget: $36,444/program
	National Youth Internet Dream Village Permanent Boarding Institute for recovery)	• Permanent Boarding Institute for recovery (2014. 8.) • 20 programs (4,000 people/year) • Budget: $1,639,942
	Family cure camps for juveniles	• 3-day family cure camp • Elementary (primary) school children and their guardian(s) • 30 families per camp (9 camps in 2013) • Budget: $13,211/camp
Ministry of Health and Welfare (MOHW)	Addiction Management Integration Supporting Center	• 55 centers (as of 2015) • Community-based screening and brief intervention, case management • 6,261 counselling cases, 581 education sessions (25,019 participants) (as of 2013)
	Social Service Center	• 54 centers (as of 2012) • Internet/game addiction treatment services for children (voucher system) • Service provision: 2,567 people (as of 2012) • Budget: $2,110,970 (as of 2012)

groups is involved in this growing business sector. Due to conflicting perspectives in regard to the public health risks and economic value, there are different attitudes toward these problems even in government agencies.

Therefore, interagency collaboration is essential to implement comprehensive interventions, including public education to increase awareness, screening to identify high-risk groups, treatment, and policies to moderate the harms caused by excessive use (see Table 8.4).

References

Ahlbom, A., Bridges, J., de Seze, R., Hillert, L., Juutilainen, J., Mattsson, M.O., Neubauer, G., Schüz, J., Simko, M., & Bromen, K. (2008). Possible effects of electromagnetic fields (EMF) on human health–opinion of the scientific committee on emerging and newly identified health risks (SCENIHR). *Toxicology, 246*(2–3), 248–50.

Andersen, J. H., Fallentin, N., Thomsen, J. F., & Mikkelsen, S. (2011). Risk factors for neck and upper extremity disorders among computers users and the effect of interventions: An overview of systematic reviews. *PLoS One, 6*(5), e19691.

Baumgartner, S. E., Sumter, S. R., Peter, J., & Valkenburg, P. M. (2012). Identifying teens at risk: Developmental pathways of online and offline sexual risk behavior. *Pediatrics, 130*(6), e1489–96.

Center for Substance Abuse Prevention. (1993). *Prevention primer: An encyclopedia of alcohol, tobacco, and other drug prevention terms.* Rockville, MD: National Clearinghouse for Alcohol and Drub Information.

Choi, J. S., Park, S. M., Lee, J., Hwang, J. Y., Jung, H. Y., Choi, S. W., . . . and Lee, J. Y. (2013). Resting-state beta and gamma activity in Internet addiction. *International Journal of Psychophysiology, 89*(3), 328–33.

Crockford, D. N., Goodyear, B., Edwards, J., Quickfall, J., & el-Guebaly, N. (2005). Cue-induced brain activity in pathological gamblers. *Biological Psychiatry, 58*(10), 787–95.

Ellickson, P. L., & Bell, R. M. (1990). *Prospects for preventing drug use among young adolescents.* Santa Monica, CA: RAND.

Ha, J. H., Kim, S. Y., Bae, S. C., Bae, S., Kim, H., Sim, M., . . . Cho, S. C. (2006). Depression and Internet addiction in adolescents. *Psychopathology, 40*(6), 424–30.

Han, D. H., Bolo, N., Daniels, M. A., Arenella, L., Lyoo, I. K., & Renshaw, P. F. (2011). Brain activity and desire for Internet video game play. *Comprehensive Psychiatry, 52*(1), 88–95.

Han, D. H., Kim, Y. S., Lee, Y. S., Min, K. J., & Renshaw, P. F. (2010). Changes in cue-induced, prefrontal cortex activity with video-game play. *Cyberpsychology, Behavior, and Social Networking, 13*(6), 655–61.

Hong Kong Department of Health, The Government of the Hong Kong Special Administrative Region. (2014). *Report of advisory group on health effects of use of internet and electronic screen products.* https://www.studenthealth.gov.hk/english/internet/report/files/e_report_wa.pdf

International Telecommunication Union. (2014). *The world in 2014. ICT facts and figures.* Geneva: International Telecommunication Union.

Institute of Medicine. (1990). *Broadening the base of treatment for alcohol problems: Report of a study by a committee of the Institute of Medicine, Division of Mental Health, and Behavioral Medicine.* Washington, DC: National Academy of Science.

Jacobs, D. F. (1986). A general theory of addictions: A new theoretical model. *Journal of Gambling Behavior, 2*(1), 15–31.

Katzer, C., Fetchenhauer, D., & Belschak, F. (2009). Cyberbullying: Who are the victims? A comparison of victimization in internet chatrooms and victimization in school. *Journal of Media Psychology: Theories, Methods, and Applications, 21*(1), 25.

Kim, J. S., Lee, B. H., Chung, S. K., & Lee, H. K. (2015). Correlates of smartphone use and Internet addiction among Korean adolescents: Public health perspective. *Journal of Behavioral Addictions, 4*(1), 1–66.

Kim, K. H., & Cha, E. J. (2012). The influence of Internet addiction on cyber delinquency among middle school students: Testing the mediating effect of Internet ethics. *Korea Institute for Health and Social Affairs, 32*(2), 364–401.

Kim, K. R., Lee, S. J., & Shin, H. S. (2008). The effects of Internet-addiction on adolescents' family communication. *Korean Home Economics Education Association, 20*(4), 187–203.

Kim, S. H., Baik, S. H., Park, C. S., Kim, S. J., Choi, S. W., & Kim, S. E. (2011). Reduced striatal dopamine D2 receptors in people with Internet addiction. *Neuroreport, 22*(8), 407–11.

Ko, C. H., Liu, G. C., Hsiao, S., Yen, J. Y., Yang, M. J., Lin, W. C., . . . Chen, C. S. (2009). Brain activities associated with gaming urge of online gaming addiction. *Journal of Psychiatric Research, 43*(7), 739–47.

Ko, C. H., Yen, J. Y., Yen, C. F., Chen, C. S., & Chen, C. C. (2012). The association between Internet addiction and psychiatric disorder: A review of the literature. *European Psychiatry, 27*(1), 1–8.

Koo, H. J., & Kwon, J. (2014). Risk and protective factors of Internet Addiction: A meta-analysis of empirical studies in Korea. *Yonsei Medical Journal, 55*(6), 1691–711.

Korn, D. A., & Shaffer, H. J. (1999). Gambling and the health of the public: Adopting a public health perspective. *Journal of Gambling Studies, 15*(4), 289–365.

Kuss, D., Griffiths, M., Karila, L., & Billieux, J. (2014). Internet addiction: A systematic review of epidemiological research for the last decade. *Current Pharmaceutical Design, 20*(25), 4026–52.

Lee, J. Y., Park, E. J., Joe, K. H., Chai, S. H., Kim, S. B., Lee, C. U., & Kim, D. J. (2010). Psychiatric comorbidities and behavioral patterns in relation to Internet addiction severity in adolescents. *Journal of Korean Academy of Addiction Psychiatry, 14*(1), 36–41.

Lee, K., Lee, H., Gyeong, H., Yu, B., Song, Y., & Kim, D. (2013). Reliability and validity of the Korean version of the Internet Addiction Test among college students. *Journal of Korean Medical Science, 28*(5), 763–68.

Lee, S. J., & Kim, H. M. (2009). Factors affecting on Internet addiction of the adolescents. *Journal of Korean Council for Children & Rights, 13*(2), 275–303.

Lee, S. K. (2010). A study on juvenile delinquency by different types of Internet addiction. *KNU Center for Social Welfare Research, 16*(2), 157–82.

Lee, S. Y., Lee, H. K., & Choo, H. (2017). Typology of Internet gaming disorder and its clinical implications. *Psychiatry and Clinical Neurosciences, 71*(7), 479–91.

McLeroy, K. R., Bibeau, D., Steckler, A., & Glanz, K. (1988). An ecological perspective on health promotion programs. *Health Education & Behavior, 15*(4), 351–77.

Messerlian, C., Derevensky, J. L., & Gupta, R. (2005). Youth gambling: A public health perspective. *Health Promotion International, 20*(1), 69–79.

Myrick, H., Anton R. F., Li, X., Henderson, S., Drobes, D., Voronin, K., & George, M. S. (2004). Differential brain activity in alcoholics and social drinkers to alcohol cues: Relationship to craving. *Neuropsychopharmacology, 29*(2), 393–401.

National Information Society Agency of Korea. (2014). *National survey of Internet addiction report.* Seoul, South Korea: Author.

Noll, J. G., Shenk, C. E., Barnes, J. E., & Haralson, K. J. (2013). Association of maltreatment with high-risk internet behaviors and offline encounters. *Pediatrics, 131*(2), e510–17.

Park, G., & Choi, Y. (2011). The effects of stress, social support and impulsiveness on adolescents' Internet addiction. *Korean Academic Society of Rehabilitation Nursing, 14*(2), 145–52.

Park, M. H., Park, E. J., Choi, J., Chai, S., Lee, J. H., Lee, C., & Kim, D. J. (2011). Preliminary study of Internet addiction and cognitive function in adolescents based on IQ tests. *Psychiatry Research, 190*(2), 275–81.

Porter, C. (2012, October 23). Calling all germs. *The Wall Street Journal, Retrieved from* http://www.wsj.com

Potenza, M. N., Steinberg, M. A., Skudlarski, P., Fulbright, R. K., Lacadie, C. M., . . . Wexler, B. E. (2003). Gambling urges in pathological gambling: A functional magnetic resonance imaging study. *Archives of General Psychiatry, 60*(8), 828–36.

Rehbein, F., Kleimann, M., & Mößle, T. (2010). Prevalence and risk factors of video game dependency in adolescence: Results of a German nationwide survey. *Cyberpsychology, Behavior, and Social Networking, 13*(3), 269–77.

Rosenberg, L., McKeon, M., & Dinero, E. (1999). Positive peer solutions: One answer for the rejected student. *Phi Delta Kappan, 81*, 114–18.

Rosenfield, M. (2011). Computer vision syndrome: A review of ocular causes and potential treatments. *Ophthalmic and Physiological Optics, 31*(5), 502–15.

Tokunaga, R. S. (2010). Following you home from school: A critical review and synthesis of research on cyberbullying victimization. *Computers in Human Behavior, 26*(3), 277–87.

Shek, D. T. L., Sun, R. C. F., & Yu, L. (2013). Internet addiction. In D. W. Pfaff & N. D. Volkow (Eds.), *Neuroscience in the 21st century* (pp. 2775–811). New York: Springer.

Skinner, H. A. (1990). Spectrum of drinkers and intervention opportunities. *Canadian Medical Association Journal, 143*(10), 1054–59.

Smahel, D., Wright, M. F., Cernikova, M. (2015). The impact of digital media on health: children's perspectives. *International Journal of Public Health, 60*(2), 131–37.

Stewart, K., & Choi, H. P. (2003). PC-Bang (Room) culture: A study of Korean college students' private and public use of computers and the Internet. *Trends in Communication, 11*(1), 63–79.

Strasburger, V. C., Hogan, M. J., Mulligan, D. A., Ameenuddin, N., Christakis, D. A., Cross, C., & Swanson, W. S. L. (2013). Children, adolescents, and the media. *Pediatrics, 132*(5), 958–61.

Young, K. S. (1999). Internet addiction: Symptoms, evaluation, and treatment. *Innovations in Clinical Practice: A Source Book, 17*, 19–31.

Young, K. S., & Rogers, R. C. (1998). The relationship between depression and Internet addiction. *CyberPsychology & Behavior, 1*(1), 25–28.

Yuan, K., Qin, W., Liu, Y., & Tian, J. (2011). Internet addiction: Neuroimaging findings. *Communicative & Integrative Biology, 4*(6), 637–39.

CHAPTER

9 Problems Relating to Internet Use in China

Status, Challenge, and Response

Wei Hao *and* Shangli Cai

Abstract

The Internet has penetrated all aspects of Chinese society and has become a crucial part of its social, economic, and cultural activities, as well as its personal life. Meanwhile, the rapid development of the Internet, along with a lag in the development of legislation and guidelines for use, has had an enormous impact on Chinese society and created unprecedented challenges. This chapter overviews the current status of Internet use in China, directing particular attention to problems that youth may encounter, and then reviews progress that the Chinese government has made in managing problems related to Internet use.

Keywords: Internet, young Internet users, Internet addiction, Internet violence, China

The Current Status of Internet Use in China

China was first permitted to access the Internet in 1994. Since then, the Internet has been integrated into diverse aspects of Chinese society, becoming a crucial platform for social, economic, and cultural activities and an integral part of personal life. According to the 34th Statistical Report on Internet Development in China (2014; http://www.cnnic.net.cn/hlwfzyj/hlwxzbg/hlwtjbg/201407/P020140721507223212132.pdf) released by the China Internet Network Information Center (CNNIC), China had 632 million Internet users as of June 2014, with a high Internet penetration rate (46.9%) and an average time spent online of 25.9 hours per week. Recent figures estimate the male:female proportion among Chinese Internet users at 55.6:44.4, consistent with figures obtained in 2013.

According to the Report on China Youth Internet Behaviour Investigation (2013; http://www.cnnic.net.cn/hlwfzyj/hlwxzbg/qsnbg/201406/P020140611557842544454.pdf), the percentage of individuals aged 10–29 years among all Internet users is 55.2%, with 41.5% aged under 25 years, thereby indicating that young people remain the largest group of Internet users in China. The percentage of Internet users with primary or lower levels of education is 48.2%. Therefore, China's Internet users tend to be relatively young individuals with relatively low levels of education, which differs from developed countries in Europe and North America. In addition, 28.2% of individuals in Chinese rural areas, or about 178 million individuals, use the Internet, leaving about 450 million individuals in these areas as non-users, the latter being a large potential population for increased future Internet use.

With the rapid development of mobile devices, mobile Internet use has promoted the development of and access to the whole Internet. According to results reported in the 2014 Newsletter of Internet Development issued by CINIC (http://www.cnnic.net.cn/hlwfzyj/hlwfzzx/qwfb/201408/W020140825417694343385.pdf), about 83.4% of Internet users access the Internet via smartphones, a dramatic shift from the 80.9% figure previously obtained for personal computers as the primary method of access. The number of mobile Internet users in China exceeds 500 million. Hence, the number of Internet users with smartphones will likely show

Table 9.1 The usage percentages of major Internet applications in China from December 2013 to June 2014

Internet applications	June 2014		December 2013		Increase ratio in 6 months (%)
	User population (in millions)	Usage percentage	User population (in millions)	Usage percentage	
Instant messenger	564.23	89.3	532.15	86.2	6.0
Search engine	507.49	80.3	489.66	79.3	3.6
Online news	503.16	79.6	491.32	79.6	2.4
Online music	487.61	77.2	453.12	73.4	7.6
Personal blog	444.30	70.3	436.58	70.7	1.8
Online video	438.77	69.4	428.20	69.3	2.5
Online game	368.11	58.2	338.03	54.7	8.9
Online shopping	331.51	52.5	301.89	48.9	9.8
Online payment	292.27	46.2	260.20	42.1	12.3
Online literature	289.39	45.8	274.41	44.4	5.5
Weibo	275.35	43.6	280.78	45.5	−1.9
E-banking	271.88	43.0	250.06	40.5	8.7
Emails	268.67	42.5	259.21	42.0	3.6
Social network	257.22	40.7	277.69	45.0	−7.4
Forum	124.07	19.6	120.46	19.5	3.0

further growth. Based on this trend, the use of instant messaging communication will likely continue to rise. Currently, China has 500 million Wechat users and nearly 300 million Weibo users, with the daily number of instant messages exceeding 20 billion.

According to the 34th Statistical Report on Internet Development in China (2014; http://www.cnnic.net.cn/hlwfzyj/hlwxzbg/hlwtjbg/201407/P020140721507223212132.pdf), Internet use continues to incease rapidly in China. Furthermore, as shown in Table 9.1, 14 major Internet applications are used by 40% or more of Internet users, with 5 of these applications used by 70% or more of users. As these figures and other data and trends indicate, in China, Internet use has come to exert a deep influence on many aspects of everyday life.

Internet Use–Related Mental Health Problems

The rapid expansion of Internet use in China seems to have led to a range of physical, mental, and social problems, especially among excessive users. Given the increasing popularity of Internet use and indications of potential adverse consequences, Chinese researchers began to study Internet addiction (IA). Investigators worked to develop definitions for Internet overuse or addiction and to create assessment tools for identifying problematic levels of use and appraising level of severity. Across these research efforts, the *Clinical Diagnostic Criteria of Internet Addiction* has come to gain considerable influence (Tao et al., 2008). These criteria define IA as a mental and behavioral disorder in which an individual repeatedly uses the Internet, shows an intense desire to continue with or return to Internet use, and experiences withdrawal reactions, including mental or physical symptoms, when Internet use is restricted or discontinued.

In China, as is the case globally, young people show the highest frequency of IA (Betül & Serkan, 2011; Mossbarger, 2008). The China Youth Association for Network Development designed a questionnaire modeled after Young's (1999) Internet Addiction Test. The questionnaire was used to conduct the China Youth Internet Addiction Survey in 2009, with the results appearing in the Report on Internet Addiction in Teenagers (2009; http://mat1.gtimg.com/edu/pdf/wangyinbaogao.pdf). The report indicated that 14.1% (about 24.0 million) of Chinese urban teenagers met criteria for IA, with an additional 12.7% (about 18.6 million) showing addictive tendencies. Urban youth in the 18-to 25-year-old age range showed the highest rate of IA (15.6%), followed in order by the 24- to 29-year-old group (14.6%) and the 13- to 17-year-old group (14.3%).

IA can harm youth in various ways, including social dysfunction, mental impairment, poor academic performance, mood disorders, and decreased life quality (Wu et al., 2013). Some users may even experience psychotic symptoms or suicidal ideation. Potential harm to physical and mental health can lead to a variety of family and social problems, including deterioration in parent–child relationships and illegal and criminal behaviors (Chou, 2001; Young, 2004). In China, the development and education of youth have always been viewed as major priorities. Thus, the types of negative impacts associated with excessive Internet use have raised widespread concerns in Chinese society and have led to considerable efforts to address the types of educational, psychological, and public health consequences that had been described or assumed.

Subsequent research on IA, however, began to raise questions or controversies about certain reported findings and assumptions. In China, the nature of IA is in dispute. Many researchers believe that IA is a new type of social disorder; therefore, its occurrence is largely attributable to psychosocial factors and shortcomings in social support and education. As such, medical treatment is not necessary; instead, what is needed is to strengthen the education of young people. In addition, the term *addiction* connotes the use of substances, such as drugs. However, the Internet is a part of the environment, and it is difficult to define or conceptualize what it means to be addicted to an aspect of the environment. Thus, some argue that it would be inappropriate to define IA as a mental illness.

An alternate view is that the manifestations of IA are surprisingly similar to substance dependence and parallel problems commonly observed by individuals with substance addictions in clinics. In addition, excessive Internet use may bring suffering to oneself and one's family and causes harm to society, in line with the definition of diseases. Therefore, some researchers argue that IA should be categorized as a psychological disorder. A third view argues that IA is merely superficial to, or a secondary symptom of, a primary mental disorder, such as a personality, anxiety, or depressive disorder.

Despite uncertainties about definition and conceptualization, a subgroup of Internet users, most commonly children and adolescents, develop increasing or escalating patterns of use, along with seemingly associated dysfunction that can substantially impact critical areas of everyday life. Therefore, the treatment of IA is of considerable interest and potential importance, although treatment strategies and services still remain at a very preliminary stage of development and often lack even basic scientific foundations. In China, treatment strategies that have been used vary widely and include psychotherapy, medication, military training, physical punishment, or even electric shock.

The most frequently used treatments include cognitive-behavioral therapy (CBT), solution-focused brief therapy (SFBT), group therapy, and family therapy, with CBT being the most common treatment of choice. CBT includes two main components (cognitive therapy and behavioral therapy) and aims to help teenagers gain insight into their addictive behaviors. CBT treatment can help excessive Internet users identify maladaptive cognitions, reconstruct adaptive cognitions, and assist them in managing their emotions and behaviors, such as the amount of time they spend on the Internet. During treatment, mental health professionals try to help addicted teenagers alter their attitudes and habitual behaviors and learn more adaptive coping patterns. A short-term controlled study involving teenagers with IA found that CBT produced significant improvements in comparison to a control group (Li & Dai, 2009). A two-stage follow-up study also yielded similar results (Wang, Dai, Li, & Li., 2011).

Some individuals with IA evidence significant depression and anxiety (Roger et al., 2014), leading to treatment approaches and studies that combine psychotropic medications with psychological therapy. The drug treatment mainly includes two categories: antidepressants and mood stabilizers (Yang, 2006). In contrast, several researchers have used other drugs for treating IA, such as scopolamine (Liu, Yang, & Yao, 2007), in order to inhibit cortical hyperexcitability, improve sleep and restorative rest, and thus interrupt obsessive online behaviors in individuals with IA. Nevertheless, IA differs from substance addiction. There is still dispute about whether drug treatment is necessary, especially for individuals who do not seem to have psychological symptoms or disorders for which drug treatment is usually targeted (e.g., excessive anxiety, significant depression); therefore, for these patients, drug treatments should be considered carefully.

In addition to receiving formal clinical treatment, many parents choose to send their children with IA to Internet Addiction Treatment Centers. Most of these centers have few professionals with a medical or mental health background. In these centers, paramilitary approaches are often emphasized, with youth housed for about a month in relatively remote regions and subjected to harsh training or even corporal punishment (Stone, 2009). This "treatment" has neither a scientific nor an evidence-based foundation and may harm children and adolescents. A few deaths have been reported from such harsh paramilitary training centers. There are also reports describing the use of electric stimulation for treating IA. (For the sake of clarity, the methods being referenced here are not electroconvulsive therapy [ECT], but simply electrical stimulation.) Although the therapists claimed that the stimulation therapy they used was very safe, the Chinese Ministry of Health issued a notice (http://www.china.com.cn/policy/txt/2009-11/05/content_18830451_2.htm) in 2009 prohibiting the use of electric stimulation for treating IA.

Internet Violence

So-called *Internet violence* mainly involves two aspects. First, perpetrators use vicious language to attack or belittle others, saying hurtful, insulting, and/or provocative things about individuals that may be untrue or unproven. Second, some individuals who are aware of or uncover the identity of virtual figures or anonymous users expose their true identity to the public. The perpetrators reveal personal information about the user that they may know or may have accessed through Internet sites. To the extent that such information is embarrasing, damaging, or intrusive, extreme distress and adverse consequences may result, not only for the victim but also for that person's relatives and friends. This second type of violence is sometimes labeled "human research engine" or "Internet mass hunting." This can transform the user's virtual world of the Internet from an online community to the real world, with serious resultant real-world consequences. The occurrence of Internet violence not only affects China's national mentality, bringing suffering to many citizens, but also disrupts the harmonious development of society. Such incidences of Internet violence also raise worldwide concern, leading the *New York Times* and European media to characterize some Chinese Internet users as an Internet Mob (see "Mob Rule on China's Internet: The Keyboard as Weapon"; http://www.nytimes.com/2006/05/31/technology/31iht-chinet.1861775.html?pagewanted=all&module=Search&mabRewa rd=relbias%3Ar%2C%7B%222%22%3A%22RI %3A12%22%7D&_r=0).

China continues to transition socially, and the occurrence of Internet violence is associated with the Internet itself and the social freedoms it creates. The Internet is a virtual world of free speech, which removes the shackles resulting from prohibitions on open expression and attenuates or eliminates personal responsibility for online communications. This so-called freedom of expression, reduced personal accountability, and group polarization of users contributes to the formation of Internet violence. Generally, *group polarization* refers to a phenomenon in which group members may have a certain inclination or fairly modest view initially, but, as group discussion proceeds, they move toward less moderate positions and may eventually adopt extreme beliefs (Cass, 2002). The proportion of group polarization among Internet users is twice as high as that found in real or nonvirtual settings (Myers, 2012).

China's Internet use is dominated by teenagers, a group that may be more susceptible to peer influences and to forming conclusions based on insufficient information and analysis; hence, under the influence of group emotion and peer pressure, they may have a decreased capacity to properly assess their actions and consequences. As a result, especially given the anonymity of the Internet, they may attack individuals who they believe to be controversial or who express views with which they disagree. Once such behaviors start, they may be fed and intensified by group participation and accompanying emotionality, leading to Internet violence. Alternatively, the rapid development of Chinese society and the fast pace of city life may create many pressures that may lead to emotional imbalance and a range of negative experiences and feelings, such as stress, anxiety, confusion, resentment, and disappointment. For individuals who lack outlets for these troubling psychological states and feelings, the Internet may become an essential tool for expressing dissatisfactions and painful emotions. Consequently, the Internet may become a platform to vent, with negative social events serving as potential fuses and group polarization effects leading to extreme, one-sided, and sometimes even paranoid ideation.

Policy Responses to Internet Use–Related Issues

Guidance for Healthy Internet Use for Minors

In 2009, the Chinese Disease Prevention and Control Bureau released a Guidance to Healthy Internet Use for Minors (draft; http://www.china.com.cn/policy/txt/2009-11/05/content_18830451.htm) to promote the physical and mental health of minors and due consideration for their rights. The purpose of this document is

- to guide minors on how to use the Internet moderately and properly;
- to provide guidance for families, schools, and society to prevent minors from Internet misuse; and
- to improve public understanding of the positive and negative consequences of Internet use on minors.

According to the Guidance, Internet misuse in adolescents can be evaluated based on levels of negative consequences, as judged by mental health professionals. The Guidance proposed the following recommendations for intervention in cases of Internet misuse:

- psychosocial interventions (with systematic and multiple components) should be provided by qualified professionals;
- the aim of intervention is to correct psychological and behavioral problems and to improve social functioning, not to restrict access to the Internet;
- restricting personal freedom or delivering physical punishment is strictly forbidden; and
- individuals with Internet misuse and comorbid mental health problems, such as anxiety, depression, or obsessive-compulsive disorders should be transferred to medical institutions, and relevant medical treatment that accords with sound clinical practice should be provided. Use of psychotropic medications should be strictly based on indications, and no surgical operation should be performed for Internet use-related problems.

In addition, in 2013, 15 national ministries and commissions, including the Ministry of Education, Ministry of Culture, Ministry of Finance, Ministry of Public Security, Ministry of Health, and Cyberspace Administration of China jointly issued the Program of Comprehensive Prevention and Intervention for Online Games Addiction among Juveniles (http://www.ccm.gov.cn/swordcms/publish/default/static/gfxwj/284303648.htm). This official program is intended to integrate almost all kinds of governmental forces dealing with online gaming addiction and related mental and behavioral disorders. The Program addresses local standards for early prediction and diagnosis in a highly visible forum. It encourages scientific research institutions and mental health service providers to develop a set of local evaluation criteria that are suitable for Mainland China and to designate proper intervention strategies. Moreover, the Program also proposes to provide a legislative and regulatory framework for prevention and treatment and thus to provide stringent regulations for all entities offering any services related to online gaming addiction. Arguably of greatest importance and a groundbreaking development, the document stipulates explicitly that all relevant government sectors and public institutions on every level should actively take part in the Program and ensure sufficient funding for its implementation. Although the Program was initiated just a few years ago and concrete achievements are at early stages, its creation and beginning implementation is a big step for Mainland China in response to ICT- related disorders.

Regulations for the Administration of Public Internet Business Premises

In order to regulate the development of the Internet, the Chinese government implemented a licensing system for business entities that provide Internet services. The State Council had promulgated the Regulations of Internet Service in Business Premises (http://www.gov.cn/banshi/2005-08/21/content_25106.htm), effective January 8, 2011. The Regulations indicates that Internet services should check and register validating documents, such as the identity cards of Internet consumers; that online information should be recorded; and that business sites that provide Internet services should be at least 200 meters away from the campuses of middle and elementary schools and should not be located in residential areas. Minors are not permitted to enter the service premises, with a sign posted at the entrance indicating such. Operating hours are to be limited to 8 AM to 12 PM.

The management of Internet development by China's government has changed from supervision to active control. Mainstream media, including China Central Television, People's Daily, have launched a massive action again Internet violence. *China Youth Daily* published a series of reports in 2012 on "Refusing Internet Violence" (http://zqb.cyol.com/html/2012-08/06/nw.D110000zgqnb_20120806_5-03.htm), which reflect the Chinese government's strengthened efforts to control Internet use.

Since August of 2013, China's police have arrested several "Internet opinion leaders"; these leaders have millions of fans on Weibo, and they have had more influence in certain emergencies and on certain public issues than government forces and media. The governance of Internet opinion leaders has included legislation intended to counter Internet rumors and slander. Nowadays, the so-called government Weibo has become an important channel for releasing official and authoritative information from the government, and such releases may actively guide public opinion. Additionally, the government is trying to use the Internet to obtain increased information about public opinion. In October 2013, the State Council issued "Opinions on Further Strengthening Government Information Disclosure in Response to Public Concerns and Increasing

Credibility of the Government" (http://www.gov.cn/zwgk/2013-10/15/content_2506664.htm). The government started to hold press conferences regularly and to take quick action in response to public opinion and demands. In September 2013, the Supreme People's Court and Supreme People's Procuratorate issued an official explanation for criminal cases involving libel, affray, blackmail, and illegal business via information networks. This explanation was based on Criminal Law of the People's Republic of China, as well as the Regulations on Internet Security. This is a sign that the government's manner of dealing with Internet issues has shifted from more passive approaches to exerting active control.

Outlook

It is predictable that, given further developments in network technology, especially the development of wearable smart devices, people may maintain continuous contact with the Internet anytime and anywhere and that the Internet's influence on Chinese society and everyday life will likely continue to deepen. It is anticipated that the Internet will be an integral part of working, living, and even human spiritual beliefs, becoming an extension of the human brain. At that time, one wonders how relevant issues involving the Internet will change and expand. The extension of informational and networking technologies is an irresistible trend; thus, a virtually created Internet community will likely become a second world to many. In this transformation, people's lifestyles, as well as their spiritual beliefs and practices, will likely be changed significantly. Anticipating such developments, the following problems should be addressed in the future from the standpoint of public health and legislation:

1. *Definition.* It is difficult to define Internet-related problems. Some researchers define excessive or problematic use of the Internet as an impulse-control disorder, similar to early classifications of pathological gambling (Young, 1999), while others view it as more closely aligned with substance addictions (Liu, Hao, & Young, 2006). Varying labels have been used for problematic Internet use: IA disorder, Internet abuse, virtual addiction, pathological Internet use, pathological computer use, and compulsive Internet use. Hence, it is necessary for the professional community to recognize the reality of IA and to respond to the potential threats related to its rapid expansion (Liu, Hao, & Young, 2004).

2. *The nature of the problem.* There may be two types of Internet-related problems. One problem involves the adverse impact that Internet use can have on psychological well-being or adjustment, and another problem involves preexisting psychiatric problems that might be closely related to or exacerbated by Internet use (Shaffer, LaBrie, & LaPlante, 2004). These psychiatric problems include personality disorders, anxiety disorders, depression, bipolar disorders, substance dependence, impulse-control disorders, pathological gambling, and eating disorders, among others (Shaffer, 1996).

3. *The extent and etiology of Internet use–related problems.* Much of the original research on Internet use and misuse was exploratory or used potentially problematic research methodology, thereby limiting conclusions, especially about possible causal pathways. Although surveys, for example, help evaluate how people feel about themselves or what problems they may have, they provide a very limited basis for drawing conclusions about the possible role of the Internet in causing such problems. Almost all surveys are based on self-selected data from websites, and few epidemiological surveys have included samples or sampling techniques that are likely to yield representative data. Most surveys also lack mechanisms to control for potential confounds, such as preexisting mental disorders (Grohol, 1999).

4. *Natural course and treatment outcomes.* Unfortunately, China lacks long-term follow-up studies on mental health or other problems potentially linked to Internet use and lacks studies providing systematic evaluation of current Chinese treatment approaches. When conducting a meta-analysis, Byun et al. (2009) uncovered only a few longitudinal studies on the natural course of IA and treatment outcomes. They noted that existing studies adopted inconsistent criteria to define IA, used recruiting methods that could generate serious sampling bias, and primarily examined data using exploratory rather than confirmatory approaches, thereby limiting the ability to go beyond appraising associations.

5. *Policy and legislation issues.* With an increasing penetration into modern society, more Internet-related problems will emerge, making it increasingly essential to guide Internet users in proper and healthy use of this technology. There is also a growing need to help guide relationships between people and people, and people and the Internet society; to clarify various rights, obligations, and responsibilities of Internet users;

and to foster sound moral and ethical values and behavioral codes. All of these efforts require the establishment of ethical guides for the Internet. In addition, the government should strengthen legal education for Internet users, refine and implement punishment guidelines for cybercrimes, and promote constructive legislation that can help prevent crimes from happening in the first place.

References

Betül, A., & Serkan, V. S. (2011). Internet addiction among adolescents: The role of self-esteem. *Procedia Social and Behavioral Sciences, 15*, 3500–05.

Byun, S., Ruffini, C., Mills, J. E., Douglas, A. C., Niang, M., Stepchenkova, S., . . . Blanton, M. (2009). Internet addiction: Metasynthesis of 1996–2006 quantitative research. *CyberPsychology & Behavior, 12*(2), 203–07.

Cass, R. S. (2002). *Republic.com*. Princeton, NJ: Princeton University Press.

Chou, C. (2001). Internet heavy use and addiction among Taiwanese college students: An online interview study. *CyberPsychology & Behavior, 4*(5), 573–85.

Grohol, J. M. (1999). Too much time online: Internet addiction or healthy social interactions? *CyberPsychology & Behavior, 2*(5), 395–401.

Li, G., & Dai, X. Y. (2009). [Control study of cognitive-behavior therapy in adolescents with Internet addiction disorder]. *Chinese Mental Health Journal, 23*(7), 457–60.

Liu, B. L., Hao, W., & Young, D. S. (2004). [The status and problems in the studies of Internet addiction disorders]. *Foreign Medicine: Psychiatry Section, 24*, 199–202.

Liu, B. L., Hao, W., & Young, D. S. (2006). [Case control study on characteristics of 65 cases with Internet addiction disorders]. The seventh national academic annual meeting of the Chinese psychiatric association. Beijing: Central South University, China. https://kns.cnki.net/KCMS/detail/detail.aspx?dbcode=CPFD&dbname=CPFD9908&filename=ZHYX200600001410&v=MDUyMjZPVUtyaWZaZVp2RWlqalVMeklKRjRRUHlYU2RyRzRIdGZNcjQ5RlplOE9EQk5LdWhkaG5qOThUbmpxcXhkRWVN&uid=WEEvREcwSlJHSldTTEYzVDhUSFJQQkppYzdEQ01yWWNIWW9nRFc3bFNPYz0=$9A4hF_YAuvQ5obgVAqNKPCYcEjKensW4IQMovwHtwkF4VYPoHbKxJw!!

Liu, Y., Yang, G. D., & Yao, X. M. (2007). [The effect of pharmacotherapy and psychotherapy with 40 IAD cases]. *Chinese Journal of Drug Abuse Prevention and Treatment, 13*(2), 88–91.

Mossbarger, B. (2008). Is Internet addiction addressed in the classroom? A survey of psychology textbooks. *Computers and Human Behavior, 24*(2), 468–74.

Myers, D. G. (2012). *Social psychology* (11th ed.). New York: McGraw-Hill.

Roger, C. H., Melvyn, W. B. Z., Tammy, Y. T., Anastasia, H. T., Fang, P., Lu, Y. X., . . . Mak, K. K. (2014). The association between Internet addiction and psychiatric co-morbidity: A meta-analysis. *BMC Psychiatry, 14*, 183–92.

Shaffer, H. J. (1996). Understanding the means and objects of addiction: Technology, the Internet, and gambling. *Journal of Gambling Studies, 12*(4), 461–69.

Shaffer, H. J., LaBrie, R. A., & LaPlante, D. A. (2004). Laying the foundation for quantifying regional exposure to social phenomena: Considering the case of legalized gambling as a public health toxin. *Psychology of Addictive Behaviors, 18*(1), 40–48.

Stone, R. (2009). China reins in wilder impulses in treatment of Internet addiction. *Science in Society, 324*(5935), 1630–31.

Tao, R., Huang, X. Q., Wang, J. N., Liu, C. Y., Zhang, H. M., Xiao, L. J., & Yao, S. M. (2008). A proposed criterion for clinical diagnosis of Internet addiction. *Med J Chin PLA, 33*, 1188–91.

Wang, Y. L., Dai, X. Y., Li, Q. L, & Li, G. (2011). [Follow-up study of cognitive behavior therapy on adolescent with Internet addiction disorder]. *Chinese Journal of Behavioral Medicine & Brain Science, 20*(3), 227–30.

Wu, X. H., Chen, X. G., Han, Meng, H., Luo, J. H., Nydegger, L., & Wu, H. R. (2013). Prevalence and factors of addictive Internet use among adolescents in Wuhan, China: Interactions of parental relationship with age and hyperactivity-impulsivity. *PLoS ONE, 8*(4), e61782.

Yang, X. (2006). The theoretical foundation of Internet addiction prevention and treatment. *Nervous Diseases and Mental Health, 04*: 314–17.

Young, K. S. (1999). Internet addiction: Symptoms, evaluation and treatment. In L. VandeCreek & T. Jackson (Eds.), *Innovations in clinical practice: A source book* (Vol. 17; pp. 19–31). Sarasota, FL: Professional Resource Press.

Young, K. S. (2004). Internet addiction: A new clinical phenomenon and its consequences. *American Behavioral Scientist, 48*(4), 402–15.

CHAPTER

10

An Overview of Prevention and Intervention Work in Hong Kong on Health Problems Relating to Internet Use

Thomas Chung

Abstract

The Internet is this era's most important new tool, allowing people to accomplish different tasks anytime, anywhere. Users are spending more time online, and the age at which children begin using Internet is becoming younger. Like many useful tools, before we can make the most benefit of it, we must avoid the dangers and risks brought on by its improper use. Young children, who use the Internet for entertainment, learning, and communicating with others, rely on parents and teachers to guide them in healthy Internet use and to execute control to prevent them from misusing it. This chapter summarizes the work of relevant government departments, nongovernmental organizations, and other institutions in Hong Kong to create a supportive environment for healthy use of the Internet and to tackle health problems relating to its use. These approaches range from education and health promotion to case identification and management of those suffering from harm. Results of these efforts allow the younger generation to make the best use of and gain the maximum benefit from Internet use.

Keywords: Internet, Hong Kong, health promotion, addiction, prevention, intervention

Introduction

Since the invention of the Internet decades ago, health problems associated with its use have been reported and studied around the world. With the increasing popularity of affordable Internet access via different handheld products like smartphones and tablets, more people will likely be affected by excessive use of the Internet and related electronic screen products. Although these new technologies have brought us much convenience and have become integral to our daily lives, they carry potential health risks, particularly when use is excessive.

Although Internet addiction (IA) is not yet classified as a disease, excessive Internet use is worrisome. More children are using the Internet and electronic screen products at younger ages and for increasing amounts of time. In Hong Kong, 93% of the households were using fixed broadband service as at August 2019 and the mobile subscriber penetration rate in the same period was 281% (Telecommunications, 2019). According to the Thematic Household Surveys conducted by the Census and Statistics Department of Hong Kong (Information Technology Usage and Penetration, 2003 & 2018), the proportion of children aged 10–14 years who spend 20–50 hours per week using the Internet increased from 16.3% in 2003 to 52.9% in 2018; with the figures for those aged 15–24 years increasing from 32.3% in 2003 to 68.3% in 2018. According to a survey conducted by the Department of Health in 2017 (Growing up Digital, 2019), the median ages at which preschool children in Hong Kong started using computers and started using tablets were 24 months and 18 months, respectively.

In Hong Kong, different sectors and disciplines in the community, including government bureaus and departments, schools, and nongovernment organizations (NGOs), are providing different programs to various target groups with the aims of preventing various adverse conditions and consequences (including IA) and helping those suspected of engaging in problematic use. The following is a brief account of the work of various government bureaus and departments, public agencies, and NGOs in Hong Kong have performed to prevent and treat health problems relating to Internet use. The list of organizations and information presented here is not exhaustive.

Government Bureaus and Departments

Department of Health

Major functions of the Department of Health (DH) include disease prevention and health promotion through partnership. In view of the increasing use of the Internet and concerns about associated health risks for children and adolescents, the DH convened the Advisory Group on Health Effects on Use of Internet and Electronic Screen Products in December 2013, inviting medical specialists and other professionals to address the issue. The Advisory Group published a report with recommendations in July 2014. Various service units within the DH are actively disseminating the information in their routine services as well as through their health promotion partners, including other government departments, schools, NGOs, and related organizations. The DH is also encouraging its partners to incorporate the recommendations into their services and programs when appropriate.

The DH has been working on this important topic through various channels (e.g., by incorporating relevant information in its health promotion activities). Guidelines for target groups, including children and parents, on such health concerns as restriction of screen time, are available in major health promotion programs, including "Change for Health" (2019) and the "StartSmart@school.hk" (2017).

Health education materials relating to the use of computers, the Internet, and IA are also circulated through various service units. These materials include Smart e-Team for primary school and secondary school students, parents, and teachers, produced by the Student Health Service (Recommendations for Parents, Teachers and Students, 2014); the health promotion articles, "Growing up Digital: Overview of Screen Media Use among Children" and "Trapped in the Net" by the Noncommunicable Disease Division (Growing up Digital, 2019; Trapped in the Net, 2013); and a newsletter for professionals and parents, "Do your 0-5 years old children need electronic screen products?" by the Family Health Service ("Do your 0-5 years old children need electronic screen products?", 2018). In addition, outreach programs by the Student Health Service, which include talks to students and parents on healthy use of the Internet, are conducted regularly, including "Balance in the Net" for Secondary 1–6 students, and "Never Lost in the Net Again" for parents. To reach younger children, animation cartoons on health tips in using the Internet and related electronic devices were produced (Health Tips, 2015) and uploaded in government and partner NGO social networking sites. A designated webpage was developed and maintained by the Student Health Service to promote this health information to the general public (Healthy Use, 2014). The webpage allows visitors to browse and download useful materials and provides relevant links.

Education Bureau

With the rapid development of information and communications technology (ICT), e-learning has become significantly integrated in educational efforts. Instead of avoiding or discouraging the use of ICT, it is more important to be aware of the potential health risks relating to its use—or more particularly its improper use—and to adopt appropriate measures to minimize risks. A significant amount of time that children spend on the Internet and with electronic screen products involves information searches and preparation of homework for academic purposes.

The Education Bureau (EDB) and schools in Hong Kong have taken note of potential adverse health effects and acted accordingly. The response includes the ongoing development of school curricula and learning/teaching resources targeted at different key learning stages, the implementation of cyberbullying awareness programs in schools as part of an anti-bullying campaign, and the provision of training to teachers on various themes like cybersafety and sex relating to digital media. Advice on the use of computer and e-books with respect to visual health has also been provided.

Starting from the Third Strategy on Information Technology in Education (2007/08), the EDB has allocated funding to promote parents' information literacy and assist them in guiding children on the use of information technology at home (Report on the Review Surveys, 2012). In the Fourth Strategy on Information Technology in Education, the EDB further worked on using the potential of Information Technology to enhance interactive learning and teaching experiences as well as to nurture students in becoming ethical users (Report on the Fourth Strategy, 2015).

The EDB has commissioned NGOs to conduct seminars for students, parents, and teachers. To address individual concerns, the EDB has also commissioned NGOs to provide a hotline service staffed by social workers to discuss potential concerns and address the needs of students, parents, and teachers. The EDB has also produced relevant guidelines and resource packages. These products include Cyberbullying and Internet Safety Resources as well as Co-creating a Harmonious School resource package for primary and secondary schools, which contains teaching kits and guidelines for students and parents (Cyberbullying, 2013; Co-creating a Harmonious School, 2013).

Home Affairs Bureau

An especially concerning form of IA is online gambling. In Hong Kong, the Home Affairs Bureau (HAB) is the governmental agency responsible for formulating gambling policy and monitoring its implementation (Gambling Policy, 2008). Current policy calls for restricting gambling opportunities to a limited number of authorized, regulated outlets. At present, such authorized gambling outlets include horse racing organized by the Hong Kong Jockey Club, the Mark Six Lottery, authorized football betting, and gaming activities authorized by the public officer appointed by the Secretary for Home Affairs under the Gambling Ordinance.

The HAB established The Ping Wo Fund in September 2003 to implement various preventive and remedial measures to address gambling-related problems. Major activities include research and studies on gambling-related issues and problems, as well as public education and other measures to prevent or alleviate problems relating to gambling (About Us: The Ping Wo Fund, 2019).

To effectively spread the message of "Say No to Gambling" to all levels of the community, the HAB has produced various television and radio announcements in the public interest (APIs). By showing the audience the potential adverse impacts of gambling on one's health, family, social status, and finances, the APIs' slogans of "Don't Gamble Your Life Away" and "Don't Gamble to Excess" have become widely known to the community.

Over the years, education campaigns by the HAB, such as those just mentioned, have repeatedly emphasized the adverse impact of excessive or illegal gambling on the community and especially on young people. The law stipulates that it is illegal for gambling operators to accept bets from individuals younger than 18 years of age or to allow them to participate in gambling. The HAB also cooperates with relevant government departments, including the EDB, the Police, and the Social Welfare Department (SWD), and with NGOs, particularly youth organizations, to launch education campaigns to remind youth not to engage in underage or illegal gambling.

Office for Film, Newspaper and Article Administration

The Office for Film, Newspaper, and Article Administration (OFNAA) is responsible for film classification, control of obscene and indecent articles, and newspaper registration in accordance with relevant legislation. Among other things, the OFNAA regulates the publication of obscene and indecent articles by enforcing the Control of Obscene and Indecent Articles Ordinance (COIAO) and organizes publicity and public education programs to promote public awareness of the provisions of the COIAO (Office for Film, Newspaper and Article Administration, 2012).

Currently, the COIAO regulates, among others, the publication of obscene and indecent articles on the Internet via Hong Kong-based servers. Such articles are dealt with under a co-regulatory approach, under which the OFNAA works with the Hong Kong Internet Service Providers Association to implement a Code of Practice. As set out in the Code of Practice, if the content under complaint is deemed indecent, the Internet Service Provider (ISP) will request the webmaster to add the required statutory warning notice or remove the indecent article. If the content under complaint is considered obscene, the ISP will block access to the article or request the webmaster to remove it. The ISP may also cancel the account of repeat offenders. The COIAO also regulates all computer and video games published in Hong Kong, with restrictions varying depending on whether obscene and/or indecent content is involved.

The OFNAA organizes publicity and educational programs to promote the COIAO to youngsters, parents, and general public. The OFNAA also conducts talks and workshops for students and parents to promote the use of filtering software.

Office of the Government Chief Information Officer

The establishment of the Office of the Government Chief Information Officer (OGCIO) provides a streamlined government structure and leadership for delivering the ICT functions with the Government and enables the Government to take a proactive, leading role in championing ICT development in the community.

"Smarter Hong Kong, Smarter Living" is the theme of the latest Digital 21 strategy (Public Consultation, 2013). It sets out the framework for Hong Kong to leverage new technologies to propel continuous economic and social development on various fronts. The strategy outlines an array of initiatives under four strategic thrusts:

- *Empowering everyone*: aim to build platforms that enable the public and businesses to realize their aspirations
- *Igniting business innovation*: aim to enhance research and development and provision of open data
- *Supporting a thriving ICT industry*: aim to recognize excellence and facilitate local ICT companies to gain a foothold in the Mainland and overseas markets
- *Transforming and integrating public services*: aim to develop intuitive, personalized, and multiplatform e-services

While the OGCIO is responsible for promoting ICT, it is also concerned about its possible adverse impacts on users. As such, the OGCIO commissioned a 1-year territory-wide "Be NetWise" Internet education campaign from September 2009 to November 2010, with a budget of HK$63 million, to promote the safe and healthy use of the Internet among students, parents, and teachers. (LCQ16: "Be NetWise" Internet Education Campaign, 2010).

The OGCIO also launched and maintains a designated webpage on Internet safety. Various guidelines and materials on the safe use of the Internet cover such topics as cybersafety and prevention of cybercrime, with this information also made available to the general public, students, youth, parents, teachers, and IT professionals (Cyber Security Information Portal, 2014). Meanwhile, year-round campaigns were organized in an ongoing effort to educate the public and increase their knowledge of IT security, such as "Build a Secure Cyberspace 2017- Smart Home, Safe Living", "Build a Secure Cyberspace 2018 –Stay Smart, Keep Cyber Scam Away", "Build a Secure Cyberspace 2019 -Phishing scams? No more!" which includes school visits, seminars and talks, radio programs, and contests (Build a Secure Cyberspace Promotional Campaign, 2020).

Social Welfare Department

Among other tasks, the SWD commissioned three NGOs to each implement the Pilot Cyber Outreaching Project and one Evaluation Study from 2011 to 2015, with funding support from the Lotteries Fund (SWD Review 2011-12 & 2012-13, n.d.). The three pilot projects were further extended in 2015 to 2018 with funding support from the Hong Kong Jockey Club Charities Trust (賽馬會網上青年外展服務, 2016).

In consideration of a wide array of cyber-related youth problems, SWD has been subsidising five NGOs (Cyber Youth Support Team, 2019; Caritas InfinityTeens, 2019; Nite Cat,n.d.; eSm^_^iley, n.d.; uTouch, 2020) to set up cyber youth support team since December 2018. They are aimed at using cyber means to reach out to youth in need, in particular those identified as at-risk/hidden youths. Social workers identify these youth through the Internet through various means, such as use of emails, mobile applications, chat rooms, and online games. Timely intervention and provision of support services will be provided to the engaged at-risk/hidden youth. Referrals are made to other services as needed if follow-up is required.

Nongovernment Organizations

The Hong Kong Federation of Youth Groups

Under the support of the OGCIO, the Hong Kong Federation of Youth Groups (HKFYG) acted as the central coordinator of a territory-wide "Be Netwise Internet Education Campaign" in 2009–2010. Engaging 13 other NGOs and additional organizations, the campaign aimed to foster a healthy Internet culture among children and youth. "Be Netwise" was intended for primary and junior secondary-level students, as well as their parents and teachers, and was designed to enhance awareness of safe and proper Internet behaviors through a wide array of activities at territory-wide and district-based levels.

Activities included massive educational programs, such as talks for students, parents, and teachers; the production of parent handbooks and educational kits; home visits; awareness activities; and developing and implementing a cybersafety portal and supportive hotline services. As part of the campaign, the "NetWise Support Centre for Families" was created to provide multidisciplinary support to youth and parents on issues associated with Internet use. Available services included hotline support, education, counseling, therapeutic treatment, and parent–child mediation. Funding for the Support Centre was later extended beyond 2010. In relation to this program, five surveys were conducted in 2009–2010 on children's behavior in Internet access, views of parents and young people about Internet risks, parenting issues, and cyberbullying among secondary school students. It was found that almost all the children had Internet knowledge, although rates were much lower among parents. There also was a large gap between parents and children in their use of the Internet, with most parents treating the Internet as a tool while children regarded it as an important part of their life (Research Study, 2010). For cyberbullying, 30% of secondary school students reported being bullied and 20% reported having bullying others, with male predominance in both groups. Close to 60% reported witnessing a cyberbullying incident; among these 15% had joined either flaming the incident by forwarding the message or pictures to others or, conversely assisted victims to attack bullies (A Study on Cyberbullying, 2010).

To enhance the service delivery, the HKFYG has launched a Wellness Mind Centre to consolidate the services of the School Social Work Unit, the Student Guidance Team, the Media Counselling Centre, the Youth Wellness Centre, Youthline 2777 8899, uTouch online outreach, stationing school social work teams and student support services to comprehensively address issues related to emotional health, relationships and sex, learning difficulties as well as media literacy (HKFYG Museum, 2013). They adopted narrative approach to help youths explore the possibility of life and minimize the risk of Internet addiction (Wellness Mind Centre, 2020).

Tung Wah Group of Hospitals

The Tung Wah Group of Hospitals (TWGHs) has run a "Say No to Cyber Addiction Project" since 2005. The project aims to enhance public awareness, especially among adolescents, parents, and teachers, on IA and to promote healthy family life through a balanced lifestyle to prevent IA. The project targets primary and secondary students, adolescents who are at risk of IA, youth workers, teachers, and parents. Services include talks, workshops, and treatment groups (Say No to Cyber Addiction, 2005).

TWGHs also launched the Integrated Centre on Addiction Prevention and Treatment (ICAPT) in October 2012, aiming to provide to the general public professional treatment services for multiple addictions, including IA, and comorbid mental health disorders. ICAPT has a multidisciplinary team consisting of psychiatrists, social workers, a clinical psychologist, and a psychiatric nurse to provide a one-stop comprehensive assessment and treatment program including hotline counseling, individual and family counseling, health assessment, and psychological and psychiatric assessment and treatment (Integrated Centre on Addiction Prevention and Treatment, 2013).

Since the launching of ICAPT, the numbers of cases experiencing problematic use of Internet have increased tremendously. To respond to this escalating issue of problem Internet use, TWGHs has funded a project, Project "COOL" since 2015, which provides hotline counseling, intensive counseling, online counseling and outreach, preventive education, treatment groups, treatment camps, and a parent's workshop (Project COOL, 2019). The project has extended until now in response to the huge service demand. The project also collaborates with the Hong Kong Polytechnic University, Interaction Design Lab and Asian Lifestyle Design Lab to design and develop omnipresent solutions including mobile application and household products in addressing IA.

Since September 2015, "COOL" has provided preventive education program to more than 50,000 youths and parents, intensive counseling to more than 300 families with 450 individuals, and more than 65,000 online counseling contacts.

Hong Kong Family Welfare Society

The Hong Kong Family Welfare Society (HKFWS) developed the "Net" Education and Counseling Service in 2004, with the dual aims of increasing public concern about Internet use–related problems, including net addiction, cyberbullying prevention, and youth net problems, and reducing the generation gap in the digital era ("Net" Education and Counselling Service, 2020). Since then, the HKFWS has trained more than 300 young people and parent ambassadors to promote healthy use of the Internet in communities and schools and has organized more than 1,000 talks and activities on healthy Internet use. Resource kits for the use of primary, junior secondary, and senior secondary students, each with an educational compact disc and booklets, are produced and distributed to schools and local groups.

In 2009 and 2012, the HKFWS conducted two studies in understanding cyberbullying among adolescents. As a follow-up to the survey findings, the HKFWS formulated training programs to promote healthy use of the Internet and a "zero tolerance" approach to deal with cyberbullying. In 2016, the HKFWS released the report "A Study on Youth's Digital Usage Habit in Relation to Family Relationships" (「青少年使用數碼產品與家庭關係研究」調查報告, 2016). It indicated that cohesive family relationship, parental involvement, and high parental confidence can facilitate healthy Internet use among adolescents. The HKFWS developed a webpage "Healthy Internet" (healthynet.hk) to promote effective learning through the Internet and to help children and young people develop constructive and healthy Internet attitudes and habits for better family harmony (Healthy Net, 2020).

Commissioned by the EDB, the HKFWS launched a counseling hotline in December 2011 on healthy Internet use, with service components including a telephone hotline and WhatsApp application. More than 1,000 calls are received each year.

Hong Kong Christian Service

To help young individuals with IA regain their self-control over computer use, the Integrated Children and Youth Service (Happy Teens Club) of the Hong Kong Christian Service (HKCS) developed the "Online New Page Project," which first appeared in February 2005 (Online New Page, 2016). This service targets young people between the ages of 6 and 24 years, as well as their parents. The project provides counseling and supportive services for those who use the Internet excessively or are found to be addicted to Internet use. Services include counseling through hotline, outreach, and online agent groups (groups for young people) as well as supportive services through talks and workshops, professional training/sharing sessions, case inquiries, online buddy alliances, and a parent support network.

Public Organization/Hospital Authority

In Hong Kong, public hospitals and medical services are provided by the Hospital Authority, a government-funded public organization. At present, public hospitals in Hong Kong offer no specific treatment services specifically targeted at problematic Internet use. However, if those with problematic Internet use present with comorbid psychiatric conditions, they may be referred to a psychiatrist on a general psychiatric service. Likewise, public hospitals in Hong Kong do not have specific medical treatment teams on pediatric or adolescent health units for Internet-related health problems. General advice may be given to parents if they raise such concerns during a medical consultation (i.e., as part of a generic parenting issue). Excessive use of portable devices may cause pain and damage to wrists, thumbs, neck, and back, and an e-book was published in 2010 to demonstrate finger, hand, and wrist stretching exercises to prevent repetitive strain injuries associated with the use of portable devices (舒筋健指法, 2010).

Conclusion

Various governmental departments, public agencies, and NGOs in Hong Kong have been providing different programs and services to prevent or treat adverse physical and mental health conditions related to problematic use of the Internet and related electronic products. Considering the rapid development and penetration of such technologies into everyday life, as well as the increasing use of the Internet and related products among the general public, there is a pressing need to monitor the public health impacts of excessive technology use closely, with a view toward fine-tuning services. Various groups in Hong Kong should pool evidence, experience, and expertise, working together to strengthen prevention and treatment services to reduce adverse health impacts that may result from use of the Internet and related electronic products.

Acknowledgments

I would like to thank my colleagues in the Department of Health who helped me to put together all relevant information. I would also like to express my gratitude to all colleagues, friends, and partners from other departments and organizations mentioned in this chapter for their contributions, support, and permission on the compilation of information in this chapter.

References

「青少年使用數碼產品與家庭關係研究」調查報告 [Internet]. (2016). Hong Kong Family Welfare Society. https://www.hkfws.org.hk/reports

舒筋健指法 [Internet]. (2010). Hospital Authority. http://www.ha.org.hk/kwh/ebooks/ebook_index.html

賽馬會網上青年外展服務. *(2016). BGCA, Caritas, & HKFYG. http://www.cyberyouthhk.org/*

A Study on Cyber-Bullying Among Hong Kong Secondary Students [Internet]. (2010, September). The Hong Kong Federation of Youth Groups. http://benetwise.hk/download/cyberbully_research.pdf

About Us: The Ping Wo Fund. (2019). The Ping Wo Fund. http://www.donotgamble.org.hk/en/about1.php

Build a Secure Cyberspace Promotional Campaign [Internet]. (2020). Office of the Government Chief Information Officer, Hong Kong Special Administrative Region. https://www.cybersecurity.hk/en/build-a-secure-cyberspace.php

Caritas Infinity Teens-Cyber Youth Support Team [Internet]. (2019). Caritas Hong Kong. http://it.caritas.org.hk/

Change for Health [Internet]. (2019). Centre for Health Protection, Department of Health, Hong Kong Special Administrative Region. https://www.change4health.gov.hk/en/whats_new/health_watch/20190430.html

Co-creating a Harmonious School. (2013). Education Bureau, Hong Kong Special Administrative Region. http://www.edb.gov.hk/en/teacher/student-guidance-discipline-services/gd-resources/co-creating-harmonious-school.html

Cyber-bullying and Internet Safety Resources (website). (2013). Education Bureau, Hong Kong Special Administrative Region. http://www.edb.gov.hk/en/teacher/student-guidance-discipline-services/gd-resources/cyber-bullying-and-internet-safety-resources/index.html

Cyber Security Information Portal [Internet]. (2014). Office of the Government Chief Information Officer, Hong Kong Special Administrative Region. https://www.cybersecurity.hk/en/index.php

Cyber Youth Support Team (Hong Kong Island) - Six Degree Hubs[Internet]. (2019). St. James' Settlement. http://cyberyouth.sjs.org.hk/

Do your 0-5 years old children need electronic screen products? [Internet]. (2018). Family Health Service, Department of Health, Hong Kong Special Administrative Region. https://www.fhs.gov.hk/english/health_info/child/30047.pdf

eSm^_^iley Cyber Youth Support Team [Internet]. (n.d.). Hong Kong Children & Youth Services. https://esmiley.hkcys.hk/

Gambling Policy. District, community and public relations [Internet]. (2008). Home Affair Bureau, Hong Kong Special Administrative Region. http://www.hab.gov.hk/en/policy_responsibilities/District_Community_and_Public_Relations/gambling.htm

Growing up Digital: Overview of Screen Media Use among Children. NCD Watch. (2019, March). Centre for Health Protection, Department of Health, Hong Kong Special Administrative Region. https://www.chp.gov.hk/files/pdf/ncd_watch_march_2019.pdf

Health Tips on Using Internet and Electronic Screen Products [YouTube]. (2015). Student Health Service, Department of Health, Hong Kong Special Administrative Region. https://www.youtube.com/watch?v=C2vuDZ-uoks&index=5&list=PLy8zN7Ql_1rb6I_FTDAWDIKtq6ODNqThN

Healthy Use of Internet and Electronic Screen Products (webpage). (2014). Student Health Service, Department of Health, Hong Kong Special Administrative Region. http://www.studenthealth.gov.hk/english/internet/health_effects.html

HealthyNet [Internet]. (2020). Hong Kong Family Welfare Society. http://healthynet.hk/?lang=en

HKFYG Museum [Internet]. (2013). The Hong Kong Federation of Youth Groups. http://museum.hkfyg.org.hk/hkfyg.php

Information Technology Usage and Penetration. Thematic Household Survey Report No. 15 (2003). Census and Statistics Department, Hong Kong Special Administrative Region. https://www.statistics.gov.hk/pub/B11302152003XXXXB0200.pdf

Information Technology Usage and Penetration. Thematic Household Survey Report No. 67 (2018). Census and Statistics Department, Hong Kong Special Administrative Region. https://www.statistics.gov.hk/pub/B11302672019XXXXB0100.pdf

Integrated Centre on Addiction Prevention and Treatment [Internet]. (2013). Tung Wah Group of Hospitals. http://icapt.tungwahcsd.org/page.aspx?corpname=icapt&i=479&locale=en-US

LCQ16: "Be NetWise" Internet Education Campaign [Internet]. (2010). news.gov.hk, Hong Kong Special Administrative Region. https://www.info.gov.hk/gia/general/201011/03/P201011030161.htm

"Net" Education and Counselling Service [Internet]. (2020). Hong Kong Family Welfare Society. https://www.hkfws.org.hk/en/how-we-help/integrated-children-and-youth-services/net-education-and-counselling-service

Nite Cat Online – Cyber Youth Support Team [Internet]. (n.d.). The Boys' & Girls' Clubs Association of Hong Kong. http://nitecat.bgca.org.hk/tc/

Office for Film, Newspaper and Article Administration, Hong Kong Special Administrative Region. (2012). [Internet] https://www.ofnaa.gov.hk/eng/home/index.htm

Online New Page - Online Addiction Counselling Centre [Internet]. (2016). Hong Kong Christian Service. http://www.hkcs.org/en/services/online

Project COOL: Internet Addiction Prevention and Treatment Service [Internet]. (2019). Tung Wah Group of Hospitals. http://internetaddiction.tungwahcsd.org/.

Public Consultation on 2014 Digital 21 Strategy: Smarter Hong Kong Smarter Living. (2013, September). Commerce and Economic Development Bureau, Hong Kong Special Administrative Region. https://www.ogcio.gov.hk/en/news/consultations/d21_submission_2013/doc/2014D21S-booklet.pdf

Recommendations for Parents, Teachers and Students. (2014). Student Health Service, Department of Health, Hong Kong Special Administrative Region. http://www.studenthealth.gov.hk/english/internet/recommendations/recommendations_parents.html

Report on the Fourth Strategy on Information Technology in Education: Realizing IT potential, unleashing learning power, a holistic approach. (2015, August). Education Bureau, Hong Kong Special Administrative Region. http://www.edb.gov.hk/attachment/en/edu-system/primary-secondary/applicable-to-primary-secondary/it-in-edu/ITE4_report_ENG.pdf

Report on the Review Surveys of the Third Strategy on Information Technology in Education. (2012, December). Education Bureau, Hong Kong Special Administrative Region. http://www.edb.gov.hk/attachment/en/edu-system/primary-secondary/applicable-to-primary-secondary/it-in-edu/RS2_Final%20Report_PUBLIC_Eng_clean%2021012013.pdf

Research Study on Internet Education (Final Report). (2010, July). Published by YMCA of Hong Kong, Department of Social Work and Social Administration, HKU, Policy 21 Limited; central coordinator: The Hong Kong Federation of Youth Groups; supported by Office of the Government Chief Information Officer. http://www.benetwise.hk/download/Final_Report_Internet_Study_5July2010.pdf

Say No to Cyber Addiction Project [Internet]. (2005). Tung Wah Group of Hospitals. http://cyberaddiction.tungwahcsd.org/

StartSmart@school.hk. (2017). Department of Health, Hong Kong Special Administrative Region. http://www.startsmart.gov.hk/en/index.aspx

SWD Review 2011-12 & 2012-13 [Internet]. (n.d.). Social Welfare Department, Hong Kong Special Administrative Region. https://www.swd.gov.hk/annualreport/swdreview2013/en/services-for-young-people.html

Telecommunications. (2019, December). Office of the Communications Authority, Hong Kong Special Administrative Region. http://www.ofca.gov.hk/filemanager/ofca/en/content_113/telecommunications.pdf

Trapped in the Net. NCD Watch. (2013, July). Centre for Health Protection, Department of Health, Hong Kong Special Administrative Region. https://www.chp.gov.hk/files/pdf/ncd_watch_jul2013.pdf

uTouch Cyber Youth Outreach Service [Internet]. (2020). The Hong Kong Federation of Youth Groups. https://utouch.hk/

Wellness Mind Centre [Internet]. (2020). The Hong Kong Federation of Youth Groups. https://wmc.hkfyg.org.hk/wmc/

CHAPTER

11 Networking and Other Social Aspects of Technology Use

Past Developments, Present Impact, and Future Considerations

Rachel Kowert, Emese Domahidi, *and* Thorsten Quandt

Abstract

From the first multiuser dungeons and rudimentary chatrooms to the vast lands of online gaming and incredibly popular social networking sites like Facebook and Twitter, the Internet continues to provide many ways to connect socially. This chapter provides a historical context to the discussion of the social aspects of technology use and their various functionalities to provide users with a sense of social connectedness or embeddedness. The aim of this discussion is to highlight the idiosyncrasies of the different social networking services available today in terms of their ability to connect or disconnect individuals. The chapter concludes with a brief discussion of future considerations for research in this area in terms of how to better understand the impact and utility of social technology in everyday life.

Keywords: technology, digital technology, social networking, social media, video games, social embeddedness

From the humble beginnings of chatrooms to the incredibly popular social networking sites like Facebook and Twitter, the Internet continues to provide endless possibilities to connect its users socially. Although social networking services are often thought of as being similar in more ways than they are different because they all provide the ability to connect socially with others in mediated spaces, the various social platforms available online today vary in their utility, scope, and range of services they provide. To highlight this variability, this chapter overviews the social functionality of several of the more popular social networking services, like social networking sites (SNSs), forums, and blogs, and discuss the variability in their potential capacity to create a sense of social connectedness or embeddedness.

In an attempt to provide a historical context for this discussion, the chapter begins with a brief overview of the rise of social networking services. From a few selected services to the thousands of platforms available today, the Internet now allows us to connect with virtually anyone "anytime, anyplace, and anywhere" (Quinn & Oldmeadow, 2013a, p. 238). Indeed, the choices for connecting with others, both near and far, continue to expand rapidly. Following this, a general overview of several of the more popular social platforms available online today will be presented. This discussion focuses on six distinct categories of Internet-based social networking services (i.e., mailing services, instant/direct messaging, SNSs, online forums and blogs, online games, and content sharing sites) and overviews their unique features, prevalence, popularity, and ability to promote socialization between users.

This broad overview will be followed by a more detailed discussion of the social utility of selected services in promoting or hindering users' sense of social embeddedness or connectedness. The aim of this discussion is to highlight the need to consider the idiosyncrasies of these different social services, particularly when one is discussing any potential positive or negative impacts they may have on individuals. Attention will be directed toward not only the similarities but especially the differences between SNSs and online video games as these two services are vastly different in terms of their perceived propensities to connect or disconnect individuals. Although anecdotal evidence suggests that the use of SNSs may be socially beneficial (e.g., Facebook contributes to a sense of belonging with one's preexisting friendship groups; Quinn & Oldmeadow, 2013b), the use of online video games is often perceived as being "all bad" in terms of their impact on the user (e.g., online game players are perceived to be reclusive, socially inept individuals; Kowert, Griffiths, & Oldmeadow, 2012). However, scientific research in this area is far more nuanced than these gross generalizations, particularly in terms of how these social networking services can impact users' everyday social lives and, more specifically, their social connectedness. Moreover, while recent meta studies could highlight the beneficial association between SNS use and social outcomes, there was no evidence for a negative association of social outcomes with online game use (Domahidi, 2018; Liu, Ainsworth, & Baumeister, 2016).

The chapter concludes with a brief discussion of future considerations for research in this area in terms of how to better understand the impact and utility of social networking technologies in one's everyday life as they continue to grow in popularity and scope.

Historical Overview

Humans are often described as having an innate desire to connect with others (Young, 2008). As such, it is perhaps unsurprising that Internet technologies have been adapted for such purposes. The development of computer-mediated communication (CMC) has freed communication across time and space and removed its traditional geographical, language, and time barriers. In addition to changing the way that individuals communicate and relate to each other (Kiesler & Sproull, 1992; Spears & Lea, 1994) by allowing users to connect with virtually anyone at any time, CMC has equalized communication in a way that was only possible through the relative anonymity and invisibility of the Internet (Spears & Lea, 1994; Suler, 2004). For example, in any particular chat room, online forum, or online game, one may find the old interacting with the young or people from opposite sides of the world engaging in a political debate. In this sense, CMC (and especially via social networking) could help to foster online communities where there is an equality of participation between users (Kiesler & Sproull, 1992; Sproull & Kiesler, 1991; Walther, 1996; Weisband, 1992).

While individuals have been interested in developing new platforms to connect socially with others via the Internet almost since its inception, the development and popularization of such platforms grew slowly. Before 1990, the Internet was primarily used for research by educational organizations (Internet Society, 2014). During this time there were very few social options available on the Internet apart from basic electronic mail (i.e., email) and chat programs or the earliest online games, such as multiuser dungeons (i.e., MUDs). However, post-1990, email and instant messaging quickly gained in popularity. This was soon followed by the popularization of other social networking services, such as SNSs and discussion forums. The propagation of social networking services has continued to demonstrate unabated growth in terms of their development and popularity. Today, one would be hard pressed to find many individuals who have not integrated some form of digital social interaction into their everyday lives (Fox & Rainie, 2014).

Perhaps because of this rapid growth, immense popularity, and generally wide scope, the distinctions between the various Internet-based social networking services have become somewhat distorted. Although they all provide a basis for promoting interaction between users via the Internet, their social utilities—or more specifically their key features and ability to connect users and provide a sense of social connectedness—vary widely. Recognizing the unique characteristics of different mediated social networking services is key to understanding what role these play in our everyday lives, how they are being utilized, and what social impact (if any) they may have on users over time.

For example, the stereotype of players of massively multiplayer online role-playing games (MMORPGs) revolves around themes of being anti-social and reclusive (Kowert & Oldmeadow, 2012). However, these generalizations often fail to recognize that online games are highly social and playful spaces that can foster a strong sense of connectedness between users (Hussain & Griffiths, 2009; Kowert, 2015; Kowert, Vogelgesang, Festl, & Quandt, 2015; Yee, 2007). In fact, the use of online games has also been found to promote social and psychological well-being, such as reduced depression (Bessiere, Kiesler, Kraut, & Boneva, 2004).

A recent but major development for the use of Internet-based social networking services can be attributed to the advent of mobile technologies and smartphones that are widely used worldwide (Taylor & Silver, 2019). Given the new possibilities, users "seem to communicate and interact almost permanently" online (Vorderer & Kohring, 2013, p. 188), particularly through social networking services.

To help clarify some of the similarities and differences across the different available social networking services, the following section provides an overview of several of the more popular available today.

Social Networking Services: A Range of Options

There are innumerable platforms belonging to various social networking services available on the Internet today. While some researchers continue to discuss these services as if they were analogous in popularity, social utility, and scope (e.g., Madden et al., 2013), others have begun to tease apart their unique features and develop categorization systems that can serve as organizational aids. For example, Grahl (2014) has identified six types of social media, including SNSs (e.g., Facebook), bookmarking sites (e.g., Delicious), social news (e.g., Reddit), media sharing (e.g., YouTube), microblogging (e.g., Twitter), and blog comments and forums. Contributors to the Pew Research Internet Project (Duggan & Smith, 2013; Madden et al., 2013) and Childnet International (http://www.childnet.com/) have also made some attempts to categorize these services; however, they have primarily invoked broad classifications focusing on the various SNSs rather than categorizing the range of Internet-based services into several unique classifications. Additionally, until today few studies examine and compare a multitude of Internet-based social networking services and are able to compare their relationship with social outcomes (Domahidi, 2018).

Drawing from previous research, we propose a more comprehensive categorization system for the various Internet-based social networking services available today (see Table 11.1). Each of the six proposed categories is discussed in more detail in upcoming sections. However, it must be noted that any proposed typology of social networking services has inherent shortcomings given the increasing convergence between different services and platforms. These kinds of social networking services are not completely independent as they often unify multiple types of services within them. For example, Facebook is not only a SNS because it is also often used for content sharing and instant messaging. The focus of the proposed categorization system is to identify the primary purpose of each social networking service while remaining mindful that the categories serve mainly analytical purposes. Additionally, as outlined earlier, the rise of mobile technologies and their corresponding applications are transforming social networking services into multifaceted platforms that include networking, content sharing, and instant messaging, among others. To what extent these services will change in the coming years is difficult to forecast although increasing convergence is possible.

Mailing Services: Electronic (E-) Mail

Some may not initially think of email as a social networking technology; however, it was among the first and most basic social service to emerge alongside the popularization of the Internet. While various definitions of email have been proposed, in its broadest form it can be defined as "mail being transmitted electronically" (Tao & Reinking, 1996, p. 3), including the exchange of text-based messages as well images and/or media files. Email grants a user almost instantaneous exchange of data with others, such as personal or institutional information. Perhaps the most distinguishing feature of email is its scope and popularity. Although it is difficult to determine just how many people use email services, a 2019 market report by the Radicati Group Inc. (a technology market research firm) generated estimates of more than 3.9 billion users (Radicati, 2019). The same report predicts that worldwide the number of email users will grow over the next 4 years to more than 4.4 billion in 2023. There are numerous email providers worldwide, including Gmail (~1 billion active users; Lardinois, 2016) and Yahoo (~227.8 million active users; Lunden, 2018).

Instant or Direct Messaging

Instant or direct messaging refers to the near-instantaneous transfer of messages between users over the Internet (Campbell, Rosenberg, Schulzrinne, Huitema, & Gurle, 2002). Typically, these kinds of messages are short and transmitted directly between two users. Depending on the particular platform, instant or direct messages can be transmitted as a whole (i.e., the whole message is sent at once) or character by character, rather than allowing for completion of the message before sending. Instant messaging can be transmitted through a stand-alone platform, such as Skype; via texting services from one's mobile phone; or can be integrated into other services (e.g., Facebook offers instant and direct

Table 11.1 Social networking services matrix

Social networking services and selected prominent platforms	Description of platform	Number of global users (millions)	Key features of platform
Mailing services			
Electronic (E-) mail	The most basic form of text communication and data sharing via the Internet.	3,930,000[1]	One-to-one or one-to-group private messaging, data sharing
Gmail	A popular email service	1,000[2]	
Yahoo Mail	A popular email service	227.8[3]	
Instant/Direct Messaging			
Skype	A platform whose basic function is to (video) telephone both one-to-one or with a group using voice over technology.	1.300[4]	Text, voice, and video conferencing, data sharing, group conferencing/calling
WhatsApp	Mobile instant messaging application. The primary function is private one to one or group chatting. Tends to be used in lieu of traditional SMS functions.	1,500[5]	Private and group instant messaging, data sharing, allows users to "text" across countries and continents via Internet networks and without additional fees
Social Networking Sites			
Facebook	The largest social networking site today. It primarily connects people who already know each other.	2,230[6]	Profile creation, interacting with small and large circles, data sharing, group and private instant messaging, public posting, file sharing
Linkedin	A business platform with the primary function to connect employers and employees.	575[7]	Business networking, recruiting, creating business profiles
Twitter	A SNS service that allows people to publicly post short messages (called "microblogging," up to 140 characters) as well as follow the messages of celebrities, colleagues, and friends.	3,330[8]	Posting texts and pictures, sending and reading private messages, follow celebrities, companies, and other users
Classmates.com	A social networking site to connect (primarily) older generations to each other and helps them to keep contact with former classmates.	70[9]	Photo uploading, group and private instant messaging, public posting, data sharing
Nextdoor	A social networking site targeted toward users in a particular neighborhood	<1 million[10]	Profile creation, recommendations, group and private messaging, data sharing
Online Forums and Blogs			
Reddit	An online forum and news site on which people can submit texts and tag them with key words (subreddits).	542[11]	Information gathering/sharing, news stream functionality, private messaging
Tumblr	A photo blogging service on which users share images with other users.	463.5[12]	Photo uploading, group and private instant messaging, public posting, real-time updates from other users, data sharing
WordPress	A blogging website where users can create text-based blogs.	172[13]	Information gathering/sharing, blogging, embedding photos or video to a site, can be integrated with other social platforms like Facebook or Linkedin

Stack Overflow	Belongs to the Stack Exchange Network, a family of more than 170 Q&A sites. The leading platform for questions and community around programming and developing.	50[14]	Posting questions and answers, having a profile, endorsements and gamified elements
Online Games			
Steam	A free platform made available by Valve that allows users to purchase computer games and network with other players.	1,000[15]	Private and group instant messaging, community building, in-game voice messaging, installation and automatic management of software
World of Warcraft	The most popular online MMORPG on the market today. Players can engage alone or with a group of people to solve missions. Communication serves primarily as an instrument to reach in-game goals.	10.2[16]	Group and private messaging, voice chatting
Content Sharing Sites			
Instagram	A photo and video sharing platform that enables users to edit photos with filters before uploading them.	1,000[15]	Photo sharing and editing, integration with other platforms (e.g., Twitter, Facebook)
Snapchat	A mobile app where users can send and receive pictures, videos, and messages. Unlike other services, the data are deleted after a designated period of time (e.g., 15 seconds).	190[17]	Video, photo, and text sharing
Pinterest	A photo sharing platform that allows users to create and follow theme-based collections of photos and images.	250[18]	Photo sharing, creation and management of theme-based image collections, ability to "follow" and repost other collections
YouTube	An extremely popular video sharing platform. Users can upload videos, create a channel, follow other users and topics.	1,900[19]	Video sharing, creation and management of theme-based channels, interaction with other users, integration with other platforms (e.g., Twitter, Facebook)

1 Radicati (2019).
2 Lardinois (2016).
3 Lunden (2018).
4 Statista (2018b).
5 Constine (2018).
6 Constine (2018).
7 Cooper (2019).
8 Osman (2019).
9 Brown (2015).
10 Nextdoor claims to have 236,000 neighborhoods connected as of June (2019).
11 Statista (2019).
12 Alexa Internet (2018).
13 Barron (2019).
14 Stackoverflow claims to have 50 million users each month as of June (2019).
15 Lanier (2019).
16 Holisky (2012).
17 Constine (2019).
18 Osman (2019).
19 YouTube claims to have 1,900 million users each month as of June 2019.

messaging between linked users). The use of instant and direct messaging is popular across age groups but more prevalent among the younger generations (Krapf, 2010).

Texting may have been the first Internet-based technology to be integrated into telephone technologies, and it remains exceedingly popular today. Mobile technologies have vastly expanded with the advent and popularization of the smartphone, and instant message services became very popular and widespread. For example, Whatsapp is a popular application that permits text messaging and data sharing across phones via Internet networks. This highly popular service (recent reports suggest that there are more than 1.5 billion monthly users; Constine, 2018) differs from traditional texting in allowing users across countries, or even continents, to message for the relatively low cost of the app rather than paying a premium rate per message to their mobile data carriers. It is important to note that through texting services, users are able to send text and multimedia messages, such as pictures and video. Group communication is often supported, too.

Social Networking Sites

SNSs are among the most prevalent (relative to numbers) and popular services available today. While SNSs can cover a range of interests and populations, their services always fall within a system of three defining characteristics: a user can "(1) construct a public or semi-public profile within a bounded system, (2) articulate a list of other users with whom they share a connection, and (3) view and traverse their list of connections and those made by others within the system" (Boyd & Ellison, 2007, p. 211). Consequently, SNSs are designed so that users can build social networks or relationships. SNSs typically also provide various ways to connect with others socially, including group and private instant messaging, public posting, and file sharing.

At present, there are numerous social networking platforms. Facebook is currently the most popular, with more than 2.23 billion monthly users (Clement 2020; Constine, 2018), including millions of new users older than 55 emerging over the last few years (Schaffel, 2018). It is likely that this expansion reflects a growing desire to use social networking services to stay in touch with younger or geographically distant family members. However, it needs to be noted that other SNSs were superseded by Facebook and even struggle to maintain their user base: For example, MySpace, one of Facebook's predecessors and the biggest SNS during the mid-2000s, is in constant decline (Garrahan, 2009). As early as 2011, MySpace was being described as no longer being socially relevant but rather framed as a space for advertisement rather than to connect with others (Kiser, 2011).

There are also several SNSs dedicated to specific kinds of networking or networking within specific locations. For example, Linkedin is primarily aimed at linking employers and employees (Utz, 2015). Consequently, as one might expect, it has a slightly older user base, with 80% of users older than 30 (Beal, 2014). In terms of location-based networking, there are several SNSs with a national, regional, or even local focus, such as Nextdoor, which is dedicated to connecting users who live in a specific neighborhood. Not surprisingly, these kinds of networks tend to be less broadly used than global networks such as Facebook. Several other popular SNSs not discussed here, such as Twitter (which can be considered a specific subtype of SNS, i.e., microblogging), are also outlined in Table 11.1.

Online Forums and Blogs

An online forum, or electronic message board, is an online discussion website where individuals hold conversations in the form of posted messages. The primary difference between online forums and chat rooms is that forum messages are often longer than a single line of text and are (at least temporarily) archived on a server. Online forums are usually organized in a hierarchical structure whereby a forum can contain a number of subforums that may cover several topics. For instance, within the subheading of "Science" there could be several subforums such as "Biology," "Chemistry," and "Physics." In addition to topical forums (e.g., forums organized around a topic, such as "Movies"), forums may revolve around discussions relating to a particular geographical location (e.g., residents of Germany) or a specific demographic (e.g., single mothers). There are now also various general forums available that cover a range of topics and communities. Reddit is one of the largest online forums, with 330 million monthly active users (Hutchinson, 2018) that engage in discussions in among various "subreddits," which are discussions focused on a specific topic of interest.

Online blogs differ from online forums in that the focus is placed on a user's or group's specific perspective, and the forums typically relate to a defined topic. When blogs (short for weblog) became popular in the late 1990s, they were primarily meant as personal diaries and a form of individual self-expression (i.e., a one-way communication device). However, over time, various options for social interaction were integrated into blogs.

Nowadays, discussions are often encouraged by the inclusion of comment sections or dedicated forums. There are also several companies that offer services and web space for easily setting up (micro) blogs. For example, Tumblr, which hosts 463.5 million blog accounts (Statista, 2019b), allows users to post short-form blogs on widely varying topics, such as science, sports, parenting, and art. In general, the user base of such services tends to be quite young: 43% of the people who blog on Tumblr are under the age of 24 (Statista, 2018a).

It is also important to recognize Q&A sites that specialize in allowing users to ask a question that will be answered by another user. One of the most popular platforms is the Stack Exchange Network to which the famous Q&A site Stack Overflow belongs. Stack Exchange Network hosts more than 170 Q&A sites on specific topics (Vasilescu, Serebrenik, Devanbu, & Filkov, 2014). While users remain anonymous, they provide each other with support and information, with the community of users being the focus, as with other online forums and blogs. Social networking is often connected with reputation systems and gamified elements in Q&A sites (Vasilescu et al., 2014).

Online Games

Video games are perhaps a surprising category when talking about social networking online—however, online (video) games are very relevant interaction and communication environments for a high number of users. Simply put, online video games are video games that are played over the Internet (Kowert, 2015). The introduction of the online element to preexisting video game technologies has vastly expanded their multiplayer functionality by allowing players to connect with others in a shared gaming space beyond the boundaries of their geographical location. As Smyth (2007) stated, the addition of this multiplayer dimension has changed video game play from "a solitary or small group activity into a large, thriving social network" (p. 178).

Social interaction in online games can take many forms. For example, players can converse in-game using a chat room–like interface. Such interactions might involve all other players in their particular region, groups of players sharing a specific area of expertise (e.g., players share the same in-game role, such as "healer"), or a smaller group of players that has formed for a specific reason (e.g., players who have formed a collective for the purposes of overcoming a particularly difficult in-game challenge). Players are typically also able to instant or direct message other players using a one-on-one private chat function, sometimes referred to as "whispering." (Players can also augment text-based chat within online games with voice-over technologies, such as Teamspeak or Skype, which allows them to talk in real-time. However, there are limited data on the use and prevalence rates of these kinds of technologies. As such, this discussion remains focused on text-based, in-game communication.)

Outside of the game context, there are further opportunities to engage with the broader game-playing community through the use of game-specific online forums. In this sense, online games are unique in that they encompass various forms of social networking (i.e., SNSs, online forums, and instant and direct messaging) within the context of a shared activity.

Online video games are very popular activities, and not just among young people as is sometimes assumed (e.g., Kowert et al., 2012; Kowert & Oldmeadow, 2012). The age range of players who engage in online video game play spans more than 60 years, with only one-quarter of game players being teenagers (Brown, 2017). There are more online players in their 30s than in their 20s (Ghuman & Griffiths, 2012; Kowert et al., 2012; Williams, Yee, & Caplan, 2008), indicating that online game play is an activity enjoyed by a wide age range.

Content Sharing Sites

The increased access to and popularity of web-based applications combined with high-speed Internet connections have made it easy for users to share a variety of content online with others (Hargittai & Walejko, 2008). While content sharing is possible on other platforms as well, these content sharing sites have a specific focus: the capability to upload user-created content and distribute it to other users. User-generated content ranges from pictures or videos to music. Content sharing platforms can be highly social: they often encourage the evaluation of shared content via endorsements and comments. Additionally, users can often follow other users, and this supports network building.

Instagram is one of the most popular content sharing sites. With a database of more than 1 billion users (Constine, 2018), Instagram allows its members to share and comment on pictures with their friends as well as with all other users of the application. Content sharing sites are utilized more frequently among younger age groups. For example, 72% of Instagram users are between the ages of 13 and 17 (West, 2019). Similarly, 69% of Snapchat users (a photo and video sharing service) are under 17 (West, 2019). While adolescence and young adulthood is the time when users show a greater use of content sharing technologies, not everyone can profit equally form these possibilities. Research showed, for example, that creative activity in an online setting and the sharing of content is associated with young users' socioeconomic status (Hargittai & Walejko, 2008).

YouTube, a popular video sharing platform, was the most used platform in the United States in 2019 (Perrin & Anderson, 2019): 73% of all US adults claimed to use the platform. Among, 18- to 29-year-olds, the rate rises to 91%. Just over half (51%) of YouTube users say they visit the site daily.

Other sites offer the sharing of other content like music (e.g., Spotify) but have a smaller user base compared to photo or video sharing sites, partly consisting of paying customers (Porter, 2019). All of the mentioned content sharing platforms offer various networking options like following other users and the possibility to comment and endorse content.

Other Social Networking Services and Platforms

The overview of Internet-based social networking services just provided is not exhaustive but rather intended to touch on some of the more popular social services and platforms available online today. We had to omit certain services for varying reasons, like popularity of the application or its scope. For example, chat rooms were not included as an independent category. The use of online chat rooms has declined significantly in popularity since 2000 (Lenhart, Madden, Smith, & Macgill, 2007), and they are no longer a central platform from which Internet users choose to socialize with other users. A discussion of online dating services was not covered in our overview of Internet-based social services either, and there are numerous other interactions that may be possible via the Internet—and that may or may not be regarded as being "social" (like online shopping, etc.).

Even within the categories presented, the list of examples and unique platforms was far from comprehensive. For instance, in reference to online games alone, there are thousands of online games available that range from the more casual browser games to the large and immersive worlds of MMORPGs. The examples mentioned here were simply intended to provide a glimpse into the variety of platforms that are currently available within the different categories of communication technologies, rather than being an all-inclusive list.

Exploring Associations Between Social Networking Site Use, Online Video Game Play, and Social Embeddedness

As evidenced from the preceding discussion, various forms of Internet-based social networking services are currently available that differ in popularity, primary user base, and main social utility and scope. Such variations influence the extent to which these outlets can impact users and promote socialization among them. The potential impact of CMC use has been widely discussed in public discourse and has been a popular research topic across disciplines (Domahidi, 2018). However, systematic evaluation of the services and platforms themselves has been lacking, leading at times to arbitrary differences in research agendas intended to address if and how these different social networking services are helpful or harmful (socially) to their users (Domahidi, 2018; Liu et al., 2016).

On the one hand, these technologies have created the greatest advancement in connecting individuals across geographical boundaries since the advent of the telephone. On the other hand, there is a growing concern that the asynchronous and text-based nature of CMC technologies, and their capacity to connect relative strangers, may be socially detrimental. For example, such use may contribute to the displacement of one's preexisting friends, who are valuable sources of social and emotional support, for more diffuse online relationships (Galston, 2000; Kowert, Domahidi, Festl, & Quandt, 2014; Kraut et al., 1998; Slouka, 1995). These concerns about adverse outcomes can be framed in terms of the impact that CMC may have on users' social embeddedness or "the connections that individuals have to significant others in their social environments" (Barrera, 1986, p. 415).

More generally, social embeddedness refers to the quantity of individuals' social relationships, including both strong and weak ties (Barrera, 1986; Granovetter, 1977). The degree to which someone is socially embedded can be quantified as the actual number of members in one's social network who can potentially lead to increases in social resources like social support (Barrera, 1986) or social capital (for an overview of social capital, see Putnam, 2000). The primary question of interest is whether CMC is impacting on one's degree of social embeddedness and, if so, the extent to which such influences are positive (through social augmentation processes; i.e., that relationships formed online add to offline relationships and enrich users sociability) or negative (secondary to social displacement; i.e., that increased time spent with online contacts almost inevitably decreases time spent with offline contacts) (Kowert, 2015; Kraut et al., 1998; Nie, 2001; Nie & Erbring, 2002; Shen & Williams, 2011). There are certainly other topics of focused research regarding CMC, like life satisfaction (Orben, Dienlin, & Przybylski, 2019), problematic use (Scharkow, Festl, & Quandt, 2014), and other social resources (Domahidi, 2018; Domahidi, Breuer, Kowert, Festl, & Quandt, 2016; Kowert et al., 2015). However, social embeddedness remains widely discussed and is a major indicator of both the positive and negative effects of CMC.

However, it would be erroneous to begin with the assumption that the use of any particular social networking service will be associated with outcomes that are either all good (e.g., social augmentation) or all bad (e.g., social displacement). As Shen and Williams (2011) explain, "The Internet is a malleable medium that allows for both social and asocial use" (p. 126). Yet research examining the impacts of CMC on its users has often framed the issue of impact dichotomously, in particular in terms of its impact on a user's social embeddedness.

We cannot discuss all of the social services mentioned in the previous section in detail. Hence, the discussion will focus on SNSs and online games because they are two of the more popular and culturally relevant services in terms of user base and public debate. Of course, the differences between other social services are equally relevant and, in some cases, have been mentioned in our overview of technologies. The following discussion should be understood as an exemplification of the argument that substantial differences exist across presently available social services.

Social Embeddedness and Online Games

Almost since their inception, the impact of online digital games on user's offline and online relationships has been a focus of research. While online games provide a social environment where users maintain old friendships as well build new ones (Cole & Griffiths, 2007; Steinkuehler & Williams, 2006), they also potentially lead to social isolation, particularly in the case of excessive or addictive play (Domahidi & Quandt, 2014; Griffiths & Hunt, 1998; Wan & Chiou, 2006). For example, researchers have found that online game players begin to neglect their preexisting offline friends (Williams, 2006) and family (Shen & Williams, 2011) as their play increases, particularly when playing with strangers. However, these concerns may be exaggerated, as Domahidi, Scharkow, and Quandt (2013) found that online game players primarily engage online with their preexisting contacts. Thus, rather than displacing offline relationships for online ones, players are embedding their social online experiences in their offline lives. As with other shared activities (such as being a member of a sports team/club), playing and talking about games can become deeply embedded within one's friendship network and improve friendship quality (De Grove, 2014).

Thus, taken together, the research in this area suggests that online games can both augment and displace friendships depending on the user and the ways in which the games are being utilized in daily life (e.g., addictive or non-addictive play, playing with preexisting contacts or relative strangers, etc.). Before continuing, it must be noted that the aforementioned research primarily employed convenience samples of highly engaged gamers. These selective samples limit the ability to generalize findings to the overall population, which consists of more active (e.g., "core") gamers and less active (e.g., "casual") gamers or players. This sampling issue is important because online video game play is a widespread phenomenon, with highly involved gamers being just one subgroup among many (Lenhart et al., 2007; Lenhart, Jones, & Macgill, 2008).

Overcoming this limitation, Domahidi, Festl, and Quandt (2014) obtained a representative sample and evaluated social embeddedness among social online game players and non-players. No significant differences were found between the two groups in regard to the number of their friends. The researchers suggested that this may have been due to high rates of "modality switching" (Ramirez & Zhang, 2007) among players, whereby they integrate their online friends in their offline environments and their offline friends into online contexts (Domahidi et al., 2014). Follow-up studies demonstrated that shy users may particularly benefit from playing social online games. Engaging in the communal and playful environments of online games can help such individuals overcome social difficulties that may have hindered friendship formation in traditional contexts

(Kowert et al., 2014). However, these effects were of small magnitude, thereby suggesting that media use has only a limited impact on friendship formation among shy users and that there may be other more important explanatory variables such as players' motivations (Domahidi, et al., 2014, Yee, 2007), personality (Lo, Wang & Fang, 2005), or social ability (Kowert & Oldmeadow, 2012).

Social Embeddedness and Social Networking Sites

Online and offline friendships have been discussed under a somewhat different viewpoint when examining the use of SNSs. Initially, SNS friends were framed as being not "real" friends, and fears were voiced that people might forget what "real" friendships are. When everyone is a "friend" (friendship provides SNS's central metaphor, as most sites call within-site connections "friends"; Baym & Ledbetter, 2009, p. 410), people may lose sight of their "real" close friends and, consequently, experience a decline in social capital.

The research community meanwhile paints a more optimistic picture, as scholars have found that users of SNS primarily employ this technology to interact with preexisting offline ties rather than to meet new people (Ellison, Steinfield & Lampe, 2007). In this sense, SNSs mirror and expand already existing social networks. In a follow-up study, Ellison, Gray, Lampe, and Fiore (2014) concluded that the total number of friends one has on one's social network (e.g., Facebook) does not significantly impact one's social capital either positively or negatively. In general, several studies have focused on the impact of online/offline contacts on users' well-being and self-esteem or life satisfaction (e.g. Orben et al., 2019; Reinecke & Trepte, 2014). Furthermore, the impact of SNS use on adolescents' sense of belonging has been of particular interest over the past decade (Cheung, Chiu, & Lee, 2011; Quinn & Oldmeadow, 2013a, 2013b). This line of research suggests that various friendship benefits are gained through the use of these sites, with non-users missing out on these opportunities.

In contrast, there is some suggestion that, among socially vulnerable populations such as children and adolescents, SNSs may have an augmenting impact. Valkenburg, Peter, and Schouten (2006) found that the use of SNSs by adolescents can stimulate the relationships formed through the site. Other researchers have found SNS use was associated with a higher quality of offline friendships in adolescents (Reich, Subrahmanyam, & Espinoza, 2012). However, the results from the longitudinal analyses of this research indicate that higher friendship quality predicts higher SNS use and not vice versa, suggesting that media multiplexity is indeed important for maintaining strong ties.

Conclusion and Future Considerations

As social uses of the Internet continue to expand in popularity and scope, concordant growth has occurred in researchers' interest in the uses, applications, and impact of Internet-based social networking services. While all of these services can be viewed as falling under the umbrella of "social networking" because all of the Internet-based social platforms connect users socially, one must remain mindful of the wide range in scope, utility, and potential positive or negative influence on those who use them and across various platforms.

As evidenced by the body of research described in this chapter, outcomes relating to the impact of CMC technologies are not uniform. Research evaluating the impact of online video game use and users' social embeddedness has concluded that playing online games can help to build social capital at best and that it does not contribute to a substantial detriment in terms of social displacement on preexisting offline networks. Conversely, the primary use of SNSs was found to be maintaining social relationships. While preexisting networks are strengthened, new relationships are rarely formed and remain mostly weak ties. However, the latter research line focused less on questioning users' social embeddedness as a result of SNSs use and more on the effects of these relationship on other concepts like well-being.

Further research in this area should remain mindful of the idiosyncrasies of these technologies. Although all Internet-based social services may share certain common features, they are unique in a wide variety of other ways. Not only do they vary greatly in terms of their primary scope, age group, and modality of use (e.g., via one's home computer, game console, or mobile devices), no two platforms are analogous in terms of the range of social services they provide. For instance, while one can text message and share photos and audio files to one or a group of people via Whatsapp, users of online games are able to do all of these same things and more through in- and out-of-game social services tailored to the online gaming community. Furthermore, users seem to use these different technologies in unique ways. While online games are often (and most likely also predominantly) played with strangers, SNS communication occurs primarily with one's preexisting social contacts. Accordingly, newer studies should focus on concepts like "affordances" that describe the qualities of a technology in conjunction with user perceptions of its utility (Treem & Leonardi, 2012).

As these technologies continue to become integrated into everyday life, we will likely see a corresponding increase in scholarship evaluating the uses of such social services. As such, we call for a more nuanced approach to evaluating these technologies, particularly when assessing their potential positive or negative social impact on the user, their social group, and society at large. One must consider the characteristics of the social services themselves as well as the unique qualities of the users who engage with them.

References

Alexa Internet. (2018). Reddit.com SiteInfo. https://www.alexa.com/siteinfo/reddit.com

Barrera, M. (1986). Distinctions between social support concepts, measures, and models. *American Journal of Community Psychology, 14*, 413–45. doi:10.1007/BF00922627

Barron, B. (2019, May 12). 25 astonishing WordPress facts that will blow your mind. www.whoishostingthis.com/compare/wordpress/stats/

Baym, N. K., & Ledbetter, A (2009). Tunes that bind? *Information, Communication & Society, 12*(3), 408–27. doi: 10.1080/13691180802635430

Beal, A. (2014). Facebook is the most visited social network; Twitter and Google+ tied for 3rd. *Marketing Pilgrim.*

Bessiere, K., Kiesler, S., Kraut, R., & Boneva, B. (2004). Longitudinal effects of internet uses on depressive affect: A social resources approach. *Unpublished manuscript, Carnegie Mellon University*, Pittsburg, PA.

Boyd, D. M., & Ellison, N. B. (2007). Social network sites: Definition, history, and scholarship. *Journal of Computer-Mediated Communication, 13*, 210–30. doi:10.1111/j.1083-6101.2007.00393.x

Brown, A. (2017). *Younger men play video games, but so do a diverse group of other Americans.* Pew Research Center. https://www.pewresearch.org/fact-tank/2017/09/11/younger-men-play-video-games-but-so-do-a-diverse-group-of-other-americans/

Campbell, B., Rosenberg, J., Schulzrinne, H., Huitema, C., & Gurle, D. (2002). Session Initiation Protocol (SIP) extension for instant messaging. *IETF.* http://www.ietf.org/rfc/rfc3428.txt

Cheung, C. M. K., Chiu, P. Y., & Lee, M. K. O. (2011). Online social networks: Why do students use Facebook? *Computers in Human Behavior*, 27(4), 1337–43. doi: 10.1016/j.chb.2010.07.028

Clement, J. (2020, February 14). Most popular social networks worldwide as of January 2020, ranked by number of active users. *Statista.* Retrieved from https://www.statista.com/statistics/272014/global-social-networks-ranked-by-number-of-users/

Cole, H., & Griffiths, M. D. (2007). Social interactions in massively multiplayer online role-playing gamers. *CyberPsychology & Behavior, 10*(4), 575–83. doi: 10.1089/cpb.2007.9988

Constine, J. (2018). *WhatsApp hits 1.5 billion monthly users. $19B? Not so bad.* TechCrunch.com. https://techcrunch.com/2018/01/31/whatsapp-hits-1-5-billion-monthly-users-19b-not-so-bad/

Constine, J. (2019). *Snapchat revives growth in Q1 beat with 190M users.* TechCrunch.com. https://techcrunch.com/2019/04/23/snapchat-q1-2019-earnings/

Cooper, C. (2019, February 27). *23 Pintrest statistics that matter to marketers in 2019.* https://blog.hootsuite.com/pinterest-statistics-for-business/

De Grove, F. (2014). Youth, friendship, and gaming: A network perspective. *Cyberpsychology, Behavior, and Social Networking, 17*(9), 603–608. doi: 10.1089/cyber.2014.0088

Domahidi, E. (2018). The associations between online media use and users' perceived social resources: A meta-analysis. *Journal of Computer-Mediated Communication, 23*(4), 181–200. doi: 10.1093/jcmc/zmy007

Domahidi, E., Breuer, J., Kowert, R., Festl, R., & Quandt, T. (2016). A longitudinal analysis of gaming- and non-gaming-related friendships and social support among social online game players. *Media Psychology, 21*(2), 288–307. doi:10.1080/15213269.2016.1257393

Domahidi, E., Festl, R., & Quandt, T. (2014). To dwell among gamers—Investigating the relationship between social online game use and gaming-related friendships. *Computers in Human Behavior.* doi:10.1016/j.chb.2014.02.023.

Domahidi, E., & Quandt, T. (2014). "And all of a sudden my life was gone . . ." A biographical analysis of highly engaged adult gamers. *New Media & Society.* doi:10.1177/1461444814521791.

Domahidi, E., Scharkow, M., & Quandt, T. (2013). Real friends and virtual life? Computer games as foci of activity for social community building. In P. Moy (Ed.), *Communication and community* (pp. 149–69). New York: Hampton Press.

Duggan, M., & Smith, A. (2013). *Social media update 2013.* http://www.pewinternet.org/2013/12/30/social-media-update-2013/

Ellison, N. B., Gray, R., Lampe, C., & Fiore, A. T. (2014). Social capital and resource requests on Facebook. *New Media & Society, 16*(7), 1104–21. doi: 10.1177/1461444814543998

Ellison, N. B., Steinfield, C., & Lampe, C. (2007). The benefits of Facebook "friends": Social capital and college students' use of online social network sites. *Journal of Computer-Mediated Communication, 12*(4), 1143–68. doi: 110.1111/j.1083-6101.2007.00367.x

Fox, S., & Rainie, L. (2014). *The Web at 25 in the US.* http://www.pewinternet.org/2014/02/27/the-web-at-25-in-the-u-s/

Galston, W. A. (2000). Does the Internet strengthen community. *National Civic Review, 89*(3), 193–202.

Garrahan, M. (2009). The rise and fall of MySpace. *Financial Times.* https://www.ft.com/content/fd9ffd9c-dee5-11de-adff-00144feab49a

Ghuman, D., & Griffiths, M. D. (2012). A cross-genre study of online gaming: Player demographics, motivation for play, and social interactions among players. *International Journal of Cyber Behavior, Psychology, and Learning, 2*(1), 13–29. doi: 10.4018/ijcbpl.2012010102

Grahl, T. (2014). The 6 types of social media. *Out:think.* http://outthinkgroup.com/tips/the-6-types-of-social-media

Granovetter, M. S. (1977). The strength of weak ties. In *Social Networks* (pp. 347–367). Academic Press. doi: 10.1016/B978-0-12-442450-0.50025-0

Griffiths, M. D., & Hunt, N. (1998). Dependence on computer games by adolescents. *Psychological Reports, 82*(2), 475–80. doi: 10.2466/pr0.1998.82.2.475

Hargittai, E., & Walejko, G. (2008). The participation divide: Content creation and sharing in the digital age. *Information, Communication & Society, 11*(2), 239–56. doi: 10.1080/13691180801946150

Holsky, A. (2012, February, 9). World of Warcraft subscriber numbers dig 100000 to 10.2 million. *WoW Insider*. Retrieved from wow.joystiq.com/2012/09/09/world-of-warcraft-subscriber-numbers/

Hussain, Z., & Griffiths, M. (2009). The attitudes, feelings, and experiences of online gamers: A qualitative analysis. *Cyberpsychology and Behavior, 12*(6), 747–53. doi: 10.1089/cpb.2009.0059

Hutchinson, A. (2018). Reddit now has as many users as Twitter, and far higher engagement rates. https://www.socialmediatoday.com/news/reddit-now-has-as-many-users-as-twitter-and-far-higher-engagement-rates/521789/

Internet Society. (2014). *A brief history of the Internet & related networks*. http://www.internetsociety.org/internet/what-internet/history-internet/brief-history-internet-related-networks

Kiesler, S., & Sproull, L. (1992). Group decision making and communication technology. *Organizational Behavior and Human Decision Processes, 52*(1), 96–123. doi: 10.1016/0749-5978(92)90047-B

Kiser, P. (2011). *Who uses Facebook, Twitter, LinkedIn, MySpace—social media update: 4th Q 2010 and 1st Q 2011*. http://paulkiser.wordpress.com/2011/04/12/who-uses-facebook-twitter-linkedin-myspace-?-social-media-update-4th-q-2010-and-1st-q-2011/

Kowert, R. (2015). *Video games and social competence*. New York: Routledge.

Kowert, R., Domahidi, E., Festl, R., & Quandt, T. (2014). Social gaming, lonely life? The impact of digital game play on adolescents' social circles. *Computers in Human Behavior, 36*, 385–90. doi: 10.1016/j.chb.2014.04.003

Kowert, R., Griffiths, M. D., & Oldmeadow, J. A. (2012). Geek or chic? Emerging stereotypes of online gamers. *Bulletin of Science, Technology & Society, 32*(6), 471–79. doi:10.1177/0270467612469078

Kowert, R., & Oldmeadow, J. A. (2012). The stereotype of online gamers: New characterization or recycled prototype? In *Nordic DiGRA: Games in Culture and Society conference proceedings* (pp. 1–13). Tampere, Finland: DiGRA.

Kowert, R., Vogelgesang, J., Festl, R., & Quandt, T. (2015). Psychosocial causes and consequences of online video game play. *Computers in Human Behavior, 45*, 51–58. doi: 10.1016/j.chb.2014.11.074

Krapf, E. (2010, August). Profiling the Skype user: Female, young, well-off. *Nojitter.com*. http://www.nojitter.com/post/226600277/profiling-the-skype-user-female-young-wellof

Kraut, R,, Patterson, M., Lundmark, V., Kiesler, S., Mukopadhyay, T., & Scherlis, W. (1998). Internet paradox: A social technology that reduces social involvement and psychological well-being? *American Psychologist, 53*(9), 1017–31.

Lanier, L. (2019, April 30). Steam now has one billion accounts (and 90 million active users). *Variety.com*. https://variety.com/2019/gaming/news/steam-one-billion-accounts-1203201159/

Lardinois, F. (2016, February 1). Gmail now has more than 1B monthly active users. *TechCruch*. https://techcrunch.com/2016/02/01/gmail-now-has-more-than-1b-monthly-active-users/

Lenhart, A., Madden, M., Smith, A., & Macgill, A. (2007). Teens' online activities and gadgets. *Pew Research Center*. http://www.pewinternet.org/2007/12/19/teens-online-activities-and-gadgets/visiting-a-chatroom-has-declined-significantly-in-popularity-since-2000

Lenhart, A., Jones, S., & Macgill, A. R. (2008). *Adults and Video Games*. Pew Internet & American Life Project.

Liu, D., Ainsworth, S. E., & Baumeister, R. F. (2016). A meta-analysis of social networking online and social capital. *Review of General Psychology, 20*(4), 369–91. doi:10.1037/gpr0000091

Lo, S., Wang, C., & Fang, W. (2005). Physical interpersonal relationships and social anxiety among online game players. *Cyberpsychology and Behavior, 8*(1), 15–20. doi: 10.1089/cpb.2005.8.15

Lunden, I. (2018, May). Yahoo mail aims at emerging markets and casual users, launches versions for mobile web and Android Go. *TechCrunch*. https://techcrunch.com/2018/06/19/yahoo-mail-go/

Madden, M., Lenhart, A., Cortesi, S., Gasser, U., Duggan, M., Smith, A., & Beaton, M. (2013). *Teens, social media, and privacy*. http://www.pewinternet.org/files/2013/05/PIP_TeensSocialMediaandPrivacy_PDF.pdf

Nie, N. (2001). Sociability, interpersonal relations, and the internet: Reconciling conflicting findings. *American Behavioral Scientist, 45*, 420–35. doi: 10.1177/00027640121957277

Nie, N., & Erbring, L. (2002). Internet and mass media: A preliminary report. *IT & Society, 1*(2), 134–41.

Orben, A., Dienlin, T., & Przybylski, A. K. (2019). Social media's enduring effect on adolescent life satisfaction. *Proceedings of the National Academy of Sciences, 116*(21), 10226–28. doi: 10.1073/pnas.1902058116

Osman, M. (2019, May 24). Mind-blowing Linkedin statistics and facts. *Kinsta*. https://kinsta.com/blog/linkedin-statistics/

Perrin, A., & Anderson, M. (2019). Share of US adults using social media, including Facebook, is mostly unchanged since 2018. *Pew Research Center*. https://www.pewresearch.org/fact-tank/2019/04/10/share-of-u-s-adults-using-social-media-including-facebook-is-mostly-unchanged-since-2018/

Porter, J. (2019). Spotify is first to 100 million paid subscribers. *The Verge*. https://www.theverge.com/2019/4/29/18522297/spotify-100-million-users-apple-music-podcasting-free-users-advertising-voice-speakers

Putnam, R. (2000). *Bowling alone: The collapse and revival of American community*. New York: Simon & Schuster.

Quinn, S., & Oldmeadow, J. (2013a). The martini effect and social networking sites: Early adolescents, mobile social networking and connectedness to friends. *Mobile Media & Communication, 1*, 237–47. doi:10.1177/2050157912474812

Quinn, S., & Oldmeadow, J. (2013b). Is the igeneration a "we" generation? Social networking use among 9–13 year-olds and belonging. *Journal of Developmental Psychology, 31*(1), 136–42. doi: 10.1111/bjdp.12007

Radicati, S. (2019). *Email Market, 2019–2023*. https://www.radicati.com/wp/wp-content/uploads/2019/04/Email-Market-2019-2023-Executive-Summary.pdf

Ramierez Jr, A., & Zhang, S. (2007). When online meets offline: The effect of modality switching on relational communication.

Communication Monographs, 74(3), 287–310. doi: 10.1080/03637750701543493

Reich, S. M., Subrahmanyam, K., & Espinoza, G. (2012). Friending, IMing, and hanging out face-to-face: Overlap in adolescents" online and offline social networks. *Developmental Psychology, 48*(2), 356. doi: 10.1037/a0026980

Reinecke, L., & Trepte, S. (2014). Authenticity and well-being on social network sites: A two-wave longitudinal study on the effects of online authenticity and the positivity bias in SNS communication. *Computers in Human Behavior, 30*, 95–102. doi: 10.1016/j.chb.2013.07.030

Schaffel, G. (2018, February, 20). It's official: Facebook is becoming the platform for you. *AARP*. https://www.aarp.org/home-family/personal-technology/info-2018/facebook-users-age-fd.html

Scharkow, M., Festl, R., & Quandt, T. (2014). Longitudinal patterns of problematic computer game use among adolescents and adults—A 2-year panel study. *Addiction, 109*(11), 1910–17. doi: 10.1111/add.12662

Shen, C., & Williams, D. (2011). Unpacking time online: Connecting Internet and massively multiplayer online game use with psychological well-being. *Communication Research, 20*(10), 1–27. doi:10.1177/0093650210377196

Slouka, M. (1995). *War of the worlds: Cyberspace and the high-tech assault on reality*. New York: Basic.

Smyth, J. (2007). Beyond self-selection in video game play. *Cyberpsychology and Behavior, 10*(5), 717–21. doi: 10.1089/cpb.2007.9963

Spears, R., & Lea, M. (1994). Panacea or panopticon? The hidden power in computer-mediated communication. *Communication Research, 21*, 427–59. doi: 10.1177/009365094021004001

Sproull, L., & Kiesler, S. (1991). *Connections: New ways of working in the networked organization*. Cambridge, MA: MIT Press.

Statista. (2018a). *Percentage of US Internet users who use Tumblr as of January 2018, by age*. https://www.statista.com/statistics/246214/share-of-us-internet-users-who-use-tumblr-by-age-group/

Statista. (2018b). *Number of estimated Skype users registered worldwide from 2009 to 2024*. https://www.statista.com/statistics/820384/estimated-number-skype-users-worldwide/

Statista. (2019a). *Number of monthly active Twitter users worldwide from 1st quarter 2010 to 1st quarter 2019*. https://www.statista.com/statistics/282087/number-of-monthly-active-twitter-users/

Statista. (2019b). *Cumulative total of Tumblr blogs from May 2011 to April 2019 (in millions)*. https://www.statista.com/statistics/256235/total-cumulative-number-of-tumblr-blogs/

Steinkuehler, C. A., & Williams, D. (2006). Where everybody knows your (screen) name: Online games as "third places." *Journal of Computer-Mediated Communication, 11*(4), 885–909. doi: 10.1111/j.1083-6101.2006.00300.x

Suler, J. (2004). The online disinhibition effect. *Cyberpsychology and Behavior, 7*(3), 321–26. doi: 10.1089/1094931041291295

Tao, L., & Reinking, D. (1996). What research reveals about email in education. In *Information analyses*. Charleston, SC: College Reading Association, p. 1–16. http://files.eric.ed.gov/fulltext/ED408572.pdf

Taylor, K., & Silver, L. (2019). Smartphone ownership is growing rapidly around the world, but not always equally. *Pew Research Report*. www.pewresearch.org/global/2019/02/05/smartphone-ownership-is-growing-rapidly-around-the-world-but-not-always-equally/

Treem, J. W., & Leonardi, P. M. (2012). Social media use in organizations: Exploring the affordances of visibility, editability, persistence, and association. *Annals of the International Communication Association, 36*(1), 143–89. doi: 10.1080/23808985.2013.11679130

Utz, S. (2015). Is LinkedIn making you more successful? The informational benefits derived from public social media. *New Media & Society*, 18(*11*), 2685–2702. doi:10.1177/1461444815604143

Valkenburg, P. M., Peter, J., & Schouten, A. P. (2006). Friend networking sites and their relationship to adolescents' well-being and social self-esteem. *CyberPsychology & Behavior, 9*(5), 584–90. doi: 10.1089/cpb.2006.9.584

Vasilescu, B., Serebrenik, A., Devanbu, P., & Filkov, V. (2014). How social Q&A sites are changing knowledge sharing in open source software communities. In *Proceedings of the 17th ACM Conference on Computer Supported Cooperative Work & Social Computing* (pp. 342–54). doi: 10.1145/2531602.2531659

Vorderer, P., & Kohring, M. (2013). Permanently online: A challenge for media and communication research. *International Journal of Communication, 7*, 188–96.

Walther, J. (1996). Computer-mediated communication: Impersonal, interpersonal, and hyperpersonal interaction. *Communication Research, 23*(1), 3–43. doi: 10.1177/009365096023001001

Wan, C.-S., & Chiou, W.-B. (2006). Psychological motives and online games addiction: A test of flow theory and humanistic needs theory for Taiwanese adolescents. *CyberPsychology & Behavior, 9*(3), 317–24. doi: 10.1089/cpb.2006.9.317

Weisband, S. P. (1992). Group discussion and first advocacy effects in computer-mediated and face-to-face decision-making groups. *Organizational Behavior and Human Decision Processes, 53*(3), 352–380. doi:10.1016/0749-5978(92)90070-N

West, C. (2019). 2019 social media demographics for marketers. *Sprout Social*. https://sproutsocial.com/insights/new-social-media-demographics/Snapchat

Williams, D. (2006). Groups and goblins: The social and civic impact of online games. *Journal of Broadcasting and Electronic Media, 50*, 651–81. doi: 10.1207/s15506878jobem5004_5

Williams, D., Yee, N., & Caplan, S. (2008). Who plays, how much, and why? Debunking the stereotypical gamer profile. *Journal of Computer Medicated Communication Monographs, 13*(4), 993–1018. doi: 10.1111/j.1083-6101.2008.00428.x

Yee, N. (2007). Motivations of play in online games. *Journal of CyberPsychology and Behavior, 9*(6), 772–75. doi: 10.1089/cpb.2006.9.772

Young, S. N. (2008). The neurobiology of human social behaviour: An important but neglected topic. *Journal of Psychiatry and Neuroscience, 33*(5), 391–92.

PART 2

Impact of Internet and Technology Use

Major Conceptual Issues

CHAPTER

12 Debates Regarding the Classification, Categorization, and Conceptualization of Problematic Internet Use and Video Gaming

Stephanie Yarnell-Mac Grory *and* Marc N. Potenza

Abstract

Worldwide Internet use has risen over the past two decades, and with it problematic use has also increased. Problematic Internet use (PIU) may occur when individuals begin to spend excessive amounts of time online, forgo important tasks and responsibilities to use the Internet, feel anxiety when use is prohibited, and experience negative impacts on other aspects of life as a result of continued use. Some studies indicate that the prevalence of PIU has increased over the past two decades; however, the extent to which PIU constitutes a unique psychiatric disorder remains debated. This chapter describes issues relating to the classification, categorization, and conceptualization of PIU. Specifically, this chapter discusses PIU as a behavioral addiction, obsessive-compulsive spectrum disorder (OCSD), impulse-control disorder (ICD), or exacerbation of another underlying comorbidity.

Keywords: PIU, behavioral addiction, Internet, technology, OCSD, ICD

Introduction

Internet usage has recently demonstrated a rapid growth worldwide, and this is expected to increase in the coming decade (Mythily, Qiu, & Winslow, 2008). At the same time, the Internet is becoming more accessible to more people through the increasing number of smartphones, tablets, and other devices and the availability of multiple websites, apps, and programs. For most, the Internet is a tool that may enhance day-to-day life, business, and information access, and use of the Internet does not lead to significant psychosocial disruption. Indeed, the ability to have readily available, easily accessible information is in many ways advantageous. The Internet provides for tremendous educational opportunities with links to books, journals, and educational sites, and its use may enhance communication between teachers and classmates (Mythily et al., 2008). However, while the Internet may be used for educational purposes, it may also be used for myriad other reasons. Some suggest that the Internet may give many young people a group with whom to confide when otherwise they would have no one around who shares common interests (LaRose, Eastin, & Gregg, 2001). Activities online may also serve as a means of coping with depression or other emotions (Ceyhan, 2008). It has been suggested that if some adolescents were not to use the Internet, they might become socially isolated and not gain acceptance into peer groups (Steinkuehler & Williams, 2006; Suler, 2007).

However, for some individuals, it appears that increased use may lead to significant distress, psychosocial decline, and physical and emotional impairment (Adler and Adler, 2008). Affected persons may have difficulties maintaining a balance in their everyday life and controlling their use, at times choosing to spend time on the Internet instead of pursuing other important activities. It has been suggested then that these individuals may be exhibiting problematic Internet use (PIU) (Yau et al., 2014).

Younger individuals may be at highest risk for PIU, perhaps given their frequencies of Internet use. A study from Singapore estimated that 84% of people aged 10–14 years used the Internet, 64% of those aged 15–59 years, and 21% of those aged

60 years or older (Infocomm, 2006). This same study suggested that 78% of families have one or more computers in the home (Infocomm Development Authority Singapore, 2006). In the United States, data suggested that 68% of individuals aged 11–14 years, 77% of those aged 15–17 years (Debell & Chapman, 2003), and more than 90% of those 18–42 years are using the Internet, with usage rates dropping significantly only after age 62 (Estabrook, Witt, & Rainie, 2007). Other studies suggest that upward of 95% of adolescents (aged 12–17) use the Internet, with half reporting use multiple times a day (Pew Research, 2011). Consistent with these usage trends, adolescents in particular appear to have higher prevalence rates of PIU than adult counterparts (Bakken, Wenzel, Götestam, Johansson, & Oren, 2009; Johansson & Götestam, 2004; Liu, Desai, Krishnan-Sarin, Cavallo, & Potenza, 2011). However, studies of PIU and efforts to treat PIU have been limited by lack of agreement on diagnostic criteria. Indeed, even the name of this entity has not been agreed upon, nor the extent to which it should represent a diagnosable condition.

Nomenclature

PIU has had a variety of names in the literature. Though not in the *Diagnostic and Statistical Manual of Mental Disorders* (DSM) or International Classification of Diseases per se (see later discussion), the terms "Internet addiction (IA)," "PIU," and "pathological computer use" have all been used. For the purposes of this chapter, PIU will be the term used, and it will be defined as use of the Internet that is poorly controlled, that leads to significant functional and psychosocial impairments, and is not better accounted for by a primary psychiatric disorder such as mania or the effects of substance use (Liu & Potenza, 2007).

PIU remains a relatively newly recognized concept. Concern regarding Internet overuse was first suggested (perhaps satirically) in 1995 by Ivan Goldberg (New Yorker Magazine, 1997); however, use of the Internet in an addictive fashion was described shortly thereafter (Griffiths, 1996; Young, 1998). At that time, using DSM-IV criteria relating to substance use disorders, it was suggested that persons demonstrating Internet overuse may fulfill dependence criteria relating to tolerance, withdrawal, craving, preoccupation, and negative consequences as a result of continued use (Griffiths, 1996; Young, 1998, 1999b). Young's criteria included preoccupation with the Internet, a need for increased time spent online to achieve the same amount of satisfaction; repeated efforts to curtail Internet use; irritability, depression, or mood lability when Internet use was limited; staying online longer than anticipated; putting a job or relationship in jeopardy to use the Internet; lying to others about how much time is spent online; and using the Internet as a means of regulating mood, and these shared similarities not only with substance dependence but also with pathological gambling (Young, 1998). Given similarities between the proposed criteria and those for substance dependence, PIU was initially termed "Internet addiction" (Young, 1998). These criteria, though not universally accepted, became the foundation for many studies and were found to demonstrate sufficient reliability (Bernardi & Pallanti, 2009; Han et al., 2009; Widyanto & McMurran, 2004; Young, 1998). Studies using Young's criteria and modifications of these for IA or PIU have suggested rates ranging from less than 1% to 80% in the general population (Bai, Lin, & Chen, 2001; Chou, 2001; Mitchell, 2000; Whang, Lee, & Chang, 2003; Young, 1998) and from 8.1% to 17.1% of the adolescent population (those aged 12–18) and possibly rising (Mythily et al., 2008; Tsai & Lin, 2001; Yang & Tung, 2007). However, the lack of a universally agreed upon name or diagnostic criteria has resulted in difficulty in making comparisons between studies (Beard, 2005).

Debated Aspects

Addiction

Arguments against IA are varied. One argument against PIU involves dissent over the idea that it is an addiction at all. Proponents of this theory argue that while words such as "tolerance" and "withdrawal" are often used, there is little to no actual physiologic effect, thereby making these subjective terms (Pies, 2009). However, neurobiological studies have demonstrated similarities between brain dysfunction in PIU and substance use disorders. In patients with suspected PIU, studies have found cue-induced gaming urges to activate the right orbitofrontal cortex, right nucleus accumbens, bilateral anterior cingulate cortex, medial frontal cortex, right dorsolateral prefrontal cortex, and right caudate nucleus (Ko, Liu, et al., 2009). Cue-induced cravings in substance-addicted persons have yielded activation of similar brain regions, leading some to postulate that similar neurobiological mechanisms may exist across conditions (Ko, Liu, et al., 2009). Furthermore, imaging studies have demonstrated gray matter differences in the brains of persons suspected of having IA. Specifically, studies suggest less gray matter volume in the left anterior cingulate cortex, left insula, left posterior cingulate cortex, left lingual gyrus, cerebellum, bilateral dorsolateral prefrontal cortex, orbitofrontal cortex, and supplementary motor area and increased homogeneity in the right cingulate gyrus and bilateral parahippocampus (Yuan et al., 2012; Zhou, Lin, Du, Qin, & Zhao, 2011). The duration of addiction correlated negatively with gray matter volumes in the right dorsolateral prefrontal cortex, left anterior cingulate cortex, and the right supplemental motor area (Yuan et al., 2012). Similar changes have been noted on imaging studies of substance abuse, where significant reduction in gray matter density has been noted in the right dorsolateral prefrontal cortex, as well as volume loss in the nucleus accumbens and orbitofrontal cortex (Thayer, Crotwell, Callahan, Hutchinson, & Bryan, 2012; Yuan et al., 2010). Functional studies of individuals with substance use disorders have further demonstrated this similarity through decreased resting connectivity of the right dorsolateral prefrontal cortex with the left inferior parietal lobe (Yuan et al., 2010) and significantly decreased functional connectivity between the nucleus accumbens, dorsal anterior cingulate cortex, dorsolateral prefrontal cortex, and frontal operculum (Motzkin, Baskin-Sommers, Newman, Kiehl, & Koenigs, 2014). Perhaps unsurprisingly, functional brain imaging has previously suggested that these areas of the brain, particularly the dorsolateral prefrontal cortex and anterior cingulate cortex, are involved in cognitive control (Barber & Carter, 2005; Krawczyk, 2002; MacDonald, Cohen, Stenger, & Carter, 2000; Wilson, Sayette, & Fiez, 2004), and neuroimaging studies of individuals with substance use disorders has revealed deactivation of these regions in individuals with opioid use (Forman, Dougherty, Casey, Siegle, & Braver, 2004; Fu, Bi, Zou, Wang, & Ye, 2008) and cocaine use (Li & Sinha, 2008) disorders. Persons with PIU, like those with substance use disorders, demonstrate impaired cognitive control (Cao, Su, Liu, & Gao, 2007; Dong, Lu, Zhou, & Zhao, 2010; Kaufman, Ross, Stein, & Garavan, 2003; Li & Sinha, 2008). Given that the dorsolateral prefrontal cortex, anterior cingulate cortex, orbitofrontal cortex, supplemental motor area, and cerebellum have all been shown to be associated with cognitive control and goal-directed behavior (Chou, Condron, & Belland, 2005; Dong et al., 2010; Ko et al., 2009; Ko, Hsiao, Liu, Yen, & Yang, 2010), differences in these areas may in part explain features of PIU (Yuan et al., 2012), although more research is needed. Furthermore, abnormal white matter properties in the parahippocampal gyrus have been postulated to be potentially responsible for observed deficits in working memory sometimes found in association with PIU and substance use disorders (Ko et al., 2009; Yuan et al., 2012).

Given some similarities in the neurobiological features of PIU and substance use disorders, it has been suggested that PIU may be classified as an addiction (Dong, Huang, & Du, 2011; Yuan et al., 2012). PIU, like gambling disorder, problematic video game playing, and compulsive shopping, has been suggested to represent a non-substance or behavioral addiction (Holden, 2010; Leeman & Potenza, 2012; Potenza, 2006, 2008; Shaffer, 2001; Widyanto & Griffith, 2006;Yau, Crowley, Mayes, & Potenza, 2012). Currently, only gambling disorder is classified as a non-substance addiction in the DSM-5 (American Psychiatric Association, 2013), but the inclusion of Internet gaming disorder in Section 3 of DSM-5 (as an entity deserving additional research) represents an important change (Potenza, 2006, 2014), and the classification of a non-substance use disorder (gambling disorder) together with substance use disorders helps fortify the existence of behavioral addictions as a group (Blanco, Moreyra, Nunes, Saiz-Ruiz, & Ibanez, 2001; Grant, Brewer, & Potenza, 2006; Ko, Yen, Chen, Yeh, & Yen, 2009; Potenza, 2014). It has been proposed that substance and non-substance addictions may represent different expressions of a common underlying etiology (Shaffer et al., 2004). Particularly, it has been suggested that most, if not all, of those diagnosed with IA may actually merely be individuals with a premorbid vulnerability toward addictive behaviors (Yellowlees & Marks, 2007) and that the Internet may represent an outlet for other forms of addiction. As this was debated in DSM-5 proceedings (Petry, 2006; Petry & O'Brien, 2013; Petry et al., 2014a, 2014b, 2014c), the focus of the Internet-related diagnostic entity in Section 3 of the DSM-5 focuses on Internet gaming (e.g., interactive video games like World of Warcraft) as this form of Internet use had the most data supporting its negative health impact and study to date (Petry et al., 2014a, 2014b, 2014c).

Classification and Categorization

It has been suggested that PIU may not represent a distinct diagnostic entity and instead that the Internet may represent a medium of communication and type of environment for the expression of another problem (e.g., related to gaming, gambling, or shopping) (Bell, 2007). To address this, some have suggested segregating PIU into smaller, behavior-specific modalities such as online gambling addiction, online gaming addiction, online shopping addiction, email addiction, pornography addiction, etc. (Davis, 2001; Davis, Flett, & Besser, 2002; Griffiths, 2000a,b; Hellman, Schoenmakers, Nordstrom, & van Holst, 2013; Tsai & Lin, 2003). Most notably, Internet gaming disorder has been introduced into the DSM-5 as an area of further research, with a focus on the specific entity of gaming. Analogously, gaming disorder has been introduced into the eleventh edition of the International Classification of Diseases (ICD-11). However, PIU and problematic Internet gaming may not carry the same health concerns (Desai et al., 2010). For this reason, some have suggested separating PIU into subtypes relating to excessive gaming, sexual preoccupation, emailing/texting, and social networking (Block, 2008; Yau et al., 2012). Others have proposed further specifying as "specific PIU" to account for problematic use toward specific ends, such as gambling, gaming, or pornography use, and "generalized PIU" to define use that is problematic but that may include but is not limited to these specific behaviors (Griffiths, 2003). This argument holds that the Internet may be used as a platform for engaging in specific behaviors with relative ease and anonymity, and either one or multiple behaviors may be problematic for specific individuals (Yau & Potenza, 2014).

Other Considerations: Problematic Internet Use as an ICD or OCSD

PIU has also been proposed to possibly represent an impulse-control disorder (ICD) or obsessive-compulsive-spectrum disorder (OCSD) (Shapira, Goldsmith, Keck, Khosla, & McElroy, 2000). Relationships between ICDs and OCD have been questioned, in part given ego-syntonic versus ego-dystonic motivations (Potenza, Koran, & Pallanti, 2009). Impulsive and compulsive behaviors were at one time considered to lie along a unidimensional spectrum (Hollander & Wong, 1995) although more recent data suggest that disorders like substance use disorders and behavioral addictions (e.g., gambling disorder) have both impulsive and compulsive features, with individuals with these disorders (as well as those with OCD) scoring higher than control comparison subjects on both dimensions (el-Guebaly, Mudry, Zohar, Tavares, & Potenza, 2012; Fineberg et al., 2014). Based on a body of literature, decisions were made in DSM-5 to group together grooming-related conditions (like excoriation [skin-picking] disorder and trichtillomania, previously classified as an ICD in DSM-IV) and OCD together, and these were separated from conduct/aggression-related ICDs and from substance-related and addictive disorders (substance use disorders and gambling disorder), each of which are in separate categories in DSM-5. The Substance Use Disorder workgroup for DSM-5 considered Internet gaming, but decided against including the disorder in the main text of the DSM-5 given the limited data on the disorder (Petry & O'Brian, 2013; Petry et al., 2014a, 2014b, 2014c). However, it remains debated whether the Internet may create conditions for distinct disordered behaviors or whether it acts to precipitate, enact, or amplify other conditions (Kirmayer, Raikhel, & Rahimi, 2013).

PIU may frequently co-occur with other psychiatric conditions, with comorbidity estimates as high as 86% (Ahn, 2007). In addition to depressive symptoms, ICDs, attention deficit hyperactivity disorder, OCD, substance use disorders, bipolar disorder, social anxiety, and personality disorders have been reported to co-occur with PIU (Anderson, 2001; Bai et al., 2001; Barry, Stefanovics, Desai, & Potenza, 2011; Beard & Wolf, 2001; Bernardi & Pallanti, 2009; Black, Belsare, & Schlosser, 1999; Davis et al., 2002; Dowling & Brown, 2010; Dowling & Quirk, 2009; Holden, 2001; Liu & Potenza, 2007; Mazhari, 2012; Mitchell, 2000; Petry, Stinson, & Grant, 2005; Shaffer, & Korn, 2002; Shapira et al., 2000; Treuer, Fabian, & Furedi, 2001). Interestingly, these relationships appear similar to those reported in pathological gambling, compulsive eating, compulsive shopping, kleptomania, substance use disorders, and other ICDs and addictions (Pratarelli & Browne, 2002). Like gambling and substance use disorders, PIU has been associated with mood disorders, legal issues, and incarceration, as well as poor physical and mental health (Ko, Yen, et al., 2009; Liu et al., 2011; Morasco, Pietrzak, Blanco, Grant, Hasin, & Petry, 2006; Milani, Osualdella, & Di Blasio, 2009; Shapira et al., 2000; Shaw & Black, 2008).

Treatment

Currently there is no uniformly agreed-upon treatment model for PIU. In China, rigid timetables, strict disciplinary action, and electric shock treatments have been used (Flisher, 2010), although testing of the efficacies and tolerabilities of these treatments has not been systematically performed. Cognitive-behavioral therapy (CBT) has been proposed as a means of treating excessive Internet use (Davis, 2001; Yellowlees, 2001). Others have suggested using risk education techniques (Young & Case, 2004). Some have suggested pharmacotherapeutic interventions. Given similarities to other behavioral addictions, it has been suggested that medications such as naltrexone and buproprion, both of which have been shown to decrease cravings, may help decrease excessive Internet use (Han, Hwang, & Renshaw, 2010; Yellowlees & Marks, 2007). However, all of these possible treatments are largely still in experimental stages.

Conclusion

There currently exists considerable debate over the classification and categorization of PIU. Some data suggest that PIU may best be classified as a non-substance/behavioral addiction based on similarities with other addictions. However, differences have also been noted, and alternate classifications (as an OCSD or ICD) have been proposed. Taken together, it remains debated whether excessive Internet use constitutes an independent disorder or whether the Internet may act more specifically to precipitate, enact, or amplify other behaviors or conditions (Kirmayer et al., 2013). Until such time as these issues are resolved, it will remain difficult to establish diagnostic criteria for the disorder and to investigate prevalence and incidence rates, as well as to determine the most appropriate treatment modalities. However, given the introduction in the DSM-5 of provisional diagnostic criteria for Internet gaming disorder and into the ICD-11 criteria for gaming disorder, there exists hope that this process may move forward in an efficient fashion.

References

Adler, P., & Adler, P. (2008). The cyber worlds of self-injurers: Deviant communities, relationships, and selves. *Symbolic Interaction. 31*(1), 33–56.

Ahn, D. H. (2007). *Korean policy on treatment and rehabilitation for adolescent's internet addiction.* Paper presented at the International Symposium on the Counseling and Treatment of Youth Internet Addictions, Seoul, Korea.

American Psychiatric Association. (2013). *Diagnostic and statistical manual of mental disorders* (5th ed). Washington, DC: Author.

Anderson, K. J. (2001). Internet use among college students: An exploratory study. *Journal of American College Health, 50*(1), 21–26.

Bai, Y. M., Lin, C. C., & Chen, J. Y. (2001). Internet addiction disorder among clients of a virtual clinic. *Psychiatric Services, 52*(10), 1397.

Bakken, I. J., Wenzel, H. G., Götestam, K. G., Johansson, A., & Oren, A. (2009). Internet addiction among Norwegian adults: A stratified probability sample study. *Scandinavian Journal of Psychology, 50*(2), 121–27.

Barber, A., & Carter, C. (2005). Cognitive control involved in overcoming prepotent response tendencies and switching between tasks. *Cerebral Cortex, 15*, 899–912.

Barry, D. T., Stefanovics, E. A., Desai, R. A., & Potenza, M. N. (2011). Gambling problem severity and psychiatric disorders among Hispanic and white adults: Findings from a nationally representative sample. *Journal of Psychiatric Research, 45*(3), 404–11.

Beard, K. (2005). Internet addiction: A review of current assessment techniques and potential assessment questions. *CyberPsychology & Behavior, 8*, 7–14.

Beard, K. W., & Wolf, E. M. (2001). Modification in the proposed diagnostic criteria for Internet addiction. *Cyberpsychology & Behavior, 4*(3), 377–83.

Bell, V. (2007). Online information, extreme communities, and Internet therapy: Is Internet good for our mental health? *Journal of Mental Health, 16*(4), 447–57.

Bernardi, S., & Pallanti, S. (2009). Internet addiction: A descriptive clinical study focusing on comorbidities and dissociative symptoms. *Comprehensive Psychiatry, 50*(6), 510–16.

Black, D., Belsare, G., & Schlosser, S. (1999). Clinical features, psychiatric comorbidity, and health-related quality of life in persons reporting compulsive computer use behavior. *Journal of Clinical Psychiatry, 60*(12), 839–44.

Blanco, C., Moreyra, P., Nunes, E. V., Saiz-Ruiz, J., & Ibanez, A. (2001). Pathological gambling: Addiction or compulsion? *Seminars in Clinical Neuropsychiatry, 6*(3), 167–76.

Block, J. (2008). Issues for DSM-V: Internet addiction. *American Journal of Psychiatry, 165*, 306–307.

Cao, F., Su, L., Liu, T., & Gao, X. (2007). The relationship between impulsivity and Internet addiction in a sample of Chinese adolescents. *European Psychiatry, 22*, 466–71.

Ceyhan, A. (2008). Predictors of problematic internet use on Turkish university students. *Cyberpsychology & Behavior, 11*(3), 363–66.

Chou, C. (2001). Internet heavy use and addiction among Taiwanese college students: An online interview study. *Cyberpsychology & Behavior, 4*(5), 573–85.

Chou, C., Condron, L., & Belland, J. (2005). A review of the research on Internet addiction. *Educational Psychology Review, 17*, 363–88.

Davis, R. (2001). A cognitive-behavioral model of pathological Internet use. *Computers in Human Behavior, 17*, 187–95.

Davis, R., Flett, G., & Besser, A. (2002). Validation of a new scale for measuring problematic internet use: Implications for pre-employment screening. *Cyberpsychology & Behavior, 5*(4), 331–45.

DeBell, M., & Chapman, C. (2003). *Computer and internet use by children and adolescents in 2001: Statistical analysis report.* Washington, DC: National Center for Education Statistics.

Desai, R., Krishnan-Sarin, S., Cavallo, D., & Potenza, M. N. (2010). Video-gaming among high school students: Health correlates, gender differences, and problematic gaming. *Pediatrics, 126*(6), 1414–24.

Dong, G., Huang, J., & Du, X. (2011). Enhanced reward sensitivity and decreased loss sensitivity in internet addicts: An fMRI study during a guessing task. *Journal of Psychiatric Research, 45*(11), 1525–29.

Dong, G., Lu, Q., Zhou, H., & Zhao, X. (2010). Impulse inhibition in people with Internet addiction disorder: Electrophysiological evidence from a Go/NoGo study. *Neuroscience Letters, 485*, 138–42.

Dowling, N., & Brown, M. (2010). Commonalities in the psychological factors associated with problem gambling and Internet dependence. *Cyberpsychology, Behavior and Social Networking, 13*(4), 437–41.

Dowling, N., & Quirk, K. (2009). Screening for Internet dependence: Do the proposed diagnostic criteria differentiate normal from dependent Internet use? *CyberPsychology & Behavior, 12*(1), 21–27.

el-Guebaly, N., Mudry, T., Zohar, J., Tavares, H., & Potenza, M. (2012). Compulsive features in behavioral addictions: The case of pathological gambling. *Addiction, 107*(10), 1726–34.

Estabrook, L., Witt, E., & Rainie, L. (2007). *Information searches that solve problems: How people use the internet, libraries, and government agencies when they need help.* Washington, DC: Pew Internet & American Life Project.

Fineberg, N., Chamberlain, S., Goudriaan, A., Stein, D., Vanderschuren, L., Gillan, C., . . . Potenza, M. (2014). New developments in human neurocognition: Clinical, genetic, and brain imaging correlates of impulsivity and compulsivity. *CNS Spectrums, 19*(1), 69–89.

Flisher, C. (2010). Getting plugged in: An overview of Internet addiction. *Journal of Paediatrics and Child Health, 46*, 557–59.

Forman, S., Dougherty, G., Casey, B., Siegle, G., & Braver, T. (2004). Opiate addicts lack error-dependent activation of rostral anterior cingulate. *Biological Psychiatry, 55*, 531–37.

Fu, L., Bi, G., Zou, Z., Wang, Y., & Ye, E. (2008). Impaired response inhibition function in abstinent heroin dependents: An fMRI study. *Neuroscience Letters, 438*, 322–26.

New Yorker Magazine. (1997). Just Click No. Talk Story about Dr. Ivan K. Goldberg and the Internet Addiction Disorder. http://www.newyorker.com/magazine/1997/01/13/just-click-no. Accessed on 15 March 2020.

Grant, J. E., Brewer, J. A., & Potenza, M. N. (2006). The neurobiology of substance and behavioral addictions. *CNS Spectrums, 11*(12), 924–30.

Griffiths, M. (1996). Nicotine, tobacco and addiction. *Nature, 384*, 18.

Griffiths, M. (2000a). Does Internet and computer "addiction" exist? Some case study evidence. *Cyberpsychology & Behavior, 3*(2), 211–18.

Griffiths, M. (2000b). Internet addiction: Time to be taken seriously? *Addiction Research, 8*, 413–18.

Griffiths, M. (2003). Internet gambling: Issues, concerns and recommendations. *CyberPsychology & Behavior, 6*, 557–68.

Han, D., Hwang, J., & Renshaw, P. (2010). Buproprion sustained release treatment decreases craving for video games and cue-based brain activity in patients with internet video game addiction. *Experimental Clinical Psychopharmacology, 18*, 297–304.

Han, D., Lee, Y., Na, C., Ahn, J., Chung, U., & Daniels, M. (2009). The effects of methylphenidate on internet video game play in children with attention-deficit hyperactivity disorder. *Comprehensive Psychiatry, 50*, 251–56.

Hellman, M., Schoenmakers, T., Nordstrom, B., & van Holst, R. (2013). Is there such a thing as online video game addiction? A cross disciplinary review. *Addiction and Research Theory, 21*(2), 102–12.

Holden, C. (2001). Behavioral addictions: Do they exist? *Science, 294*(5544), 980–82.

Holden, C. (2010). Behavioral addictions debut in proposed DSM-V. *Science, 327*(5968), 935.

Hollander, E., & Wong, C. (1995). Obsessive-compulsive spectrum disorders. *Journal of Clinical Psychiatry, 56*, 53–55.

Infocomm Development Authority Singapore. (2006). *Annual survey on Infocomm usage in households and by individuals for 2006.* http://www.ida.gov.sg/doc/Publications/Publications_Level2/2006_hh_exec%20summary.pdf.

Johansson, A., .& Götestam, K. (2004). Internet addiction: Characteristics of a questionnaire and prevalence in Norwegian youth (12–18 years). *Scandinavian Journal of Psychology, 45*(3), 223–29.

Kaufman J., Ross, T., Stein, E., & Garavan, H. (2003). Cingulate hypoactivity in cocaine users during a GO-NOGO task as revealed by event-related functional magnetic resonance imaging. *Journal of Neuroscience, 23*, 7839–843.

Kirmayer, L., Raikhel, E., & Rahimi, S. (2013). Cultures of the Internet: Identity, community, and mental health. *Transcultural Psychiatry, 50*(2),165–91.

Ko, C., Hsiao, S., Liu, G., Yen, J., & Yang, M. (2010). The characteristics of decision making, potential to take risks, and personality of college students with Internet addiction. *Psychiatry Research, 175*, 121–25.

Ko, C., Liu, G., Hsiao, S., Yen, J., Yang, M., & Lin, W. (2009). Brain activities associated with gaming urge of online gaming addiction. *Journal of Psychiatric Research, 43*(7), 739–47.

Ko, C., Yen, J., Chen, C., Yeh, Y., & Yen, C. (2009). Predictive values of psychiatric symptoms for Internet addiction in adolescents: A 2-year prospective study. *Archives of Pediatrics & Adolescent Medicine, 163*(10), 937–43.

Krawczyk, D. (2002). Contributions of the prefrontal cortex to the neural basis of human decision making. *Neuroscience & Biobehavioral Reviews, 26*, 631–64.

LaRose, R., Eastin, M., & Gregg, J. (2001). Reformulating the Internet paradox: Social cognitive explanations of Internet use and depression. *Journal of Online Behavior,1*, 2.

Leeman, R., & Potenza, M. (2012). Similarities and differences between pathological gambling and substance use disorders: A focus on impulsivity and compulsivity. *Psychopharmacology, 219*(2), 469–90.

Li, C., & Sinha, R. (2008). Inhibitory control and emotional stress regulation: Neuroimaging evidence for frontal-limbic dysfunction in psycho-stimulant addiction. *Neuroscience & Biobehavioral Reviews, 32*, 581–97.

Liu, T., Desai, R., Krishnan-Sarin, S., Cavallo, D., & Potenza, M. (2011). Problematic Internet use and health in adolescents: Data from a high school survey in Connecticut. *Journal of Clinical Psychiatry, 72*(6), 836–45.

Liu, T., & Potenza, M. (2007). Problematic internet use: Clinical implications. *CNS Spectrums, 12*(6),453–66.

MacDonald, A., Cohen, J., Stenger, V., & Carter, C. (2000). Dissociating the role of the dorsolateral prefrontal and anterior cingulate cortex in cognitive control. *Science, 288*, 1835–38.

Mazhari, S. (2012). Association between problematic Internet use and impulse control disorders among Iranian university students. *Cyberpsychology, Behavior and Social Networking, 15*(5), 270–73.

Milani, L., Osualdella, D., & Di Blasio, P. (2009). Quality of interpersonal relationships and problematic Internet use in adolescence. *CyberPsychology & Behavior, 12*(6), 681–84.

Mitchell, P. (2000). Internet addiction: Genuine diagnosis or not? *Lancet, 355*(9204), 632.

Morasco, B., Pietrzak, R., Blanco, C., Grant, B., Hasin, D., & Petry, M. (2006). Health problems and medical utilization associated with gambling disorders: Results from the National Epidemiological Survey on Alcohol and Related Conditions. *Psychosomatic Medicine, 68*, 976–84.

Motzkin, J., Baskin-Sommers, A., Newman, J., Kiehl, K., & Koenigs, M. (2014). Neural correlates of substance abuse: Reduced functional connectivity between areas underlying reward and cognitive control. *Human Brain Mapping, 35*(9), 4282–92.

Mythily, S., Qiu, S., & Winslow, M. (2008). Prevalence and correlates of excessive Internet use among youth in Singapore. *Annals of the Academy of Medicine Singapore, 37*(1), 9–14.

Petry, N. (2006). Should the scope of addictive behaviors be broadened to include pathological gambling? *Addiction, 101*(s1), 152–60.

Petry, N., & O'Brien, P. (2013). Internet gambling disorder and the DSM-5. *Addiction, 108*, 1186–87.

Petry, N., Rehbein, F., Gentile, D., Lemmens, J., Rumpf, H., Moble, T., . . . O'Brien, C. (2014a). An international consensus for assessing internet gaming disorder using the new DSM-5 approach. *Addiction, 109*(9), 1399–406.

Petry, N., Rehbein, F., Gentile, D., Lemmens, J., Rumpf, H., Moble, T., . . . O'Brien, C. (2014b). Internet gaming and addiction: A reply to King and Delfabbro. *Addiction, 109*(9), 1567–68.

Petry, N., Rehbein, F., Gentile, D., Lemmens, J., Rumpf, H., Moble, T., . . . O'Brien, C. (2014c). Moving internet gaming disorder forward: A reply. *Addiction, 109*(9), 1412–13.

Petry, N., Stinson, F., & Grant, F. (2005). Comorbidity of DSM-IV pathological gambling and other psychiatric disorders: Results from the National Epidemiologic Survey on Alcohol and Related Conditions. *Journal of Clinical Psychiatry, 66*(5), 564–74.

Pew Research. (2011). *Who's online: Internet user demographics (Teens)*. http://pewinternet.org/Trend-Data-(Teens)/Whos-Online.aspx

Pies, R. (2009). Should DSM-V designate "Internet Addiction" as a mental disorder? *Psychiatry, 6*(2), 31–37.

Potenza, M. (2006). Should addictive disorders include non-substance-related conditions? *Addiction, 101*(1), 142–51.

Potenza, M. (2008). The neurobiology of pathological gambling and drug addiction: An overview and new findings. *Philosophical Transactions of the Royal Society B, 363*(1507), 3181–89.

Potenza, M. (2014). Non-substance addictive behaviors in the context of DSM-V. *Addictive Behaviors, 39*, 1–2.

Potenza, M., Koran, L., & Pallanti, S. (2009). The relationship between impulse control disorder and obsessive-compulsive disorder: A current understanding and future research directions. *Psychiatry Research, 170*(1), 22–31.

Pratarelli, M., & Browne, B. (2002). Confirmatory factor analysis of internet use and addiction. *Cyberpsychology & Behavior, 5*(1), 53–64.

Shaffer, H. (2001). Strange bedfellows: A critical view of pathological gambling and addiction. *Addiction, 94*, 1445–48.

Shaffer, H., & Korn, D. (2002). Gambling and related mental disorders: A public health analysis. *Annual Review of Public Health, 23*, 171–212.

Shaffer, H., LaPlante, D., LaBrie, R., Kidman, R., Donato, A., & Stanton, M. (2004). Toward a syndrome model of addiction: Multiple expressions, common etiology. *Harvard Review Psychiatry, 12*, 367–74.

Shapira, N., Goldsmith, T., Keck, P., Khosla, U., & McElroy, S. (2000). Psychiatric features of individuals with problematic internet use. *Journal of Affective Disorders, 57*(1–3), 267–72.

Shaw, M., & Black, D. (2008). Internet addiction. *CNS Drugs, 22*(5), 353–65.

Steinkuehler, C., & Williams, D. (2006). Where everybody knows your (screen) name: Online games as "third places." *Journal of Computer-Mediated Communication, 11*(4), article 1.

Suler, J. (2007). Computer and cyberspace addiction. *International Journal of Applied Psychoanalytic Studies, 1*, 359–362.

Thayer, R., Crotwell, S., Callahan, T., Hutchinson, K., & Bryan, A. (2012). Nucleus accumbens volume is associated with frequency of alcohol use among juvenile justice-involved adolescents. *Brain Science, 2*(4), 605–18.

Treuer, T., Fabian, Z., & Furedi, J. (2001). Internet addiction associated with features of impulse control disorder: Is it a real psychiatric disorder? *Journal of Affective Disorders, 66*(2–3), 283.

Tsai, C., & Lin, S. (2001). Analysis of attitudes toward computer networks and Internet addiction of Taiwanese adolescents. *Cyberpsychology & Behavior, 4*, 373–76.

Tsai, C., & Lin, S. (2003). Internet addiction of adolescents in Taiwan: An interview study. *Cyberpsychology & Behavior, 6*(6), 649–52.

Whang, L., Lee, S., & Chang, G. (2003). Internet over-users' psychological profiles: A behavior sampling analysis on internet addiction. *Cyberpsychology & Behavior, 6*(2), 143–50.

Widyanto, I., & McMurran, M. (2004). The psychometric properties of the internet addiction test. *Cyberpsychology & Behavior, 7*, 443–50.

Widyanto, L., & Griffith, M. D. (2006). Internet addiction: A critical review. *International Journal of Mental Health and Addiction, 4*, 31–51.

Wilson, S., Sayette, M., & Fiez, J. (2004). Prefrontal responses to drug cues: A neurocognitive analysis. *Nature Neuroscience, 7*, 211–14.

Yang, S., & Tung, C. (2007). Comparison of Internet addicts and non-addicts in Taiwanese high school. *Computers in Human Behavior, 23*, 79–96.

Yau, Y., Crowley, M., Mayes, L., & Potenza, M. (2012). Are Internet use and video-game-playing addictive behaviors? Biological, clinical and public health implications for youths and adults. *Minerva Psichiatrica, 53*, 153–70.

Yau, Y., Pilver, C., Steinberg, M., Rugle, L., Hoff, R., Krishnan-Sarin, S., & Potenza, M. (2014). Relationships between problematic Internet use and problem-gambling severity: Findings from a high-school survey. *Addictive Behaviors, 39*, 13–21.

Yau, Y., & Potenza, M. (2014). Problematic Internet use and behavioral addictions. *Psychiatric Annals, 44*(8), 365–67.

Yellowlees, P. (2001). *Your guide to e-Health, third millennium medicine on the Internet.* Brisbane, Australia: University of Queensland Press.

Yellowlees, P., & Marks, S. (2007). Problematic Internet use or Internet addiction? *Computers in Human Behavior, 23,* 1447–53.

Young, K. (1998). Internet addiction: The emergence of a new clinical disorder. *Cyberpsychology & Behavior, 1,* 25–28.

Young, K. (1999). Internet addiction: Evaluation and treatment. *Student BMJ, 7,* 351–52.

Young, K. (1999). Internet addiction: Symptoms, evaluation and treatment. *Innovations in Clinical Practice: A Source Book, 17,* 19–31.

Young, K., & Case, C. (2004). Internet abuse in the workplace: New trends in risk management. *Cyberpsychology & Behavior, 7*(1), 105–11.

Yuan, K., Qin, W., Dong, M., Liu, J., Sun, J., Liu, P., . . . Tian, J. (2010). Gray matter deficits and resting-state abnormalities in abstinent heroin-dependent individuals. *Neuroscience Letters, 482*(2), 101–105.

Yuan, K., Qin, W., Wang, G., Zeng, F., Zhao, L., Yang, X., . . . Tian, J. (2012). Microstructure abnormalities in adolescents with Internet addiction. *Plos One, 7*(1), e30253.

Zhou, Y., Lin, F., Du, Y., Qin, L., & Zhao, Z. (2011). Gray matter abnormalities in Internet addiction: A voxel-based morphometry study. *European Journal of Radiology, 79*(1), 92–95.

CHAPTER

13 Digital Technology Use and Overuse

Neurobiology, Neuropsychology, and Genetics

Yvonne H. C. Yau *and* Marc N. Potenza

Abstract

Digital technologies are rapidly gaining in popularity and impact. Discussions continue on whether excessive engagement in digital technologies, such as problematic Internet use and video game playing, merit consideration as behavioral addictions. The recent inclusion of Internet gaming disorder as a condition for further study in the DSM-5 invigorated a new wave of research into the potential impact of technology use on psychological well-being. Akin to individuals with substance use disorders, these individuals show tendencies for increased risk-taking, novelty-seeking, and impulsivity. Corroborating evidence comes from neuroimaging studies suggesting that neurocircuitries and neurotransmitter systems implicated in reward and executive control are altered. However, our understanding of the neural underpinnings of problematic engagement in digital technologies is limited and requires further study. A better understanding of the development and maintenance of problematic engagement in digital technologies is important in facilitating the development of improved treatments efforts.

Keywords: neurobiology, neuropsychology, genetics, impulsivity, frontal-striatal network, dopamine

Introduction

The past two decades have bore witness to an explosion in digital technology. For many individuals, access to computers and Internet connection is now an integral part of daily life. What once could only be accessed through a desktop computer connected through a dial-up connection is now almost ubiquitously available, is typically high-speed, and can be accessed seemingly everywhere in the form of mobile devices such as smartphones and tablets. The Internet is used to complete schoolwork, access information, find relationships, and communicate for work and other reasons. According to the US Census Bureau (2013), 83.8% of American households own a computer and 63.6% own a portable handheld device with capabilities of connecting to the Internet. Despite this "Digital Revolution" and its high proliferation in daily life, little is known about the potential impact of such technology use on psychological well-being. Even less is known about the neurobiological and genetic underpinnings of excessive use of the Internet. The striking dearth of empirically based knowledge stands in stark contrast to the popular interest in the impact of digital technologies.

In tandem with the Digital Revolution, there is increasing recognition by addiction professionals and the public that certain behaviors bear resemblance to alcohol and drug dependence. Data have been forwarded that these behaviors warrant consideration as non-substance or "behavioral" addictions (Frascella, Potenza, Brown, & Childress, 2010; Karim & Chaudhri, 2012; Potenza, 2006). Aided by data from neurobiological studies, this view has gained traction. In this setting, the American Psychiatric Association renamed a diagnostic category "Substance Use and Addictive Disorders" in the fifth edition of the *Diagnostic and Statistical Manual of Mental Disorders* (DSM-5). This category includes both substance- and non-substance–related addictions (American Psychiatric Association, 2012). While disordered gambling is currently the only behavioral addiction included in this new diagnostic category, there was discussion to include Internet-related behaviors in this category.

There exist data suggesting that problematic patterns of engagement in digital technologies, such as Internet use and video game playing, merit consideration as a behavioral addiction (Yau, Crowley, Mayes, & Potenza, 2012). Clinical evidence suggests that individuals with "Internet addiction (IA)" or problematic Internet use (PIU) experience multiple symptoms and consequences that mirror those reported in the substance use disorder (SUD) literature (Beutel, Hoch, Wolfling, & Muller, 2011). PIU may represent a heterogeneous construct that may include online gaming, gambling, shopping, or social networking, and these activities may carry varying degrees of associated harm. To date, online gaming has been the most widely studied specific form of PIU (Kuss & Griffith, 2012), Internet gaming disorder (IGD) was proposed for inclusion in the DSM-5, and gaming disorder has been included in the eleventh edition of the International Classification of Diseases (ICD-11) as released in June 2018. The DSM-5 Substance Use Disorder Work Group concluded that there was not sufficient evidence to merit the inclusion of IGD in the main section of DSM-5. However, IGD was added to Section 3 of the DSM-5, a section in which conditions that require further research are located. On the other hand, the World Health Organization determined that gambling disorder should be included in ICD-11 as a disorder due to addictive behaviors.

The neurobiological correlates of substance addiction have been investigated for decades using neuropsychological, biochemical, pharmacological, neuroimaging, and genetic approaches. In the past decade, neural mechanisms underlying PIU and IGD have begun to be examined, often within an addiction framework (Kuss & Griffith, 2012; Weinstein & Lejoyeux, 2013). This chapter discusses recent developments in our understanding of the neurobiological correlates of PIU and IGD.

Neuropsychology

Neuropsychological investigations have implicated certain cognitive-control functions in substance addictions. *Cognitive control* is a construct that refers to the ability to control one's own actions and the management of other cognitive processes. The executive system is theorized to encapsulate processes including manipulation of information in working memory, goal orientation, task flexibility, problem solving, planning and organization, and decision-making. These functions are strongly linked, but not limited, to parts of the prefrontal cortex (Niendam et al., 2012). The prefrontal cortex is connected with the basal ganglia, with the main component being the striatum (which is comprised of the caudate and putamen). This connection is commonly referred to as the *fronto-striatal circuitry* and links the striatum with the dorsolateral section of the prefrontal cortex and the limbic circuitry connecting the amygdala and other structures (thalamus, globus pallidus, hypothalamus, hippocampus and others) influencing motivational aspects of behavior. Models for conceptualizing PIU within a cognitive-behavioral neural framework have been proposed (Dong & Potenza, 2014).

There has been a growing, albeit limited, number of studies published on neuropsychological function in individuals with PIU and/or IGD. Diminished control over Internet use and sustained engagement despite knowledge of negative consequences may relate importantly to characteristics such as risk-taking personality and impairments in decision-making. Poor performance on the Iowa Gambling Task, which has been widely used to assess decision-making under ambiguous conditions and ability to use feedback information, has been associated with various SUDs and addictive behaviors (Bechara, Damasio, Tranel, & Damasio, 2005). The poor performance has been termed a "myopia for the future" in that individuals often fail to modify behavior in response to feedback about negative payoffs and appear hypersensitive to wins and hyposensitive to losses (Garavan & Stout, 2005). Several studies have replicated these findings with PIU (Sun et al., 2009), although there is also evidence indicating the opposite pattern—that individuals reporting PIU symptoms tended to select more advantageous cards in the Iowa Gambling Task and overall perform better than healthy comparison subjects (Ko et al., 2010). Others have also adapted the Iowa Gambling Task to include pornographic and neutral pictures on the card decks. Individuals who reported more frequent access to online pornography were found to continue selection of cards from decks with pornographic pictures despite the decks' association with high losses (Laier, Pawlikowski, & Brand, 2014).

Other tasks have also been used to study PIU. For example, individuals who endorsed more PIU symptoms and frequently played online games made riskier and more disadvantageous choices on the Game of Dice task than did healthy comparison subjects (Pawlikowski & Brand, 2011). College students who met criteria for PIU discounted rewards on the Kirby Delay Discounting task faster than did matched comparison subjects, suggesting that they may be more impulsive and less willing to wait for larger, delayed rewards (Saville, Gisbert, Kopp, & Telesco, 2011). Interestingly, data suggest that individuals with PIU tend to perform normally on Go/No-Go tasks which assess the inhibition of responses when certain stimuli are presented (Dong, Lu, Zhou, & Zhao, 2010; Sun et al., 2009). In addition, the classic Stroop Task that assesses selective attention and response inhibition has yielded mixed results, with some studies suggesting normal (Dong, Hu, & Lin, 2013) and others suggesting impaired (Dong, Zhou, & Zhao, 2011) performance. One possible explanation is that individuals with PIU may only have trouble inhibiting responses to Internet-related cues, as has been seen with cocaine abuse (Pike, Stoops, Fillmore, & Rush, 2013), and that generic tasks used to assess response inhibition function may fail to capture this difference. Further research on this area is needed to more fully understand these phenomena.

Questionnaires assessing characteristics such as risk-taking, novelty-seeking, and impulsivity-related personality tendencies have been used to characterize individuals with PIU. These constructs typically refer to the potential to seek new experiences and engage in risky behaviors despite knowledge of potential negative outcomes. Individuals with SUDs and disordered gambling often score highly on scales measuring these constructs (Leeman & Potenza, 2012). Adolescents with PIU similarly demonstrate high levels of novelty-seeking (Ko et al., 2006) and score high on the Barratt Impulsiveness Scale (Cao, Su, Liu, & Gao, 2007). However, in contrast to individuals with SUDs, those with PIU tend to be harm-avoidant (Ko et al., 2006). Taken together, these studies suggest that, although there exist similarities between PIU and SUDs, there also appear to be features unique to PIU.

Neuroimaging

Functional Imaging Studies

As discussed earlier, fronto-striatal circuitry has been implicated in addictive behaviors. Hyperactivation of the nucleus accumbens, dorsal striatum, and limbic and paralimbic regions (e.g., the orbitofrontal cortex) have been linked to elevated craving and increased desire to engage in substance use (Morein-Zamir & Robbins, 2014; Volkow, Wang, Fowler, Tomasi, & Telang, 2011). Hypoactivation of the dorsolateral prefrontal cortex, an area associated with higher order cognitive functions, has been observed and may reflect diminished executive function (Goldstein, Moeller & Volkow, 2011). Dysfunction in these brain regions and their connections may play an important role in the development and maintenance SUDs (Everitt et al., 2008). It is hypothesized that these neural correlates may also underlie PIU.

To date, most studies investigating neural correlates of PIU with functional neuroimaging techniques have focused on IGD. These studies have aimed to identify and investigate brain regions and circuits involved in cue-reactivity, craving, and other cognitive processes in individuals engaging excessively in online video game playing. In one of the first studies of potential brain correlates of craving in IGD participants, Ko et al. using a functional magnetic resonance imaging (fMRI) task, examined World of Warcraft players who played at least 30 hours a week compared to infrequent players (Ko et al., 2009). Participants were presented with ingame screenshots; frequent, compared to infrequent players, demonstrated stronger activations in the nucleus accumbens, orbitofrontal cortex, and caudate in response to these stimuli. Moreover, these activations were positively correlated with self-reported gaming urges. In another study, individuals who played World of Warcraft excessively were found to demonstrate greater activation in response to World of Warcraft pictures in areas including the dorsolateral prefrontal cortex, bilateral temporal cortex, cerebellum, and caudate nucleus compared to infrequent gamers (Sun et al., 2012). Additionally, among excessive players, the bilateral prefrontal cortex, anterior cingulate cortex, and right inferior parietal lobe activations were positively correlated with subjective craving during viewing of World of Warcraft pictures. Other studies employing cue-exposure craving tasks with measures of cue-reactivity and gaming urges in excessive video game players have reported similar results (Han, Hwang, & Renshaw, 2010; Lorenz et al., 2013). These results parallel those reported in the SUD literature (Papachristou et al., 2012) and suggest that, on a neuronal level, individuals with IGD may react with craving to Internet gaming–related cues in the same way as individuals with SUDs to substance-related cues. Consistent with this, a study found that individuals with co-occurring IGD and nicotine dependence showed higher cue-induced activation of fronto-striatal and parahippocampal regions in response to both gaming and smoking cues, which suggests overlaps in the mechanisms involved in IGD and nicotine dependence (Ko et al., 2013).

Studies have also investigated potential decision-making impairments in individuals with PIU. Behaviorally, individuals with PIU have been reported to take longer to deliberate and to make more errors on the classic Stroop task (Dong, Hu, Lin, & Lu, 2013). Corresponding neuroimaging data indicate that, compared to individuals without PIU, those with PIU demonstrated increased brain activity in the inferior frontal gyrus and decreased activity in the posterior cingulate cortex when faced with continuing losses during task performance. The authors reasoned that this suggests PIU participants may have trouble considering previous selections and relevant outcomes and may need to engage more cognitive resources to complete decision-making tasks. In another publication from the same research group, it was reported that individuals with PIU showed impaired error monitoring with increased activation in the anterior cingulate cortex and decreased activation in the orbitofrontal cortex following error responses when performing the Stroop task (Dong, Shen, Huang, & Du, 2013). The research group also reported that individuals with PIU showed decreased posterior cingulate activation compared to healthy comparison subjects after continuing losses (Dong, Hu, & Lin, 2013). Taken together, these findings suggest that individuals with PIU may demonstrate hypersensitivity to wins and hyposensitivity to losses, although this hypothesis warrants further investigation. Problems in decision-making may contribute to the continued engagement in Internet-related activities despite knowledge of the adverse consequences.

Electroencephalography (EEG) studies have demonstrated impairments in response inhibition in PIU, particularly in relation to monitoring negative feedback. Recordings of event-related potentials (ERPs) of the N2 amplitudes (implicated in response inhibition and conflict monitoring) and P3 amplitudes (implicated in inhibitory processes and response valuation) via EEG found that individuals with PIU, compared to the comparison group without, had lower N200 and higher P300 amplitudes during a Go/No-Go Task. Based on these findings, the authors concluded that PIU participants may have had to use more cognitive resources to complete the inhibition task, were less efficient with information processing, and had poorer impulse control (Dong et al., 2010). Similarly, another research group investigating error-processing and response inhibition found that individuals with excessive video game playing displayed reduced error-related negativity ERP amplitudes following incorrect trials during performance of a Go/No-Go task (Littel et al., 2012).

Preliminary evidence suggests that there may exist gender differences in brain activations in relation to PIU and IGD. During the playing of a novel video game, female and male participants demonstrated increased activation of brain regions implicated in reward and addiction (e.g., nucleus accumbens, dorsolateral prefrontal cortex, and orbitofrontal cortex) (Hoeft, Watson, Kesler, Bettinger, & Reiss, 2008). However, results also suggest that male relative to female participants in this study had greater activation and increased functional connectivity between these areas.

Functional neuroimaging studies have often, but not uniformly, supported the view that cognitive-control processes and executive function are impaired in individuals with PIU. From cue-related research, it appears that such impairments may be particularly pertinent to Internet-related stimuli. Given the immersion of the Internet into daily life for many individuals, it is clinically relevant to understand how the brain reacts toward these stimuli in interaction with cognitive-control functioning.

Resting State Imaging Studies

Resting-state fMRI is a promising tool by which to study the relationships between spontaneous brain activity and other features. Differences in resting-state functional connectivity between specific brain regions have been reported in multiple psychiatric illnesses including addictions, depression, and schizophrenia (Raichle, 2010). Functional connectivity can help elucidate baseline differences between individuals with and without PIU. Adolescents with PIU have been reported to show reduced functional connectivity in multiple cortical/subcortical networks, including prefrontal, parietal, and posterior cingulate cortices (Hong, Zalesky et al., 2013). Moreover, reduced connectivity between the posterior cingulate gyrus and right precuneus, thalamus, caudate, ventral striatum, supplementary motor area, and lingual gyrus was correlated with the severity of IGD (Ding et al., 2013). These findings indicate a widespread and significantly reduced resting functional connectivity in fronto-striatal circuits which may link to

IGD or specific features thereof, although this requires more direct testing.

Regional homogeneity is a complementary method for investigating spontaneous brain activity. Regional homogeneity measures the temporal synchronization of the time series of neighboring regions and can provide information about the local activities of separate brain regions. It has been reported that individuals with IGD demonstrate enhanced regional homogeneity in the brainstem, inferior parietal lobule, left posterior cerebellum, and left middle frontal gyrus, regions that have been linked to sensory-motor coordination. In addition, IGD participants showed decreased regional homogeneity in temporal, occipital, and parietal brain regions, areas that have been linked to visual and auditory functioning (Dong, Huang, & Du, 2012). The authors suggest that prolonged engagement in online video game playing may enhance brain synchronization in regions involved with sensory–motor coordination but decrease excitability in regions involved in visual and auditory processing, although longitudinal studies are needed to examine this possibility directly.

Structural Imaging Studies

Structural MRI (sMRI) provides a relatively stable brain measure that can identify structural brain alterations. Among 62 healthy male adults, a significant positive correlations between lifetime amount of video game playing and gray matter volumes in the parahippocampus/entorhinal cortex and left occipital cortex were observed. Genre of video games played appears to moderate this effect with logic/puzzle games and platform games contributing positively, while action-based role-playing games contributed negatively (Kuhn & Gallinat, 2014). This result parallels regional homogeneity findings and may reflect adaptive neural plasticity related to navigation and visual attention. In a study involving 154 healthy adolescents, the same research group found that adolescents reporting frequent video game playing (median 9 hours/week) had greater left striatal gray matter volume in comparison to those reporting infrequent video game playing. Moreover, left striatal gray matter volume was negatively correlated with deliberation time in the Cambridge Gambling Task (CGT), a decision-making task that assesses risk-taking propensity (Kühn et al., 2011). In a smaller sample of 18 adolescents with PIU, decreased gray matter volume was found in several prefrontal regions, including the bilateral dorsolateral prefrontal, orbitofrontal and cingulate cortices, and supplementary motor area, as well as in the cerebellum (Yuan et al., 2011). In separate studies, reductions in gray matter density were also found in the anterior and posterior cingulate cortices, as well as in the insula (Zhou et al., 2011) and the orbitofrontal cortex (Hong, Kim et al., 2013). In addition, volumes in the orbitofrontal region were correlated with performance on the Stroop Task (Yuan et al., 2013). These findings again highlight the involvement of fronto-striatal regions in PIU.

There exist studies investigating white matter integrity in PIU. Using a tract-based spatial statistical analysis of fractional anisotropy (FA) in a study employing diffusion tensor imaging (DTI), Lin et al. observed widespread reductions of FA in major white matter pathways among adolescents with PIU as compared to those without PIU, reflecting a disruption in the organization of white matter tracts (Lin et al., 2012). A more recent study identified lower white matter densities in individuals with PIU, as compared to those without, in the amygdala, insula, inferior frontal gyrus, and anterior cingulate (Lin, Dong, Wang, & Du, 2015). As noted by the authors, these findings suggest that white matter differences may exist in PIU in regions previously linked to decision-making, response inhibition, and emotional regulation.

Neurotransmitter Systems

Multiple neurotransmitters (e.g., serotonin, dopaminergic, noradrenergic, opioidergic) have been implicated in the pathophysiology of substance addictions (Koob & Volkow, 2010; Potenza, 2008). Of these, the dopaminergic system has arguably received the most research attention. A reward deficiency syndrome that includes blunted dopaminergic activity has been proposed to underlie addictive behaviors (Blum et al., 1996). Changes in dopaminergic functioning may partially explain diminished control over a behavior. As mentioned earlier, the prefrontal cortex, in particular the dorsolateral prefrontal cortex, may contribute importantly to cognitive control, and this region contains a large number of dopamine receptors and is highly sensitive to dopaminergic projections from the basal ganglia and the nucleus accumbens (Cools & D'Esposito, 2011; D'Ardenne et al., 2012). Changes in the dopaminergic system may also impact other neurotransmitter systems (e.g., glutamate, gamma aminobutyric acid [GABA]) and influence the function of fronto-striatal circuits. However, the extent to which dopamine contributes centrally to behavioral addictions (e.g., gambling disorder) has also been questioned (Potenza, 2013). As such, direct examination into neurochemical features of PIU is warranted.

Although findings are preliminary, there is some evidence for dopaminergic involvement in video game playing and PIU and/or IGD. Koepp et al. identified striatal dopamine release in eight young adult males while they played a video game that involved navigating a tank for monetary incentive (Koepp et al., 1998). Using positron emission tomography (PET) with the radioligand [^{11}C]raclopride, they reported increased release of dopamine in the ventral striatum following 50 minutes of video game playing. A more recent study using single-photon emission computed tomography (SPECT) similarly observed dopamine release in the caudate during a motorbike racing computer game, compared to baseline measures, among healthy adult males (Weinstein, 2010). Findings of dopamine release during video game play complement findings of increased gray matter volume (Kühn et al., 2011) and activation of striatal regions (Ko et al., 2009) in PIU. Striatal release of dopamine as measured by PET has been shown to correlate with blood oxygen level dependent (BOLD) response measured by fMRI in the striatum (Schott et al., 2008), suggesting a link between neurochemical and fMRI findings.

There also exists evidence for baseline changes in dopaminergic systems. For example, a SPECT study found that the level of dopamine transporter expression in the striatum is decreased in individuals with PIU and that volume, weight, and uptake ratio of the corpus striatum were reduced relative to control subjects (Hou et al., 2012). A study employing [^{11}C]raclopride PET techniques observed reduced availability of D_2-like receptors in the striatum among individuals with PIU (Kim et al., 2011).

Beyond the investigation of the dopaminergic system, other studies have addressed resting-state brain function in individuals with PIU. Using ^{18}F-FDG PET techniques to measure glucose metabolism, Park et al. observed that excessive online video game players had increased glucose metabolism in the right orbitofrontal cortex and also in parts of the basal ganglia (left caudate, right insula), though decreased metabolism was observed in posterior regions (e.g., parietal and occipital areas) (Park et al., 2010).

Genetic Studies

The genetic mechanisms underlying PIU and IGD have only been preliminarily examined to date. Han et al. reported that the presence of the Taq1A1 allele of the DRD2 gene (associated with the dopaminergic system and the ANKK1 gene) and the low activity Val158Met variant of the catecholamine-O-methyltransferase (COMT) gene (coding for the protein that degrades dopamine, epinephrine, and norepinephrine) were more prevalent among IGD adolescent males with IGD than those without IGD (Han et al., 2007). A second Korean study found that homozygosity of the short allelic variant of the 5HTTLPR (SS-5HTTLPR) gene (coding for the serotonin transporter) may be particularly frequent among male PIU adolescents (Lee et al., 2008). PIU subjects expressing SS-5HTTLPR showed higher harm avoidance and scored higher on Young's Internet Addiction Scale than PIU individuals who expressed other variants of the gene (Lee et al., 2008). The nicotinic acetylcholine receptor subunit alpha 4 gene (CHRNA4) may also relate to PIU. The T-variant (CC genotype) of the rs1044396 polymorphism of the CHRNA4 gene occurred more frequently among PIU (vs. control) participants; further analyses revealed that this finding was driven by females, suggesting sex-specific genetic effects (Montag, Kirsch, Sauer, Markett, & Reuter, 2012). However, these preliminary studies warrant more verification in larger samples and the use of additional methodologies (e.g., genome-wide association studies).

Conclusion and Future Directions

Neuropsychological and neuroimaging research on excessive and addictive use of the Internet, and in particular online video game playing, is an emerging field of scientific study. Though the topic remains debated, functional and structural imaging results suggest that PIU is linked to fronto-striatal circuitry, including regions that have been frequently implicated in SUDs (Koob & Volkow, 2010). However, it is important to consider the limitations of existing studies. First, the samples used are often very small, and findings may not be generalizable. Second, most studies have based their criteria for PIU on the frequency of engagement in online activities and not on symptoms endorsed. This may not accurately capture PIU because frequency does not necessary equate to problematic engagement. Third, there is a sampling bias in the reported data, with many samples consisting mainly of adolescent males in Asian countries. Developmental, gender-related, and cultural differences are important to consider and may potentially be variables that influence the underlying mechanisms of PIU. Fourth, while there is a sizeable amount of research on IGD, other subtypes of PIU (e.g., gambling, shopping, pornography use, or social networking) are relatively understudied. Further study of potential common and specific neural correlates of these different subtypes will help better understand the correlates of a seemingly heterogeneous grouping of behaviors and possibly lead to improved prevention and treatment strategies. Future studies should address these important limitations in order to systematically address and better understand PIU.

A better understanding of the neural features associated with the development and maintenance of addictive behaviors related to using the Internet is important for the development of specific and effective treatments. Neurobiological measures incorporated into randomized clinical trials for PIU and IGD may provide insight into the mechanisms underlying effective treatments for these conditions, as have been proposed for behavioral treatments for behavioral addictions like gambling disorder (Potenza et al., 2013). Ultimately, such knowledge may facilitate the development of improved treatments for IGD and other forms of PIU.

References

American Psychiatric Association. (2012). Proposed revisions - Substance Use and Addictive Disorders. http://www.dsm5.org/proposedrevision/pages/substanceuseandaddictivedisorders.aspx.

Bechara, A., Damasio, H., Tranel D., & Damasio A. R. (2005). The Iowa Gambling Task and the somatic marker hypothesis: Some questions and answers. *Trends in Cognitive Sciences, 9*(4), 159–62.

Beutel, M. E., Hoch, C., Wolfling, K., & Muller, K. W. (2011). Clinical characteristics of computer game and internet addiction in persons seeking treatment in an outpatient clinic for computer game addiction. *Zeitschrift für Psychosomatische Medizin und Psychotherapie, 57*(1), 77–90.

Blum, K., Sheridan, P. J., Wood, R. C., Braverman, E. R., Chen, T. J. Cull, J. G., & Comings, D. E. (1996). The D2 dopamine receptor gene as a determinant of reward deficiency syndrome. *Journal of the Royal Society of Medicine, 89*(7), 396–400.

Cao, F., Su, L., Liu, T., & Gao, X. (2007). The relationship between impulsivity and Internet addiction in a sample of Chinese adolescents. *European Psychiatry, 22*(7), 466–71.

Cools, R., & D'Esposito, M. (2011). Inverted-u–shaped dopamine actions on human working memory and cognitive control. *Biological Psychiatry, 69*(12), e113–25.

D'Ardenne, K., Eshel, N., Luka, J., Lenartowicz, A., Nystrom, L. E., & Cohen, J. D. (2012). Role of prefrontal cortex and the midbrain dopamine system in working memory updating. *Proceedings of the National Academy of Sciences, 109*(49), 19900–09.

Ding, W. N., Sun, J. H., Sun, Y. W., Zhou, Y., Li, L., Xu, J. R., & Du, Y. S. (2013). Altered default network resting-state functional connectivity in adolescents with Internet gaming addiction. *PLoS One, 8*(3), e59902.

Dong, G., Hu, Y., & Lin, X. (2013). Reward/punishment sensitivities among internet addicts: Implications for their addictive behaviors. *Progress in Neuro-Psychopharmacology and Biological Psychiatry, 46*(0), 139–45.

Dong, G., Hu, Y., Lin, X., & Lu, Q. (2013). What makes Internet addicts continue playing online even when faced by severe negative consequences? Possible explanations from an fMRI study. *Biological Psychology, 94*(2), 282–89.

Dong, G., Huang, J., & Du, X. (2012). Alterations in regional homogeneity of resting-state brain activity in internet gaming addicts. *Behavioral and Brain Functions, 8*(1), 41.

Dong, G., Lu, Q., Zhou, H., & Zhao, X. (2010). Impulse inhibition in people with Internet addiction disorder: Electrophysiological evidence from a Go/NoGo study. *Neuroscience Letters, 485*(2), 138–42.

Dong, G., & Potenza, M. N. (2014). A cognitive-behavioral model of Internet gaming disorder: Theoretical underpinnings and clinical implications. *Journal of Psychiatric Research, 58*, 7–11.

Dong, G., Shen, Y., Huang, J., & Du, X. (2013). Impaired error-monitoring function in people with Internet addiction disorder: An event-related fMRI study. *European Addiction Research, 19*(5), 269–75.

Dong, G., Zhou, H., & Zhao, X. (2011). Male Internet addicts show impaired executive control ability: Evidence from a color-word Stroop task. *Neuroscience Letters, 499*(2), 114–18.

Everitt, B. J., Belin, D., Economidou, D., Pelloux, Y., Dalley, J. W., & Robbins, T. W. (2008). Review. Neural mechanisms underlying the vulnerability to develop compulsive drug-seeking habits and addiction. *Philosophical Transactions of the Royal Society of Lond B Biological Sciencs, 363*(1507), 3125–35.

Frascella, J., Potenza, M. N., Brown, L. L., & Childress, A. R. (2010). Shared brain vulnerabilities open the way for nonsubstance addictions: Carving addiction at a new joint? *Annals of the New York Academy of Sciences, 1187*(1), 294–315.

Garavan, H., & Stout, J. C. (2005). Neurocognitive insights into substance abuse. *Trends in Cognitive Sciences, 9*(4), 195–201.

Goldstein, R. Z., Moeller, S. J., & Volkow, N. D. (2011). Cognitive disruptions in drug addiction: A focus on the prefrontal cortex. *Neuroimaging in Addiction*, 177–207.

Han, D. H., Hwang, J. W., & Renshaw, P. F. (2010). Bupropion sustained release treatment decreases craving for video games and cue-induced brain activity in patients with Internet video game addiction. *Experimental and Clinical Psychopharmacology, 18*(4), 297–304.

Han, D. H., Lee, Y. S., Yang, K. C., Kim, E. Y., Lyoo, I. K., & Renshaw, P. F. (2007). Dopamine genes and reward dependence in adolescents with excessive internet video game play. *Journal of Addiction Medicine, 1*(3), 133–38.

Hoeft, F., Watson, C. L., Kesler, S. R., Bettinger, K. E., & Reiss, A. L. (2008). Gender differences in the mesocorticolimbic system during computer game-play. *Journal of Psychiatric Research, 42*(4), 253–58.

Hong, S. B., Kim, J. W., Choi, E. J., Kim, H. H., Suh, J. E., Kim, C. D., . . . Yi, S. H. (2013). Reduced orbitofrontal cortical thickness in male adolescents with internet addiction. *Behavioral and Brain Functions, 9*, 11.

Hong, S.-B., Zalesky, A., Cocchi, L., Fornito, A., Choi, E.-J., Kim, H.-H., . . . Yi, S.-H. (2013). Decreased functional brain connectivity in adolescents with Internet addiction. *PLoS One, 8*(2), e57831.

Hou, H., Jia, S., Hu, S., Fan, R., Sun, W., Sun, T., & Zhang, H. (2012). Reduced striatal dopamine transporters in people with Internet addiction disorder. *Journal of Biomedicine and Biotechnology, 2012*, 854524.

Karim, R., & Chaudhri, P. (2012). Behavioral addictions: An overview. *J Psychoactive Drugs, 44*(1), 5–17.

Kim, S. H., Baik, S.-H., Park, C. S., Kim, S. J., Choi, S. W., & Kim, S. E. (2011). Reduced striatal dopamine D2 receptors in people with Internet addiction. *NeuroReport, 22*(8), 407–11.

Ko, C. H., Hsiao, S., Liu, G. C., Yen, J. Y., Yang, M. J., & Yen, C. F. (2010). The characteristics of decision making, potential to take risks, & personality of college students with Internet addiction. *Psychiatry Research, 175*(1–2), 121–25.

Ko, C.-H., Liu, G.-C., Hsiao, S., Yen, J.-Y., Yang, M.-J., Lin, W.-C., . . . Chen, C.-S. (2009). Brain activities associated with gaming urge of online gaming addiction. *Journal of Psychiatric Research, 43*(7), 739–47.

Ko, C. H., Liu, G. C., Yen, J. Y., Yen, C. F., Chen, C. S., & Lin, W. C. (2013). The brain activations for both cue-induced gaming urge and smoking craving among subjects comorbid with Internet gaming addiction and nicotine dependence. *Journal of Psychiatric Research, 47*(4), 486–93.

Ko, C.-H., Yen, J.-Y., Chen, C.-C., Chen, S.-H., Wu, K., & Yen, C.-F. (2006). Tridimensional personality of adolescents with internet addiction and substance use experience. *Canadian Journal of Psychiatry, 51*(14), 887–94.

Koepp, M. J., Gunn, R. N., Lawrence, A. D., Cunningham, V. J., Dagher, A., Jones, T., . . . Grasby, P. M. (1998). Evidence for striatal dopamine release during a video game. *Nature, 393*(6682), 266–68.

Koob, G. F., & Volkow, N. D. (2010). Neurocircuitry of addiction. *Neuropsychopharmacology, 35*(1), 217–38.

Kuhn, S., & Gallinat, J. (2014). Amount of lifetime video gaming is positively associated with entorhinal, hippocampal and occipital volume. *Molecular Psychiatry, 19*(7), 842–47.

Kühn, S., Romanowski, A., Schilling, C., Lorenz, R., Morsen, C., Seiferth, N., . . . Gallinat, J. (2011). The neural basis of video gaming. *Translational Psychiatry, 1*, e53.

Kuss, D. J., & Griffith, M. D. (2012). Internet gaming addiction: A systematic review of empirical research. *International Journal of Mental Health and Addiction, 10*(2), 278–96.

Laier, C., Pawlikowski, M., & Brand, M. (2014). Sexual picture processing interferes with decision-making under ambiguity. *Archives of Sexual Behavior, 43*(3), 473–82.

Lee, Y. S., Han, D., Yang, K. C., Daniels, M. A., Na, C., Kee, B. S., & Renshaw, P. F. (2008). Depression like characteristics of 5HTTLPR polymorphism and temperament in excessive internet users. *Journal of Affective Disorders, 109*(1–2), 165–9.

Leeman, R. F., & Potenza, M. N. (2012). Similarities and differences between pathological gambling and substance use disorders: A focus on impulsivity and compulsivity. *Psychopharmacology, 219*(2), 469–90.

Lin, F., Zhou, Y., Du, Y., Qin, L., Zhao, Z., Xu, J., & Lei, H. (2012). Abnormal white matter integrity in adolescents with Internet addiction disorder: A tract-based spatial statistics study. *PLoS One, 7*(1), e30253.

Lin, X., Dong, G., Wang, Q., & Du, X. (2015). Abnormal gray matter and white matter volume in 'Internet gaming addicts.' *Addictive Behaviors, 40*, 137–43.

Littel, M., van den Berg, I., Luijten, M., van Rooij, A. J., Keemink, L., & Franken, I. H. A. (2012). Error processing and response inhibition in excessive computer game players: An event-related potential study. *Addiction Biology, 17*(5), 934–47.

Lorenz, R. C., Kruger, J. K., Neumann, B., Schott, B. H., Kaufmann, C., Heinz, A., & Wustenberg, T. (2013). Cue reactivity and its inhibition in pathological computer game players. *Addiction Biology, 18*(1), 134–46.

Montag, C., Kirsch, P., Sauer, C., Markett, S., & Reuter, M. (2012). The role of the CHRNA4 gene in Internet addiction: A case-control study. *Journal of Addiction Medicine, 6*(3), 191–95.

Morein-Zamir, S., & Robbins, T. W. (2014). Fronto-striatal circuits in response-inhibition: Relevance to addiction. *Brain Research, 1629*, 117–129.

Niendam, T., Laird, A., Ray, K., Dean, Y. M., Glahn, D., & Carter, C. (2012). Meta-analytic evidence for a superordinate cognitive control network subserving diverse executive functions. *Cognitive, Affective, & Behavioral Neuroscience, 12*(2), 241–68.

Papachristou, H., Nederkoorn, C., Havermans, R., van der Horst, M., & Jansen, A. (2012). Can't stop the craving: The effect of impulsivity on cue-elicited craving for alcohol in heavy and light social drinkers. *Psychopharmacology (Berl), 219*(2), 511–18.

Park, H. S., Kim, S. H., Bang, S. A., Yoon, E. J., Cho, S. S., & Kim, S. E. (2010). Altered regional cerebral glucose metabolism in internet game overusers: A 18F-fluorodeoxyglucose positron emission tomography study. *CNS Spectrums, 15*(3), 159–66.

Pawlikowski, M., & Brand, M. (2011). Excessive Internet gaming and decision making: Do excessive World of Warcraft players have problems in decision making under risky conditions? *Psychiatry Research, 188*(3), 428–33.

Pike, E., Stoops, W. W., Fillmore, M. T., & Rush, C. R. (2013). Drug-related stimuli impair inhibitory control in cocaine abusers. *Drug and Alcohol Dependence, 133*(2), 768–71.

Potenza, M. N. (2006). Should addictive disorders include non-substance-related conditions? *Addiction, 101*(1), 142–51.

Potenza, M. N. (2008). The neurobiology of pathological gambling and drug addiction: An overview and new findings. *Philosophical Transactions of the Royal Society B, 363*(1507), 3181–89.

Potenza, M. N. (2013). How central is dopamine to pathological gambling or gambling disorder? *Frontiers in Behavioral Neuroscience, 7*, 206.

Potenza, M. N., Balodis, I. M., Franco, C. A., Bullock, S., Xu, J., Chung, T., & Grant, J. E. (2013). Neurobiological considerations in understanding behavioral treatments for pathological gambling. *Psychology of Addictive Behaviors, 27*(2), 380–92.

Raichle, M. E. (2010). Two views of brain function. *Trends in Cognitive Science, 14*(4), 180–90.

Saville, B. K., Gisbert, A., Kopp, J., & Telesco, C. (2011). Internet addiction and delay discounting in college students. *The Psychological Record, 60*(2), 5.

Schott, B. H., Minuzzi, L., Krebs, R. M., Elmenhorst, D., Lang, M., & Winz, O. H. (2008). Mesolimbic functional magnetic resonance imaging activations during reward anticipation correlate with reward-related ventral Striatal dopamine release. *Journal of Neuroscience, 28*, 14311–319.

Sun, D.-L., Chen, Z.-J., Ma, N., Zhang, X.-C., Fu, X.-M., & Zhang, D.-R. (2009). Decision-making and prepotent response inhibition functions in excessive internet users. *CNS Spectrums, 14*(2), 75–81.

Sun, Y., Ying, H., Seetohul, R. M., Xuemei, W., Ya, Z., Qian, L., . . . Ye, S. (2012). Brain fMRI study of crave induced by cue pictures in online game addicts (male adolescents). *Behavioral Brain Research, 233*, 563–76.

US Census Bureau. (2013). *Computer and Internet access in the United States: 2013*. http://www.census.gov/content/dam/Census/library/publications/2014/acs/acs-28.pdf.

Volkow, N. D., Wang, G.-J., Fowler, J. S., Tomasi, D., & Telang, F. (2011). Addiction: Beyond dopamine reward circuitry. *Proceedings of the National Academy of Sciences, 108*(37), 15037–42.

Weinstein, A., & Lejoyeux, M. (2013). New developments on the neurobiological and pharmaco-genetic mechanisms underlying internet and videogame addiction. *American Journal on Addictions, 2013*, 1521–0391.

Weinstein, A. M. (2010). Computer and video game addiction-a comparison between game users and non-game users. *American Journal of Drug and Alcohol Abuse, 36*, 268–76.

Yau, Y. H. C., Crowley, M. J., Mayes, L. C., & Potenza, M. N. (2012). Are Internet use and video-game-playing addictive behaviors? Biological, clinical and public health implications for youths and adults. *Minerva Psichiatrica, 53*, 153–70.

Yuan, K., Cheng, P., Dong, T., Bi, Y., Xing, L., Yu, D., Zhao, L., . . . Tian, J. (2013). Cortical thickness abnormalities in late adolescence with online gaming addiction. *PLoS One, 8*(1), e53055.

Yuan, K., Qin, W., Wang, G., Zeng, F., Zhao, L., Yang, X., . . . Tian, J. (2011). Microstructure abnormalities in adolescents with internet addiction disorder. *PLoS One, 6*(6), e20708.

Zhou, Y., Lin, F. C., Du, Y. S., Qin, L. G., Zhao, Z. M., Xu, K. R., & Lei, H. (2011). Grey matter abnormalities in Internet addiction: A voxel-based morphometry study. *European Journal of Radiology, 79*, 92–95.

CHAPTER

14 Selecting and Refining Measures for Assessing Digital Gaming Use and Misuse in Clinical and Research Settings

Kyle A. Faust, David Faust, Joseph F. Meyer, *and* Nathan E. Cook

Abstract

Throughout the years, various terminologies have been used to describe problematic digital gaming use. Due to differing definitions and criteria, there have similarly been a large number of measurement tools developed. Although the DSM-5 term "Internet gaming disorder" has recently become the most commonly used, it is likely that the ICD-11 could replace it with the term "gaming disorder." This chapter provides a brief review of measurement tools and provides recommendations to strengthen future problematic gaming measurements. Recommendations include an agreed-upon definition of the problem; accounting for positive effects of gaming; accounting for careless and random responding; strengthening reliability; improving norms and reference groups; improving positive and negative predictive powers by strengthening sensitivity and specificity; utilizing additional longitudinal studies; producing more studies examining risk factors and course of problem gaming; comparing and contrasting various measurement tools; adjusting for age, language, and cultural factors; measuring time frame, outcome, and severity; and establishing proper balance in brevity and comprehensive measurement for ease of use in research and clinical practice.

Keywords: measurement, digital technology, gaming disorder, refining methodology, Internet gaming disorder

Introduction

The enormous expansion of digital technology has led to considerable interest in potential positive and negative consequences and their measurement. In this chapter, we focus on measurement within a critical subdomain of digital technology that potentially impacts millions of individuals and has captured the interest of numerous investigators and the public as well: *digital gaming*. By "digital gaming," we refer to any type of game that can be played on an electronic source (e.g., video games, computer games, mobile phone games, etc.).

We first briefly overview measures designed to assess problematic digital game use and their underlying conceptual framework. We then present detailed suggestions that may assist in the further refinement or development of measures. Some of these suggestions also have potential application to measures designed to assess positive and negative consequences of other types of digital technology or to appraise other behavioral addictions. For instance, our definition of digital gaming does not include problematic or addictive Internet use (aside from games played on the Internet). Internet addiction tools have also been the subject of scholarly reviews (Lortie & Guitton, 2013), and some of our recommendations will also (but not fully) apply to these measures. Our suggestions are not intended as negative commentary on existing measures, a variety of which possess multiple favorable qualities and have created a foundation for assessing key constructs and advancing the field. Rather, they are intended to offer possible avenues for enhancing the clinical and research utility of measures.

A word on terminology is in order before proceeding. Certain terms in this chapter refer to diagnostic categories that have been or are in general use, such as "Internet gaming disorder" (IGD), "pathological gambling" (PG), and its revised form, "gambling disorder" (GD). Other terms as used here, such as "addictive" or "problematic game use," are not intended as references to formal diagnostic categories, but rather as descriptors or qualifiers. Given the intent and purpose of this chapter, we will not cover the potential pros and cons of using the label "addiction" when addressing excessive digital gaming. Thus, whether we use such a term as "problematic use" *or* "addiction," we are not taking a position on this issue. At times we do prefer "problematic digital game use" (PDG) over "addiction" because the former is broader and includes types of excessive use that seemingly do not fit well with common conceptions of addiction.

An additional, important note is regarding the recent inclusion of gaming disorder in the ICD-11 (World Health Organization, 2018). This diagnosis is provided for a gamer who meets all of the following criteria: (1) impaired control over gaming (e.g., onset, frequency, intensity, duration, termination, context), (2) increasing priority given to gaming to the extent that gaming takes precedence over other life interests and daily activities, and (3) continuation or escalation of gaming despite the occurrence of negative consequences. The behavior pattern is of sufficient severity to result in significant impairment in personal, family, social, educational, occupational, or other important areas of functioning. The pattern of gaming behavior may be continuous or episodic and recurrent. The gaming behavior and other features are normally evident over a period of at least 12 months in order for a diagnosis to be assigned, although the required duration may be shortened if all diagnostic requirements are met and symptoms are severe (World Health Organization, 2018). This recent addition of gaming disorder will likely be quite valuable in future research and treatment methods and will likely become the diagnosis most frequently provided in future literature until a diagnosis is created in the *Diagnostic and Statistical Manual of Mental Disorders* (DSM). Even so, as will shortly be presented, these criteria all come from those that have been used elsewhere. We believe that, much as is true for other measures, refinements can be made to improve future measurements of all types of problematic gaming.

Methods and Criteria for Assessing Problematic Digital Game Use

There is broad agreement that a subgroup of individuals who play digital games develop patterns of problematic use that may have serious negative consequences (Sim, Gentile, Bricolo, Serpelloni, & Gulamoydeen, 2012). For example, concerns have been raised about an increased tendency to act violently (Anderson et al., 2010). Other concerns include the belief that escalation toward extreme levels of use could compromise many areas of everyday functioning, such as social or occupational activities (King, Delfabbro, & Zajac, 2014). Epidemiological studies have provided widely differing estimates of frequency (Ferguson, Coulson, & Barnett, 2011; Gentile, Coyne, & Bricolo, 2013), but even working with the lower range estimates such as 2% or 3% of gamers, multiplying such a percentage by the hundreds of millions of individuals who engage in digital gaming worldwide generates a large, if not massive, figure.

Concerns about digital gaming, and especially its potential for extreme or addictive use and resultant adverse impacts, have led to concentrated efforts to develop measurement tools. Many of these investigators have turned to the DSM for foundational guidance. We thus begin by examining how the conceptualization of PDG, particularly as described in the DSM, has shaped the development of most measures, and then discuss advantages and potential limitations of these and other conceptual approaches.

Use of DSM-IV-TR as a Foundational Tool

Most initial efforts to develop measurement tools for PDG used criteria that largely paralleled or adapted DSM-IV-TR criteria for pathological gambling or general substance dependence (King, Haagsma, Delfabbro, Gradisar, & Griffiths, 2013). Examples include the Problem Videogame Playing Scale (Salguero & Moran, 2002), the Game Addiction Scale (Lemmens, Valkenberg, & Peter, 2009), and the Problematic Online Game Use Scale (Kim & Kim, 2010). We will examine these criteria in some detail later. King et al. (2013) provided a scholarly review of such measures, and it is instructive to describe their conclusions in some detail.

King et al. (2013). covered 18 instruments, all of which used criteria quite similar to those contained within DSM-IV-TR's categories for pathological gambling or general substance dependence (American Psychiatric Association, 2000). King et al. (2013) concluded that most of the measures possess multiple positive qualities, such as brevity, ease of scoring, strong internal consistency, and strong convergent validity. In addition, various measures seem suited to collecting important information for a range of purposes, such as developing normative databases.

King et al. (2013) identified areas of concern, including inconsistent coverage of diagnostic criteria, differing cutoff scores (thereby compounding problems discerning true pathologic use or comparing rates across studies using contrasting measures), lack of a temporal dimension, and inconsistent dimensionality. For example, factor analysis yielded a single common dimension for a number of measures which seemed to represent PDG, but two or more dimensions for other measures, such as compulsive use, withdrawal, and tolerance. The authors also provided suggestions for improving measurement, such as adding time scales and validity checks (e.g., examining whether the gamer or the gamer's family believe their gaming is problematic), obtaining data from expanded or more representative samples, and studying the sensitivity and specificity of various tools. In this chapter, we hope to add to King et al.'s useful suggestions.

Publication of DSM-5 and Changes in Diagnostic Categories and Criteria

King et al.'s (2013) review appeared shortly before DSM-5 (American Psychiatric Association, 2013) was published and thus did not cover revisions in the manual, in particular the creation and introduction of the category "Internet Gaming Disorder" under the section "Conditions for Further Study." In response to this revision, some researchers directly adopted the DSM-5 criteria for IGD to assess PDG. It might be assumed that IGD only applies to online games, but the "Subtypes" section of DSM-5 indicates that IGD "could also involve non-Internet computerized games as well, although these have been less researched" (American Psychiatric Association, 2013).

The IGD diagnostic criteria are quite similar to both the old DSM-IV-TR criteria for pathological gambling and DSM-5's modified version of these criteria under the renamed category, "Gambling Disorder." Under DSM-5, the only major difference between IGD and GD comes down to a single diagnostic criterion: IGD does not include one of the diagnostic criterion for GD ("Relies on others to provide money or relieve desperate financial situations caused by gambling"), and instead uses "Loss of interests in previous hobbies and entertainment as a result of, and with the exception of, Internet games."

Recently, Pontes and Griffiths (2015) published a brief measure called the Internet Gaming Disorder Scale. This questionnaire uses the nine DSM-5 IGD criteria in a 5-point Likert scale format. Pontes and Griffiths (2015) studied a sample of 1,060 gamers and indicated that the measure, along with IGD, could provide a unified method of assessing video game addiction.

Those using DSM-5 might assume that IGD potentially encompasses a range of Internet activities, such as online gambling disorder (because online poker could debatably be considered a digital game). Hence, a key clarification is in order: DSM-5 states that IGD does not include use of the Internet for purposes other than gaming, such as recreational or social Internet use (American Psychiatric Association, 2013). It further states that Internet gambling is not included in IGD.

Further Consideration of Diagnostic Criteria and Categories

At this point, it might seem as if these various criteria for PDG are very similar. After all, the IGD criteria differ minimally from DSM criteria for pathological gambling or GD. Furthermore, most alternatives, such as a well-known addiction model developed by Brown and modified by Griffiths (2005), appear to overlap considerably with these other diagnostic criteria. Consequently, it might be assumed that so long as the various assessment tools cover such criteria, they are all likely to measure about the same thing. It may also seem to follow that the IGD criteria should become the new, preferred method for assessing digital gaming problems, especially because they were proposed in the latest DSM. Indeed, some researchers (Petry et al., 2014; Pontes & Griffiths, 2015) have recommended that future measurement should consist of items that best reflect the nine IGD criteria.

Unfortunately, the situation is probably not that simple as these measures are not free from some limiting or problematic features. For example, it is not clear that all pertinent criteria or constructs of PDG have been properly captured to date, and some of the criteria and constructs that apply to GD may have limited or minimal value for identifying PDG and vice versa. As such, it is important that we stay open to modifying existent criteria or adopting new criteria for PDG and IGD given the rapid evolution of digital technology and emerging research findings.

Improving/Refining Measures

The following sections provide recommendations that might further improve existing measures or lead to the development of even stronger measures.

Need for a Specific Definition of Problem Gaming

Regardless of what the problem is called (PDG, IGD, or gaming addiction), a term needs to be established that properly includes all types of digital games. We believe that "digital gaming" achieves this goal, but numerous researchers use the term "video games" when they intend to refer to all types of digital games, whereas other researchers use this term when they are referring exclusively to video console games (which is why we have also used "video games" when citing certain researchers in this chapter).

Another important consideration in achieving a concrete definition of PDG is deciding what counts as digital game play. For a researcher with less background in this area, this may seem like a foolish question, but many digital gamers spend significant amounts of time *watching* digital games. Similar to professional sports viewers, some players likely spend more time watching or talking about digital games than they do playing them. These gamers may watch their friends play, or they may watch videos of game playing online, where they are often able to interact with skilled players. Skilled gamers may also spend time watching recorded videos to analyze their gameplay or use chat programs to communicate with other players about different games. It remains unclear if research on the various 18 assessment tools that King et al. (2013) reviewed accounted for this type of digital game use. If not, it is likely that some respondents did, and some did not, count time spent watching digital games when answering questions, as some gamers would consider watching games different from playing them. Attempting to appraise and reduce these ambiguities is a worthwhile goal.

The question of what type of gaming activities to count raises additional questions. Should researchers count time gamers spend talking about digital games among their friends in a social situation as digital game use? If not, would it count as digital game use time if the gamer instead had a conversation over the Internet? Why, or in what way, should online social interaction be viewed differently from real-life social interaction? The implications of these questions are very important, particularly because researchers and clinicians might disagree on answers, and the availability of scientific data to resolve differences in viewpoint may be scant. For the time being, perhaps all of these differing modes of involvement in digital gaming should be captured in some way. It remains unclear how different the effects of *watching* or *analyzing* digital games are from playing them, but beginning to study these differences and incorporating the differences into questionnaires would likely be beneficial.

Adequate Coverage of Content: Accounting for Positive Effects

A factor that makes PDG an especially interesting issue is the benefits that digital gaming may produce (Connolly, Boyle, MacArther, Hainey, & Boyle, 2012; Wouters, van Nimwegen, van Oostendorp, & van der Spek, 2013). Examples include improvements in reaction time (Dye, Green, & Bavelier, 2009), spatial resolution and visual processing (Green & Bavelier, 2007), working memory (Thorell, Lindqvist, Nutley, Bohlin, & Klingberg, 2009), cognitive flexibility (Glass, Maddox, & Love, 2013), strategic problem solving (Hong & Liu, 2003; Shaffer, 2006), and prosocial behavior (Carlo & Randall, 2002). Even PDG, despite its adverse impacts, may simultaneously produce these or other benefits.

Although a central reason to assess PDG is to determine if digital games are impacting a person's life negatively, it may be a mistake to disregard benefits that could also be occurring. This is not to fault current measures for focusing on adverse impacts, which often are of central interest and concern. That said, it should be possible to create questionnaires that evaluate both the potential pros and cons of digital gaming. Such a questionnaire would likely be regarded far more positively by gamers, as many gamers (regardless of whether their digital game use is problematic) are frequently bothered by responding to questionnaires they perceive as having a strong negative bias toward gaming. Researchers have sometimes described challenges in recruiting gamers to participate in studies, and the presence of positive items on questionnaires and interest in potential positive impacts might go a fair distance in increasing involvement and improving the representativeness of samples. In addition, measurement of positive and negative features could prove very helpful in longitudinal studies that examine crossover from benign or relatively benign patterns of use to more problematic ones, or subsequent movement from problematic to less problematic use.

As a specific example, the evaluation of treatment programs might benefit from measurement that attends to not only negative impacts but also more benign and even positive impacts. Weighing both the pros and cons of gaming could also be particularly useful in developing treatment plans. If a gamer is experiencing both positive and negative effects from gaming activities, treatment could first involve reducing gaming use to more moderate levels, particularly if a gamer is unwilling to immediately quit gaming entirely. Ideally, lowering gaming time would reduce or remove some of the more negative impacts of gaming, while the positive impacts could continue. If the gamer is an extremely problematic user and is unable to moderate his or her use in this manner, setting more extreme limitations may be necessary.

Currently, a standard method of measuring the positive impact of digital gaming seems to be lacking. When assessing positive gaming impact, researchers have typically used measures that do not involve digital games. For example, in a study assessing the potential influence of both prosocial and violent video games, Saleem, Anderson, and Gentile (2012) used the 25-item Prosocial Tendencies Measure to examine whether participants had more prosocial tendencies after gaming. Other researchers, such as Glass, Maddox, and Love (2013), have used various neuropsychological measures prior to and after exposing participants to digital games to determine if the games led to cognitive improvements.

Based on these previous approaches, some suggestions can be provided for the development of positive-impact item content and topics. These include asking gamers or respondents (a) how often they engage in games that involve a lot of physical activity, such as Dance Dance Revolution; (b) if they make a financial living off of gaming, such as being a professional gamer or a professional gaming commentator; (c) how often they engage in social activity while gaming; (d) the different types of games they engage in (as some games appear to have more pros or more cons than other games); and (f) some of a gamer's perceived benefits of gaming (which might prove useful for developing treatment plans for gamers in need of intervention). It would likely also prove informative to use a brief prosocial measure, such as the Prosocial Tendencies Measure by Saleem, Anderson, and Gentile (2012), and one or more brief cognitive measures that cover areas in which research has demonstrated improvements.

Accounting for Careless and Random Responding

The value of a self-report measure can be seriously compromised when respondents fail to cooperate sufficiently with procedures and engage in careless or random responding. Some respondents, for example, wish to complete questionnaires as quickly as possible, and, in many situations, the anonymity of research creates almost no barriers to careless or random responding. Investigations show that careless and random responding to questionnaires is more common than may be assumed, with rates sometimes running as high as 20% (Charter & Lopez, 2002; Crede, 2010). Furthermore, even a relatively small proportion of careless or random responders may have a surprisingly robust impact on research data and may cause paradoxical effects (e.g., not only impeding the detection of true relationships, but even creating artifactual associations between variables that are actually unrelated, as shown by Faust, Faust, Baker, & Meyer, 2012).

It fortunately turns out that often just a few items can achieve a high level of accuracy in identifying random responding and moderate to high accuracy in detecting careless responding. Such a small item set should take most respondents well under a minute to complete. In addition, random and careless response items may well retain effectiveness when applied to or adapted across measures, or can easily be modified to blend into the content of questionnaires. Thus, an effective and simple method of improving current PDG assessment tools is to include a few careless or random response questions, which would allow researchers to identify and remove most of these non-cooperating individuals and hence attenuate their potentially damaging impact considerably.

Reliability

Reliability is sometimes used as synonymous with accuracy, but that is not its intended meaning in the field of measurement or psychometrics. Rather, it refers to consistency of measurement in its varying forms (e.g., over time or across different individuals scoring the same test items). In this context, reliability is generally viewed as a necessary but not sufficient condition for accurate or valid measurement. To illustrate this point, suppose one has a bathroom scale that provides widely varying results for the same person (even when that person's weight has not changed). Given this lack of consistency, one would say that the scale lacks reliability. It follows that if the scale cannot even predict itself, it will not be effective in predicting another thing, such as whether the weight indicated is conducive to health. In contrast, if the scale yields a consistent result, it can be said to be reliable. However, even if the scale produces consistent results, it may still produce outcomes with a large margin of error (e.g., if a person who truly weighs 225 pounds obtains a recorded weight of about 85 pounds each time he or she steps on the scale). Consequently, the scale will be reliable but not *valid.*

Studies on the reliability of measures for assessing digital gaming or problematic use tend to primarily examine what is termed *internal consistency.* Internal consistency reflects the uniformity or relative uniformity of items designed to measure some characteristic, such as math aptitude. For example, one might find that 14 of the 15 test items tend to produce interrelated results (e.g., if a person passes one item, he or she is also likely to pass another item), but that the last item yields results that do not converge with any of the other test items. This last item may contain such complex language that, rather than assessing mathematical ability, performance relates more to verbal intelligence.

This is not the forum to discuss just how highly items should be interrelated or other technical aspects of internal consistency. It is worth noting, however, that when items designed to measure presumably distinctive dimensions nevertheless show a high association with one another, that is not necessarily a good thing. For example, presume a questionnaire is designed to measure five diagnostic criteria for digital gaming disorder that are assumed to have some degree of independence from one another, but one finds that most or all of the items show high correlations with one another. Such a result suggests that one might instead be measuring a single common factor rather than multiple dimensions or distinct criteria.

In many clinical and research applications, consistency over time, or what is often referred to as *test-retest reliability,* is as or more important than internal consistency, or, to put the matter another way, a test that has good internal consistency but lacks sufficient temporal stability is likely to be of little or no use. When a measure has high test-retest reliability or temporal stability (and the person being assessed has not changed), the test should yield a similar result if administered over time. For example, if a person with extreme IGD obtains a highly elevated score on a measure designed to identify the disorder of IGD and that disorder has changed minimally over the course of 3 months, then readministration of the measure should yield a similar result.

If a measure lacks temporal stability, then one does not know whether changes in results over time reflect true change in the individual (e.g., the beneficial effects of treatment) or measurement artifact. Without temporal stability, longitudinal research, which is so important in advancing knowledge about digital gaming, is partly or completely enfeebled. To make matters worse, when measures lack temporal stability, it is often also the case that *both* the initial measurement and the subsequent measurement or measurements are inaccurate as well. This "double jeopardy" occurs because low test-retest reliability often signals a high degree of error in the results that the measure generates. That, in turn, interferes, sometimes gravely, with efforts to link the measure's results with other phenomena. For example, suppose one is attempting to study potential differences between those with and without problematic use. If the measure used to identify status is flawed in the first place, study results may reflect measurement error more than anything else.

In short, most conceivable uses of measure require at least adequate levels of test-retest reliability, although high levels of reliability are more ideal. Consequently, if the test-retest reliability of the measure has not been studied, one might as well be guessing about whether it is adequate for the intended research purposes. Hence, having at least one well conducted background study on temporal stability or test-retest reliability seems essential and provides a critical basis for evaluating whether measures should be used in clinical settings or research endeavors. It should be added that assessment of internal consistency, which can have value for a number of important purposes, is not a substitute for the assessment of temporal stability.

If temporal stability has not been studied (which unfortunately is often the case for measures) but one feels compelled to go ahead nevertheless, there are certain test qualities that increase the likelihood of reliable results. The more dimensions one tries to measure and the fewer items one uses to do so, then, all else being equal, there is a greater risk of insufficient reliability. In contrast, if measures primarily assess a single dimension and contain a greater number of items (within limits), the greater the likelihood of adequate or greater reliability. For example, some measures attempt to assess half a dozen dimensions or more, with only one or two items dedicated to each dimension, in which case reliability problems are likely to result. In contrast, other measures contain 15 or 20 items designed to measure some type of common factor (e.g., level of problem game use), making the odds of achieving adequate reliability considerably brighter. For the former type of measure, there may be a sensible rationale or procedure for pooling the items into a summary score. It may be far better to place primary reliance on that summary score and far less or negligible reliance on the multiple subdimensions, considering the strong possibility that much of what the latter produces is measurement error or chance outcomes that do more to detract from rather than add to the scientific knowledge base.

Improved Norms and Reference Groups

It is often difficult to interpret the outcome of a measure if appropriate normative or reference groups are lacking. In this context, by "normative groups," we are referring to members of the general population who presumably are not addicted or problem users. Alternatively, one might prefer a more stringently defined normative group that is comprised of general population members who are free of psychiatric disorder. The term "reference group" is broader than "normative group" and can be used to refer to any comparison group that might be informative relative to the group of interest (which in this domain is likely to be problem digital gamers).

Normative groups and reference groups often provide crucial information, such as the frequency with which characteristics used to identify individuals within a diagnostic category occur in other groups. For example, some proposed criteria for problematic digital gaming refer to types of dysfunction that are not specific to this activity (e.g., academic or occupational dysfunction) but are observed among a certain percentage of the general population and perhaps many individuals with certain clinical disorders. Relative frequency of occurrence across these various groups provides valuable guidance on the usefulness of proposed diagnostic criteria, such as whether or how successfully they distinguish affected individuals from members of the general population, or to assist in differential diagnosis. For example, a characteristic that is common among problematic video gamers but rare among the general population likely has some utility, but if these same characteristics occur as often or more often among various clinical groups they may have little or no utility for differential diagnosis. Obviously, determining whether potential signs and indicators separate out individuals with PDG from those without PDG, how accurately they do so, and whether or the extent to which they help with differential diagnosis can provide invaluable assistance to clinical and research efforts. For example, deriving effective or optimal cutoff scores requires such information.

As noted in the previous discussion of content domain and the potential advantages of adding positive items, recruiting gamers to participate in studies has posed challenges. For example, problematic or frequent users may distrust researchers and suspect a negative agenda. Given the considerable value of developing quality normative and reference group data, the effort seems worth it. There is much to be gained by expanding normative data bases, making it a clear priority in measurement design, development, and selection.

Studies on Sensitivity, Specificity, Positive Prediction, and Negative Prediction

Sensitivity refers to the frequency with which a disorder that is present is detected, and *specificity* refers to the accuracy with which the absence of disorder is identified. Both qualities need to be studied because there is an inevitable tradeoff between the two (unless a diagnostic method is perfect). Ill-derived cutoff scores may produce very impressive results for sensitivity but abysmal results for specificity and vice versa. A measure has limited or no value (and marked potential for harm) if it almost always identifies a disorder but almost always misidentifies normal individuals as abnormal, or if the reverse occurs. Such outcomes are functionally similar to discarding the measure and identifying almost everyone as abnormal or almost everyone as normal.

Sensitivity and specificity also provide the basis for determining *positive predictive power* and *negative predictive power*, which adjust figures for sensitivity and specificity in accord with the base rate for a disorder in the population of interest. In this context, adjusting sensitivity and specificity in relation to base rates allows one to determine how often a positive or negative result on a diagnostic indicator will identify PDG or lack of PDG correctly. Clinicians and researchers use assessment measures in conditions and settings in which base rates can vary considerably, and hence reporting not only sensitivity and specificity but also positive and negative predictive power could offer essential practical guidance for developing, evaluating, and applying PDG measures.

Studies Examining Risk Factors and Course

For questions pertaining to onset, course, and prognosis, there is often no replacement for longitudinal studies. Longitudinal studies are rarely easy to conduct, but these troubles are often more than offset by the value of such research (Gentile et al., 2011; Lam & Peng, 2010), including the generation of information that may be difficult or nearly impossible to capture through cross-sectional designs. Using longitudinal studies to expand knowledge about onset and course could provide substantial assistance in advancing the understanding of causal pathways, identifying factors that foster resilience or increase risk, determining if and when preventative steps are warranted, and evaluating the need for therapeutic intervention. For example, better understanding of risk and protective factors could be especially beneficial for preventing PDG before such difficulties exert a truly detrimental impact on a person's life. It is for these reasons that we suggest, when selecting or developing questionnaires, serious consideration be given to including items that address potential risk and protective factors for PDG, such as the risk factors that Rehbein, Kleimann, and Mossle (2010) and other researchers, such as Hyun et al. (2015) have uncovered.

A newly emerging and increasingly prevalent risk factor involves games that allow players to spend actual money while gaming to improve the game or their gaming characters (Cleghorn & Griffiths, 2015). It seems probable that engagement with such games overlaps with, but is distinguishable from, GD, and that the amount of money spent gaming will become a good predictor of PDG. Although these purchases may have a positive impact on a player's sense of enjoyment or well-being when used in moderation (Cleghorn & Griffiths, 2015), the purchases could quickly get out of hand for a gamer who struggles with impulse control. Those developing assessment tools may wish to examine real-life money spent for "in-game" purchases as a potential predictor (or criteria) of problematic use. However, this predictor would require critical analysis because a gamer with substantial financial resources could spend considerably more money on in-game purchases without experiencing any significant adverse consequences in comparison to a gamer with less monetary resources.

Comparative Studies

Thanks to the efforts of talented researchers, various measures are now available with differing degrees of supportive validation evidence. Given the array of measures, proper selection for clinical and research uses would be greatly assisted by knowing more about how they compare to one another. For example, some PDG measures may exceed others in identifying problem users, others may be superior for treatment planning, and still others may be better suited for certain age groups. To identify the measure or measures most effective for intended applications in research and clinical settings, comparative studies are needed.

Measures Adjusted for Age, Language, and Cultural Factors

PDG measures designed for adults have often been used with children and adolescents without examining the need for modification. In addition, language factors and cultural differences may exert a major impact on the utility of measures and the extent of generalization across groups. Terms and phrases may have nonequivalent connotations across cultures, and translation or interpretation may inadvertently change the meaning of test items. For example, a term of endearment in one culture may reflect dislike in another culture. Cultural and linguistic considerations are particularly important in the area of digital gaming, given its international reach and applicability across broad sociodemographic strata. Consequently, cross-cultural research on measures would be of great potential value. For those who may be interested, Hambleton, Merenda, and Spielberger (2006) provide an excellent source on adapting measures across cultures.

Measurement of Time Frame, Severity, and Outcome

PDG measures that incorporate temporal dimensions would increase their value. Even one or two questions addressing when someone first engaged in digital gaming, and whether, for example, level of play has decreased, increased, or remained stable over the past year would provide some indication of duration and trajectory of usage. Inquiring about patterns of use over time cannot substitute for longitudinal studies, but it at least expands the snapshot of usage across a longer time frame. As noted previously, research that incorporates temporal patterns can assist in identifying risk and protective factors, exposing potential causative factors, predicting course over time, and distinguishing between pathology that is partly or largely independent of engagement in digital gaming and pathology that is accelerated or caused by use.

Combining Brevity with Comprehensive Measurement in Research and Clinical Practice

Some research and clinical applications call for brief assessment of digital gaming. For example, it could be argued that, in most intake interviews with youth, at least a few questions should be asked about involvement with digital gaming, but given the totality of topics that usually need to be covered, unless the youth's responses raise concern, further coverage of gaming would usually not be indicated. Likewise, in epidemiological studies that cover many forms of pathology, including more than a few questions about digital gaming can be hard to justify. Obviously, in other circumstances, such as when there are strong reasons to believe a client is engaged in patterns of extreme maladaptive use, more comprehensive information gathering likely should be performed.

We strongly recommend the design of measures with varying formats and length depending on the application of interest and, in many cases, responses to a core set of items. For example, as is commonly done in structured interviews, it should be feasible to design a set of screening items, to be followed by more detailed items when a certain threshold is surpassed. In fact, it might be wise to incorporate such designs for a wide range of problems seen with Internet use (e.g., pathological gambling; excessive shopping; cyberbullying) and across a range of behavioral addictions given their frequency of occurrence. When designing screening procedures, it is important to keep in mind that, to a point, false-negative errors are often worse than false-positive errors simply because a negative result ends the procedure and thus a false-negative error may never be caught or corrected. In contrast, an initial false-positive error may be detected and corrected when in follow-up as a more detailed assessment procedure is performed.

Another important recommendation would be for future studies to consider keeping track of the type of digital games an individual is spending most of his or her time playing. Various studies, such as a longitudinal study by Rehbein, Kleimann, and Moble (2010) have indicated that certain types of digital games, such as massively multiplayer online role-playing games (MMORPGs) may have more problematic impacts than other types of games.

Finally, and although perhaps stating the obvious, in clinical settings it will often be helpful to supplement use of digital gaming measures with other measures of psychological status. Given the seeming frequency of comorbid conditions and the somewhat narrow scope of many measures of digital technology use, adding measures in such areas as mood and everyday functional capacity should provide a more rounded picture of clinical status and needs.

Conclusion

Most measures used to assess PDG have incorporated or relied heavily on DSM criteria, with recent extension by some researchers to the measurement of IGD using criteria set forth in DSM-5. Although various measures developed to date have a number of positive features and one or multiple supportive studies, there are some limitations to these approaches. Fortunately, there are a number of ways in which measurement can be further strengthened. Some of the suggestions we provided (e.g., accounting for careless/random responding, incorporating data from longitudinal studies, etc.) can also be applied to improving a wide range of assessment tools. It is strongly recommended that more measures include appraisal of both the positive and negative impacts of digital gaming as this will create a more balanced picture of how these activities impact lives and should provide information helpful to treatment planning and monitoring. As digital gaming continues to become more prevalent across many different countries and cultures, so, too, will it become increasingly important to further refine the state of measurement and the assessment of PDG. With improved measurement, it will become far more feasible to properly assess and provide assistance to individuals who are at risk for or are currently engaged in problematic digital game use.

References

American Psychiatric Association. (2000). *Diagnostic and statistical manual of mental disorders* (4th ed., text rev.). Washington, DC: Author.

American Psychiatric Association. (2013). *Diagnostic and statistical manual of mental disorders* (5th ed., text rev.). Washington, DC: Author.

Carlo, G., & Randall, B. A. (2002). The development of a measure of prosocial behaviors for late adolescents. *Journal of Youth and Adolescence, 3*, 31–44.

Charter, R., & Lopez, M. (2002). Millon clinical multiaxial inventory (MCMI-III): The inability of the validity conditions to detect random responders. *Journal of Clinical Psychology, 58*(12), 1615–17.

Cleghorn, J., & Griffiths, M. D. (2015). Why do gamers buy "virtual assets"? An insight in to the psychology behind purchase behavior. *Digital Education Review, 27*, 98–117.

Connolly, T., Boyle, E., MacArthur, E., Hainey, T., & Boyle, J. (2012). A systemic literature review of empirical evidence on computer games and serious games. *Computers and Education, 59*(2), 661–86.

Crede, M. (2010). Random responding as a threat to the validity of effect size estimates in correlational research. *Journal of Educational and Psychological Measurement, 70*, 596–612.

Dye, M., Green, S., & Bavelier, D. (2009). Increasing speed of processing with action video games. *Current Directions in Psychological Science, 18*, 321–26.

Faust, K., Faust, D., Baker, A., & Meyer, J. (2012). Refining video game use questionnaires for research and clinical application: Detection of problematic response sets. *International Journal of Mental Health and Addiction, 10(6)*, 936–47.

Ferguson, C. J., Coulson, M., & Barnett, J. (2011). A meta-analysis of pathological gaming prevalence and comorbidity with mental health, academic and social problems. *Journal of Psychiatric Research, 45*, 1573–78.

Gentile, D. A., Choo, H., Liau, A. K., Sim, T., Li, D., Fung, D., & Khoo, A. (2011). Pathological video game use among youths: A two-year longitudinal study. *Pediatrics, 127*, 319–29.

Gentile, D. A., Coyne, S. M., & Bricolo, F. (2013). Pathological technology addictions: What is scientifically known and what remains to be learned. In K. E. Dill (Ed.), *The Oxford handbook of media psychology* (pp. 382–402). New York: Oxford University Press.

Glass, B., Maddox, T., & Love, B. (2013). Real-time strategy game training: Emergence of a cognitive flexibility trait. *Plos One 8*(8): e70350. doi:10.1371/journal.pone.0070350

Green, C. S., & Bavelier, D. (2007). Action-video-game experience alters the spatial resolution of vision. *Psychological Science, 18*, 88–94.

Griffiths, M. D. (2005). A components model of addiction within a biopsychosocial framework. *Journal of Substance Use, 10*, 191–97.

Hambleton, R. K., Merenda, P. F., & Spielberger, C. D. (Eds.). (2006). *Adapting psychological and educational tests for cross-cultural assessment.* Mahwah, NJ: Erlbaum.

Hong, J.-C., & Liu, M.-C. (2003). A study on thinking strategy between experts and novices of computer games. *Computers in Human Behavior, 19*, 245–58. doi:10.1016/S0747-5632(02)00013-4

Hyun, G. J., Han, D. H., Lee, Y. S., Kang, K. D., Yoo, S. K., Chung, U.-S., & Renshaw, P. F. (2015). Risk factors associated with online game addiction. A hierarchical model. *Computers in Human Behavior, 48*, 706–13.

Kim, J., & Kim, M. G. (2010). Cross-validation of reliability, convergent and validity for the problematic online game use scale. *Computers in Human Behavior, 26*, 389–98.

King, D., Delfabbro, P., & Zajac, I. (2014). The cognitive psychology of internet gaming disorder. *Clinical Psychology Review, 34*, 298–308.

King, D., Haagsma, M., Delfabbro, P., Gradisar, M., & Griffiths, M. (2013). Towards a consensus definition of pathological video game playing: A systemic review of psychometric assessment tools. *Clinical Psychology Review, 33*, 331–42.

Lam, L. T., & Peng, Z. W. (2010). Effect of pathological use of the Internet on adolescent mental health: A prospective study. *Archives of Pediatrics and Adolescent Medicine, 164*(10), 901–906.

Lemmens, J., Valkenberg, P., & Peter, J. (2009). Development and validation of a game addiction scale for adolescents. *Media Psychology, 12*, 77–95.

Lortie, C. L., & Guitton, M. J. (2013). Internet addiction assessment tools: Dimensional structure and methodological status. *Addiction 108*, 1207–16.

Petry, N., Rehbein, F., Gentile, D., Lemmens, J., Rumpf, H., Moble, T., . . . O'Brien, C. (2014). An international consensus for assessing internet gaming disorder using the new DSM-V approach. *Addiction, 109*, 1399–406.

Pontes, H., & Griffiths, M. (2015). Measuring DSM-5 internet gaming disorder: Development and validation of a short psychometric scale. *Computers in Human Behavior, 45*, 137–43.

Rehbein, F., Kleimann, M., & Mossle, T. (2010). Prevalence and risk factors of video game dependency in adolescence: Results of a German nationwide survey. *Cyberpsychology, Behavior, and Social Networking, 13(3)*, 269–77.

Saleem, M., Anderson, C. A., & Gentile, D. A. (2012). Effects of prosocial, neutral, and violent video games on college students' affect. *Aggressive Behavior, 38*, 263–71.

Salguero, R., & Moran, R. (2002). Measuring problem video game playing in adolescence. *Addiction, 97*, 1601–06.

Shaffer, D. W. (2006). *How computer games help children learn.* New York: Palgrave Macmillan. doi:10.1057/9780230601994

Sim, T., Gentile, D., Bricolo, F., Serpelloni, G., & Gulamoydeen, F. (2012). A conceptual review of research on the pathological use of computers, video games, and the internet. *International Journal of Mental Health Addiction, 10*, 748–69.

Thorell, L., Lindqvist, S., Nutley, S. B., Bohlin, G., & Klingberg, T. (2009). Training and transfer effects of executive functions in preschool children. *Developmental Science, 12*(1), 106–13.

World Health Organization. (2018). *International statistical classification of diseases and related health problems* (11th rev.). https://icd.who.int/browse11/l-m/en

Wouters, P., van Nimwegen, C., van Oostendorp, H., & van der Spek, E. (2013). A meta-analysis of the cognitive and motivational effects of serious games. *Journal of Educational Psychology, 105*(2), 249–66.

PART 3

Potential Positive Impacts of Internet and Technology Use

CHAPTER

15 Positive Effects of Video Gaming on Human Behavior

Aaron Cochrane, Sara Prot, Jorge Blanco, C. Shawn Green, *and* Douglas A. Gentile

Abstract

The enormous rise in the popularity of video games can be accounted for, at least in part, by their engaging and enjoyable nature. Interestingly, from the perspective of psychological science, the same basic mechanics that give rise to these motivating and pleasure-provoking attributes also make games powerful environments for inducing behavioral change. Indeed, it is easy to identify mechanics in video games that are known to facilitate learning (e.g. feedback, reinforcement, adaptive difficulty). It is therefore unsurprising that video game play has been linked with differences in a host of core psychological processes. Research has included several types of converging methods. This includes correlational methodology, where individuals who play certain types of video games are contrasted against individuals who do not play those types of games; longitudinal methodology, in which players are followed over an extended period of time; and true experiments, in which individuals are randomly assigned to be trained on certain video games. Reported game-related improvements range from heightened visual perception to increased pro-social behaviors to enhanced ability to perform surgery. Although these effects are wide-ranging, it must be emphasized that not all games are equal with respect to the psychological changes they induce. Instead the observed changes are clearly linked to the dynamics, mechanics, and content inherent in individual games. Future work treating video games as rich learning environments will improve our understanding of the interplay between humans and designed dynamic environments.

Keywords: video games, learning, reinforcement, education, general learning model

Introduction

Over the past 40 years, the ranks of individuals who play video games regularly have swollen dramatically. The first recognizable commercial home video game system, the Magnavox Odyssey (1972), sold only around 300,000 units. In contrast, the most popular systems released in the mid to late 2000s (e.g., the XBox 360, the PlayStation 3, the Nintendo DS, and the Nintendo Wii) have together sold more than 400 million units. Around three-quarters of all households in the United States today have at least one video game player, and consumers spend more than $43 billion per year on video games (Entertainment Software Association, 2019). Gaming is also consuming an increasing amount of time. A substantial number of players now report playing games for more than 20 hours per week (Pryor et al., 2012). The total estimated amount of time that has been spent playing just one popular game franchise—the *Call of Duty* series—is more than 25 billion hours. This increase in gaming time has led to a concomitant reduction in other leisure activities such as watching TV or movies (Entertainment Software Association, 2019).

As video games have played an increasingly large role in society, this has spurred significant scientific interest in the possible effects that gaming has on cognition and behavior. Although much of this research has focused on the negative effects (e.g., the effects of violent video games on aggression [Anderson et al., 2010] or the possibility that games can be addictive [Chiu, Lee, & Huang, 2004; Fisher, 1994]), there exists a significant body of research demonstrating that gaming can have positive effects as well. This chapter reviews the theory and empirical research surrounding positive effects of video game playing on cognitive functioning, social functioning, creativity, educational outcomes, and health outcomes.

Why Games Might Be Particularly Good at Changing Behavior

Before discussing the effects of video games on human behavior, it is worth briefly considering why we might expect video games to have any effects at all. This expectation may be surprising, as many individuals consider video gaming to be little more than entertainment. Simply put, good video games are, at their core, good learning environments. After all, no one would play a game where success is immediate and total, and neither would one play a game where success is forever unattainable. It is perhaps not surprising, then, to find that modern video games have come to instantiate many principles and practices long known to reflect effective pedagogy (Gentile & Gentile, 2008; Green & Bavelier, 2008). This includes promoting high levels of motivation via intrinsic and extrinsic reinforcement, employing individually appropriate and highly adaptable levels of difficulty, relying on active learning with immediate and informative feedback, producing significant physiological arousal, ensuring a proper balance of massed versus distributed practice, and utilizing a high degree of stimulus and response variety.

Intrinsic and Extrinsic Reinforcement

Perhaps the single best predictor of learning is simply the amount of time an individual spends practicing on a learning task (Greenwood, Horton, & Utley, 2002). For more than a century, behavioral scientists have known that one of the simplest ways to promote time on task is to utilize reinforcement; humans, like all animals, are hardwired to perform actions that result in reward.

Video games employ a wide variety of types of extrinsic reinforcement to promote time on task (points, badges, achievements, etc.; Lorenz, Gleich, Gallinat, & Kühn, 2015). These reward systems have been successful enough in altering behavior that they have spawned an entire field built around the concept of "gamifying" real-life behaviors in various domains (e.g., providing "points" to office staff for successfully collaborating on projects; see Hamari, Koivisto, & Sarsa, 2014, for a review). Research has also shown that video games can involve substantial intrinsic reinforcement, providing for certain basic psychological needs such as autonomy (the belief that one has control over his or her own actions and decisions), competence (the belief that one has the level of skill necessary to achieve goals), and relatedness (the feeling that one is socially connected with other human beings; Przybylski, Rigby, & Ryan, 2010). Finally, at the level of the brain, there is research showing that neurotransmitters related to reward processing, such as dopamine, are released in abundance when individuals play video games. These are the same chemicals released when individuals receive food or water when they are hungry or thirsty, as well as when individuals take many common drugs of abuse. In fact, the magnitude of the dopamine release seen as a result of game playing is similar to that seen when individuals take recreational doses of some drugs (Koepp et al., 1998).

Task Difficulty

Individuals tend to learn best when the demands of a task just barely exceed their level of ability. Such a circumstance ensures not only that errors are made frequently, but that the errors are informative and can thus be used to drive learning. If tasks are too easy, no errors will be made (thus there is nothing to learn). If tasks are too difficult, errors will obviously be made in abundance; however, the individual may lack the ability to interpret the errors and use them to improve performance (e.g., consider a fourth-grade student taking a graduate-level chemistry exam; it is unlikely that the feedback he or she receives could be used to improve subsequent performance). The basic idea that learning is most efficient at intermediate levels of difficulty has been recognized in a number of guises throughout the field of psychology but is perhaps best known as the *zone of proximal development* (Vygotsky, 1978).

Video games utilize a number of methods to ensure players are consistently challenged. For instance, nearly all video games have an adaptable initial level of difficulty (e.g., "novice," "normal," "expert"). This guarantees that no player will be immediately overwhelmed. Then, as the game progresses and the player's skills improve, the level of difficulty is increased. In some games this takes the form of distinct "levels"—where each additional level indicates an increase in difficulty. In other games, the level of difficulty is titrated online as a function of player aptitude. For instance, in the video games Resident Evil 5 and Left 4 Dead, player performance is measured continuously, and this measure is used to alter elements that control game difficulty (e.g., the number of enemies that appear and the extent of enemy resistance).

Active Learning with Immediate and Informative Feedback

There is a rich literature demonstrating that active learning, wherein individuals attempt to perform a given task and then are provided immediate feedback, far outpaces more passive forms of learning (Hogarth, Gibbs, McKenzie, & Marquis, 1991; Ivancic & Hesketh, 2000; Moreno, 2004). Essentially every theory of learning operates on the basis of error signals—signals that only exist when a response has been made and feedback has been provided. Active learning can take myriad forms such as actively attempting a tennis serve rather than passively watching an instructor serve, or actively taking quizzes rather than passively reviewing course material (Hattikudur & Postle, 2011; James et al., 2002). In video games there is very little passive instruction. Instead, even in introductory levels, the player is tasked with completing actions, and, if the player fails in completing the action, he or she is then provided with immediate and informative feedback.

Arousal

For more than a century psychologists have recognized that learning performance is an inverse U-shaped function of arousal level (Yerkes & Dodson, 1908). Learning environments that lead to very low levels of arousal (i.e., are "boring") tend to result in poor learning, as do environments that lead to exceedingly high levels of arousal (Frankenhaeuser & Gardell, 1976). Between these extremes is a level of arousal that leads to a maximum amount of learning. Video games clearly elicit a degree of physiological arousal (i.e., "fight-or-flight" response—pupil dilation, increase in heart rate/breathing, etc.; see Hebert, Beland, Dionne-Fournelle, Crete, & Lupien, 2005; Segal & Dietz, 1991; Shosnik, Chatterton Jr., Swisher, & Park, 2000) and are associated with a sustained optimal level of arousal which facilitates learning (Lorenz et al., 2015).

Massed Versus Distributed Practice

Since the seminal work by Baddeley and Longman (1978), showing that practicing typing skills for a half hour per day over many days leads to much more effective learning than practicing typing skills for several hours per day over a shorter number of days, there have been literally hundreds of studies throughout the field of psychology demonstrating that "massed practice" (i.e., accumulating many hours of training in a short amount of time) will greatly reduce the efficiency of learning as compared to "distributed practice" (i.e., shorter practice sessions spaced over greater amounts of time; Cepeda, Pashler, Vul, Wixted, & Rohrer, 2006).

While the level of "video game play" practice may at times seem somewhat massed (i.e., individuals who play for hours on end), proper video game design involves ensuring that the actual skills that are being practiced are distributed across time. In other words, even if an individual plays a video game for 3 hours straight, it does not mean that she is using and refining the exact same skill for the entirety of those 3 hours. Instead, situations designed to improve individual abilities are spread out over time—with an initial learning opportunity followed by many later temporally dispersed opportunities to relearn the skill. This structure is known to be optimal for preventing forgetting and for developing *automatized* structures of knowledge, or *schemas* (e.g., Anderson, 1983; Ellis & Hunt 1993; Glaser, 1984).

Variety

The learning principles just discussed—task difficulty, motivation engendered via reinforcement, active learning, arousal, distributed practice—are all critical in producing effective learning on a task itself. *Variety*, in contrast, is essential to producing learning that generalizes beyond just the trained context (Schmidt & Bjork, 1992), known as *skill transfer* in the education literature. Indeed, it is typically the case that when humans learn to perform a task, they show improvements only on the trained task, with little to no benefits being observed on even very similar tasks. For instance, individuals trained on certain types of "brain trainers" will show massive improvements on the training tasks themselves, but then show no benefits on tests of more general cognitive function (Owen et al., 2010). Greater amounts of stimulus and response variety tend to overcome this tendency toward task-specific learning (Brady & Kersten, 2003; Gómez, 2002; Onnis, Monaghan, Christiansen, & Chater, 2004; Reeder, Newport, & Aslin, 2013). Video games very naturally instantiate substantial stimulus and task variety. In fact, in most video games it is rarely the case that an individual will perform exactly the same action in exactly the same context twice (even if playing the same game a second time).

The General Learning Model

Video games clearly employ a number of techniques known to produce effective learning, but how then do we consider the overall structure of how video games alter behavior? The General Learning Model

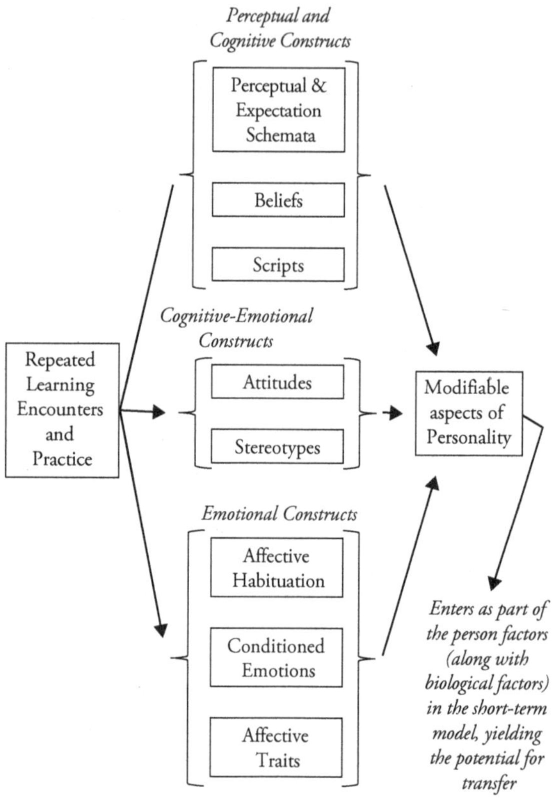

Figure 15.1 Long-term processes in the General Learning Model.

(GLM; Gentile, Groves & Gentile, 2014; Maier & Gentile, 2012) integrates a number of more specific learning theories and provides a broad framework for understanding video game effects on different outcomes. The GLM holds that people learn from experiences (including from video game play) via many learning mechanisms (such as classical conditioning, habituation, reinforcement, and social learning). Different types of learning work both serially and in parallel to produce learning outcomes (Gentile, Groves, & Gentile, 2014).

According to the GLM, video games affect players in the short term by influencing their internal state, including their current thoughts, emotions, and arousal. These changes, in turn, shape a person's interpretation of events, decision-making processes, and behaviors in the current situation. For example, playing pro-social games that portray characters acting in kind, caring, and helpful ways primes pro-social behavioral scripts and positive affect (Gentile et al., 2009; Greitemeyer, 2011). These changes lead players to demonstrate increased pro-social behavior outside the game immediately after playing.

Repeated experiences lead to more lasting changes in cognition, affect, and behavior—in particular if the repeated experiences occur in slightly different contexts. The GLM proposes that, in the long term, different experiences affect behavior through effects on perceptual and cognitive constructs, cognitive-emotional constructs, and emotional constructs (shown in Figure 15.1). For instance, pro-social video game play has been found to lead to long-term changes in helping via its effects on trait empathy (a cognitive-emotional construct; Prot et al., 2014).

The GLM has been applied predominantly to study effects of pro-social media (including pro-social video games) on empathy and pro-social behavior (Gentile et al., 2009; Greitemeyer, 2011; Greitemeyer & Mügge, 2014; Saleem, Anderson, & Gentile, 2012). However, this model provides a broad framework that can be used to understand any learning opportunity. Such learning opportunities include mediated learning through video games, such as effects of educational video games on educational outcomes, effects of "exergames" and health games on health outcomes, and effects of games portraying counter-stereotypical characters on reductions in prejudice and stereotyping.

How Do We Study the Effects of Games?

The mass popularity of video games allows for a much more varied set of viable methodological approaches than in many other domains. In particular, cross-sectional approaches and longitudinal approaches are possible, rather than only experimental methods. The various methods employed in the field each have a unique set of advantages and disadvantages.

Cross-Sectional Approaches

Perhaps the most common design in the literature on video gaming is the cross-sectional design. Individuals who play certain types of video games or play video games in a particular way as part of their natural life are compared with individuals who do not play those games as often. This method has the advantage that it is typically easy to recruit participants with specific types of experience, and it can assess "real-life" consequences and situations. It has the distinct disadvantage, however, that it cannot be used to draw causal inferences, although it can provide tests for causal theories. For instance, if one observes that individuals who commonly play violent video games score higher on measures of aggression, this cannot be used to infer that the act of playing violent video games *causes* increases in aggression as it could just as easily be the case that individuals who are naturally aggressive tend to disproportionately play violent video games (although it does refute the null hypothesis that there is no relation between them). Because of this limitation, studies often include both a cross-sectional design and one of the alternative designs discussed later to address the question of causation.

Longitudinal Approaches

Like a cross-section design, a longitudinal design can take advantage of natural variations in gaming behavior. However, rather than measuring gaming experience and the behaviors of interest at a single point in time, these measurements are made at several points over the course of multiple months or years. This allows for certain confounds present in cross-sectional studies to be controlled for. For instance, one might ask whether individuals who play violent video games over the course of several years show a disproportionate increase in aggression after controlling for their initial levels of trait aggression. However, again, because longitudinal methods rely on natural variations in behavior, they again cannot rule out all possible confounds related to the causal relationship between gaming and behavior.

Short-Term Experimental Approaches

In a short-term experimental study, individuals are randomly assigned to play either an experimental video game or a control video game (see later discussion for considerations that determine proper experimental and control game selection). The behaviors of interest are measured directly before and directly after a short amount of video game play (e.g., 20–30 minutes), with the critical question being whether the behavior changes more from pre-test to post-test in the group that played the experimental game than in the group that played the control game. For example, prior to gaming experience, the accessibility of aggressive thoughts may be measured via a word completion task (i.e., participants may be asked to fill in the word "k i _ _"—with completions such as "kick" or "kill" being indicative of more easily accessible aggressive thoughts than completions of "kilt" or "kiss"). Individuals then play either a violent video game (predicted to increase the accessibility of aggressive thoughts) or a control game (predicted to lead to no change in aggressive thoughts but matched in other visual/motor/motivational dimensions) and immediately after training undergo the same behavioral measure as during pre-test (in the case of word completion with different words). The key question is thus whether the group that played the violent video game showed an increase in aggressive thoughts as compared to the group that played the control game. While such short-term experimental studies have the benefit that they can be used to demonstrate a *causal* relationship between gaming and changes in behavior, because of the short-term nature of the effects (depending on the domain, the effects of 20–30 minutes of gaming persist for approximately 5 minutes and thus are more accurately described as "priming" rather than "learning"), they do not necessarily imply a long-term change in behavior.

Long-Term Experimental Approaches

To demonstrate conclusively that video gaming causes long-term changes in behavior, long-term training studies are performed. The basic design is similar to the short-term experimental approach just described, with two key differences. The first, and most obvious, is that the amount of gaming time is considerably longer in a long-term experimental study (the majority of the literature using durations of between 10 and 50 hours spaced over the course over many days and/or weeks). The second key difference is that the pre-test and post-test are temporally separated from the video game experience. In other words, rather than completing the post-test immediately after the final session of gaming, the post-test occurs at least 1 day after the final gaming session. This ensures that any effects that are observed are related to a stable change in behavior (i.e., "learning") rather than a reflection of transient effects (i.e., priming effects or effects related to temporary changes in arousal state, etc.).

Other Considerations

Scientific investigations into the effects of gaming today nearly always differentiate games by content, dynamics, and/or mechanics (see Gentile, 2011, for a review). This is because the term "video game" is a superordinate category label that encompasses an incredibly broad range of experiences—from extremely simple games that can be played on a smartphone or tablet through highly complex, elaborately designed multimillion dollar games on the newest consoles; from games that are solitary single-player activities through games that involve a network of hundreds of other players; from games with a rich narrative structure grounding the goals of the gameplay to games that are little more than a set of rules and rewards. Thus, in a cross-sectional or longitudinal study, because of the enormous variety in the content, dynamics, and mechanics that exist between different types of games, there is virtually no predictive value in knowing that an individual plays "video games." Instead, it is critical to consider the *types* of games an individual plays (as we will see later, only certain types of games are associated with certain changes in behavior). Similarly, in experimental settings, investigators contrast games with certain features that they believe are critical in driving changes in the behavior of interest (e.g., games with violent content driving changes in aggression) with games that lack those critical features (while matching the experimental game on as many other potentially confounding dimensions as possible—visual demands, motor demands, interest, arousal, engagement, etc.). Finally, the context in which video games are played can moderate effects of video game play on different outcomes. For example, recent research suggests that playing violent video games in a cooperative context can reduce detrimental effects of violent video game play on aggression and increase positive effects of video game play on empathy (Greitemeyer, 2013). Thus, in every section to come we will not be discussing the effects of "video games" on various aspects of human behavior but will instead be discussing the effects of a very limited set of well-specified video games and game situations.

Perceptual, Attentional, and Cognitive Effects of Video Games

Much of the pioneering initial research into the cognitive effects of video game playing was cross-sectional in nature and did not clearly differentiate between types of gaming experience (partially because, in the 1980s and 1990s, there was simply less variety in terms of the types of games available; Greenfield, Brannon, & Lohr, 1994; Griffith, Voloschin, Gibb, & Bailey, 1983; Kuhlman & Beitel, 1991). However, this research did convincingly demonstrate that video games have the potential to alter basic perceptual, attentional, and cognitive abilities.

Over the past decade, one particular genre of video games—known as "action video games"—has been the subject of the most study in the perceptual and cognitive domains. Action games differ from other types of games by including a fast pace (both in terms of the velocity of moving objects and many transient events), complex motor response demands, significant load on peripheral processing, and multiple possible objects to track and outcomes to consider. Games such as first-person shooters and third-person shooters are the most common types that encompass these features, although other types of games—such as certain car driving games—have similar features (and effects).

Effects on Perceptual Skills

Performance on perceptual tasks has repeatedly been associated with video game playing. For instance, one core aspect of visual perception is *contrast sensitivity*, the ability to detect slight variations in the luminance of adjacent stimuli. In cross-sectional work comparing individuals who play substantial amounts of action video games as part of their normal life—known as "action video game players" or AVGPs—with individuals who play no action games as part of their daily life—known as "non-video game players" or NVGPs—AVGPs were found to have significantly better contrast sensitivity than NVGPs. Then, in a long-term experimental training study, where NVGPs were trained for 50 hours on either an action video game or a non-action video game, action video game playing was associated with an improvement of roughly 50% percent on contrast sensitivity. This was significantly greater than any changes observed in the non-action video game playing control group (Li, Polat, Makous, & Bavelier, 2009).

Similar results have been found in many measures of basic perceptual skills. For instance, performance in visual crowding tasks (where a target surrounded by nearby distracting items must be identified) is indicative of an individual's visual spatial resolution. Green and Bavelier (2007) found that AVGPs had better performance in crowding tasks (i.e., could identify targets even when distracting items were placed very close to the targets) than did NVGPs. Then, in a long-term experimental study, NVGPs who trained for 30 hours on an action video game (Unreal Tournament 2004) had a decreased crowding threshold when compared to NVGPs who were trained for 30 hours on a non-action video game (Tetris). This decrease indicates a substantial improvement in this basic visual perceptive ability. Together, improvements in contrast resolution and crowded acuity indicate that video game playing enables individuals to experience and act in the world with more precision than without video games.

Although the majority of effects seen in the perceptual domain have been visual, some effects have also been seen in audition. For example, Donohue, Woldorff, and Mitroff (2010) found that, when asked to determine whether a visual stimulus or an auditory stimulus was presented first, video game players were able to distinguish the stimulus order with greater temporal resolution than were NVGPs. This finding indicates a relationship between video game playing and an increased ability to perceptually associate or dissociate multisensory stimuli, which is crucial for success at daily tasks ranging from driving to conversation.

Effects on Visual Attentional Skills

In addition to perceptual changes due to playing action video games, visual attentional processes are also improved. These include various subdomains of visual attention, such as spatial selective attention, temporal resolution, and attentional capacity. One measure used to determine individuals' performance on spatial selective attention is the Useful Field of View (UFOV) task. A modification of visual search methods, in the UFOV task participants must locate a peripheral target (presented either 10, 20, or 30 degrees from fixation) from among a field of distracting objects. Multiple studies have now shown both that AVGPs outperform NVGPs on this task and that long-term training on action video games produces significantly greater improvements on the task than training on non-action video games (Dye & Bavelier, 2010; Feng, Spence, & Pratt, 2007; Green & Bavelier, 2003, 2006; Wu et al., 2012). Similar results have been seen in numerous other measures of spatial visual attention including more standard visual search tasks (Castel, Pratt, & Drummond, 2005; Hubert-Wallander, Green, Sugarman, & Bavelier, 2011; Wu & Spence, 2013).

In terms of measuring temporal visual selective attention, the *attentional blink task* is commonly employed. The "attentional blink" refers to the fact that, for a short period after attending to a stimulus, individuals are not able to attend to a subsequent stimulus (Raymond, Shapiro, & Arnell, 1992). In the attentional blink task, participants view a series of rapidly presented black letters. Somewhere in the stream, one white letter is presented. At the end of the stream the participant is asked to indicate the identity of this letter. Additionally, 50% of the time, a black "X" is presented somewhere after the white letter. The participant is also asked to indicate whether or not an "X" appeared. When these two targets are presented within around 400 ms of each other, participants have difficulty detecting the second of the two targets (i.e., the "X"). As time between the targets increases, accuracy in attending to the second target also increases. Playing action video games is associated with a consistent reduction in the presence of attentional blink (Oei & Patterson, 2013). Green and Bavelier (2003) demonstrated that, with only 10 hours of action video game training over the course of 10 days, the period of attentional blink decreases in comparison to the benefits from playing a non-action video game. Similar results have been seen in various other measures of temporal attention such as in temporal masking (Li, Polat, Makous, & Bavelier, 2006).

Finally, the capacity of visual attention has been shown to change as a result of action video gaming. One measure of attentional capacity, the Multiple Object Tracking (MOT) paradigm, requires individuals to view several moving distinctive targets (e.g., red dots) among a field of moving distractors (e.g., blue dots). After a short period of tracking the distinctive targets, the targets change to become identical to the distractors. The goal of the task, then, is to continue tracking the targets even when they are perceptually identical to the distractors. At the end of each trial, the viewer must identify which items are targets. As with attentional blink and UFOV, both adult and child AVGPs have repeatedly demonstrated improved performance on

MOT tasks (Boot, Kramer, Simons, Fabiani, & Gratton, 2008; Dye & Bavelier, 2010; Trick, Jaspers-Fayer, & Sethi, 2005), and action video game playing improvements in MOT performance have also been observed experimentally (Green & Bavelier, 2006).

It is worth noting that the word "attention" is used here to refer to very specific aspects of visual perception and information detection. This is different from what parents and teachers often mean by "attention," where they tend to mean focused and sustained attention. In fact, some studies have found that amount of video game play predicts poorer attention in the classroom (e.g., Gentile, Swing, Lim, & Khoo, 2012; Swing, Gentile, Anderson, & Walsh, 2010). These results make sense when combined. As a child plays action games, he or she learns to widen his or her useful field of view, detect small changes and movements, and quickly reorient attention to the detected change. Yet, in the classroom, this same child is expected to be able to ignore the student fidgeting in the seat next to him or her. It is critical, therefore, to be careful to note what we mean when talking about attention.

Effects on Cognitive Skills

Various cognitive abilities that are goal-oriented and under effortful control, commonly called *executive functions*, are also demonstrably related to action video game playing. For instance, the fast-paced environment of action video games, combined with their constant decision-making demands, makes a relationship between them and the ability to rapidly switch between tasks seem quite natural. Indeed, AVGPs have demonstrated an increased speed in switching between tasks (Cain, Landau, & Shimamura, 2012; Colzato, van Leeuwen, van den Wildenberg, & Hommel, 2010; Karle, Watter & Shedden, 2010). Although there are many individual versions of task-switching tasks, they all share a common structure. On every trial, participants perform one of two tasks. For instance, they may be shown a digit from 1 to 9 (5 excluded) and be asked to either indicate whether the digit is even/odd (Task 1) or whether the digit is greater than or less than 5 (Task 2). Or they may be shown both a digit and a letter and be asked to indicate either whether the letter is a vowel or a consonant (Task 1) or whether the digit is odd or even (Task 2). On some trials they will be asked to perform the same task as on the previous trial, while on other trials they will be asked to switch tasks. What has been consistently found in the literature is that reaction times in the former case (perform the same task as was performed on the previous trial) are considerably faster than in the latter case (switch to the other task), with the difference in reaction time between these two types of trials being known as the *switch cost.*

Several groups have now seen reduced switch costs both in cross-sectional studies comparing AVGPs and NVGPs (Cain, Landau, & Shimamura, 2012; Colzato, van Leeuwen, van den Wildenberg, & Hommel, 2010; Karle, Watter, & Shedden, 2010) and in long-term experimental studies. For instance, Strobach, Frensch, and Schubert (2012) found that NVGPs had a reduction in switch cost after training on an action video game (Medal of Honor) for 15 hours and that this reduction was larger than that seen in a group that played a control non-action video game. In this study, the improved task switching performance was present even in the absence of an overall difference in reaction times between AVGPs and non-action video game players. This indicates that the specific task demands of action video games are related to an improved ability to switch between goal-oriented tasks, but not related to enhanced ability to react. In the same study, NVGPs trained on the action video game also improved more than a control group in their ability to perform a dual-task assessment. A dual-task test measures the ability to concurrently respond to two different stimuli, which corresponds well with both the heightened demands of action video game environments and the complex world that humans must successfully navigate on a daily basis (Wu & Spence, 2013). Other effects in the cognitive domain include changes in mental imagery and in visual memory (Boot et al., 2008; McDermott, Bavelier, & Green, 2014; Nikolaidis, Voss, Lee, Vo, & Kramer, 2014; Sungur & Boduroglu, 2012).

Effects in the Real World

Given the size, breadth, and reliability of the action gaming effects that have been observed in the perceptual, attentional, and cognitive domains, a number of groups have started to explore whether these off-the-shelf games could be used to make positive impacts in the real world.

One of the most promising applications for action video game–related perceptual and/or cognitive improvements is in the area of rehabilitation. Research has shown that action video games have the potential to help individuals with various disorders, such as amblyopia or dyslexia. *Amblyopia,* colloquially known as "lazy eye," is a relatively common disorder in which perceptual information is favored from one eye while being disregarded from the other eye. Although amblyopia is resistant to behavioral rehabilitation after childhood, Li, Ngo, Nguyen, and Levi (2011) demonstrated that training with either action video games or non-action video games helped adults with amblyopia improve their vision beyond the standard eye patching rehabilitation procedure, with the effects of action games being larger and persisting longer than non-action games.

Dyslexia, remediation-resistant reduced literacy independent of other deficits (Shaywitz, Shaywitz, Pugh, & Fulbright, 2001), is another promising area for positive video game effects. Individuals with this condition have distinct learning and livelihood disadvantages (McNulty, 2003; Mortimore & Crozier, 2006), and an effective remediation for dyslexic children would improve millions of lives. Franceschini, Gori, Ruffino, Viola, Molteni, and Facoetti (2013) trained 10-year-old dyslexic children on either action or non-action video games and found that children who had played action video games had improved on reading assessments significantly more than children who had played non-action video games. Together, these rehabilitative applications of action video game playing are promising, and indicate that other forms of action video game therapy may be possible as well.

In addition to rehabilitative applications of action video games, several studies have demonstrated that the benefits can help improve individuals' cognitive abilities even beyond normal levels and that these improvements transfer into enhanced performance in cognitively demanding professions. Evidence of improved performance of pilots after video game training has been present for more than two decades (Gopher, Weil, & Bareket, 1994). The relationship between video game training and flying is becoming increasingly relevant as flight controls are becoming more digitized and drone flight more common. Indeed, McKinley, McIntire, and Funke (2011) found that AVGPs performed similarly to experienced manned-aircraft pilots on assessments of the ability to fly drones and even outperformed these pilots on measures requiring heavy demands on visual attention.

Another profession that is cognitively taxing is that of surgeons. Endoscopic surgeons in particular must perform extremely precise medical procedures under very tight time restraints with difficult-to-utilize screen-based visual input and surgical tools. In an assessment of laparoscopic surgeons, Rosser et al. (2007) found that surgeons playing more than 3 hours of video games per week performed about 40% better in a simulated surgery than NGVP surgeons. Additionally, video game playing was more predictive of increased speed and decreased errors than experience with surgery. In a follow-up study, surgeons who had just played a video game performed better on surgical drills than those who hadn't. Furthermore, specific training on an action game led to increased endoscopic surgical skill (on a simulator) than training on a control game (Rosser, Gentile, Hannigan, & Danner, 2012). These and other findings have reliably shown action video game playing to be associated with better surgical performance, including lower risk to patients, and to demonstrate one of the potential social benefits of action video games (Lynch, Aughwane, & Hammond, 2010; Schlickum, Hedman, Enochsson, Kjellin, & Fellander-Tsai, 2009).

Underlying Brain Changes

Given the robust behavioral evidence for cognitive improvements related to video games, it is no surprise that there is also interest in the underlying neural changes that subserve these behavioral changes (Krishnan, Kang, Sperling, & Srinivasan, 2013). Mishra, Zinni, Bavelier, and Hillyard (2011) used EEG recordings over parietal-occipital sites to measure visually evoked potentials in AVGPs and NVGPs. Participants viewed a screen with three simultaneous streams of changing letters. They were asked to attend to just one of the streams (ignoring the other two) and report whenever a digit was presented instead of a letter in the attended stream. AVGPs performed this selective attention task better than NVGPs with regard to both speed and accuracy. Furthermore, because the three streams of letters were presented at slightly different temporal frequencies, it was possible to examine the amount of neural processing being devoted both to the attended stream and the ignored streams. While AVGPs and NVGPs showed similar enhancements in the neural processing of the attended stream, AVGPs showed a greater degree of suppression of the to-be-ignored streams. In addition, video game players displayed greater event-related potential (ERP) magnitudes in response to targets than NVGPs. These results provide a compelling starting point for understanding the neural basis for video game–related improvements in attentional abilities, and further ERP research has revealed a training-related causal relationship between action video game playing and neural activity related to visuospatial selective attention (Wu et al., 2012).

Similar patterns of enhanced distractor inhibition in AVGPs was found by Bavelier, Achtman, Mani, and Focker (2011) using functional magnetic resonance imaging (fMRI). In this study, distractors were associated with lower activity in an attention-related neural area (MT/MST) for AVGPs than for NVGPs. This provides further support for the role of video games' positive influence on neural mechanisms of selective attention and a possible relationship to many other improvements.

Other Types of Games

The majority of research findings on the cognitive effects of video game playing have involved action video games such as first-person shooters. However, in the past two decades, video games have changed considerably. As such, the extent to which "action video games" is synonymous with "shooter" video games may be disappearing. Indeed, many games that would be best categorized as "real-time strategy" or "role-playing" games now include a large number of the dynamics and mechanics that are characteristic of action games (including the need to attend to multiple independent sources of information, to make precise motor responses to targets in clutter, etc.). As such, recent work suggests that games, such as some car driving games, real-time strategy games, and role-playing games, may have similar effects (Basak, Boot, Voss, & Kramer, 2008; Glass, Maddox, & Love, 2013; Mayas, Parmentier, Andres, & Ballesteros, 2014; Oei & Patterson, 2013; Wu & Spence, 2013).

Pro-social Behavior and Empathy

The types of games considered in the literature on pro-social behavior and empathy are obviously very different from those considered in the literature on perception, visual attention, and cognition. In the pro-social behavior/empathy literature, the games of interest are those that give players an opportunity to act in helpful, kind, and cooperative ways toward other players and game characters and without exhibiting aggression to other players. For example, in the game Zoo Vet, the player is tasked with treating sick or injured animals. Or, in the game Lemmings, the player is tasked with saving as many characters (the "lemmings") as possible. Conversely, a game such as Gears of War—where a player can rescue injured teammates but can also kill enemies—would not be considered a strictly pro-social game, although it could be played in a pro-social manner.

Pro-Social Behavior

Numerous short-term experimental studies have found that playing a pro-social game increases cooperation and helping immediately after game play among both children and adults (Greitemeyer, 2011; Greitemeyer & Mügge, 2014; Saleem, Anderson, & Gentile, 2012). For instance, in a study by Greitemeyer and Osswald (2010), participants who had just played the pro-social game Lemmings were more willing to help a female experimenter who was seemingly harassed by her ex-boyfriend. Children in a study by Saleem, Anderson, and Gentile (2012) were more likely to help a supposed partner by assigning them easy puzzles to complete if they had just played a pro-social game. It seems that the main mediating mechanism of such short-term effects is accessibility of pro-social cognitions (Greitemeyer, 2011; Greitemeyer & Osswald, 2010). Playing a pro-social video game primes pro-social thoughts that in turn make players more likely to help others.

The existence of significant effects of pro-social video game use on pro-social outcomes is also supported by meta-analytic evidence. A recent meta-analytic review by Greitemeyer and Mügge (2014) combined effect sizes from 119 experimental, correlational and longitudinal studies that explored effects of pro-social and violent video games. Pro-social video game use was found to increase pro-social outcomes and decrease aggressive outcomes consistently across different types of studies. Violent video game use had opposite effects and increased aggression while decreasing pro-social outcomes. These findings underscore the fact that video game effects depend on content—whereas violent video games increase aggression and decrease helping, pro-social games have equally strong positive effects.

Empathy

Habitually playing pro-social video games predicts stable increases in empathy, cooperation, and helping over time (Gentile et al., 2009; Prot et al., 2014). For example, Gentile and colleagues (2009) found that playing pro-social video games predicts helpful and pro-social behaviors over time, even when statistically controlling initial levels of pro-social behavior. Recent research suggests that empathy is a key mediating mechanism of such long-term effects—pro-social video game use predicts increases in trait empathy over time, which, in turn, predicts more pro-social behavior (Prot et al., 2014). These findings generalize across culture, gender, and age groups. It is unclear at this time, however, what other mediating psychological mechanisms may underlie the effects as very few mechanisms other than empathy have been measured.

Stereotype Reduction

The majority of studies that have examined video games and stereotyping have focused on negative effects. Such studies demonstrate that stereotypical portrayals of racial groups, ethnic groups, and gender groups in video games contribute to stereotyping and prejudice in real life (Saleem & Anderson, 2013; Yang, Gibson, Lueke, Huesmann, & Bushman, 2014). This research interest makes sense given the frequency of negative stereotype portrayals in video games (Dill, Gentile, Richter, & Dill, 2005). However, the same learning processes through which video games create and reinforce negative stereotypes could also be used to reduce them. For instance, a recent study successfully used immersive virtual reality to reduce racial prejudice (Peck, Seinfeld, Aglioti, & Slater, 2013). Caucasian participants who used a black avatar in virtual reality subsequently showed lower implicit racial bias. Apart from video games, another line of research examining effects of music lyrics showed that listening to songs with pro-equality lyrics (such as "Respect" by Aretha Franklin) reduces prejudice toward women (Greitemeyer, Hollingdale, & Traut-Mattausch, 2015). These results are promising and suggest that playing video games that include prosocial content or promote identification with stereotyped groups could be used to fight stereotyping and prejudice.

Other Positive Effects of Gaming

Creativity

There is a growing interest in the video game effects literature on potential positive effects of video game play on creativity. Most parents believe that video games affect the development of their children's creativity (Stošić & Stošić, 2014), and a small number of studies support this belief. Cross-sectional research demonstrates significant positive associations between habitual video game play and creativity (Gackenbach & Dopko, 2012; Jackson et al., Zhao, 2012). For instance, Jackson and colleagues (2012) found that video gaming habits predict higher performance on different measures of creativity regardless of age, sex, race, or type of games played. A diary study by Gackenbach and Dopko (2012) found that time spent playing video games is linked with both figural creativity (nonverbal, graphic creativity measured using picture-based exercises) and dream bizarreness.

Although much of the research in this domain is cross-sectional, there is some evidence that the link between video game use and creativity is causal. Fard, Asgary, Sarami, and Zarekar (2014) applied game elements to a traditional math instruction software to create an effective method of improving creative problem-solving. Game elements included instant feedback, positive reinforcement for correct responses, progression inhibition for incorrect responses, high interactivity, multiple possible forms of responses, and personal instruction and pacing. Participants who were randomly assigned to complete the computer-based instruction that included game elements subsequently outperformed participants in the control condition on several components of creativity. Further experimental research is needed in this area to show evidence of causal effects of video game play on different aspects of creativity. In addition, more research is needed to explore the mechanisms through which such effects occur and possible moderating variables (such as game type).

Health

A number of empirical studies and several narrative reviews show that video games can be used to improve health-related knowledge, attitudes, and behaviors (Lieberman, 2001; Parisod et al., 2014). For example, the video game Re-Mission was designed as an educational intervention for young cancer patients. The game has been found to improve self-efficacy, knowledge, and adherence to medication among adolescent and young adult cancer patients (Kato, Cole, Bradlyn, & Pollock, 2008). Playing a video game designed to improve self-care among diabetics for 6 months reduced emergency room visits by 77% among diabetic youth (Lieberman, 2001).

A newer line of research has explored positive effects of active video games (exer-games), which require players to move and exercise. Such active games have been found to increase physical activity and energy expenditure among children and adults (Biddiss & Irwin, 2010; Parisod et al., 2014).

Education

Video games are highly effective teachers. Game features such as clear goals, quick feedback, reinforcement, distributed practice, and active involvement make video games excellent instructional tools (Gentile & Gentile, 2008). Unfortunately, most video games do not contain educational content, so overall amount of video game play tends to be a negative predictor of school achievement (Anderson, Gentile, & Buckley, 2007). On the other hand, educational video games that are designed to teach specific content can have significant beneficial effects on players. A number of studies demonstrate positive effects of educational video games on academic achievement in different school subjects, such as history, biology, and language learning (Corbett, Koedinger, & Hadley, 2001; Murphy, Penuel, Means, Korbak, & Whaley, 2001; Young et al., 2012). In addition, there is growing evidence that physically active video games (exer-games) may contribute to physical education (Young et al., 2012).

Conclusion

The public discussion of video games tends to oversimplify the issue—asking whether games are "good" or "bad." Ironically, even the research on violent video game effects on aggression demonstrates valuable aspects of learning and transfer. When examined in more detail, however, we find that games have many effects at many different levels of analysis. Furthermore, the ultimate effects themselves may not be as interesting as defining the specific game aspects that lead to changes in specific psychological mechanisms and how those changes (i.e., learning) can influence other psychological processes. As shown in this review, games have both intentional effects (e.g., educational and health games) and unintentional effects (e.g., action games influencing perception skills). What is clear is that games are excellent teaching tools even if not specifically designed to be such. The implication, therefore, is that we have barely begun to scratch the surface of the benefits that games can have.

References

Anderson, J. R. (1983). *The architecture of cognition*. Cambridge, London: Harvard University Press.

Anderson, C. A., Gentile, D. A., & Buckley, K. E. (2007). *Violent video game effects on children and adolescents: Theory, research, and public policy*. New York: Oxford University Press.

Anderson, C. A., Shibuya, A., Ihori, N., Swing, E. L., Bushman, B. J., Sakamoto, A., . . . Saleem, M. (2010). Violent video game effects on aggression, empathy, and prosocial behavior in Eastern and Western countries. *Psychological Bulletin, 136*, 151–73.

Baddeley, A. D., & Longman, D. J. A. (1978). The influence of length and frequency of training session on the rate of learning to type. *Ergonomics, 21*, 627–35.

Basak, C., Boot, W. R., Voss, M. W., & Kramer, A. F. (2008). Can training in a real-time strategy video game attenuate cognitive decline in older adults? *Psychology and Aging, 23*(4), 765–77.

Bavelier, D., Achtman, R. L., Mani, M., & Focker, J. (2011). Neural bases of selective attention in action video game players. *Vision Research, 61*, 132–43.

Biddiss, E., & Irwin, J. (2010). Active video games to promote physical activity in children and youth. *Archives of Pediatrics and Adolescent Medicine, 164*(7), 664–72.

Boot, W. R., Kramer, A. F., Simons, D. J., Fabiani, M., & Gratton, G. (2008). The effects of video game playing on attention, memory, and executive control. *Acta Psychologica, 129*, 387–98.

Brady, M. J., & Kersten, D. (2003). Bootstrapped learning of novel objects. *Journal of Vision, 3*(6), 413–422. doi: 10.1167/3.6.2

Cain, M. S., Landau, A. N., & Shimamura, A. P. (2012). Action video game experience reduces the cost of switching tasks. *Attention, Perception, & Psychophysics, 74*(4), 641–47.

Castel, A. D., Pratt, J., & Drummond, E. (2005). The effects of action video game experience on the time course of inhibition of return and the efficiency of visual search. *Acta Psychologica. 119*, 217–30.

Cepeda, N. J., Pashler, H., Vul, E., Wixted, J. T., & Rohrer, D. (2006). Distributed practice in verbal recall tasks: A review and quantitative synthesis. *Psychological Bulletin, 132*(3), 354–80.

Chiu, S.-I., Lee, J.-Z., & Huang, D.-H. (2004). Video game addiction in children and teenagers in Taiwan. *CyberPsychology & Behavior, 7*(5), 571–81.

Colzato, L. S., van Leeuwen, P. J., van den Wildenberg, W. P. M., & Hommel B. (2010). DOOM'd to switch: Superior cognitive flexibility in players of first person shooter games. *Frontiers in Psychology, 1*(8), 1–5.

Corbett, A. T., Koedinger, K. R., & Hadley, W. (2001). Cognitive tutors: From the research classroom to all classrooms. In P. S. Goodman (Ed.), *Technology enhanced learning* (pp. 235–63). Mahwah, NJ: Erlbaum.

Dill, K. E., Gentile, D. A., Richter, W. A., & Dill, J. C. (2005). Violence, sex, race and age in popular video games: A content analysis. In E. Cole & J. Henderson Daniel (Eds.), *Featuring females: Feminist analyses of the media*. Washington, DC: American Psychological Association.

Donohue, S. E., Woldorff, M. G., & Mitroff, S. R. (2010). Video game players show more precise multisensory temporal processing abilities. *Attention, Perception, & Psychophysics, 72*(4), 1120–29.

Dye, M. W., & Bavelier D. (2010). Differential development of visual attention skills in school-age children. *Vision Research, 50*(4), 452–59.

Ellis, H. C., Hunt, R. R., & Ellis, H. C. (1993). *Fundamentals of cognitive psychology* (5th ed). Madison, WI: Brown & Benchmark.

Entertainment Software Association. (2019). 2019 Essential Facts About the Computer and Video Game Industry. https://www.theesa.com/wp-content/uploads/2019/05/ESA_Essential_facts_2019_final.pdf

Fard, A., Asgary, A., Sarami, G. R., & Zarekar, A. (2014). Comparative study of the effect of computer-based instruction and problem-solving instruction on the students' creativity. *Journal of Education and Training Studies, 2*(2), 105–13.

Feng, J., Spence, I., & Pratt, J. (2007). Playing an action video game reduces gender differences in spatial cognition. *Psychological Science, 18*(10), 850–855. doi:10.1111/j.1467-9280.2007.01990.x

Fisher, S. (1994). Identifying video game addiction in children and adolescents. *Addictive Behaviors, 19*(5), 545–53.

Franceschini, S., Gori, S., Ruffino, M., Viola, S., Molteni, M., & Facoetti, A. (2013). Action video games make dyslexic children read better. *Current Biology, 23*(6), 462–66.

Frankenhaeuser, M., & Gardell, B. (1976). Underload and overload in working life: Outline of a multidisciplinary approach. *Journal of Human Stress, 2*, 35–46.

Gackenbach, J. I., & Dopko, R. (2012). The relationship between video game play, dream bizarreness, and creativity. *International Journal of Dream Research, 5*(1), 23–36.

Glaser, R. (1984). Education and thinking: The role of knowledge. *American Psychologist, 39*(2), 93–104. doi:10.1037/0003-066X.39.2.93

Gentile, D. A. (2011). The multiple dimensions of video game effects. *Child Development Perspectives, 5*, 75–81.

Gentile, D. A., Anderson, C. A., Yukawa. S., Ihori, N., Saleem, M., Ming, L. K., . . . Sakamoto, A. (2009). The effects of prosocial video games on prosocial behaviors: International evidence from correlational, experimental, and longitudinal studies. *Personality and Social Psychology Bulletin, 35*, 752–63.

Gentile, D. A., & Gentile, J. R. (2008). Video games as exemplary teachers: A conceptual analysis. *Journal of Youth and Adolescence, 37*, 127–41.

Gentile, D. A., Groves, C., & Gentile, J. R. (2014). The general learning model: Unveiling the learning potential form video games. In F. C. Blumberg (Ed.), *Learning by playing: Frontiers of video gaming in education* (pp. 121–142). New York: Oxford University Press.

Gentile, D. A., Swing, E. L., Lim, C. G., & Khoo, A. (2012). Video game playing, attention problems, and impulsiveness: Evidence of bi-directional causality. *Psychology of Popular Media Culture, 1*, 62–70.

Glass, B., Maddox, W., & Love, B. (2013). Real-time strategy game training: Emergence of a cognitive flexibility trait. *PLoS One, 8*(8), e0070350.

Gómez, R. L. (2002). Variability and Detection of Invariant Structure. *Psychological Science, 13*(5), 431–436. doi:10.1111/1467-9280.00476.

Gopher, D., Weil, M., & Bareket, T. (1994). Transfer of skill from a computer game trainer to flight. *Human Factors, 36*, 387–405.

Green C. S., & Bavelier, D. (2003). Action video game modifies visual selective attention. *Nature, 423*(6939), 534–37.

Green, C. S., & Bavelier, D. (2006). Enumeration versus multiple object tracking: The case of action video game players. *Cognition, 101*(1), 217–45.

Green, C. S., & Bavelier, D. (2007). Action video game experience alters the spatial resolution of attention. *Psychological Science, 18*(1), 88–94.

Green, C. S., & Bavelier, D. (2008). Exercising your brain: A review of human brain plasticity and training-induced learning. *Psychology and Aging*, 23(4), 692–701.

Greenfield, P. M., Brannon, G., & Lohr, D. (1994). Two-dimensional representation of movement through three-dimensional space: The role of video game expertise. *Journal of Applied Developmental Psychology, 15*(1), 87–103.

Greenwood, C., Horton, B., & Utley, C. (2002). Academic engagement: Current perspectives on research and practice. *School Psychology Review, 31*, 328–49.

Greitemeyer T., & Osswald S. (2010). Effects of prosocial video games on prosocial behavior. *Journal of Personality and Social Psychology, 98*, 211–21.

Greitemeyer, T. (2011). Effects of prosocial media on social behavior: When and why does media exposure affect helping and aggression. *Current Directions in Psychological Science, 20*, 251–55.

Greitemeyer, T. (2013). Playing video games cooperatively increases empathic concern. *Social Psychology, 44*, 408–13.

Greitemeyer, T., Hollingdale, J., & Traut-Mattausch, E. (2015). Changing the track in music and misogyny: Listening to music with pro-equality lyrics improves attitudes and behavior toward women. *Psychology of Popular Media Culture, 4*(1), 56–67.

Greitemeyer, T., & Mügge, D. O. (2014). Video games do affect social outcomes: A meta-analytic review of the effects of violent and prosocial video game play. *Personality and Social Psychology Bulletin, 40*, 578–89.

Griffith, J. L., Voloschin, P., Gibb, G. D., & Bailey, J. R. (1983). Differences in eye-hand motor coordination of video-game users and non-users. *Perceptual and Motor Skills, 57*(1), 155–58.

Hamari, J., Koivisto, J., & Sarsa, H. (2014). *Does gamification work? A literature review of empirical studies on gamification.* Proceedings of the 47th Hawaii International Conference on System Sciences, Hawaii, USA.

Hattikudur, S., & Postle, B. R. (2011). Effects of test-enhanced learning in a cognitive psychology course. *Journal of Behavioral and Neuroscience Research, 9*(2), 151–57.

Hebert, S., Beland, R., Dionne-Fournelle, O., Crete, M., & Lupien, S. J. (2005). Physiological stress response to video-game playing: The contribution of built-in music. *Life Sciences, 76*(20), 2371–80.

Hogarth, R. M., Gibbs, B. J., McKenzie, C. R., & Marquis, M. A. (1991). Learning from feedback: Exactingness and incentives. *Journal of Experimental Psychology: Learning, Memory, and Cognition, 17*(4), 734–52. http://doi.org/10.1037/0278-7393.17.4.734

Hubert-Wallander, B., Green, C. S., Sugarman, M., & Bavelier, D. (2011). Changes in search rate but not in the dynamics of exogenous attention in action videogame players. *Attention, Perception, & Psychophysics, 73*, 2399–412.

Ivancic, K., & Hesketh, B. (2000). Learning from errors in a driving simulation: Effects on driving skill and self-confidence. *Ergonomics, 43*(12), 1966–84.

Jackson, L. A., Witt, E. A., Games, A. I., Fitzgerald, H. E., von Eye, A., & Zhao, Y. (2012). Information technology use and creativity: Findings from the children and technology project. *Computers in Human Behavior, 28*(2), 370–76.

James, K. H., Humphrey, G. K., Vilis, T., Corrie, B., Baddour, R., & Goodale, M. A. (2002). "Active" and "passive" learning of three-dimensional object structure within an immersive virtual reality environment. *Behavior Research Methods, Instruments, & Computers, 34*(3), 383–90.

Karle, J. W., Watter, S., & Shedden, J. M. (2010). Task switching in video game players: Benefits of selective attention but not resistance to proactive interference. *Acta Psychologica, 134*(1), 70–78.

Kato, P. M., Cole, S. W., Bradlyn, A. S., & Pollock, B. H. (2008). A video game improves behavioral outcomes in adolescents and young adults with cancer: A randomized trial. *Pediatrics, 122*, e305–17.

Koepp, M. J., Gunn, R. N., Lawrence, A. D., Cunningham, V. J., Dagher, A., Jones, T., & Grasby, P. M. (1998). Evidence for striatal dopamine release during a video game. *Nature, 393*(6682), 266–68.

Krishnan, L., Kang, A., Sperling, G., & Srinivasan, R. (2013). Neural strategies for selective attention distinguish fast-action video game players. *Brain Topography, 26*(1), 83–97.

Kuhlman, J. S., & Beitel, P. A. (1991). Videogame experience: A possible explanation for differences in anticipation of coincidence. *Perceptual and Motor Skills, 72*(2), 483–88.

Li, R. W., Ngo, C., Nguyen, J., & Levi, D. M. (2011). Video-game play induces plasticity in the visual system of adults with amblyopia. *PloS Biology, 9*(8).

Li, R., Polat, U., Makous, W., & Bavelier, D. (2009). Enhancing the contrast sensitivity function through action video game training. *Nature Neuroscience, 12*(5), 549–51.

Lieberman, D. A. (2001). Management of Chronic Pediatric Diseases with Interactive Health Games: Theory and Research Findings. *The Journal of Ambulatory Care Management, 24*(1), 26–38. https://journals.lww.com/ambulatorycaremanagement/Fulltext/2001/01000/Management_of_Chronic_Pediatric_Diseases_with.4.aspx

Lorenz, R. C., Gleich, T., Gallinat, J., & Kühn, S. (2015). Video game training and the reward system. *Frontiers in Human Neuroscience, 9*(40), 1–9.

Lynch, J., Aughwane, P., & Hammond, T. M. (2010). Video games and surgical ability: A literature review. *Journal of Surgical Education, 67*(3), 184–89.

Mayas, J., Parmentier, F. B., Andres, P., & Ballesteros, S. (2014). Plasticity of attentional functions in older adults after non-action video game training: A randomized controlled trial. *PLoS One, 9*(3), e0092269.

McDermott, A. F., Bavelier, D., & Green, C. S. (2014). Memory abilities in action video game players. *Computers in Human Behavior, 34*, 69–78.

McKinley, A., McIntire, L., & Funke, M. (2011). Operator selection for unmanned aerial systems: Comparing video game players and pilots. *Aviation, Space, and Environmental Medicine, 82*, 635–42.

McNulty, M. A. (2003). Dyslexia and the life course. *Journal of Learning Disabilities, 36*(4), 363–81.

Mishra, J., Zinni, M., Bavelier, D., & Hillyard, S. A. (2011). Neural basis of superior performance of action videogame players in an attention-demanding task. *Journal of Neuroscience, 31*(3), 992–98.

Moreno, R. (2004). Decreasing cognitive load for novice students: Effects of explanatory versus corrective feedback in discovery-based multimedia. *Instructional Science, 32*(1/2), 99–113.

Mortimore, T., & Crozier, W. R. (2006). Dyslexia and difficulties with study skills in higher education. *Studies in Higher Education, 31*(2), 235–51.

Murphy, R., Penuel, W., Means, B., Korbak, C., & Whaley, A. (2001). *E-Desk: A review of recent evidence on the effectiveness of discrete educational software.* Menlo Park, CA: SRI International.

Nikolaidis, A., Voss, M. W., Lee, H., Vo, L. T., & Kramer, A. F. (2014). Parietal plasticity after training with a complex video game is associated with individual differences in improvements in an untrained working memory task. *Frontiers in Human Neuroscience, 8*, 169.

Oei, A. C., & Patterson, M. D. (2013). Enhancing cognition with video games: A multiple game training study. *PLoS One, 8*(3), e58546.

Onnis, L., Monaghan, P., Monaghan@psych, P., York, A., Uk, Christiansen, M., & Chater, N. (2004). Variability is the spice of learning, and a crucial ingredient for detecting and generalizing in nonadjacent dependencies. *Proceedings of the Annual Meeting of the Cognitive Science Society.*

Owen, A. M., Hampshire, A., Grahn, J. A., Stenson, R., Dajani, S., Burns, A. S., & Ballard, C. G. (2010). Putting brain training to the test. *Nature, 465*(7299), 775–78.

Parisod, H., Pakarinen, A., Kauhanen, L., Aromaa, M., Leppänen, V., Liukkonen, T.,...Salanterä, S. (2014). Promoting children's health with digital games: A review of reviews. *Games for Health Journal, 3*(3), 145–56.

Peck, T. C., Seinfeld, S., Aglioti, S. M., & Slater, M. (2013). Putting yourself in the skin of a black avatar reduces implicit racial bias. *Consciousness and Cognition, 22*(3), 779–87.

Prot, S., Gentile, D. G., Anderson, C. A., Suzuki, K., Swing, E., Lim, K. M.,...Lam, C. P. (2014). Long-term relations between prosocial media use, empathy and prosocial behavior. *Psychological Science, 25*, 358–68.

Pryor, J. H., Eagan, K., Blake, L. P., Hurtado, S., Berdan, J., & Case, M. H. (n.d.). *The American Freshman: National Norms Fall 2012.*

Przybylski, A. K., Rigby, C. S., & Ryan, R. M. (2010). A motivational model of videogame engagement. *Review of General Psychology, 14*, 154–66.

Raymond, J. E., Shapiro, K. L., & Arnell, K. M. (1992). Temporary suppression of visual processing in an RSVP task: An attentional blink? *Journal of Experimental Psychology: Human Perception and Performance, 18*(3), 849–60.

Reeder, P. A., Newport, E. L., & Aslin, R. N. (2013). From shared contexts to syntactic categories: The role of distributional information in learning linguistic form-classes. *Cognitive Psychology, 66*(1), 30–54. doi:10.1016/j.cogpsych.2012.09.001.

Rosser, J. C., Gentile, D. A., Hannigan, K., & Danner, O. K. (2012). The effect of video game "warm-up" on performance of laparoscopic surgery tasks. *Journal of the Society of Laparoendoscopic Surgeons, 16*, 3–9.

Rosser, J. C., Lynch, P. J., Cuddigy, L., Gentile, D. A., Klonsky, J., & Merrell, R. (2007). The impact of video games on training surgeons in the 21st century. *Archives of Surgery, 142*, 181–86.

Saleem, M., & Anderson, C. A. (2013). Arabs as terrorists: Effects of stereotypes within violent contexts on attitudes, perceptions and affect. *Psychology of Violence, 3*, 84–99.

Saleem, M., Anderson, C. A., & Gentile, D. A. (2012). Effects of prosocial, neutral, and violent video games on children's helpful and hurtful behaviors. *Aggressive Behavior, 38*, 281–87.

Schlickum, M. K., Hedman, L., Enochsson, L., Kjellin, A., & Fellander-Tsai, L. (2009). Systematic video game training in surgical novices improves performance in virtual reality endoscopic surgical simulators: A prospective randomized study. *World Journal of Surgery, 33*, 2360–67.

Schmidt, R. A., & Bjork, R. A. (1992). New conceptualizations of practice: Common principles in three paradigms suggest new concepts for training. *Psychological Science, 3*, 207–17.

Segal, K. R., & Dietz, W. H. (1991). Physiological responses to playing a video game. *American Journal of Diseases of Children, 145*(9), 1034–36.

Shaywitz, B. A., Shaywitz, S. A., Pugh, K. R., & Fulbright, R. K. (2001). The neurobiology of dyslexia. *Clinical Neuroscience Research, 1*(4), 291–99.

Shosnik, P. D., Chatterton, R. T. Jr, Swisher, T., & Park, S. (2000). Modulation of attentional inhibition by norepinephrine and cortisol after psychological stress. *International Journal of Psychophysiology, 36*(1), 59–68.

Stošić, L., & Stošić, I. (2014). Impact of computers on the creativity of children. *International Journal of Cognitive Research in Science, Engineering and Education, 2*(2), 29–34.

Strobach, T., Frensch, P., & Schubert, T. (2012). Video game practice optimizes executive control skills in dual-task and task switching situations. *Acta Psychologica, 140*(1), 13–24.

Sungur, H., & Boduroglu, A. (2012). Action video game players form more detailed representation of objects. *Acta Psychologica, 139*(2), 327–34.

Swing, E., Gentile, D. A., Anderson, C. A., & Walsh, D. A. (2010). Television and video game exposure and the development of attention problems. *Pediatrics, 126*, 214–21.

Trick, L. M., Jaspers-Fayer, F., & Sethi, N. (2005). Multiple-object tracking in children: The "Catch the Spies" task. *Cognitive Development, 20*, 373–87.

Vygotsky, L. S. (1978). *Mind and society: The development of higher psychological processes.* Cambridge, MA: Harvard University Press.

Wu, S., Cheng, C. K., Feng, J., D'Angelo, L., Alain, C., & Spence, I. (2012). Playing a first-person shooter video game induces neuroplastic change. *Journal of Cognitive Neuroscience, 24*(6), 1286–93.

Wu, S., & Spence, I. (2013). Playing shooter and driving videogames improves top-down guidance in visual search. *Attention, Perception, & Psychophysics, 75*(4), 673–86.

Yang, G. S., Gibson, B., Lueke, A. K., Huesmann, L. R., & Bushman, B. J. (2014). Effects of avatar race in violent video games on racial attitudes and aggression. *Social Psychological and Personality Science, 5*(6), 698–704.

Yerkes, R. M., & Dodson, J. D. (1908). The relation of strength of stimulus to rapidity of habit-formation. *Journal of Comparative Neurology and Psychology, 18*, 459–82.

Young, M. F., Slota, S., Cutter, A. B., Jalette, G., Mullin, G., Lai, B., . . . Yukhymenko, M. (2012). Our princess is in another castle: A review of trends in serious gaming for education. *Review of Educational Research, 82*(1), 61–89.

Further Reading

Ball, K., & Sekuler, R. (1982). A specific and enduring improvement in visual motion discrimination. *Science, 218*(4573), 697–98.

Bavelier, D., Green, C. S., Schrater, P., & Pouget, A. (2012). Brain plasticity through the life span: Learning to learn and action video games. *Annual Reviews of Neuroscience, 35*, 391–416.

Bejjanki, V. R., Zhang, R., Li, R., Pouget, A., Green, C. S., Lu, Z.-L., & Bavelier, D. (2012). Action video game play facilitates the development of better perceptual templates. *Proceedings of the National Academy of Sciences of the United States of America, 111*(47), 16961–66.

Brashers-Krug, T., Shadmehr, R., & Bizzi, E. (1996). Consolidation in human motor memory. *Nature, 382*(6588), 252–55.

Cohen, J. E., Green, C. S., & Bavelier, D. (2007). Training visual attention with video games: Not all games are created equal. In H. O'Neil & R. Perez (Eds.), *Computer games and adult learning.* Amsterdam: Elsevier.

Destefano, M., Lindstedt, J. K., & Gray, W. D. (2011). Use of complementary actions decreases with expertise. In L. Carlson, C. Hölscher, & T. Shipley (Eds.), *33rd Annual Conference of the Cognitive Science Society* (pp. 2709–2014). Austin, TX: Cognitive Science Society.

Erickson, K. I., & Kramer, A. F. (2009). Aerobic exercise effects on cognitive and neural plasticity in older adults. *British Journal of Sports Medicine, 43*, 22–24.

Fahle, M. (2004). Perceptual learning: A case for early selection. *Journal of Vision, 4*(10), 879–90.

Fahle, M. (2005). Perceptual learning: Specificity versus generalization. *Current Opinion in Neurobiology, 15*(2), 154–60.

Fiorentini, A., & Berardi, N. (1980). Perceptual learning specific for orientation and spatial frequency. *Nature, 287*, 43–44.

Fulvio, J. M., Green, C. S., & Schrater, P. R. (2014). Task-specific response strategy selection on the basis of recent training experience. *PLoS Computational Biology, 10*(1), e1003425.

Gagnon, D. (1985). Videogames and spatial skills: An exploratory study. *Educational Communication and Technology Journal, 33*(4), 263–75.

Gandolfo, F., Mussa-Ivaldi, F. A., & Bizzi, E. (1996). Motor learning by field approximation. *Proceedings of the National Academy of Science, 93*, 3843–46.

Green, C. S., & Bavelier, D. (2012). Learning, attentional control, and action video games. *Current Biology, 22*, R197–206.

Green, C. S., Sugarman, M., Medford, K., Klobusicky, E., & Bavelier, D. (2012). The effect of action video game experience on task-switching. *Computers in Human Behavior, 28*(3), 984–94.

Greenfield, P. M., deWinstanley, P., Kilpatrick, H., & Kaye, D. (1994). Action video games and informal education: Effects on strategies for dividing visual attention. *Journal of Applied Developmental Psychology, 15*, 105–23.

Li, R., Polat, U., Makous, W., & Bavelier, D. (2006). Temporal resolution of visual processing in action video game players. *Journal of Vision, 6*(6), 1008.

Mackrous, I., & Proteau, L. (2007). Specificity of practice results from differences in movement planning strategies. *Experimental Brain Research, 183*, 181–93.

Maier, J. A., & Gentile, D. A. (2012). Learning aggression through the media: Comparing psychological and communication approaches. In L. J. Shrum (Ed.), *The psychology of entertainment media: Blurring the lines between entertainment and persuasion* (2nd ed., pp. 267–99). New York: Taylor & Francis.

Melby-Lervåg, M., & Hulme C. (2013). Is working memory training effective? A meta-analytic review. *Developmental Psychology, 49*(2), 270–91.

Mollon, J. D., & Danilova, M. V. (1996). Three remarks on perceptual learning. *Spatial Vision, 10*(1), 51–58.

Ou, Y., McGlone, E. R., Camm, C. F., & Khan, O. A. (2013). Does playing video games improve laparoscopic skills? *International Journal of Surgery, 11*(5), 365–69.

Overney, L. S., Blanke, O., & Herzog, M. H. (2008). Enhanced temporal but not attentional processing in expert tennis players. *PLoS One, 3*(6), e2380.

Plerhoples, T. A., Zak, Y., Hernandez-Boussard, T., & Lau, J. (2011). Another use of the mobile device: Warm-up for laparoscopic surgery. *Journal of Surgical Research, 170*(2), 185–88.

Ramachandran, V. S., & Braddick, O. (1973). Orientation-specific learning in stereopsis. *Perception, 2*, 371–76.

Rauscher, F. H., Shaw, G. L., Levine, L. J., Wright, E. L., Dennis, W. R., & Newcomb, R. L. (1997). Music training causes long-term enhancement of preschool children's spatial–temporal reasoning. *Neurological Research*, *19*(1), 2–8.
Rideout, V. J., Foehr, U. G., & Roberts, D. F. (2010). *Generation M2—media in the lives of 8- to 18-year olds.* Menlo Park CA: Kaiser Family Foundation.
Sowden, P. T., Rose, D., & Davies, I. R. (2002). Perceptual learning of luminance contrast detection: Specific for spatial frequency and retinal location but not orientation. *Vision Research*, *42*, 1249–58.
Vandewater, E. A., Shim, M. S., & Caplovitz, A. G. (2004). Linking obesity and activity level with children's television and video game use. *Journal of Adolescence*, *27*(1), 71–85.
White-Schwoch, T., Carr, K. W., Anderson, S., Strait, D. L., & Kraus, N. (2013). Older adults benefit from music training early in life: Biological evidence for long-term training-driven plasticity. *Journal of Neuroscience*, *33*(45), 17667–674.

CHAPTER

16 Professional and Competitive Gaming

Discussing Potential Benefits of Scientific Study

Kyle A. Faust, Joseph F. Meyer, *and* Mark D. Griffiths

Abstract

Gamers are now capable of making a living from playing digital games through competing in tournaments and sponsorships. These gamers, known as *professional gamers* or *e-sports competitors*, are able to earn large amounts of money by playing certain types of digital games, such as League of Legends and Fortnite. Professional gaming, despite existing for almost two decades, has still received little study. This chapter focuses on five key ways in which professional gaming impacts research on both positive and negative aspects of digital technology, including skills development, career choice, prosocial behavior, excessive use, and perception of negative stereotypes. Perspectives of a number of professional and competitive players illustrating unique insights into professional and competitive gaming are also provided. Last, ideas for future studies are given that could provide valuable contributions in the field of digital technology use.[1]

Keywords: professional gaming, e-sports, digital technology, expertise, positive gaming effects, gaming disorder

Introduction

Some readers may not know that it is possible to make a very comfortable living by competing in digital gaming (also known as any type of game played electronically) tournaments, but this is exactly what professional gamers do. Some of these professional gamers make large sums of money from their tournament winnings. In a recent Defense of the Ancients 2 tournament run by the gaming company Valve, the first-prize team of five players was awarded more than US$9 million (E-Sports earnings, 2016). Although this sum of money is unusual, professional gaming prizes are growing each year as professional gaming generates more money and sponsors (E-Sports earnings, 2016). The term "competitive gamer," which is related to professional gaming, usually refers to a skilled player who regularly competes in gaming tournaments. On the other hand, "professional gaming" refers to players who can make a living solely from playing their digital game of choice. These professional gamers may share much in common with top professional chess players in the sense that they exhibit a dedication to mastering a difficult set of skills; freely teach these skills to others; demonstrate persistence, discipline, and intelligence; perform with keen competence under intense pressure and scrutiny; work cooperatively with fellow team mates; and achieve a high level of financial success (Reeves, Brown, & Laurier, 2009). These positive qualities often characterize successful professional gamers.

However, in contrast to the extensive literature on professional chess players, professional and competitive gaming has not been widely researched or recognized in the scientific and professional literature on digital games. Although "competitive gaming" has occasionally been mentioned in the psychological literature, the majority of researchers define it as any game that involves competition. However, this is not how most gamers themselves define it. To avoid confusion, this chapter will refer to "competitive gamers" by the definition provided in the first paragraph. This chapter will also argue that professional and competitive gaming is a fruitful area of future study. Although we ideally prefer to anchor descriptions and hypotheses in established scientific evidence, peer-reviewed research is often lacking, which is motivating the current call for further research. Currently, the professional and competitive gaming fields primarily depend on research in closely related or allied areas while also drawing from less rigorous, non–peer-reviewed articles (e.g., statistics available from websites, responses from a number of professional and competitive gamers, and the personal observations of one of the authors with first-hand experience in this area). Although the nature and combination of these sources often call for tentative conclusions and positions, it will be argued that they provide a strong basis for arguing the merits of initiating research in this area.

Professional Gaming Tournaments

Professional gaming and competitive gaming tournaments exist for a wide variety of games. Some of the games that generate the largest prize pools and the most professional players are currently multiplayer online battle arena games (e.g., Defense of the Ancients 2 and League of Legends), real-time strategy games (e.g., Starcraft 2), as well as many free-person shooter games (e.g., Counter-Strike and Halo 3). There are many other types of games played both professionally and competitively, including role-playing games (e.g., World of Warcraft), fighting games (e.g., Smash Brothers Melee or Dead or Alive 4), racing games (e.g., Forza Motorspot 2), sports games (e.g., FIFA 08 or Madden NFL 13), and even online collectible card games, such as Hearthstone (E-sports earnings, 2016). It would be difficult to list every professional digital game, but there are even more game genres with tournaments and competitive players. Despite the number of professional and competitive gamers, there are only a small number of games that generate enough money for players to make a comfortable financial living.

The various digital game tournaments at the professional level are often run by companies that host the events at large convention centers in major cities (e.g., New York City, Los Angeles, Seoul, etc.). At present, many "grass-root" tournaments are hosted by the players themselves. In particular, the smaller game tournaments depend on a select few players who can organize these events on a regular basis. According to *Electronic Games Magazine* (1982), gaming tournaments have been organized since the 1980s, beginning as far back as games played on the Atari console (the first home game console system), which ran competitive tournaments as soon as the games were released in the United States. Digital game tournaments reached mass popularity in South Korea, where Starcraft began to garner tremendous fandom, and professional players developed fan bases comparable to those of professional athletes in the United States (Taylor, 2012). This was in part due to massive sponsors supporting professional gaming in South Korea. Even as early as 2000, the World Cyber Games, a tournament organizer, began developing in South Korea, obtaining sponsors like Samsung Electronics, Coca-Cola, and Microsoft (Taylor, 2012).

Currently, little scientific investigation has catalogued professional and competitive gaming. One fairly recent study explored a digital game called Counter-Strike, noting that it had more than 3 million players and an annual prize of US$150,000 (Reeves et al., 2009). However, these numbers pale in comparison to games such as DOTA2, League of Legends, or Starcraft 2. Although the massive earnings of DOTA2 were mentioned earlier, tournaments around the world awarded more than US$92 million in prizes in 2016, which is a substantial increase from around US$65 million in 2015, and around US$36 million in 2014 (E-Sports earnings, 2016). Although League of Legends has a large number of players (27 million players on average play the game every day), only a small number of these players are professionals (DiChristopher, 2014). Professional gaming tournaments also attract many spectators. For instance, Major League Gaming—a large video game league that hosts professional gaming tournaments—reported 54 million viewer hours of videos of professional matches watched in 2013 (Silady, 2014). Studies have also noted that professional and competitive games now use Internet radio coverage with play-by-play commentaries, large-screen televised projections of game footage, sizeable live audiences, and significant cash prizes (e.g., Hutchins, 2008).

Many of the games played on a professional and competitive level appear to demonstrate high levels of sophistication in strategizing, planning, multitasking, and timing to master, as has been indicated by studies on games like Counter-Strike (Reeves et al., 2009). As with other sports played professionally, professional gamers must develop a wide set of skills (e.g., rapid reflexes, refined hand-eye coordination, and fluid game control) to excel in professional circles. Starcraft and Starcraft 2, that emphasize strategy and are among the most popular professional and competitive games in the Major League Gaming circuit, have certain parallels to a blitz game of chess (i.e., they require rapid decision-making skills). The two games involve building an army to defeat an opponent's army by gathering resources with "harvester" units. Each offensive unit has various strengths and weaknesses, and a player must attempt to predict which units their opponent is building in order to defeat them. A player also must decide among various courses of action contingent on their resources and in response to their opponent's behavior. Emphasis is placed on rapid decision-making—spending even a second without issuing a command or building a unit could mean a loss to a skilled opponent. Furthermore, the game can be played simultaneously with multiple players, allowing for cooperative team play.

Having briefly overviewed some of the key themes and skills involved in professional and competitive gaming, those in and outside the gaming studies field may wonder how scientific research on the profession can contribute to our knowledge of the positive and negative effects of digital technology. Therefore, the remainder of this chapter elaborates five key reasons why professional and competitive gaming merit further scientific attention, including skills development, career choice, prosocial behavior, excessive use, and perception of negative stereotypes. Additionally, the views of a number of professional and competitive players illustrating unique insights into professional and competitive gaming are provided.

Professional/Competitive Gaming/ Cognitive Development

Numerous studies have demonstrated the benefits of gaming, particularly in relation to improved spatial cognitive benefits (e.g., Green & Bavilier, 2007; Spence & Feng, 2010). Other studies (e.g., Anguera et al., 2013; Basak, Boot, Voss, & Kramer, 2008) have evaluated the potential beneficial impact of video game playing on executive functions in elderly populations. Additionally, studies have suggested that video games can provide an enriched medium for strategic problem-solving (Hong & Liu, 2003; Shaffer, 2006). A study by Glass, Maddox, and Love (2013) also found that playing 40 hours of Starcraft appeared to develop cognitive flexibility when comparing participants who instead played a more neutral game called The Sims. A groundbreaking recent study in this area found that video game players who played the online protein-folding game Foldit facilitated solving an intricate biochemical puzzle that had previously eluded scientific researchers. More specifically, they discovered the correct molecular structure essential for designing antiretroviral drugs whereas other attempts to model the structure had failed (Khatib et al., 2011). A recent paper by Granic, Lobel, and Engels (2013) summarized other studies on the benefits of gaming. The paper reported that numerous studies indicate gaming may enhance cognitive development. The authors also discussed other correlational studies indicating that digital games may help develop problem solving and creativity.

From these studies, it appears likely that specific video games can potentially promote cognitive development more than other types of games. It has been demonstrated that expert chess players think far more deeply about their decision-making than do novices (Charness, 1981) and have the ability to ignore irrelevant stimuli to make faster and more precise decisions (Bilalic, Langer, Erb, & Grodd, 2010). Given these findings, professional gamers likely also engage in much deeper thinking and rapid decision-making than do intermediate or novice players. As further discussed in a later section, professional success in gaming seemingly requires persistent practice and sophisticated skill sets. It is likely that these positive effects are more substantial than the effects of games played on a casual level. For instance, it can be argued that a professional or competitive Starcraft player operates on a very different level than a novice player. More specifically (and again using the chess analogy), novices and intermediate players are unlikely to use the same level of planning or strategy as more advanced players. Novice Starcraft players typically employ simple strategies and act slowly, whereas advanced players often think multiple steps ahead and are much faster and time-efficient in their decisions. Another example can be seen in Super Smash Brothers Melee, another game played professionally and competitively. In this game, novice players lack the ability or knowledge to perform more advanced techniques that are essential even at intermediate levels of play. In contrast, the professional players can complete these moves with ease and with little or no thought, similarly to how an experienced driver does not need to think about the motor controls necessary to use the brakes or gas.

Additional studies support the differences between novice and advanced levels of play in digital games. For instance, research has demonstrated measurable differences between novice and expert game players, the latter group often demonstrating enhanced short-term memory, executive control/self-monitoring, pattern recognition, visual-spatial abilities (e.g., object rotation), and task-switching efficiency, along with more efficient problem-solving skills (Andrews & Murphy, 2006; Boot, Kramer, Simons, Fabiani, & Gratton, 2008; Hong & Liu, 2003; Van Deventer, & White, 2002). In Hong and Liu's (2003) study of problem-solving abilities, 76 Taiwanese elementary school students were recruited to play the video game Klotski with player status (i.e., novice or expert) determined on the basis of operating time and number of steps taken to solve block puzzles. Results from five expert players and five novice players who played the game while participating in a video-recorded think-aloud protocol (i.e., verbalization of working memory content) indicated (a) a weaker relationship between operating time and number of steps for the novice group ($r = -0.03$) relative to the expert group ($r = 0.54$) and (b) significant divergence in thinking types as a function of player status (i.e., expert gamers evidenced more analogical reasoning, whereas novice gamers engaged in more trial-and-error thinking). Thus, expert gamers utilized more efficient problem-solving strategies.

Considering such exemplars from the broad literature on skill development in playing digital games, it seems reasonable to hypothesize that professional gamers may experience greater cognitive benefits than those commonly observed by more casual gamers. Potential differential benefits may apply to both spatial cognition and executive functions. For example, a professional gamer playing a shooting game (e.g., Counter-Strike) almost certainly faces considerably greater perceptual and/or cognitive demands in these areas than novices or intermediate-level players. Reeves et al. (2009) provided evidence that even nonprofessional Counter-Strike players demonstrate high levels of manual dexterity (e.g., skillfully synchronizing avatar movements and actions), a keen anticipatory sense of other players' movements and strategies, and rapid (albeit calculated) reactions to opponents' tactics. It could therefore be speculated that professional Counter-Strike players would have even greater skills in these areas than nonprofessional players. More broadly, studying the development of advanced gaming proficiencies may provide insight into designing games and educational programs that foster skill acquisition across various important domains. The value of examining skill development and transfer appears to be supported by empirically published research (e.g., Day, Arthur & Gettman, 2001).

Professional Gaming as a Career Choice

Professional gaming has become a legitimate but arguably challenging career choice. This statement likely changes some of the previously perceived notions on the productivity of digital games, as digital gaming can now serve as a profession. This also raises interesting questions about the role of context in excessive gaming and potential addiction. Although there is ongoing scientific debate on the nature and extent of adverse consequences associated with excessive digital technology use, experts have noted that long hours of video game use alone do not necessarily indicate video game addiction (i.e., heavy use is a necessary but not sufficient criterion for addiction; Griffiths, 2010). Therefore, in order to evaluate problematic video game use, researchers must consider possible negative consequences players are experiencing in their lives (Griffiths, 2010). When video game players (or any digital game players) are capable of financially supporting themselves from their play, this matter becomes more complex. For example, how would one categorize a professional digital game player who was making more than US$500,000 per year playing digital games, but this player does not experience any major negative consequences as a result of seemingly excessive digital game use? This point is not meant to imply that a successful professional gamer is incapable of suffering pathological effects from game use, but rather to raise the possibility that professional gamers will view their use as nonproblematic due to the success they experience, even if the gaming has had some negative impacts on them. It is possible for professional gamers to endorse few negative consequences from their gaming use, but it is also likely that they will have to sacrifice certain areas of their lives to remain top players. However, this does not necessarily mean they are addicted to playing the games (i.e., excessive game playing is a by-product of their job). However, for those who do appear to have a problem moderating their digital game use, it could perhaps be argued that they are addicted to their work (and in this case, their work comprises video game playing).

Workaholics have been conceptualized in different ways. For instance, a recent review by Griffiths

(2011) noted that workaholics are typically viewed as one (or a combination) of the following. They (a) are viewed as hyper-performers, (b) work as a way of stopping themselves from thinking about their emotional and personal lives, and (c) are overly concerned with their work to the point of neglecting other areas of their lives. Some of these may indeed be applied to professional or competitive gamers (particularly the reference to "hyper-performers" and the fact that other areas of their lives may be neglected in pursuit of their ultimate goal). Some authors note that there is both a behavioral component and a psychological component to workaholism. The behavioral component comprises working excessively hard (i.e., a high number of hours per day and/or week), whereas the psychological (dispositional) component comprises being obsessed with work (i.e., working compulsively and being unable to detach from work). Again, these behavioral and psychological components could potentially be applied to professional gamers.

Being a professional or competitive gamer often requires a large time commitment. Many professional or competitive players will play excessively and spend countless hours every day either practicing or competing. For some of these gamers, their whole life is dominated by their game (or games) of choice, which may impact their relationships and family life. Since a competitive gaming player is not making enough money to financially support themselves solely from gaming, their educational or occupational performance might decline if the player places a greater importance on spending time to become a professional gamer. Many competitive gaming players may be able to effectively balance their gaming life with their other responsibilities, especially those who do not desire to become professional gaming players. However, the competitive gaming players who desire to become professionals will almost certainly have to make sacrifices if they hope to become as good as the professional players.

It is important to add that professional gamers may not necessarily need to rely solely on tournament winnings or sponsorships to support themselves financially. Researchers studying the economics of synthetic worlds (e.g., digital gaming environments) have observed that gamers also procure income by marketing virtual objects in massively multiplayer online role-playing games (MMORPGs) (Castronova, 2005; Lee & Lin, 2011). These digital objects often include *avatars*, or characters controlled by players who interact with gaming environments and other players. Each avatar has unique physical attributes and skills that a player may select, purchase, and/or develop over many hours of game play (e.g., the gradual enhancement of strength, speed, weapon-wielding abilities, etc.). Consequently, avatars may be viewed as "bundles of attributes" (Castronova, 2003, p. 2) with monetary value, and many play a crucial role in certain competitive games (e.g., EverQuest and World of Warcraft). With the emergence of virtual markets and increased economic interplay within and between digital and real-life settings as humans spend increasing amounts of time in computer-generated environments (Castronova, 2003, 2005; Castronova et al., 2009; Kurzweil, 1999), professional gamers may encounter cutting-edge, revenue-generating opportunities without having to excel at defeating other players. A gamer might also be able to make a living from commentating on professional matches or "streaming" their game matches online. Streaming involves allowing an audience to watch gaming matches live on the Internet. Depending on the number of stream viewers, the player receives money each time one of the viewers watches advertisements. Some players or companies that stream matches receive a large number of viewers and can generate substantial financial revenues. This indicates that there are numerous methods for becoming a professional gamer, and these methods may continue to evolve as interest for gaming continues to grow.

Professional and Competitive Gaming as a Prosocial Behavior

Two frequently discussed negative consequences of playing video games are increased aggressive behavior (e.g., Anderson et al., 2008) and increased social isolation, which may result from heavy video game playing at the expense of spending leisure time with friends and family (Jansz & Martens, 2005). Although some video and other digital games can be played alone, the same cannot be said for most digital games played competitively or professionally. As the majority of tournaments take place at an external venue (rather than at home), professional and competitive gamers frequently interact with other players in real-life, face-to-face situations (as opposed to online virtual spaces). Furthermore, the community aspect of professional/competitive gaming may do more to foster social skill development than impede it. The professional and competitive gaming communities reward social competence and encourage gamers to spend time with others who have similar interests and aspirations.

Players may perform better in tournaments if they are well liked, respected, and admired by other players. Likable players are more likely to receive advice from other players, and they are also more likely to find other skilled players to practice against. If players befriend a professional gamer, the professional gamer may be willing to help them improve their skills. Under these circumstances, certain professional gaming communities may increase cooperation rather than increase aggression.

Many large professional and competitive gaming tournaments include cooperative team events. In fact, some of the most popular games, like DOTA2 and League of Legends, cannot be played without a full team of players working and collaborating effectively together. This collaborative element is particularly worth highlighting in light of research by Sheese and Graziano (2005) showing that cooperation in video games may encourage prosocial behaviors. It has also been hypothesized that the teamwork used in various professional games may transfer to other settings where teamwork is essential, such as business or management (Wagner, 2006). Although most professional and competitive games are adversarial, they may similarly encourage prosocial behaviors, particularly during team events. Professional and competitive gamers are likely to experience better tournament performance if they show consideration toward their teammates and learn to anticipate how their partners think. Digital game players who lack the ability to understand their teammates or develop friendships will be less likely to find good gamers willing to work with them. Reeves, Brown, and Laurier's (2009) work also supports the importance of Counter-Strike players anticipating the actions of their teammates. This anticipation likely applies to most professional or competitive gamers as there is far less margin for error among top players. Specific professional and competitive gaming communities have also engaged in fundraising activities, which raised awareness in helping larger communities outside of gaming and encouraged many community players to donate money for charities. One example is a group of fighting gaming communities raising more than US$200,000 for breast cancer research for the chance to hold a tournament for their games of choice at EVO, the largest fighting game tournament (Shreier, 2013). Another example are events run by the speed running communities that have raised millions of dollars for charities like the Prevent Cancer Foundation and Doctors Without Borders (Li, 2014).

Although professional and competitive gaming may foster prosocial development, it is important to note that each gaming community should be viewed as a separate, unique entity. Each community has its own rules and regulations as to what is considered socially acceptable, and some communities engage in behavior that would not be considered acceptable in other settings. For this reason, it is important for professional and competitive gamers to learn which behaviors and norms are acceptable or unacceptable in settings outside of their community. As long as they cultivate this awareness and can differentiate acceptable and unacceptable behaviors in other settings, professional and competitive players should be able to transfer the skills they used to develop friendships, teamwork, and connections in their own community to other settings as well.

Professional/Competitive Gaming and Excessive Use

As noted in a previous section, professional and competitive gaming players are more likely to play for extended periods of time and sacrifice other areas of their lives than casual gamers because they have the potential to make a living from gaming. This focused dedication may become problematic for some competitive gaming players, as the goal of becoming a professional gamer is often unrealistic. There are currently no robust statistics relating to the number of professional or competitive game players. This is primarily because gamers and researchers differ in their definitions of "professional" and "competitive." Numerous gamers will call themselves "professionals" in reference to their gaming skill rather than their ability to make a financial living from gaming. Websites such as E-sports Earnings suggest that only a small percentage of gamers generate sufficient income to support themselves financially. Although viability may change in the future, at present, the majority of competitive gamers will have a very hard time becoming successful and financially independent professionals. This may strike readers as a similarity to poker, as the majority of players will also have a difficult path if they desire to become a financially independent professional. Some digital games played professionally generate much more money (such as DOTA2, League of Legends, and Starcraft 2) and can therefore financially support many more players than less popular games. For this reason (i.e., the motivation to become a professional), competitive gamers may be more susceptible to excessive use than the average digital game player. Additionally, successful professional gamers are also likely to play for extended periods of time as playing less than 8 hours each day could mean that they are not practicing enough compared to other professional players. It is important to note that some professional and competitive gamers will be able to balance their other responsibilities and manage their time effectively, but the chances are high that they will need to sacrifice certain areas of their lives if they are to succeed at the highest levels. Those who work with (and treat) problematic digital game players should keep this factor in mind (King, Delfabbro, & Griffiths, 2012; King, Delfabbro, Griffiths, & Gradisar, 2011), especially given that excessive digital game use may increase as professional gaming receives more bona fide recognition as a possible career choice.

Professional/Competitive Gaming and Negative Stereotypes

Professional and competitive gaming has arguably assisted in reducing some of the negative stigma associated with gaming. For years, gamers in many countries have experienced an exceptionally negative perception of their psychological traits and behavioral characteristics (Griffiths & Hunt, 1998; Kowert, Griffiths, & Oldmeadow, 2012). It seems that many individuals label gaming as a waste of time, played most frequently by individuals who are socially inept, childish, unpopular, and/or unsuccessful. Examples of common stereotypical images associated with video game playing include the isolated adolescent "nerd" who plays video games for countless hours at the expense of social and familial relationships (Griffiths & Hunt, 1998; Roberts, Foehr, Rideout, & Brodie, 1999) and the isolated, physically unhealthy, teenage male "couch potato" (Kowert et al., 2012; Williams, 2008). These stereotypes have led many gamers to feel embarrassed of their game play and to resist participation in research studies (King, Delfabbro, & Griffiths, 2009).

Harmful stereotypes may be exacerbated by specific research findings interpreted out of context. These include associations of game play with negative outcomes, such as poor attention (Swing, Gentile, Anderson, & Walsh, 2010), low school performance (Sharif & Sargent, 2006), and increased risk of physical aggression (Anderson et al., 2008). Although some studies show that specific negative stereotypical features (e.g., low social competence) may be risk factors for pathological levels of gaming (Gentile et al., 2011), recent studies have not found consistent or strong associations between hours of game play and poor functioning (Ferguson & Meehan, 2010; Valadez & Ferguson, 2012), and the link between violent video games and hostility is being called into question (Ferguson & Rueda, 2010; Ferguson, San Miguel, Garza, & Jerabeck, 2012). Unfortunately, these nuances become clouded in media headlines and lay psychology publications, where video games are often portrayed as a slippery slope to psychopathology (Sojourner, 2011) and even outright antisocial and criminal behavior (Gye, Keneally, & Bates, 2012). Professional and competitive gaming has the capacity to challenge and overcome some of the aforementioned negative stereotypes and overgeneralizations, as well as stimulate further research on positive outcomes associated with disciplined and professional game play.

As previously mentioned, professional and competitive gamers are rewarded for strong social skills and success. For instance, a socially immature professional or competitive gamer will probably not make as many friends in the gaming community, and they will likely develop a negative reputation among peers. This negative reputation will make it far more difficult to find opponents with whom to practice. It will also make it more difficult for them to collaborate with skilled teammates. Ideally, these gamers will learn to overcome their shortcomings in order to become better players. A shy or socially anxious gamer will also have a more difficult time, and they will likely need to learn to overcome these difficulties if they are to reach professional status. In contrast, a likable, friendly, and socially skilled competitive gamer will more likely befriend other gamers, allowing for more opportunities to find skilled teammates and practice partners. Additionally, professional gaming companies are working toward changing the cultural stigma of gaming by marketing professional games like sports. The term "e-sports" (electronic sports) has recently started to catch on. The term refers to professional gaming as a sport played electronically, noting that there are virtually no differences between professional athletes and "cyberathletes," another term for professional gamers (Hutchins, 2008). Gaming has continued to become more culturally accepted in the United States, but there is still quite a bit of negative stigma. As the acceptance of gaming continues to grow in the United States and across the world, fewer gamers will feel the need to underreport the amount of time they spend playing digital games. It is our opinion that, out of embarrassment or denial, frequent gamers likely underreport their digital game use.

Perspectives from Professional and Competitive Gamers

This chapter would not be complete without some insight from professional and competitive players themselves. The first author—due to previous involvement in a few competitive gaming communities—was able to send out 15-item questionnaires to 12 professional or competitive players in various gaming communities. Although the majority of players are from the various Smash Brothers communities, two well-known professional players from DOTA 2 and Starcraft 2 were also interested in helping with the research. Although the sample size is small, the goal of these survey questions was to begin providing some insight into how professional and competitive players approach both their lives and gaming. (A number of the gamers' responses are provided in the chapter, but there was not enough room to provide them all. If the reader is interested in reading all of the responses, we plan to either make them available online or via e-mail requests.)

Gamer Responses

1. Can you provide a brief introduction of yourself (i.e., a little about your background and your competitive/professional game of choice).

"I've been playing games since I was 3 years old, starting with the classic Super Mario Bros. From then I've loved games my whole life, everything from console games to computer games to board games. The first big competition I played was the Swedish championships in Nintendo which was in 2000—I was almost 12 years at the time. I managed to finish second and continued to compete in that every year until 2006 when they stopped having it (with the exception of an additional event they had in 2012). Throughout the eight competitions I got 1st place 3 times, 2nd place 3 times, 5th place once, and 9th place once. Other than that I've competed in DOTA, which I started playing in 2004. I've always been playing mostly for fun (but always loved to compete and aimed to win) at the same time as I have been studying or doing something else, but when I started playing DOTA 2, it's when it became more serious. There is so much money and tournaments that you actually can live out of playing, and if you are good and win a lot, you can also make a lot of money. We were very lucky last year (2013) and managed to win the biggest e-sports tournament at the same with a 1st prize of US$1.4 million to split on five (the team)."

—Joakim Akterhall, aka "Akke,"
Professional DOTA 2 player

2. What do you feel you've gotten out of your professional or competitive gaming career?

"My competitive gaming career has done so much for me. I firmly believe it has been one of the most meaningful endeavors in my life, with the only thing that comes close being formal education. First and foremost, competitive gaming has made me a better learner. School teaches you a lot of things, but ironically, it doesn't emphasize how to be a better learner most of the time. On top of that, school isn't very individualized, and it's extremely spoon-fed. Nobody really has a sense of individual decision-making since everyone is just learning the same curriculum without any trial, error, or personal investment. Gaming is your own project. You do all the work yourself. You do your own research, you seek out players, you put in the time, you make your own mistakes, and learn your own lessons. This is *huge*. Competitive gaming has made me a much more confident and social person. It presented me with a huge, diverse community of people from all walks of life, and these people became my close friends. Also, because I was involved in a community outside of my high school, I wasn't as obsessed and absorbed in the trivial minutiae of high school like some of my peers were. I could honestly go on for hours about the life lessons that competitive gaming has taught me, but I'll spare you the lecture."

—Andrew Vo, aka "Tai," Professional Level Super
Smash Brothers Melee player

3. What are some of the main things going through your mind during a game or match?

"It depends: sometimes you go complete autopilot and don't have any conscious thoughts at all. Your subconscious takes over and executes everything you've been learning over the past years. But when you think, you try to remind yourself of what you've been training lately to stick to your strengths. You also need to keep in mind what your opponent can do to you to gain an upper hand as well as how to prevent that from happening. Maybe the most important thing to consciously think about is evaluating the current situation of the match. Am I ahead or am I behind? And if so how to either stay that way, finish the game, or figure out what you need to do to make up for a disadvantage. You have to extrapolate a lot because sc2 is a game of incomplete information. Gathering intelligence or denying it is one of the most important aspects to the game."

—Dario Wuensch, aka "TLO,"
Professional Starcraft 2 player

4. What do you believe are the skills or mental thought processes you possess that allow you to excel in professional/competitive gaming?

"My ability to never give up or be overwhelmed by a situation is what allows me to succeed at the top level. The positive psychology behind my mindset and approach to competing has allowed me to only focus on the match and be able to play at my full potential without any distractions. For me personally, the main skill you need to excel at the highest level is to believe in yourself and stay calm; every professional knows what to do in a match, but only those with the right mindset can execute these things when thousands of people are watching, or an entire room is cheering against you."
—Joe Cribari, aka "Toronto Joe," Professional Smash Brothers player and Tournament Organizer

5. What led to your interest in professional/competitive gaming?

"My brothers and relatives competed in game tournaments all the time and I always envied them. When I was in high school, I discovered Smash Brothers and felt that I could excel in that particular game. I wanted to become the best, but the competition was scarce in my region so I started to travel around the USA to compete. I find that the competitive atmosphere and feeling of accomplishment is what drives my interest in the sport."
—Sarath San, aka "Hayato" Former top-level Super Smash Brothers Melee player

6. Do you feel you have experienced any positive benefits resulting from your professional/competitive gaming?

"I have experienced many positive results from gaming. I feel as though I think more quickly now. I have been exposed to many high-end philosophies relating to martial art and how to be a fair but successful person, which allowed me to succeed not just in the game. I also succeed in my scholastic endeavors and my physical health understanding, as well as my sense of time management after having this experience."
—Kevin Nanney, aka "Dr. PP," Former #1 ranked Super Smash Brothers Melee player

7. Have you had to sacrifice from other areas in your life because of professional/competitive gaming?

"Oh yes, immensely. But that was more in the past, before I learned how to navigate the often complicated waters. When I was competing heavily in college it was no secret that my gaming career came first, and that was destructive to other relationships in my life. It was especially difficult to try and live in two separate worlds—I eventually learned that it is much easier to be open and honest, and let them combine."
—Chris Fabiszak, Former top-level Super Smash Brothers Melee player

8. Have you experienced any other problems resulting from professional or competitive gaming?

"Physical wear and tear of the body is something a lot of people don't realize they're doing to themselves when they're obsessively gaming. Just like any other sport, with heavy practice comes heavy use of the body. I know I am not the only one who has ever suffered wrist or thumb pain from endlessly playing Melee, trying to nail ridiculous combos until I could do it in my sleep. My friend, East Coast Eddie, wears a brace on his hand because, coupled with his job where he uses a mouse all day, Smash has damaged the nerves in his hands. I have had poor posture and back problems for as long as I can remember, most likely due to hours of being hunched over in front of TVs."
—Mike Micale, aka "Laizhensil," World of Warcraft and Smash Brothers Competitive player

9. If you were having a conversation with someone who knew nothing about professional/competitive gaming, but wanted to know why it was appealing, what would you tell them?

"I explain professional gaming through metaphors in sports or any passionate activity I know that they identify with and understand. On a fundamental level, all levels of professional competition involve a dedication toward self-improvement and becoming the 'best' at the thing you love to do. People are able to relate to the fact that professional gaming has fostered global communities of people who share a similar passion and love for the game they play. By explaining to them the relatable aspect of community and competition they are able to understand the bigger picture; making sure I avoid using technical jargon is imperative for them to idealize the environment because the most mutually understood part of pro-gaming is the fact that it pins a huge amount of people against each other with a desire to win, who share the same passion for the activity, and are immensely dedicated to refining their craft."
—Joe Cribari, aka "Toronto Joe," Professional Smash Brothers player and Tournament Organizer

10. How much time do you typically spend playing your professional/competitive game of choice (including the time you spend training via analyzing videos or training in other ways)? Additionally, how much time do you spend playing other games?

"I spend about 6–7 hours on average playing strarcraft 2 but there's more things to do as a pro-gamer than just playing the game. Organizational work, networking, promotional work etc that also needs to be done."

—Dario Wuensch, aka "TLO," professional Starcraft 2 player

11. Do you feel like your time spent with professional/ competitive gaming has allowed you to more effectively succeed in other areas of your life?

"It's hard to tell whether the skills I gained are just from professional gaming or growing older and having more experience. However the self-reflection and critique you need to apply to yourself to improve in Starcraft definitely helps in other areas of life, too. It is much easier to make progress when you can identify what you're doing wrong or right and how to proceed from there."

—Dario Wuensch, aka "TLO," Professional Starcraft 2 player

12. Where do you see professional gaming in the next 10 years?

"Professional gaming in the next 10 years is going to be huge across the world. As of right now, electronic sports or eSports, are growing at a rapid rate. Games including Super Smash Bros. Melee, DOTA 2, StarCraft II, League of Legends, and numerous more are growing incredibly. These games are achieving new heights of success that many wouldn't even imagine, such as League of Legends being an Olympic event in the 2016 Olympics Games in Rio de Janeiro. In countries such as Korea, their professional gamers are treated with very high respect from the public. In the United States and many other countries, professional gamers aren't treated like athletes because the public doesn't accept them as athletes. In the next 10 years, with events such as the Olympics spreading the word about professional gaming, maybe we will get the long-awaited respect we deserve. With all the gaming communities together in unison, the possibilities are endless."

—Kapil Mangrolia, aka "Kapzillion," Competitive Super Smash Brothers Melee player

13. What made you decide to pick up your professional/competitive game of choice over other games?

"Because it's a team game. I get very bored from playing alone which makes DOTA perfect to me. It revolves about team play, and it's also what I consider my best strength—to play and understand your teammates and make the best out of the situation."

—Joakim Akterhall, aka "Akke," Professional DOTA2 player

14. Anything else you would like to tell people about professional/competitive gaming, including those who may or may not be familiar with it?

"It's just as much of a feat to succeed in competitive gaming as it is to succeed in any high-level sport. It's just a different set of skills that are needed."

—Hugo Gonzales, aka "HugS," Professional Super Smash Brothers Melee player

15. Anything else you would like to add about yourself that you feel is important for readers to know?

"Before competitive gaming I was a regular kid who fit the typical mould for every fear a parent would have if their child became invested in video-games; I was lazy, unmotivated, and unable to socially connect with others. Now reflecting on the past 6 years of my professional gaming career, I am proud to say that I am the exact opposite of those features you would be lead to believe you earn through competitive gaming. I am the most confident, social, and motivated to succeed in life I have ever been thanks to my involvement in professional gaming, and have made meaningful connections with people across the world who I can depend on for anything inside and outside of the game."

—Joe Cribari, aka "Toronto Joe," Professional Smash Brothers player and Tournament Organizer

Summary and Thoughts on Professional/ Competitive Gamer Responses

After reviewing all of the professional and competitive gaming responses, several general themes are clearly evident. Most of the professional and competitive players expressed many perceived benefits from their gaming. Some of the most common benefits listed were financial, increased self-confidence, opportunities to learn new languages, opportunities to see new areas of the world (while traveling), improved focus/attention, increased patience, developing business/marketing skills, improved social skills, opportunities for personal growth, improved time-management, personal meaningfulness, enhanced learning/academic skills, and a method of avoiding self-destructive behaviors (e.g., excessive drug and/or alcohol use).

The professional and competitive gamers also listed some downsides to their gaming, including relationship strain due to busy travel schedules, less time for academic and occupational settings, occasional physical pain (e.g., severe wrist strain, nerve damage, and poor posture), occasional distress stemming from the behavior of other gamers, lack of social and familial support, and dealing with negative social stigma. The professional and competitive gamers occasionally articulated differing opinions on specific advantages and disadvantages, particularly when it came to social skills, eating habits, and exercise. Although most of the gamers felt their social skills had improved from interactions with other players at tournaments, a couple of gamers felt that these interactions had hindered their social skills, stating that it was hard for them to engage in non-gaming–related conversations. Some gamers also felt that their exercise and eating habits had improved because they learned the importance of these areas for optimal professional performance. In contrast, one or two gamers felt like they were more inclined to neglect these areas and instead spend more time practicing.

Participating professional gamers also identified specific skills that they felt were responsible for their success. Examples included taking time to evaluate mistakes and weaknesses (vs. placing external blame), studying the top players, engaging in good teamwork, learning to play to their greatest strengths, getting ample practice, and enjoying their game of choice. A number of professional and competitive gamers began playing games because their family members also played, indicating that family and social settings could be strong predictors of professional and competitive play. In other words, gamers are more likely to become professional or competitive if their social supports value gaming or also engage in gaming.

Although some competitive players noted they were actively thinking while playing, the majority of competitive and professional players stated they "went into autopilot" or focused on more basic tactics during a match. The only professional teams player who completed the questionnaire also felt the majority of his focus was on effective communication with his teammates, which the team had practiced routinely. The "autopilot" mode is similar to what is described among many professional athletes as "flow" (Csíkszentmihályi, 1996) and has also been reported in studies of slot machine players (Griffiths, 1991, 1994).

Gamer responses varied significantly on the amount of time spent gaming, thus rendering gaming time estimates difficult. Although the professionals stated they needed to spend a large amount of time gaming or doing other activities related to their work (i.e., promotion, networking, etc.), they mostly felt they had a good life balance. Some of the competitive gamers stated that they did not practice too much during the school year, but played for much longer periods of time during school breaks or on weekends. This information is very important to keep in mind, as a competitive gamer may be playing two or three times more on weekends or on vacations than they are during school or work days. Their gaming use may also greatly increase shortly before an important tournament takes place.

Due to the small number of participants and the nonrandomly sampled nature of this small qualitative study, it is not possible to generalize these perceived benefits and shortcomings to all professional and competitive gamers. Furthermore, the majority of these gamers focused their game play on the Smash Brothers series. Responses would likely vary across unique gaming communities focusing on different genres. Nevertheless, some of this information is valuable for illustrating the variability across professional and competitive gamers' perspectives. It also provides insight into the minds of these gamers, including responses from some gamers who are the best in the world in their respective games of choice.

Implications for Professional/Competitive Gaming and Future Research

The field of digital technology and gaming is constantly evolving. As such, specific areas, such as professional and competitive gaming, may prove fruitful for further scientific investigation. As the study of digital games and other forms of digital technology expands, researchers would benefit from consensus on criteria for identifying both problematic and beneficial game use. There is also a need for more studies assessing treatment interventions for individuals who have been negatively impacted by gaming (King et al., 2011, 2012). The gaming studies field also stands to gain from further research on how digital games may be used to promote the development of specific skills that may benefit individuals and society.

Professional and competitive gaming, as with digital game playing more generally, has psychosocial advantages and disadvantages and is thus an important area to consider when evaluating gaming as a whole. It may be critical to include questions about professional and competitive gaming (and context more generally) in measures evaluating the degree, extent, and "addictive" potential of digital game use (Griffiths, 2010). Furthermore, it remains essential for psychologists to inquire about professional and competitive gaming during clinical interviews in which clients report playing digital games. If clients turn out to be professional or competitive gamers, this will likely distinguish them in many ways from those who play video games excessively for fun and/or escape.

Various approaches and strategies could be used to stimulate research into professional and competitive gaming. For example, studies might compare the abilities of professional or high-level competitive gamers with casual or less experienced gamers to better understand similarities and contrasts in benefits and determine if skills learned through professional gaming can transfer to other important areas. The earlier described study examining transfer of skills to scientific problem-solving (i.e., Khatib et al., 2011) parallels these research aims and raises the intriguing possibility that high-level gamers' exceptional capacities and skill development may be applicable to important problems in multiple areas.

Another possibility is to study the characteristics and skill sets of highly successful professional gamers. Such in-depth studies would generate information for formulating hypotheses about potential differences between these individuals and nonprofessional gamers. How and why are some professional gamers able to succeed while many other players try and fail? Are some of these characteristics and skills (e.g., persistence and speed of mental processing) similar to those seen in professional athletes or others who are highly successful in their occupations, such as professional poker players (McCormack & Griffiths, 2012)?

Other research studies could examine the social abilities of professional and competitive gamers to gauge the degree to which greater social awareness is related to overall tournament performance. Researchers may also wish to evaluate whether professional and competitive digital game players are more vulnerable to certain negative effects compared to noncompetitive players given such factors as exceptionally high levels of time devoted to play and potential neglect of other important activities, such as schoolwork.

This chapter has attempted to convey the importance of further studying professional and competitive digital game playing. It has discussed the great popularity that these games are beginning to receive around the world as the number of professional and competitive gamers continues to grow rapidly (E-Sports earnings, 2016). This is due in large part to the continuously increasing prize money (sometimes more than US$ 1 million for first place) and important corporate sponsors. Incorporating these two types of gamers would be likely to benefit research examining both the positive and negative effects of digital technology. Professional and competitive gaming may offer numerous benefits that could be more pronounced than the positive effects found when games are played casually. It may also be problematic, as competitive gamers might be more likely to sacrifice other areas of their lives if they believe they can become professional players. Most importantly, researchers in the gaming studies field should keep in mind that competitive and professional gamers comprise a distinct population and may differ considerably (both psychologically and/or behaviorally) from casual gamers.

Note

1. Note that some of the material in this chapter was previously published in an article from 2013, which was also written by the same three authors.

References

Anderson, C. A., Sakamoto, A., Gentile, D. A., Ihori, N., Shibuya, A., & Yukawa, S. (2008). Longitudinal effects of violent videogames on aggression in Japan and the United States. *Pediatrics, 122*, 1067–72. doi:10.1542/peds.2008-1425

Andrews, G., & Murphy, K. (2006). Does video game playing improve executive functioning? In M. A. Vanchevsky (Ed.), *Frontiers in cognitive psychology* (pp. 145–61). Hauppauge, NY: Nova Science Publishers.

Anguera, J., Boccanfuso, J., Rintoul, J., Al-Hashimi, O., Faraji, F., Janowich, J., . . . Gazzaley, A. (2013). Video game training enhances cognitive control in older adults. *Nature, 501*, 97–103.

Basak, C., Boot, W., Voss, M., & Kramer, A. (2008). Can training in a real-time strategy video game attenuate cognitive decline in older adults? *Psychology and Aging, 23*, 765–77. doi:10.1037/a0013494 PMID:19140648

Bilalic, M., Langer, R., Erb, M., & Grodd, W. (2010). Mechanisms and neural basis of object and pattern recognition: A study with chess experts. *Journal of Experimental Psychology, 139*(4), 728–42.

Boot, W. R., Kramer, A. F., Simons, D. J., Fabiani, M., & Gratton, G. (2008). The effects of video game playing on attention, memory, and executive control. *Acta Psychologica, 129,* 387–98. doi:10.1016/j. actpsy.2008.09.005 PMID:18929349

Castronova, E. (2003, June). *The price of "man" and "woman": A hedonic pricing model of avatar attributes in a synthetic world* (CESifo working paper No. 957). http://www.cesifo-group.de/portal/pls/portal/docs/1/1189752.pdf

Castronova, E. (2005). *Synthetic worlds: The business and culture of online games.* Chicago, IL: The University of Chicago Press.

Castronova, E., Williams, D., Shen, C., Ratan, R., Xiong, L., Huang, Y., & Keegan, B. (2009). As real as real? Macroeconomic behavior in a large-scale virtual world. *New Media & Society, 11,* 685–707. doi:10.1177/1461444809105346

Charness, N. (1981). Search in chess: Age and skill differences. *Journal of Experimental Psychology, 7*(2), 467–76.

Csíkszentmihályi, M. (1996). *Finding flow: The psychology of engagement with everyday life.* New York: Basic Books.

Day, E., Arthur, W., Jr., & Gettman, D. (2001). Knowledge structures and acquisition of a complex skill. *The Journal of Applied Psychology, 86,* 1022–33. doi:10.1037/0021-9010.86.5.1022 PMID:11596796

DiChristopher, T. (2014, February 3), Pro gamers story: Get big, burn out, retire young. http://www.cnbc.com/id/101380550

E-sports earnings. (2016). The international 2016 Dota 2 championships. http://www.esportsearnings.com/tournaments/19287-the-international-2016

Ferguson, C. J., & Meehan, D. C. (2010). Saturday night's alright for fighting: Antisocial traits, fighting, and weapons carrying in a large sample of youth. *The Psychiatric Quarterly, 81,* 293–302. doi:10.1007/s11126-010-9138-y PMID:20405321

Ferguson, C. J., & Rueda, S. M. (2010). The Hitman study: Violent video game exposure effects on aggressive behavior, hostile feelings, and depression. *European Psychologist, 15,* 99–108. doi:10.1027/1016-9040/a000010

Ferguson, C. J., San Miguel, C., Garza, A., & Jerabeck, J. M. (2012). A longitudinal test of video game violence influences on dating and aggression: A 3-year longitudinal study of adolescents. *Journal of Psychiatric Research, 46,* 141–6. doi:10.1016/j. jpsychires.2011.10.014 PMID:22099867

Gentile, D. A., Choo, H., Liau, A., Sim, T., Li, D., Fung, D., & Khoo, A. (2011). Pathological videogame use among youths: A two-year longitudinal study. *Pediatrics, 127,* 319–29. doi:10.1542/peds.2010-1353

Glass, B., Maddox, T., & Love, B. (2013). Real-time strategy game training: Emergence of a cognitive flexibility trait. *Plos One, 8*(8): e70350. doi:10.1371/journal.pone.0070350

Goodale, G. (2003, August 8). Are video games a sport? They may not break a sweat, but these competitors say they are tomorrow's athletes. *The Christian Science Monitor.* https://www.csmonitor.com/2003/0808/p13s01-alsp.html

Granic, I., Lobel, A., & Engels, R. (2013). The benefits of playing video games. *American Psychologist, 69*(1), 66–78.

Green, C. S., & Bavilier, D. (2007). Action-video-game experience alters the spatial resolution of vision. *Psychological Science, 18,* 88–94. doi:10.1111/j.1467-9280.2007.01853.x PMID:17362383

Greitemeyer, T., & Osswald, S. (2010). Effects of prosocial video games on pro social behavior. *Journal of Personality and Social Psychology, 98,* 211–21. doi:10.1037/a0016997 PMID:20085396

Griffiths, M. D. (1991). The observational study of adolescent gambling in UK amusement arcades. *Journal of Community and Applied Social Psychology, 1,* 309–20.

Griffiths, M. D. (1994). The role of cognitive bias and skill in fruit machine gambling. *British Journal of Psychology, 85,* 351–69.

Griffiths, M. D. (2010). The role of context in online gaming excess and addiction: Some case study evidence. *International Journal of Mental Health and Addiction, 8,* 119–25. doi:10.1007/s11469-009-9229-x

Griffiths, M. D. (2011). Workaholism: A 21st century addiction. *The Psychologist: Bulletin of the British Psychological Society, 24,* 740–4.

Griffiths, M. D., & Hunt, N. (1998). Dependence on computer games by adolescents. *Psychological Reports, 82,* 475–80. doi:10.2466/pr0.1998.82.2.475 PMID:9621722

Gye, H., Keneally, M., & Bates, D. (July 2012). Dark Knight gunman faced eviction and "broke up with girlfriend" just before killing spree. *Daily Mail.* http://www.daily mail.co.uk/news/article-2177294/James-Holmes-broke-girlfriend-just-Dark-Knight-Rises-shooting-spree-Colorado.html

Hong, J.-C., & Liu, M.-C. (2003). A study on thinking strategy between experts and novices of computer games. *Computers in Human Behavior, 19,* 245–58. doi:10.1016/S0747-5632(02)00013-4

Hutchins, B. (2008). Signs of meta-change in second modernity: The growth of e-sport and the World Cyber Games. *New Media & Society, 10,* 851–69. doi:10.1177/1461444808096248

Jansz, J., & Martens, L. (2005). Gaming at a LAN event: The social context of playing video games. *New Media & Society, 7,* 333–55. doi:10.1177/1461444805052280

Khatib, F., & DiMaio, F., Foldit Contenders Group, Foldit Void Crushers Group, Cooper, S., Kazmierczyk, M., . . . Baker, D. (2011). Crystal structure of a monomeric retroviral protease solved by protein folding game players. *Nature Structural & Molecular Biology, 18,* 1175–7. doi:10.1038/nsmb.2119 PMID:21926992

King, D., Delfabbro, P., & Griffiths, M. (2009). The psychological study of video game players: Methodological challenges and practical advice. *International Journal of Mental Health and Addiction, 7,* 555–62. doi:10.1007/s11469-009-9198-0

King, D. L., Delfabbro, P. H., & Griffiths, M. D. (2012). Clinical interventions for technology-based problems: Excessive Internet and video game use. *Journal of Cognitive Psychotherapy, 26,* 43–56. doi:10.1891/0889-8391.26.1.43

King, D. L., Delfabbro, P. H., Griffiths, M. D., & Gradisar, M. (2011). Assessing clinical trials of Internet addiction treatment: A systematic review and CONSORT evaluation. *Clinical Psychology Review, 31,* 1110–6. doi:10.1016/j.cpr.2011.06.009 PMID:21820990

Kowert, R., Griffiths, M. D., & Oldmeadow, J. (2012). Geek or chic? Emerging stereotypes of online gamers. *Bulletin of Science, Technology & Society, 32,* 371–9. doi:10.1177/0270467612469078

Kurzweil, R. (1999). *The age of spiritual machines: When computers exceed human intelligence.* New York: Viking.

Lee, Y.-H., & Lin, H. (2011). "Gaming is my work": Identity work in internet-hobbyist game workers. *Work, Employment and Society, 25,* 451–67. doi:10.1177/0950017011407975

Li, R. (2014, January 9) Making money as a Zelda speedrunner. http://www.polygon.com/features/2014/1/9/5280786/making-money-zelda-speed-runner

McCormack, A., & Griffiths, M. D. (2012). What differentiates professional poker players from recreational poker players? A qualitative interview study. *International Journal of Mental Health and Addiction, 10,* 243–57.

Reeves, S., Brown, B., & Laurier, E. (2009). Experts at play: Understanding skilled expertise. *Games and Culture, 4*, 205–27. doi:10.1177/1555412009339730

Roberts, D. F., Foehr, U. G., Rideout, V. J., & Brodie, M. (1999). *Kids and media @ the new millennium*. Menlo Park, CA: Kaiser Family Foundation.

Shaffer, D. W. (2006). *How computer games help children learn*. New York: Palgrave Macmillan. doi:10.1057/9780230601994

Sharif, I., & Sargent, J. D. (2006). Association between television, movie, and video game exposure and school performance. *Pediatrics, 118*, 1061–70. doi:10.1542/peds.2005-2854 PMID:17015499

Sheese, B. E., & Graziano, W. G. (2005). Deciding to defect: The effects of video-game violence on cooperative behavior. *Psychological Science, 15*, 354–57. doi:10.1111/j.0956-7976.2005.01539.x PMID:15869692

Shreier, J. (2013, February 1). Fighting gamers raise $225,744 for breast cancer research. http://kotaku.com/5980896/fighting-gamers-raise-225744-for-breast-cancer-research

Silady, A. (2014, April 18). The economics of competitive video game playing. *Smartasset*. http://www.smartasset.com/blog/economics-of/the-economics-of-competitive-video-gaming/

Sojourner, M. (2011, January 26). Video gaming can cause depression, anxiety, and socialphobia: 2. *Psychology Today*. http://www.psychologytoday.com/blog/she-bets-her-life/201101/video-gaming-can-cause-depression-anxiety-and-social-phobia-2

Spence, I., & Feng, J. (2010). Video games and spatial cognition. *Review of General Psychology, 14*, 92–104. doi:10.1037/a0019491

Swing, E. L., Gentile, D. A., Anderson, C. A., & Walsh, D. A. (2010). Television and video game exposure and the development of attention problems. *Pediatrics, 126*, 214–21. doi:10.1542/peds.2009-1508 PMID:20603258

Taylor, T. L. (2012). *Raising the stakes: E-sports and the professionalization of computer gaming*. Cambridge, MA: MIT Press.

Valadez, J. J., & Ferguson, C. J. (2012). Just a game after all: Violent video game exposure and time spent playing effects on hostile feelings, depression, and visuospatial cognition. *Computers in Human Behavior, 28*, 608–16. doi:10.1016/j.chb.2011.11.006

Van Deventer, S. S., & White, J. A. (2002). Expert behavior in children's video game play. *Simulation & Gaming, 33*, 28–48. doi:10.1177/10468781020 33001002

Wagner, M. G. (2006). On the scientific relevance of eSports. *International Conference on Internet Computing*, 437–42.

Williams, D. (2008). Who plays, how much, and why? Debunking the stereotypical gamer profile. *Journal of Computer-Mediated Communication, 13*, 993–1018. doi:10.1111/j.1083-6101.2008.00428.x

PART 4

Potential Negative Impacts of Internet and Technology Use and Patterns of Use

CHAPTER 17

Violent Video Games Do Not Contribute to Societal Violence and Crime

Jonathan Zachariah Gallar *and* Christopher J. Ferguson

Abstract

When mass shootings and other acts of violence occur, video games are still often blamed. Yet evidence has become clearer that video games, in fact, play no substantial role in violent behaviors in society. More debate remains regarding the impact of games on milder prank-level aggression but, here too, evidence is mixed at best. Laboratory studies are often limited by methodological flaws, and results appear to have been inflated by publication bias. From longitudinal studies, evidence for long-term effects suggests that game effects are minimal, with studies often limited by the use of unstandardized aggression measures and survey self-report. Societal violence has declined substantially even as video games have increased in popularity. With the evidence examined across data sources, it appears that several decades of research has failed to identify violence in video games as a substantial contributor to societal aggression or violence.

Keywords: violence, aggression, video games, pranking, crime

> Controlling the use of violent video games is one step we can take to help protect our society from violence.
>
> —Brad Bushman (2013)

> [H]igh exposure to media violence is a major contributing cause of the high rate of violence in modern US society.
>
> —Craig Anderson (2000), testimony before the US Senate Commerce Committee on the Impact of Interactive Violence on Children

Just outside Littleton, Colorado, two teenage boys perpetrated a shooting massacre that left more than a dozen dead before taking their own lives at Columbine High School in 1999. Eight years later, the deadliest shooting incident in US history by a lone gunman was perpetrated by a university student at Virginia Tech. After another five years, another gunman shot and killed 20 children at his old elementary school, Sandy Hook. The eyes of the world watched these horrors, and one unlikely link was echoed: violent video games.

Following the events at Sandy Hook, some pundits declared, "The brutal, merciless, savage mass murder of first-graders in Connecticut was another in a long line of avid videogame players who turned their sick fantasy into our tragic reality" (Grossman, 2013). After these shocking crimes wracked the country, news outlets immediately suggested video games may be to blame. Eric Harris and Dylan Klebold, the Columbine shooters, were cast as addicts of the violent first-person shooter computer game Doom. Seung-Hui Cho, the mass murderer responsible for the Virginia Tech massacre, was said to have been fueled by the violent first-person shooter computer game Counterstrike, although the official investigation report concluded he had played no games more violent than Sonic the Hedgehog (Virginia Tech Review Panel, 2007). After Adam Lanza, the Sandy Hook shooter, was arrested for his repulsive crime, news media was quick to report he had a basement "full" of violent video games. Once more, an official investigation report concluded that, although Lanza did play both violent and nonviolent games, he was more interested in nonviolent games such as Dance Dance Revolution (State's Attorney for the Judicial District of Dansbury, 2013). Even Eric Rodgers, the UCSB shooter, declared being an obsessive World of Warcraft player in his manifesto. Few issues in criminology have been so hotly debated and have captured the public's attention as prominently as violent video games. In the face of mass shootings that trigger many prominent issues, violent video games may seem a trivial concern. However, consistently throughout the past two decades, mass shootings and other shocking crimes have been attributed to video games and other violent media.

In the two decades since violent video games were first implicated in mass shootings, they have garnered much attention from the public, with politicians rallying against shameful violent media, and family groups condemning the "murder simulators" being peddled to their children (Grossman, 2013). Despite the focus of the public, comparatively little attention had been paid to violent video games by the scientific community until the 2000s. While psychologists, sociologists, and criminologists have begun to explore the relationship between violent video games and criminal behavior, their work is not done. Scientific inquiry has been stymied by politicization and ideology. The polarization between two competing sides in the debate over causation has slowed progress in the field. In two decades of scientific inquiry regarding the relationship between media such as violent video games and real-life violence and crime, very little understanding has been reached. Despite some attempts by causationist scholars to declare a "consensus" for their side (Bushman, Gollwitzer & Cruz, 2015), these claims have since been revealed to be problematic and the result of questionable researcher practices (Etchells & Chambers, 2014). Particularly on the issue of whether media violence contributes to societal violence, evidence is accumulating that no current scientific consensus exists either for or against such beliefs (Figure 17.1).

The scientific community has been divided into two groups, labeled *causationalists* and *anti-causationalists* (Grimes, Anderson, & Bergen, 2008). As the names would suggest, causationalist researchers seek to prove the hypothesis that violent video games and other media cause or contribute to real-world violence and crime. Conversely, anti-causationalists test the hypothesis that fictional or simulated violence such as video games do not significantly contribute to real-world violent or criminal behavior.

Those who claim video games contribute to societal violence and crime are not without research findings to back their arguments. A number of prominent researchers in the field of video game violence have concluded that violent video game exposure causes aggression and violent behavior (Anderson, 2004; Boxer, Huesmann, Bushman, O'Brien, & Moceri, 2009; Cantor, 2000; Dill, Redding, Smith, Surette, & Cornell, 2011). However, scientific scrutiny, review of a wider body of literature, and methodological flaws complicate the relationship between violent media such as video games and violent or criminal behavior. This chapter seeks to explore the many problems with the causal argument and to illustrate that no causal conclusions can be drawn between violent media and actual societal violence and crime. It will explore the lack of scientific consensus in the field of media violence, statistical data on youth violence and crime, and competing interpretations of scientific research performed on violent media. It is important to clarify that this chapter does not purport to defend that violent media in the form of video games are positive for young children or even that violent video games are without negative effects. This essay simply argues that violent video games do not significantly contribute to societal violence and crime, especially to the extent that many have represented.

Lack of Consensus

The first obstacle to exploring the relationship between violent media and its effects on its consumers has been a lack of consensus in the scientific community. The polarization between two competing hypotheses, both of which consist of interpretations of scientific data, has led to much stagnation in the production of new research, particularly in the study of violent media effects. While some researchers may contend that a growing body of evidence indicates fantasy violence in the form of video games and other media contributes to real-world

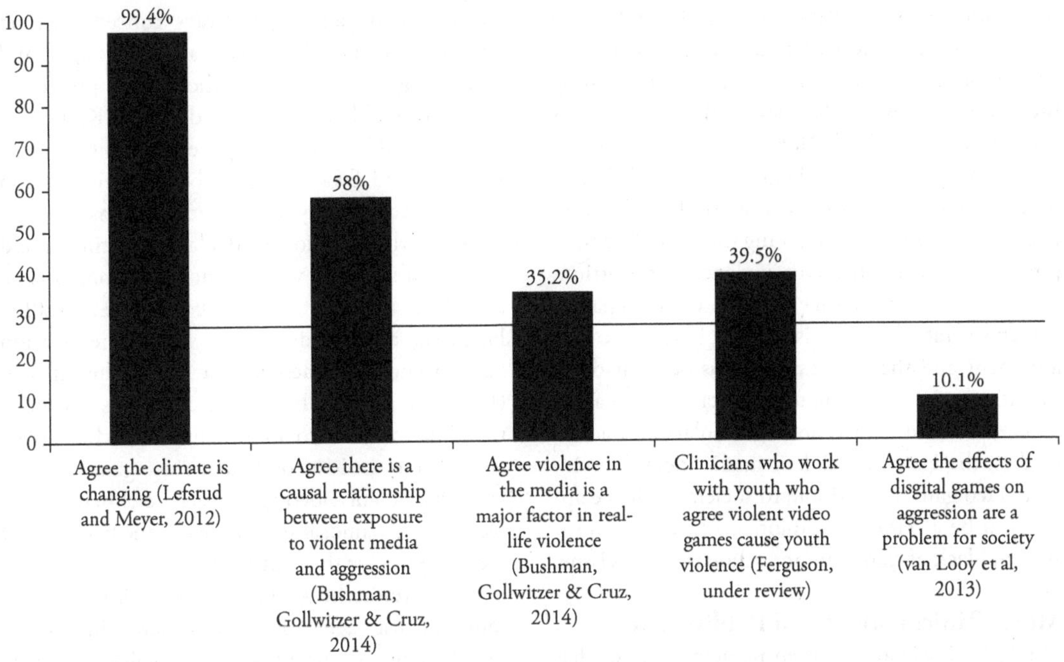

Figure 17.1 Lack of consensus among scholars on media violence.

violence (Anderson, 2004), these claims have not effected any real-world policy change. When the US Supreme Court reviewed the threat of youth violence and its relation to violent video games in *Brown, Governor of California v. Entertainment Merchants Association* in 2011, it specifically cited the lack of scientific consensus in striking down a California law that would have made selling violent video games to minors a criminal offense. In the majority opinion, Justice Scalia concluded, "Psychological studies purporting to show a connection between exposure to violent video games and harmful effects on children do not prove that such exposure causes minors to act aggressively" (*Brown v. Entertainment Merchants Assn.*, 2011). The Justices in their opinion note that the research available is not enough to infringe upon First Amendment rights, and the majority opinion was critical of the existing research, noting "These studies have been rejected by every court to consider them and with good reason," although the minority opinion did express concern about the potential negative impact of violent video games. Despite the Supreme Court ruling, many scientists maintain that sufficient evidence exists to prove a causal link between violent video games and aggressive or violent behavior. Causationalist researcher Craig Anderson, in his monograph *Violent Video Game Effects on Children and Adolescents* (2007), laments that the general public and non-researchers do not properly understand the debate and states that there is, in fact, enough evidence to support that violent video games cause long-term and significant increases in aggression. Other researchers, such as Christopher Ferguson, emphatically disagree. In a published response to Anderson's work, Ferguson and Kilburn (2010) noted that, "The influence of VVGs [violent video games] on serious acts of aggression or violence is minimal, and publication bias is a problem in this research field." The polarization between both sides, causationalists and anti-causationalists, has led to a lack of objectivity and potential publication bias against studies that have demonstrated no effect. In a meta-analysis of studies with supportive, nonsupportive, and inconclusive results in testing the causal argument, Ferguson and Kilburn noted that a majority of nonpublished studies were nonsupportive, while a majority of published studies were supportive. Their review suggests that more attention needs to be paid to the anti-causationalist argument and that publishers must ignore the politicized nature of this field and put emphasis not only on studies that confirm the causal argument, but also on those that produce no or mixed results.

The lack of consensus in the research community is perhaps the most important problem facing those who would claim that violent video games and real-world crime or violence are linked. While some researchers have declared that the debate is over (Anderson, 2004), other recent reviews of existing literature and new studies have indicated that this claim is premature (Colwell & Kato, 2003; Ferguson & Olson, 2014, Puri & Pugliese, 2012). In 2013, more than 230 scholars wrote to the American Psychological Association asking them to retire their policy statements on media violence (Consortium of Scholars, 2013). Latter sections of this chapter will enumerate the many issues that beset the causal argument and the progress that has been made in recent years in advancing the anti-causational argument. As noted earlier, among scholars and across studies, the view that violent media including violent video games contribute to societal violence appears to be a *minority* opinion, with much confusion and lack of clarity among scholars on this issue.

Moral Panic: Politics and Publication

The lack of scientific consensus demonstrates that the public response to the violent video game "threat" is disproportionate. To this end, the current outrage over violent video games has been compared to the "moral panic" phenomenon. Although earlier used to describe the panic that gripped America regarding child molesters and sex offenders (Jenkins, 1998), moral panic theory has since become a lens through which to view any moral outrage on the part of society, fueled by media and often mistaken conceptions about the subject. The aspect of media-fueled hysteria is certainly reminiscent of the violent video games panic that still exists in public discourse. When Jenkins (1998) explores the moral panic regarding child molestation throughout the 20th century, striking parallels become apparent. Politicians were quick to focus on the problem of child molesters in a disproportionate response to curry public favor, religious and family groups rallied behind child-protection rhetoric, and moral outrage fueled decisions more than did rational information. The same could be witnessed in the moral panic following Sandy Hook in 2012, when most of the debate on video game violence occurred *before* the official investigation report was released indicating that the shooter Adam Lanza was not a particularly avid gamer. Jenkins is also clear to illustrate that moral panics do not rely on science or rationalism, but rather are often punctuated by a lack of true scientific understanding of the issue and politicization. In these respects, the current scrutiny of violent video games certainly fits the description of moral panic. The fears regarding the ill effects of violent video games are always concentrated on children, with politicians, family groups, and religious groups using the rhetoric of protecting innocent children in their debates (Kutner & Olson, 2008). Even the governor of California (then Arnold Swartzenegger, both previously and since a star of many violent action films) became involved when he pioneered a law that criminalized the sale of a violent video game to a minor (*Brown v. Entertainment Merchants Assn.*, 2011). Furthermore, the addition of scientific evaluation has not ended the debate, but rather intensified it (Ferguson, 2013). The lack of consensus just illustrated has only led to a more divisive and polarized approach to the issue of violent video games. On its face, the violent video games debate closely resembles a moral panic, and they are not the first form of media to receive this treatment.

Many researchers, both causationalist and anti-causationalist, agree that this violent video game moral panic is part of a cycle involving all new media. In fact, the relationship between media and crime is much older than the wave of mass shootings that shocked America in the past few decades. In his exploration of criminogenic media, Surette (2011) argues that concerns over media, juvenile delinquency, and crime originated as early as 1908. Concerns that newspapers and books caused juvenile delinquency and even criminal behavior were present during the turn of the 20th century and are present still with the advent of visual, digital, and interactive media. Kutner and Olson (2008) review the history of media censorship and moral panics in the United States and find that the same concerns can be found for every form of "new" media—dime novels, comic books, radio, cinema, television, and finally video games. This repetitive cycle contains all the hallmarks reminiscent of these moral panics in that their focus is primarily on children and adolescents, family groups and politicians are quick to condemn the new media, and objective scientific evaluation is sparse. In Gauntlett's (1995) formulation of moral panic, he notes that scientific research promoting the moral panic is easily accepted by the public while research critical of the moral panic's subject is largely ignored. While much more scientific focus has been directed toward the moral panic regarding violent video games, the bias that Gauntlett describes is still apparent. In their review of publication bias in violent video games research, Ferguson and Kilburn (2010) note that unpublished studies on violent video game effects were more likely to support the null hypothesis and that even meta-analyses tended to selectively ignore unpublished studies supporting null results (e.g., Anderson et al., 2010). Studies that reported no causal link between video games and violence were far more likely to remain unpublished.

In the wake of shocking crimes, especially those committed by adolescents and young adults in school, many observers have claimed that serious violent crimes such as mass shootings are on the rise. From the 1999 Columbine shootings to the 2012 Newtown and Aurora shootings, mass media has sensationalized these horrible crimes to a point never before experienced. However, mass shootings have not increased in number of incidents or in number of killings over the past several decades (Fox & Delateur, 2014). Despite the public fervor in finding answers and stopping mass shootings, including the restriction of violent video games, objective data have been ignored.

The backdrop of this debate reinforces the idea that the video game panic is undeserved. US government data tracking serious violent crimes perpetrated by youths from 1980 to 2010 shows that youth violence declined greatly in the first part of the 21st century, with its peak in the early 1990s (Childstats.gov, 2019). Youth violent crime rates in 2010 were lower than in 1980. Conversely, violent video games have reached exponential new amounts of violent content, realistic graphics, and have become far more widespread during this time. In the early 1980s, arcade classics such as Pacman (1980) and Tron (1982), featuring 8- or 16-bit resolution with no gore and no human violence were the best-selling video games. In 2010, two of the three best-selling video games were the latest installments in the Halo and Call of Duty franchises; namely, violent first-person shooters featuring blood, gore, and immersive violent action (*The Independent*, 2011). The Call of Duty franchise became infamous in 2009 when Call of Duty: Modern Warfare 2 included a level in which the player aids foreign terrorists indiscriminately killing civilians in an international airport; a far cry from a grouping of yellow pixels eating pellets. Not only did video games increase in violent content during this period, but the ratio of players in the population also rose. In 1980, a minority of the population played violent video games; in the late 2000s, the majority of youths played video games, even violent ones (Kutner & Olson, 2008). A 2013 study by Ferguson found that only 11% of the juveniles he studied did not play violent video games. A national study of US adolescents showed that 97% play video games (Lenhart et al., 2008). Based on this information, anti-causationalists have asked: If video games are played by more youths, are more violent, and are more realistic, why has youth crime not experienced a dramatic rise or at least maintained a steady high level? If video games and other forms of violent media are responsible for an increase in real violence and crime, why do government statistics show just the opposite effect? If violent video games were to significantly contribute to societal violence and crime, these statistics are the opposite of the expected outcome. As the focus on violent video games as potential causes of crime and delinquency increases, actual youth violence has declined precipitously. Although causationists often speculate that crime statistics may mask smaller violent video game effects due to the multidetermined nature of aggression and violence, this seems a convenient "theory saving" rationalization, particularly when causationist scholars have pointed to past rising societal violence rates when these appeared to suit their theories (e.g., Bushman & Anderson, 2001).

The current public and scientific debate over violent video games bears an uncomfortable resemblance to historical moral panics. While public outrage in itself is not a negative phenomenon, the distortion inherent to a moral panic is certainly detrimental to society. The emotionally charged, politicized argument as to whether violent video games produce real-life violence is an important one. Unfortunately, the argument remains largely uninformed by balanced and reasonable discourse and instead has relied on emotional rhetoric and increasingly hostile discourse, at times even in academia.

Aggression: Measurement

A litany of published studies, both experimental and observational, have concluded that there exists a causal link between violent video game exposure and increased aggression (Anderson, 2004; Boxer et al., 2009; Cantor, 2000; Dill et al., 2011; Surette, 2011). Opponents argue that none of these studies proves violent games can lead to any real-life violence or crime and that their effects on aggression have been overstated. This issue has become more pronounced as an increasing number of null studies regarding violent video games and aggression have begun to be published (e.g., Ballard, Visser, & Jocoy, 2012; Charles, Baker, Hartman, Easton, & Kretzberger, 2013; Puri & Pugliese, 2012; Przybylski, Deci, Rigby, & Ryan, 2014; Tear & Nielson, 2013).

Overall, the most elementary problem with literature exploring the link between violent media and real-life violence is *measurement*. Experimental laboratory research using violent and criminal behavior is impossible in an ethical setting; researchers cannot expose subjects to harm. Therefore, experiments testing the effects of violent media and video games have turned to surrogate measurements, particularly through measuring relatively mild forms of aggression. There are, however, several problems that plague the notion of using aggression at all in scientific research. Aggression itself is a concept that is extremely difficult to operationally define, and, as such, studies examining it have often used conflicting or differing definitions of aggression. Many studies have defined aggression as thoughts, feelings, and emotions. Others have designed opportunities for participants to act in ways that could be perceived as aggressive behavior, although sometimes it is unclear whether aggression or competitiveness is being measured. While causationalist researchers argue that all of these measurements strengthen the finding that violent video games cause aggression in players (Anderson, 2004), anti-causationalists argue that these competing measures of aggression decrease the reliability of findings and lead to exaggerated effects, particularly when they have been used in an unstandardized manner (Ferguson, 2013). The inconsistency in measuring aggression is a pervasive problem confronting the causal argument, and validated consistent measures have not been implemented in empirical evaluation. This raises the concern that many outcomes related to aggression may be due to researcher expectancies and questionable researcher practices rather than "true" effects.

Research involving violent video games and behavior has been classified into two separate categories: experimental and correlational/longitudinal. *Experimental designs* involve participants playing a violent or nonviolent game while researchers observe, followed by a post-test. These post-tests can involve survey measurements or observation of aggressive actions. Survey measurements often measure cognitive aggression through the use of word-completion surveys exercises (Carnagey & Anderson, 2005), vignette completion (Bushman & Anderson, 2002), and other written scales in surveys. Aggressive actions have been measured in the laboratory through a number of surrogates, but the most notorious have been delivering punishing noise blasts (Anderson & Dill, 2000; Anderson & Carnagey, 2009) and the addition of hot sauce to other players' food (Adachi & Willoughby, 2011). In particular, these laboratory experiments involving video game play and behavioral aggression have often been targeted by researchers as methodologically flawed (Ferguson et al., 2008). While some of these studies may statistically demonstrate that players who engaged in a violent video game were more likely to ascribe a mild punishment to their opponent, they fall short of providing conclusive evidence that a violent video game could inspire violent action. While experiments involving these aggressive actions are those that garner the most criticism, it is also important to note that cognitive surveys such as word-completion exercises are also inconclusive. Cognitive surveys do not have any way of differentiating between individuals who are merely recollecting the aggressive game they just played and those who may act on those thoughts; therefore, it is difficult to claim that they predict any real-life violence or crime. The US Supreme Court acknowledged this limitation in *Brown, Governor of California v. Entertainment Merchants Association* (Ferguson, 2013). Cognitive thoughts about aggression that do not indicate intent are a poor surrogate for real-world violence, and these studies cannot be used as causal evidence of violent behavior. Overall, laboratory studies are nonstandardized and do not use validated measures of aggression (Ferguson, 2013). As a result, their conclusions about the effects of violent video games cannot be properly compared. Post-tests used to measure surrogates for aggression are often invented and tailored toward their particular study and are not reused to establish reliability as a clinical scale. Despite these issues with experimental research, these studies are relied on in building the causationalist argument. The largest effect sizes in research on violent video games have been from these often-contradictory laboratory experiments using surrogate measurements, although this may be a product of their unstandardized use and researcher expectancies more than any "real" effect (Elson, Mohseni, Breuer, Scharkow, & Quandt, 2014).

The Gulf Between Aggression and Violence

The most critical failure in using cognitive aggression measures to illustrate the potential for real-world violence and crime is addressing the gulf between thinking about violence (that is to say simply the topic of violence rather than having any intent) and violent action. Perhaps none has illustrated that gulf between the fantasy violence of violent media and true criminal violence as eloquently as

Lieutenant Colonel David Grossman in his work *On Killing* (1996), "For those who have never experienced it, the depiction of battle that Hollywood has given us, and the cultural mythology that Hollywood is based upon, appear to be as useful in understanding killing as pornographic movies would be in . . . [understanding sex] . . . he or she could never hope to understand the intimacy and intensity of the . . . experience." Grossman argues that it takes training to bridge the gap between normative human aggression and violent or criminal action such as killing. While Grossman himself equates some violent video games to military training in his work *Stop Training Our Kids to Kill* (1999), these claims are not founded on empirical research. Aggression, both cognitive and emotional, is part of normal human behavior and does not necessarily lead to violence. Researchers have not been able to predict when aggressive thoughts or feelings, or even emotional hostility, will become violent action. Therefore, it is impossible to make the claim that any amount of increased aggression, even should it be consistently demonstrated in research—which it has not—will produce an increase in real-world violence. For more reliable and accurate ways to predict violent behavior, many researchers have instead foregone laboratory studies and performed cross-sectional and longitudinal studies measuring real-world aggressive action.

Correlational and Longitudinal Research

The relationship between violent media and crime has arguably been more precisely measured through correlational cross-sectional study designs, although these studies also have methodological limitations. These studies correlate violent video games and aggression or even violent acts but, for the most part, abandon surrogate measures and instead target aggressive acts on the part of subjects. Unlike laboratory setting experiments in which subjects are allowed to punish opponents with noise blasts or hot sauce, some correlational studies measure aggression in the forms of bullying, verbal aggression, and aggressive or violent acts. These measures, of course, make the results from these studies far more generalizable to real-world violence and crime. However, as these studies move closer to measuring the target variables of violence and crime, the results are far less consistent and effect sizes shrink (Ferguson et al, 2008). For example, in a 2001 meta-analysis of studies measuring violent video game exposure and aggression, Anderson and Bushman reviewed 33 cross-sectional and experimental studies using several different measures. The strongest effect observed was when aggression was measured by "aggressive cognition" or by simple physiological arousal. These measures suffer the same weaknesses discussed earlier in laboratory studies: they cannot accurately capture potential for violence or deviance. Ultimately, including laboratory studies with severe methodological flaws only skews the understanding of how violent media influences real-world criminal behavior. In a follow-up analysis, Anderson and colleagues (2010) found that controlling for only gender in correlational studies and only gender and time 1 aggression in longitudinal studies shrunk correlational effect sizes to trivial levels. These findings are particularly important because this was the only meta-analysis to consider children and youth samples specifically (Ferguson, 2015).

Many methodologically sound studies employ far better measures of criminal or violent behavior. Ferguson and Olson (2014) measured the impact of violent video games on criminal delinquency and bullying behavior. Rather than implementing a surrogate measure, the investigators employed self-report of delinquency and the empirically validated Olweus Bully/Victim Questionnaire (Ferguson & Olson, 2014). Using these measures, they found that exposure to video game violence was *not* predictive of delinquent criminality or bullying behavior. Furthermore, only 11.4% of children involved in the study reported no exposure to violent video games in their homes.

Several studies have been done with correctional populations. One such study by Surette and Maze (2015) found that violent video game exposure did not correlate with criminal behavior among adult inmates. In another cross-sectional study that involved delinquent juveniles in a correctional setting, DeLisi, Vaughn, Gentile, Anderson, and Shook (2013) concluded that violent video game preference and exposure was significantly correlated with juvenile delinquency and histories of violence, though with less extreme effect sizes than that reported by earlier researchers. Importantly, they also acknowledged that current data are limited by research cross-sectional design and that such data could not demonstrate causal relationship without longitudinal study (DeLisi et al., 2013). Furthermore, their study was limited by several methodological issues known to be problematic in correlational research. The first is relying on youth to rate the violence of the games they play themselves, then asking about aggressive acts the youth may have committed. Such a pattern of responses potentially sets up demand characteristics which can result in spurious correlations. Second, the authors did not include multiple potential control variables in their analyses despite these variables apparently being available in the dataset from which the study was drawn (e.g., Shook, Vaughn, Goodkind, & Johnson, 2011). Third, the survey did not test for mischievous responding or the tendency for juveniles to give false answers that could result in spurious correlations (Robinson-Cimpian, 2014).

While researchers have begun to address the dearth of longitudinal research in studying violent video games, a key weakness of the causal argument is proving long-term increases in aggression and violent behavior. Even causationalist researchers agree that longitudinal studies are extremely important in clarifying the link between video games and violence (Anderson, 2004). Longitudinal studies have proved especially useful in demonstrating whether violent media can elicit a long-term effect on its consumers as opposed to a short-term effect. They are also able to evaluate the staying power of violent media and increased levels of aggression. Results, however, are far more inconclusive than those involving measures of immediate increases in aggression. In a 2005 longitudinal study involving a month-long exposure to a violent computer role-playing game, Williams and Skoric reported no measurable effect on aggression from habitual exposure to violent video games. Based on these findings, these researchers have questioned the effects of laboratory and cross-sectional studies that involve an immediate post-test after 1 or 2 hours of exposure to violent media. While longitudinal analysis has so far been limited in comparison to cross-sectional study, the current results suggest that the relationship between violent video games and aggression is more complex than laboratory approaches have suggested. In his own longitudinal study of adolescent boys and girls, Ferguson (2011) reports that he found no link between violent video game play and youth aggression. A German study led by Maria von Salisch, Vogelgesang, Kristen, and Oppl (2011) solidified these findings in an international setting, confirming that violent video game play was not predictive of aggressive, violent, or criminal behavior. Overall, results from longitudinal analyses indicate that long-term links are weak and usually attributable to other variables (Anderson et al., 2010; Ferguson, 2015).

Theoretical Perspective

While many in the past viewed media-inspired aggression or violence as a simple act of imitation (Surette, 2011), further evaluation has shown that the relationship between these two variables is far more complex. Most of the research conducted on violent media has used a cognitive or social learning theoretical framework, and the majority utilized the General Aggression Model (GAM). The GAM (Bushman & Anderson, 2002) as applied to video games was initially developed by causationalist researchers seeking to further elucidate the cognitive psychological process in forming aggression and later to explain how violent media increases aggression. In brief, the GAM posits that aggression is produced by cognitive scripts or schemas that are learned and activated (Bushman & Anderson, 2002). One of the ways for aggression to be learned and primed is through exposure to violent media, usually over long periods of time.

The GAM has recently garnered criticism from anti-causationalists as it has found less support in empirical evaluation by longitudinal study (Ferguson, 2011; von Salisch et al., 2011; Williams & Skoric, 2005) and theoretical development (Przybylski, Rigby, & Ryan, 2010). As discussed earlier, longitudinal studies should closely parallel the GAM showing that long-term, repeated exposure to violent video games increases aggression and leads to outbursts such as violent behavior. Empirical investigations have found just the opposite: longitudinal analysis of long-term and repeated violent video game exposure report lesser effects on aggression and indicators of violent behavior than short laboratory experiments. The suitability of the GAM has been questioned on theoretical grounds as well (e.g., Ferguson & Dyck, 2012) particularly regarding problematic assumptions of the model, such as how it assumes the brain treats real-life and fictional media violence in a similar manner. It is borrowed from earlier theories of passive media exposure, such as television or cinema, and many researchers on both sides of the causal argument have noted that video games differ from such passive viewing due to their interactive element (Anderson & Dill, 2000). While many contend that this makes video games more dangerous in terms of influencing their audience, this difference has yet to be addressed through empirical investigation, and, if anything, evidence suggests the opposite (Sherry, 2001). If interactivity does indeed make violent video games different, the GAM would not be an appropriate framework in which to study them. Some causationalist researchers have cited the body of background research on television and movies and aggression as strengthening the causal argument

(Bushman & Anderson, 2002) as part of its theoretical background. Meanwhile, these same researchers have argued that violent video games are far more dangerous than other types of media and that the extreme violence and realism that video games present differ from that of television and movies. Anti-causationalists and other researchers have argued that there is no research to date that has even begun to test the hypothesis that interactive media are more dangerous than noninteractive media (*Brown v. Entertainment Merchants Assn.*, 2011) although the few studies to have examined this thus far have generally not been encouraging for this assumption.

Recent empirical research, employing best practices including longitudinal study design and true measures of aggressive or violent actions, has painted a far more complex picture of the violent video games debate than laboratory studies. The addition of more diverse research groups, refinements in study design, and meta-analysis of a growing body of literature have cast doubt on the causal argument. Some research groups have even widened the lens of focus on violent video games to measuring more variables relevant to the experience, and the addition of these so-called third variables has complicated the vision of the violent video gamer further.

Aggression and Competition: The "Z" Variable

Recently, many researchers have criticized the majority of studies involving violent media for their simplistic view of media content. Characteristics of media other than violent content, which have largely been ignored by earlier research, must be measured to determine whether violence is truly the problem. Most studies evaluating aggression are designed to control only for violent and nonviolent content but fail to take into account other important aspects of the video game experience. Some video games are more difficult than others, some take longer to learn, and some are more competitive. One group of researchers has advanced the hypothesis that it is competition, not violence or simple media exposure in video games, which causes aggression (Adachi & Willoughby, 2010, 2013). In their review of studies testing aggression levels in violent media consumers, they noted a failure to address competitiveness, action content, and difficulty as potential third variables in the relationship between violent video games and consumer aggression. In studies that employ nonviolent video games as a control, they note that the violent ones are often more competitive than their nonviolent comparisons. Adachi and Willoughby (2011) also argue that the "noise blasts" employed by previous researchers may in fact be a measure of competitiveness in the video game players and not aggression. Furthermore, they discovered competitiveness was a significant predictor for aggression, as opposed to violent content. Ferguson (2011) also argues that many violent video games take longer to learn and are more difficult than their nonviolent counterparts, and this may explain some of the aggressive effects found in laboratory study, due to the frustration at not being allowed to properly learn the game during a brief (often 10–15 minutes) laboratory exposure. When college students, who are the typical participants in a laboratory experiment, are introduced to an unfamiliar game but not given time to learn the controls or become familiar, these aspects of the game may increase aggression far more than any violent content (Przybylski et al., 2014).

Time-Order: The Chicken and the Egg

As reviewed earlier, recent longitudinal and cross-sectional studies have cast doubt on the causal relationship between violent video games and violent media. They have demonstrated smaller correlations between violent content and aggression (DeLisi et al., 2013; Ferguson & Olson, 2014; Williams & Skoric, 2005) and provided doubt that other confounding variables have been adequately controlled (Adachi & Willoughby, 2011, 2013; Ferguson, 2011). Longitudinal analysis has also identified another weakness in the causal argument: time-order. The causal argument has long maintained that violent video game exposure comes before increases in aggression, and in short-term laboratory experiments this has appeared to hold true. Recent longitudinal studies have found just the opposite. Maria von Salisch and colleagues (2011) not only concluded that violent video game play was not predictive of aggression, but also observed the opposite effect. German schoolchildren who were initially rated as aggressive were more likely to prefer and spend more time with violent video games. Von Salisch's group contrasts the traditional "media socialization effects" theory (that violent games cause aggression) with their own "selection effects" theory (in which aggressive individuals select violent games). Similar results were found by Breuer, Vogelgesang, Quandt, & Festl (2015). Adachi and Willoughby (2013) found support for the selection hypothesis in their longitudinal study, where aggression predicted competitive video game play over time. Copycat crime research has also echoed support for the selection hypothesis in suggesting that individuals with existing psychopathology and violent tendencies are attracted to violent media (Grimes et al., 2008; Surette, 2011). The directionality of the relationship between video games/violent content and aggression has been a point of contention from the beginning of their study. When the US Supreme Court struck down the constitutionality of California's law, they specifically cited that the current research literature could not show that violent video games caused aggression and not vice versa (*Brown v. Entertainment Merchants*, 2011).

Conclusion

Violent video games have stolen the stage in the public and scientific debate over media effects. The ensuing moral panic during the tragic school shootings of the 1990s and 2000s that targeted isolated young men fixated on shoot-'em-up violent video games left the United States with fear, politics, and a distinct lack of scientific understanding. The past few decades have seen spirited debate but little advancement. Those who claimed that video games caused aggression and violence in the 1990s still do so today, but any causal argument must prove three points. First, the two variables at hand must be significantly correlated. Second, other third variables need to be isolated to demonstrate that the effects of one are truly caused by the other (e.g., DeCamp, 2015). Third, a time order in which one variable comes before the other must be established. Studies have failed to demonstrate that the relationship between violent video games and aggression, violence, or crime is a causal one. Indeed, research literature demonstrating violent video games correlating with even mild aggression has become decidedly mixed. Investigators have failed to isolate violent content as the cause of increased aggression or violent behavior. Additionally, many researchers have found evidence that aggressive personalities predict preoccupation with violent media, not the other way around. Given the current state of evidence, violent video games cannot be said to cause aggressive behavior, violent behavior, or criminal behavior. The simplistic view of exposure to violent video games causing aggression increasingly appears to be erroneous.

Much research remains to be done. Even though a causal statement cannot be made, recent research suggests that people with aggressive and violent personalities may become preoccupied with violent media (Grimes et al., 2008; Surette, 1990, 2011; von Salisch et al., 2011). Some speculate that violent media may then serve to inspire or intensify otherwise violent urges in those suffering from mental illness or with other criminal risk factors, although what little evidence currently exists has not supported this (Ferguson & Olson, 2014). Much of the past decades of research has been preoccupied with either proving or disproving a hypothesis that has become wholly unhelpful to society and to science. During that decade consumption of violent video games in society has been associated with a nearly 90% decline in youth violence, not an increase, as presented in Figure 17.2. Ray Surette perhaps puts it most matter-of-factly: "An assessment offered nearly half a century ago remains valid: For some children under some conditions some media is harmful. For other children under the same conditions, or for the same children under other conditions, it may be beneficial. For most children under most conditions, most media is probably neither particularly harmful nor particularly beneficial" (Surette, 2011). In that half century, our capabilities have changed. It is time to focus research forward on identifying vulnerable populations and risk factors for violent media exposure. Moving beyond the scope of negative effects, many groups have already turned to exploring how video games can be used positively on youth (Przybylski et al., 2010). Video games have seen considerable scrutiny for their ability to teach aggression. New avenues of research should be developed to instead examine pro-social learning opportunities and to explore positive effects of video gaming, even those with violent content.

Nonetheless some psychologists continue to blame video games for violence, including murder. As one example, in May 2013, Christopher Harris went on trial for the murder of a family of five in Beason, Illinois. With overwhelming forensic evidence, as well as testimony by his own brother indicating he was guilty, Harris's defense chose an unusual tactic. Harris claimed it was not he, in fact, who committed the murders, but the family's 14-year-old son Dillen Constant. Dillen, the defense claimed, had a history of attention deficit disorder, school problems, and had several violent video games in his bedroom. According to Harris, it was Dillen who killed his family. Harris happened to walk in on the multiple murders and had to defend himself from Dillen by beating Dillen 52 times with a tire iron, only incurring a blister himself. Harris was supported in his defense by a video game violence researcher who agreed that Dillen's history of

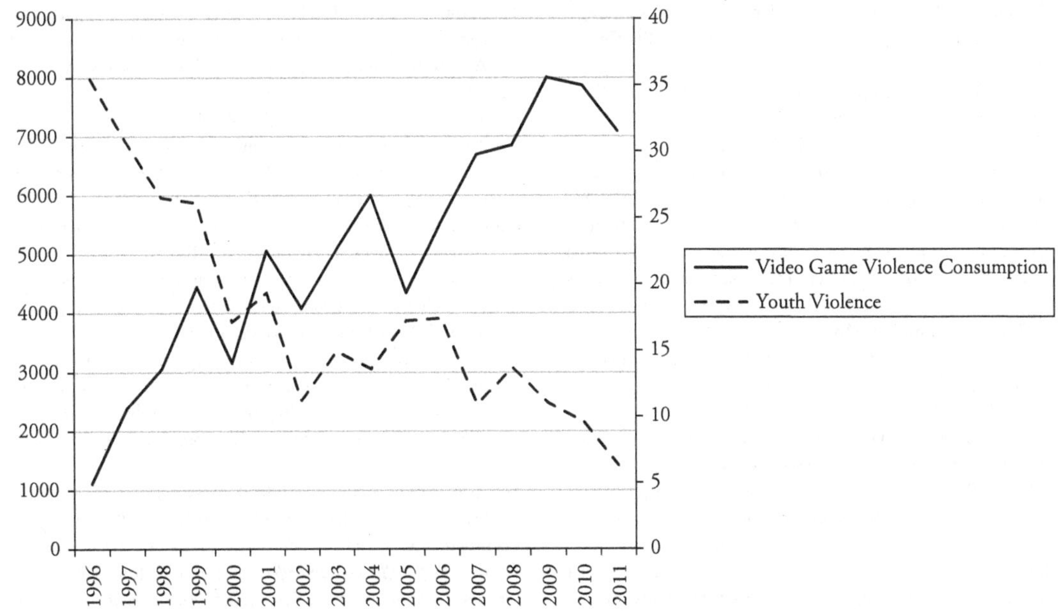

Figure 17.2 Association between violent video game consumption and youth violence in the United States.

attention deficit disorder, school problems, and possession of violent video games placed him at risk for aggressive and violent behavior (Rushton, 2013).

During cross-examination, however, the expert in question acknowledged that he was not a clinical psychologist, held no license, was not trained in risk assessment, had not verified information given to him by the defense, and had not questioned Dillen's surviving family or other witnesses. Related to video games, the expert acknowledged he did not know how often Dillen played violent video games (an analysis of the game console's saved games suggested play was infrequent), acknowledged most young boys play violent video games, acknowledged research cannot document links between video games and violent behavior, and, at one point, stated that even games such as Pac Man could be considered violent video games under some definitions. One of the assistant district attorneys was later overheard to say "The most offensive testimony I've ever heard in my life, I think" (Rushton, 2013). Harris was convicted. Psychology, as a science, needs to do better than this or risk permanent damage to its credibility (Hall, Day, & Hall, 2011).

References

Adachi, P. J. C., & Willoughby, T. (2010). The effect of violent video games on aggression: Is it more than just the violence? *Aggression and Violent Behavior, 16*, 55–62.

Adachi, P. J. C., & Willoughby, T. (2011). The effect of video game competition and violence on aggressive behavior: Which characteristic has the greatest influence? *Psychology of Violence, 1*(4), 259–74. doi:10.1037/a0024908

Adachi, P. J. C., & Willoughby, T. (2013). Demolishing the competition: The longitudinal link between competitive video games, competitive gambling, and aggression. *Journal of Youth & Adolescence, 42*, 1090–104.

Anderson, C. (2000). Violent video games increase aggression and violence: Senate Commerce Committee hearing on the impact of interactive violence on children. http://www.psychology.iastate.edu/faculty/caa/abstracts/2000-2004/00Senate.html. Accessed on: 20/01/2015.

Anderson, C. A. (2004). An update on the effects of playing violent video games. *Journal of Adolescence, 27*, 113–22.

Anderson, C. A., & Carnagey, N. L. (2009). Causal effects of violent sports video games on aggression: Is it competitiveness or violent content? *Journal of Experimental Social Psychology, 45*, 731–9.

Anderson, C. A., & Dill, K. (2000). Video games and aggressive thoughts, feelings and behavior in the laboratory and in life. *Journal of Personality and Social Psychology, 78*, 772–90.

Anderson, C. A., Ihori, N., Bushman, B. J., Rothsetin, H. R., Shibuya, A., . . . Saleem, M. (2010). Video game effects on aggression, empathy, and prosocial behavior and eastern and western countries: A meta-analytic review. *Psychological Bulletin, 136*, 151–73.

Ballard, M., Visser, K., & Jocoy, K. (2012). Social context and video game play: Impact on cardiovascular and affective responses, *Mass Communication and Society, 15*(6), 875–98.

Boxer, P., Huesmann, L. R., Bushman, B. J., O'Brien, M., & Moceri, D. (2009). The role of violent media preference in cumulative developmental risk for violence and general aggression. *Journal of Youth & Adolescence, 38*, 417–28.

Breuer, J., Vogelgesang, J., Quandt, T., & Festl, R. (2015). Violent video games and physical aggression: Evidence for a selection effect among adolescents. *Psychology of Popular Media Culture, 4*(4), 305–328. doi:10.1037/ppm0000035.

Brown v. Entertainment Merchants Association, 131 S. Ct. 2729 (CA, 2011). http://www.supremecourt.gov/opinions/10pdf/08-1448.pdf

Bushman, B. (2013). Do video games play a role in shootings? CNN.com. http://www.cnn.com/2013/09/18/opinion/bushman-video-games/

Bushman, B., & Anderson, C. (2001). Media violence and the American public. *American Psychologist, 56*, 477–89.

Bushman, B., & Anderson, C. (2002). Violent video games and hostile expectations: A test of the generalized aggression model. *Personality and Social Psychology Bulletin, 28*, 1679–86.

Bushman, B. J., Gollwitzer, M., & Cruz, C. (2015). There is broad consensus: Media researchers agree that violent media increase aggression in children, and pediatricians and parents concur. *Psychology of Popular Media Culture, 4*(3), 200–14. doi:10.1037/ppm0000046

Cantor, J. (2000). Conference proceedings: Media violence. *Journal of Adolescent Health, 27*, 30–4.

Carnagey, N. L., & Anderson, C. A. (2005). The effects of reward and punishment in violent video games on aggressive affect, cognition, and behavior. *Psychological Science, 16*, 882–9.

Charles, E., Baker, C., Hartman, K., Easton, B., & Kretzberger, C. (2013). Motion capture controls negate the violent video game effect. *Computers in Human Behavior, 29*, 2519–23.

Childstats.gov. (2019). America's children: Key national indicators of well-being, h2007. https://www.childstats.gov/americaschildren/beh5.asp

Colwell, J., & Kato, M. (2003). Investigation of the relationship between social isolation, self-esteem, aggression, and computer game play in Japanese adolescents. *Asian Journal of Social Psychology, 6*, 149–58.

Consortium of Scholars. (2013). Scholar's open statement to the APA Task Force on Violent Media. http://www.christopherj-ferguson.com/APA%20Task%20Force%20Comment1.pdf

Decamp, W. (2015). Impersonal agencies of communication: Comparing the effects of video games and other risk factors on violence. *Psychology of Popular Media Culture, 4*(4), 296–304. doi: 10.1037/ppm0000037.

DeLisi, M., Vaughn, M. G., Gentile, D. A., Anderson, C. A., & Shook, J. J. (2013). Violent video games, delinquency, and youth violence: New evidence. *Youth Violence and Juvenile Justice, 11*(2), 132–42.

Dill, K. E., Redding, R. E., Smith, P. K., Surette, R., & Cornell, D. G. (2011). Recurrent issues in efforts to prevent homicidal youth violence in schools: Expert opinions. *New Directions for Youth Development, 129*, 113–28.

Elson, M., Mohseni, R., Breuer, J., Scharkow, M., & Quandt, T. (2014). Press CRTT to measure aggressive behavior: The unstandardized use of the competitive reaction time test in aggression research. *Psychological Assessment, 26*(2), 419–432. doi:10.1037/a0035569.

Etchells, P., & Chambers, C. (2014). Violent video games research: Consensus or confusion? *The Guardian*. http://www.theguardian.com/science/head-quarters/2014/oct/10/violent-video-games-research-consensus-or-confusion

Ferguson, C. J. (2011). Video games and youth violence: A prospective analysis in adolescents. *Journal of Youth and Adolescence, 40*(4), 377–91.

Ferguson, C. J. (2013). Violent video games and the Supreme Court: Lessons for the scientific community in the wake of Brown v. Entertainment Merchants Association. *American Psychologist, 68*(2), 57–74.

Ferguson, C. J. (2015). Do angry birds make for angry children? A meta-analysis of video game Influences on children's and adolescents' aggression, mental health, prosocial behavior and academic performance. *Perspectives on Psychological Science, 10*(5), 646–666. doi:10.1177/1745691615592234.

Ferguson, C. J., & Dyck, D. (2012). Paradigm change in aggression research: The time has come to retire the General Aggression Model. *Aggression and Violent Behavior, 17*(3), 220–8. doi:10.1016/j.avb.2012.02.007

Ferguson, C. J., & Kilburn, J. (2010). Much ado about nothing: The misestimation and overinterpretation of violent video game effects in Eastern and Western nations: Comment on Anderson et al. (2010). *Psychological Bulletin, 136*(2), 21–137.

Ferguson, C. J., & Olson, C. K. (2014). Video game violence use among "vulnerable" populations: The impact of violent games on delinquency and bullying among children with clinically elevated depression or attention deficit symptoms. *Journal of Youth and Adolescence, 43*(1), 127–36.

Ferguson, C. J., Rueda, S., Cruz, A., Ferguson, A., Fritz, D., & Smith, S. (2008). Violent video games and aggression: Causal relationship or byproduct of family violence and intrinsic violence motivation? *Criminal Justice and Behavior, 35*, 311–32.

Fox, J. A., & DeLateur, M. J. (2014). Mass shootings in America: Moving beyond Newtown. *Homicide Studies, 18*(1), 125–45.

Gauntlett, D. (1995). *Moving experiences: Understanding television's influences and effects*. Luton, UK: John Libbey.

Grimes, T., Anderson, J., & Bergen, L. (2008). *Media violence and aggression: Science and ideology*. Thousand Oaks, CA: Sage.

Grossman, D. (1996). *On killing: The psychological cost of learning to kill in war and society*. Boston, MA: Back Bay Books.

Grossman, D. (1999). *Stop teaching our kids to kill: A call to action against TV, movie & video game violence*. New York: Crown Publishers.

Grossman, D. (2013). Video games as "murder simulators." *Variety*. http://www.variety.com/2013/voices/opinion/grossman-2640

Hall, R., Day, T., & Hall, R. (2011). A plea for caution: Violent video games, the Supreme Court, and the role of science. *Mayo Clinic Proceedings, 86*(4), 315–21.

Jenkins, P. (1998). *Moral panic: Changing concepts of the child molester in modern America*. New Haven, CT: Yale University Press.

Kutner, L., & Olson, C. (2008). *Grand theft childhood: The surprising truth about violent video games and what parents can do*. New York: Simon & Schuster.

Lenhart, A., Kahne, J., Middaugh, E., MacGill, A., Evans, C., & Mitak, J. (2008). *Teens, video games and civics: Teens gaming experiences are diverse and include significant social interaction and civic engagement.*

Przybylski, A. K., Deci, E., Rigby, C. S., & Ryan, R. M. (2014). Competence-impeding electronic games and players' aggressive feelings, thoughts, and behaviors. *Journal of Personality and Social Psychology, 106*(3), 441–457. doi:10.1037/a0034820.

Przybylski, A. K., Rigby, C. S., & Ryan, R. M. (2010). A motivational model of video game engagement. *Review of General Psychology, 14*(2), 154–66.

Puri, K., & Pugliese, R. (2012). Sex, lies, and video games: Moral panics or uses and gratifications. *Bulletin of Science, Technology & Society*. doi: 10.1177/0270467612463799

Robinson-Cimpian, J. (2014). Inaccurate estimation of disparities due to mischievous responders: Several suggestions to assess conclusions. *Educational Researcher, 43*, 171–85.

Rushton, B. (2013). Backdooring it: Defense maneuvers around setback. *Illinois Times*. http://www.illinoistimes.com/Springfield/article-11440-backdooring-it.html

Sherry, J. L. (2001). The effects of violent video games on aggression: A meta-analysis. *Human Communication Research, 27*(3), 409–31. doi:10.1093/hcr/27.3.409

Shook, J. J., Vaughn, M., Goodkind, S., & Johnson, H. (2011). An empirical portrait of youthful offenders who sell drugs. *Journal of Criminal Justice, 39*, 224–31.

State's Attorney for the Judicial District of Dansbury. (2013). *Report of the State's Attorney for the Judicial District of Danbury on the Shootings at Sandy Hook Elementary School and 36 Yogananda Street, Newtown, Connecticut on December 14, 2012.* Danbury, CT: Office of the State's Attorney Judicial District of Danbury.

Surette, R. (Ed.) (1990). *The media and criminal justice policy: Recent research and social effects.* Springfield, IL: Charles C. Thomas.

Surette, R. (2011). *Media, crime and criminal justice: Images, realities and policies.* Belmont, CA: Wadsworth.

Surette, R. (2013). Cause or catalyst: The interaction of real world and media crime models. *American Journal of Criminal Justice, 38*, 392–409.

Surette, R., & Maze, A. (2015). Video game play and copycat crime: An exploratory analysis of an inmate population. *Psychology of Popular Media Culture, 4*(4), 360–374. doi:10.1037/ppm0000050.

Tear, M., & Nielson, M. (2013). Failure to demonstrate that playing violent video games diminishes prosocial behavior. *PLoS One, 8*(7), e68382.

Virginia Tech Review Panel. (2007). *Report of the Virginia Tech Review Panel.* http://www.governor.virginia.gov/TempContent/techPanelReport.cfm.

von Salisch, M., Vogelgesang, J. L., Kristen, A., & Oppl, C. (2011). Preference for violent electronic games and aggressive behavior among children: The beginning of the downward spiral? *Media Psychology, 14*(3), 233–58.

Williams, D., & Skoric, M. (2005). Internet fantasy violence: A test of aggression in an online game. *Communication Monographs, 72*, 217–33.

CHAPTER

18 Violent Media Use and Violent Outcomes

Christopher L. Groves, Sara Prot, *and* Craig A. Anderson

Abstract

Electronic media is an omnipresent form of entertainment in contemporary society. A large body of empirical evidence provides support for the notion that violent media use (e.g., television, films, video games) increases the likelihood of low-level everyday forms of physical, verbal, and relational aggression. Less work has been conducted on the effects of violent media on more extreme forms of aggression that can be considered violent. This chapter provides a review of the theoretical frameworks for understanding the potential effects of violent media use on violent outcomes. It follows this discussion with a selective review of the relevant literature regarding the effects of violent media use on violent outcomes, with a focus on the effects of violent video games. Conclusions are drawn regarding the state of the literature, current debate, and future directions needed for research.

Keywords: violent media, video games, television, aggression, risk factors, violent behavior, criminal behavior

There is no doubt that the past few decades have brought about dramatic changes in the ways in which individuals entertain themselves. The public now has unprecedented access to media with the introduction of tablets, smartphones, and smart televisions. This shift in entertainment is marked most clearly by the rise in video game play, which continues to grow. In 2013, consumers spent nearly US$21 billion on video games and video game equipment (Entertainment Software Association, 2014). Nearly 90% of American children and teenagers report playing video games (Gentile, 2009) and do so for an average of 2 hours a day (Rideout, Foehr, & Roberts, 2010). This level of popularity has fostered concern among policymakers, parents, and researchers alike regarding one of the most prevalent themes of video game play: its violent content.

Research regarding violent media effects has a rich history. Analyses of violent television and film effects have consistently found modest but significant effects on a wide range of aggression-related outcomes (for reviews, see Anderson et al., 2003; Strasburger & Wilson, 2014). Recently, the field has experienced renewed interest in these effects, fostered by the increasing popularity of video games. Scholarly interest in video game effects has produced hundreds of studies that are perhaps best summarized in meta-analyses on the subject. In the largest meta-analysis on the subject to date, Anderson et al. (2010) concluded that violent video game play serves as a causal risk factor for aggressive behavior. While disagreements over specific details in the field exists, meta-analyses conducted by both proponents for and against violent media effects demonstrate a consistent relationship between violent media use and aggressive behavior even when employing overly conservative statistical controls (Boxer, Groves, & Docherty, 2015).

Much of the research on violent video game use has focused on subcriminal levels of aggression, such as the administration of hot sauce to someone participant who is known to dislike spicy foods (Barlett, Branch, Rodeheffer, & Harris, 2009), administering unpleasant noise blasts to a competitor (Anderson et al., 2004), and rating another person as less deserving of financial support (Cicchirillo &

Chory-Assad, 2005). We will label these examples of aggression *low-level aggression*. Such laboratory measures of aggression are frequently used in experimental studies designed to test the causal role of media violence. The use of these techniques has produced a thorough and methodologically sound literature that can speak to the causal nature of these relationships and to the underlying psychological processes. However, the administration of hot sauce and aversive noise blasts are far cries from the real-world extreme forms of violence that the general public and news media sometimes implicate as resulting from media violence.

This difference between the types of aggression that can ethically be used in laboratory experiments versus extreme real-world violence does not exonerate violent media use as a potential source of criminal-level aggressive outcomes. It does, however, indicate that before making strong claims about violent media effects on violent behavior, one must look beyond laboratory experiments of media violence effects on aggressive behavior. Specifically, we must consider basic theoretical processes that link media violence to aggressive and violent behavior, both directly and through media violence effects on known risk factors for violence. We also must look to nonexperimental studies of media violence effects, as these are studies that can ethically examine more extreme forms of aggression as outcome variables. Next, we briefly discuss the theoretical processes responsible for violent media effects and conclude this section by describing a useful theoretical framework for understanding how criminal-level or violent outcomes may transpire. Finally, we summarize the literature specific to such outcomes and provide directions for future research.

Theory and Definitions

Aggression is a behavior enacted with the intent to cause harm to a person who does not want to be harmed (Bushman & Anderson, 2001; Bushman & Huesmann, 2010). It is an observable behavior, not an emotion, a thought, or a fantasy that occurs inside the person. This definition excludes accidental hurtful actions (e.g., unintentionally tripping someone) as well as intentional actions that are not done with the intent to cause harm (e.g., a dentist administering a painful medical procedure). Aggression can take several forms, including physical aggression (e.g., punching someone), verbal aggression (e.g., cursing at someone), and relational aggression (e.g., harming someone's relationships by spreading a rumor behind his or her back).

Violence refers to more extreme forms of physical aggression that pose a significant risk of injury to the victim (such as assault and murder; Huesmann & Taylor, 2006). All violent behaviors are aggressive behaviors, but many aggressive behaviors are not violent (e.g., a kindergartner poking an annoyed classmate). Violent and aggressive behaviors can be viewed as a part of a continuum of severity, ranging from mild aggressive acts (e.g., poking) to severe aggressive acts which constitute violence (e.g., shooting; Anderson et al., 2003; Anderson & Huesmann, 2003). In support of the idea that aggression and violence exist on a continuum, research demonstrates strong associations between mildly aggressive behavior earlier in life and risk of violent behavior later (Huesmann, Lagerspetz, & Eron, 1984). In addition, aggressive cognitions and affect are significant predictors of aggression and violence (Anderson & Bushman, 2002; Bushman & Huesmann, 2010). Therefore, research studies measuring mild forms of aggressive behavior, thoughts, or emotions can provide valuable insight into understanding violent behavior. Of importance for the current discussion, violence is defined by the World Health Organization as "the intentional use of physical force or power, threatened or actual, against another person or against a group or community that results in or has a high likelihood of resulting in injury, death, physiological harm, maldevelopment, or deprivation" (Zwi, Krug, Mercy, & Dahlberg, 2002). This definition is important to consider as it does not require that outcomes of violent acts include injury or harm, merely that the act itself is highly capable of producing injury. This is perhaps one of the clearest differences between violent acts and criminal violence. By definition, criminal violence possesses a lower frequency compared to violent acts as violent actions do not always lead to injury and are (perhaps consequently) reported to authorities less frequently. For this reason, research benefits from the use of *violent behavior* as an outcome rather than *criminal behavior* because such actions are more common, possess more variability to explain, and can be researched with somewhat smaller samples.

The General Aggression Model

The General Aggression Model (GAM; Anderson & Bushman, 2002; DeWall, Anderson, & Bushman, 2011) provides a comprehensive framework for understanding aggression and violence. GAM describes the personal and situational factors and their resultant processes that influence an individual's aggressive behavior in the current situation as well as forces that influence the long-term development of aggressive tendencies. The GAM has guided a wealth of research in the media violence domain (Anderson et al., 2010; Anderson & Dill, 2000; Möller & Krahe, 2009) but also has been applied to numerous other aggression domains. Although GAM includes various biological processes (e.g., genetic, hormone), our present focus is on the social-cognitive aspects. It provides a basis for understanding how violent media influence aggression and violence both in short- and long-term contexts.

An overview of the key processes proposed by GAM is shown in Figure 18.1. The likelihood that a person will act aggressively in a current social encounter is influenced both by person factors (e.g., trait aggression, hostility, and psychoticism) and situation factors (e.g., provocation, heat, violent media). Media violence increases the likelihood of aggressive behavior in a current social encounter through its influence on a person's present internal state (their current thoughts, affect, and arousal level). For example, watching a violent television show primes aggressive cognition, increases hostile affect, and leads to physiological arousal. These changes in internal state variables affect appraisal and decision making. They guide a person's perception, interpretation of events, decision making, and behavior. For example, a person whose aggressive thoughts and affect have been primed by watching a violent television show is more likely to decide to act aggressively in response to provocation.

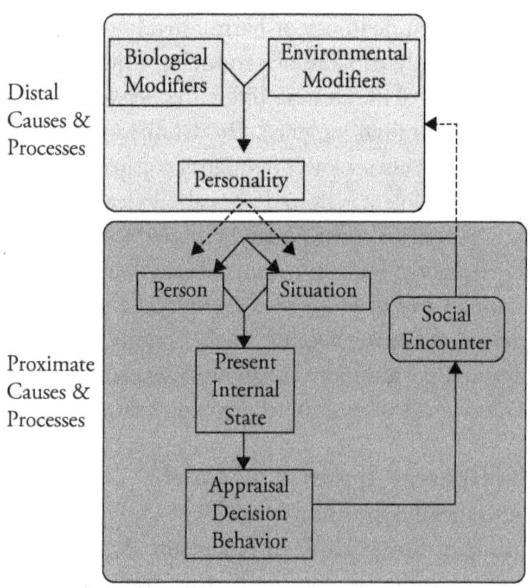

Figure 18.1 The General Aggression Model: overall view. From Anderson & Carnagey (2004).

Once a behavioral response has been chosen, it influences the ongoing social encounter, creating a feedback loop. Over time, repeated aggressive encounters (such as bullying, rejection, or habitual violent video game use) strengthen a person's habitual patterns of responding and can lead to the development of an aggressive personality. Repeated exposure to violence (in real life or in the media) involves recurring rehearsal of aggressive knowledge structures. Over time, habitual violent media consumers can become more aggressive in outlook by developing hostile perceptual biases, attitudes, beliefs, and behaviors (Bartholow, Sestir, & Davis, 2005; Gentile, Li, Khoo, Prot, & Anderson, 2014).

Risk Factor Approach

Research shows that violent actions are rarely the result of a single cause (Huesmann & Taylor, 2006). Instead, aggression and violence are caused and moderated by a large number of interacting factors, such as genetic predispositions (Hudziak et al., 2003), parenting practices (Eron, Huesmann, & Zelli, 1991), personality (Schmeck & Poustka, 2001), accessibility of guns (O'Donnell, 1995), cultural norms (Nisbett & Cohen, 1996), even climate change (Anderson & DeLisi, 2011). No reputable researcher would claim that media violence is "the cause" of violent behavior: it is one of many contributing factors (Huesmann & Taylor, 2006).

A useful approach for understanding how multiple causes contribute to violent behavior is the *risk and resilience approach* (Anderson, Gentile, & Buckley, 2007; Gentile & Bushman, 2012; Gentile & Sesma, 2003; Masten, 2001). This approach focuses on life experiences that put people at risk for future maladaptation (risk factors) and factors that protect from this risk exposure (protective factors). Effects of different risk and protective factors accumulate; the cumulative risk model posits that the likelihood of problematic functioning is increased by every risk factor present and is decreased by each protective factor present (Masten, 2001; Wright, Masten, & Narayan, 2013). Cumulative risk is expected to have a bigger role in disrupting functioning than any single risk factor (Belsky & Fearon, 2002; Gentile & Sesma, 2003). For example, Gentile and Bushman (2012) explored effects of six risk and protective factors for aggression (media violence use, physical victimization, sex, hostile attribution bias, parental monitoring, and prior aggression). Each risk factor increased the likelihood of aggression over a 6-month period, while each protective factor decreased it. Furthermore, the overall number of risk factors present was a better predictor of aggression than any single variable, showing evidence of cumulative risk.

Taking multiple risk factors into account is especially important when attempting to predict extreme and rare behaviors, such as violent behavior. After hearing about media violence effects, nonscientists sometimes give comments such as "I play violent video games, but I've never shot anyone" (Anderson et al., 2007). In fact, "shooting someone" is a severe form of physical aggression which most people will never engage in. Media violence, by itself, is unlikely to bring about extremely violent behavior (as is any single risk factor). However, it may increase the likelihood of more common or subtle forms of aggression (e.g., verbally aggressive responses like swearing at someone). It can also increase the risk of violent behavior for those individuals who have multiple risk factors (Anderson et al., 2007). In populations that have multiple risk factors and few protective factors, media violence effects on violent and criminal behaviors can be clearly observed (DeLisi, Vaughn, Gentile, Anderson, & Shook, 2013).

These processes can be illustrated using the metaphorical "aggression thermometer" (shown in Figure 18.2). People at the lowest end of the thermometer always act respectfully and nonaggressively. People at the highest end frequently engage in extremely aggressive and violent acts. Each risk factor may heat up the thermometer and increase a person's aggression level by several notches but is not powerful enough to change someone's behavior from being routinely respectful to others to being violent. If, however, the person already has other risk factors (e.g., poverty, being bullied, living in a violent neighborhood, etc.), regular media violence use may contribute enough additional risk to push them to the top of the aggression thermometer, resulting in physical aggression and violence.

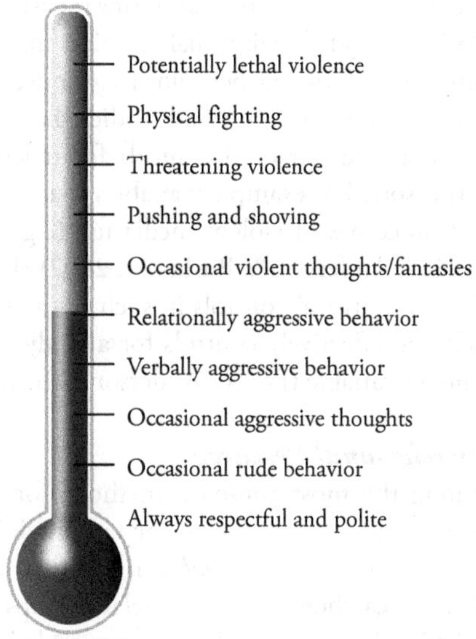

Figure 18.2 The aggression thermometer.
From Gentile & Bushman (2012).

Selective Review of Empirical Evidence

A central tenet of the risk-factor approach to understanding violent outcomes is that high-level aggression (such as assaults and murders) requires multiple risk factors to be present if it is to occur. The details of such interactions require more research in order to be fully understood. For example, future research could focus on the relative contribution of specific risk factors or determine whether specific risk factors must be present in order for certain outcomes to occur, and work to better understand the potentially curvilinear relationship between risk factor possession and such outcomes (Gentile & Bushman, 2012).

A resultant prediction from this approach is that the effect of any single risk factor should provide a progressively smaller impact on increasingly severe forms of aggression. As noted previously, the relationship between violent video game use and low-level aggressive outcomes is small but robust (Anderson et al., 2010). The predicted effect of violent video game use alone on high-level aggressive outcomes is therefore likely to be much smaller and, as measured by many research designs, statistically undetectable.

A good example of this is the oft-repeated claim that there are no studies demonstrating that media violence causes an increase in homicides. Statements such as these are rarely accompanied with the appropriate caveat that there are numerous risk factors at multiple levels (such as prenatal malnutrition, physical and psychological abuse, exposure to violence, provocation, access to guns, culture of honor) that conjunctively influence violent crimes. Furthermore, it is both practically and ethically impossible to conduct experimental studies of media violence effects on homicide rates. For this reason, we focus on studies using methods suited to answering research questions about media violence effects on violent behavior that actually are answerable. For the most part, that means focusing on correlational and longitudinal studies that include some type of violent behavior as an outcome variable. Furthermore, we avoid studies that employed inappropriate statistical controls for investigations of this sort. For example, variables that are considered outcomes of violent media use (e.g., trait aggression; Anderson & Bushman, 2002) should not serve as statistical controls in such research as their inclusion effectively controls for a study's own dependent variable (Prot & Anderson, 2013).

Correlational Research

Among the most common methods for studying the effect of violent video game use on violent outcomes is the *correlational design*. This approach allows researchers to examine relationships between variables that are typically unmeasurable in a laboratory and derive the large sample that is likely needed to observe the effects of violent video game use on violent outcomes.

In one large study by Denniston, Swahn, Hertz, and Romero (2011) of a nationally representative sample of students in grades 9–12 (n = 14,041), media use (television, video game, and computer) was dichotomized by clustering individuals who reported spending more than versus less than 3 hours per day consuming either television or video games/computer games/general computer use. Similarly, violent outcome variables were also dichotomous and included whether students had carried a weapon, a gun, or a weapon on school property within the 30 days prior to the survey. They also recorded whether students had been in a physical fight or been in a physical fight on school property within the last 12 months. They found that frequent television and video game/computer use was associated with all of these outcomes. Furthermore, the relationships including outcomes such as physical fighting and carrying a weapon on school property remained significant even when controlling for race, gender, and grade. Of important note is that media use did not include the more specific measure of violent content and therefore the effects of violent content may be underestimated when considering these findings.

In another large-scale study by Boxer, Huesmann, Bushman, O'Brien, and Moceri (2008), 820 youth (390 of which were juvenile delinquents), as well as their parents and teachers, completed measures of violent media use (reported by youth) and a number of aggression and violence-related outcomes including frequency of punching or beating another individual, throwing rocks or bottles at others, fights/bullying (reported by teachers and guardians), and several other related outcomes. Several additional risk factors for aggression were also measured including general (low-level) aggressiveness, psychopathology, callous-unemotional traits, exposure to neighborhood violence, academic skills, and exposure to low-level aggression. A composite of the violence-related measures was significantly related to violent media use even after controlling for sex, age, and these other risk factors. Violent media use was also related to delinquency status, though this is a bivariate relationship in which gender and age were not controlled.

In a recent study by Ybarra, Huesmann, Korchmaros, and Reisner (2014), longitudinal data were collected from 9-to 18-year-olds (n = 1,489). This sample was analyzed as a cross-sectional set due to the rarity of youth reporting carrying a weapon in the past month across all three time points. They asked youth to report whether they had carried a weapon to school in the past month (such as a gun, knife, or club). They found that individuals who reported playing at least some games with violent content were five times more likely to report having carried a weapon to school compared to those who reported playing games with little to no violent content.

In an additional correlational study, DeLisi et al. (2013) collected data from 227 juvenile offenders. Predictors included measures of violent video game play, prosocial video game play, sex, age, race, and antisocial personality. The primary dependent variable was self-reported serious violence as measured by gang fighting, hitting a teacher/parent/peers, and attacking another person. Despite the use of statistical controls that are considered overly conservative (antisocial personality), violent video game use was significantly associated with more violent acts.

Experimental Research

As noted previously, experimental research regarding the effects of violent media use on violence-related outcomes is rare due to the ethical considerations of eliciting seriously aggressive behavior in the laboratory. Experimental studies provide the strongest method for testing causality and ruling out potential confounding variables due to the use of random assignment. One experimental study by Konijn, Bijvank, and Bushman (2007) was able to examine violent behavior (as defined by the World Health Organization) using a modified version of Taylor's Competitive Reaction Time Task. This task involves asking participants to compete in reaction time trials against another, ostensible participant. Prior to each trial, participants select a noise volume and duration to administer to their opponent if the trial is won. Crucial to the violent outcome hypothesis, participants were told that high noise volume levels could cause permanent hearing damage to their opponent, which therefore meets the definition of violent behavior. As expected, they observed a significant main effect of violent content on the selection of noise volume levels capable of producing damage. Furthermore, this tendency was exacerbated among those who expressed desires to be like the main character of the violent games.

Longitudinal Research

Longitudinal studies are among the strongest in providing evidence for the effect of violent media use on violent behavior. They allow examination of violent behavioral change over time by measuring all key variables at two or more points in time. They also allow the testing of causal mechanisms by controlling for violent behavior at the onset of the study, thereby ruling out attraction effects that may occur if violent individuals gravitate toward violent media use. Importantly, effect sizes obtained when controlling for initial levels of violent behavior should not be considered measures of the "true" effect size as such a procedure effectively only captures the influence of violent media use on change in violent behavior between the two time periods measured and therefore ignores any prior influence of media violence that occurred before the study began.

In a short-term, longitudinal study by Gentile, Coyne, and Walsh (2011), children in the third, fourth, and fifth grades (total n = 430), their parents, and teachers completed surveys at two time points within the school year (average lag between measurements was 5 months). Violent media use was measured by asking participants to report what their three favorite video games, television shows, and movies were; how violent each was; and how often they used each. The researchers then took the product of the frequency of use and the violent content for each show/video game/movie and summed these products together to produce a total violent content use measure. Of particular interest for the current review, the measure was significantly related to a composite measure of child physical fighting as reported by the child, their teachers, and other forms of physical aggression reported by peers. Several studies have produced similar findings in which violent media use is related to physical fights among youth (Anderson et al., 2007; DuRant, Champion, & Wolfson, 2006; Gentile & Bushman, 2012). Considering this particular outcome as violent behavior, however, may be debatable given that physical fighting among youth is arguably less likely to lead to serious outcomes such as physical injury requiring medical attention. However, longitudinal work by Huesmann, Eron, Lefkowitz, & Walder (1984) indicates that aggression levels early in life (age 8) are related to serious aggressive behaviors later in life (age 30) including spousal abuse and antisocial and criminal behavior.

In other work by Huesmann et al. (Huesmann, Moise-Titus, Podolski, & Eron, 2003), individuals were followed for 15 years between the ages of 6–8 and 21–23. Data collection began in 1977–1978 and completed in 1992–1995. It is worth noting that only violent television use was measured in the current sample. When considering this limitation, it is important to note that the psychological processes involved in both violent television and violent video game effects are thought of as highly similar (Anderson et al., 2003), and therefore results from work on violent television use should be considered relevant to questions regarding the influence of violent video game play on violent outcomes. The authors found that high violent television use as a child was significantly related to adulthood pushing, grabbing, or shoving one's spouse for males; throwing items at one's spouse for females; shoving others for males and females; punching, beating, or choking another adult for females; and state-reported convictions for non-traffic violations among males.

In a study by Johnson, Cohen, Smailes, Kasen, and Brook (2002), children (n = 707) were followed over a 17-year interval. They found that television viewing among individuals (mean age 14) was associated with assault or physical fights resulting in injury, robbery, threats to injure someone, or using a weapon to commit a crime and other aggressive acts years later (mean ages 16 or 22). Furthermore, these associations continued when examined at the time these individuals were an average of 30 years old. Most critically, these associations persisted even when controlling for a variety of factors including previous aggressive behavior, childhood neglect, family income, neighborhood violence, parental education, and psychiatric disorders.

Contrasting Findings

Despite the seemingly strong findings of these studies, other investigations have found less support. One study by Gunter and Daly (2012) used a propensity score matching technique in which individuals who reported playing mature-rated (M-rated) games were individually matched with others who did not play such games but held similar scores on a large battery of control variables. They found that without using the matched sample, M-rated (mature) game players were significantly more likely to engage in all violent outcomes including hitting another person, participating in a group fight, carrying a weapon, or carrying a gun and produced a higher overall violent score. When examining the matched sample, however, these relationships were reduced to nonsignificance for all measures except for participating in a group fight and carrying a weapon. Female matched participants scores were not reduced to nonsignificance but still showed fewer and weaker overall effects.

One issue worth noting in this study is that the use of playing M-rated games as an indicator is not the best method for measuring violent video game use because such ratings take into account the presence of profanity and nudity in games—not solely the violent content. Previous research indicates that this difference in measuring violent video game exposure can lead to meaningful decrements in observed effect sizes (Busching et al., 2013). More importantly, however, the use of propensity score matching dramatically reduces the sample size used and thus the power to detect true but small effects. Given that the theoretical effect size of violent video game use on violent outcomes should be quite small, the statistical power required to detect such effects demands very large sample sizes. In fact, examination of the group differences between M-rated game players and nonviolent game players in the matched samples indicates that M-rated players scored higher on every metric of violent outcomes except for gun-carrying among males, suggesting a larger sample is needed.

A cross-sectional study by Ybarra et al. (2008), of youth aged 10–15 years (n = 1,588) included measures of violent video game, violent music, violent television use, and exposure to depictions of real violence online using the Youth Internet Safety Survey. They measured seriously violent behaviors such as stabbing or shooting someone, aggravated assault, robbery, and sexual assault. Their primary dependent variable was whether individuals had engaged in one or more of these behaviors in the previous year. They found that violent television, video game play, and even music use were each associated with increased likelihoods of engaging in at least one seriously violent act within the past year. Individuals consuming such violent media were between 2.6 and 7.2 times more likely to engage in violent acts depending on the type of violent media used. These relationships, however, dropped to nonsignificance for all forms of media except for the depiction of real-life violence on Internet websites when a large battery of covariates including race, socioeconomic status, substance use, violence in the home and community, a number of indices of poor parental care, academic performance, and delinquent peers were added to the statistical model. Those who viewed instances of real violence on online websites, however, remained five times more likely to engage in seriously violent behavior within the past year compared to those who did not view such websites. The authors note that the explanations for the disparity between these effect sizes are unknown and require further research.

In another contrasting study, Robertson, McAnally, and Hancox (2013) assessed a group of individuals (n = 1,037) from birth to 26 years of age beginning in 1972–1973. Importantly, they assessed television viewing throughout a large portion of the participants' childhood (ages 5–15 years) and also measured several covariates during this time. They found that television viewing throughout childhood was related to the likelihood of being diagnosed with antisocial personality disorder, aggressive personality traits, and the likelihood of criminal conviction. These effects occurred even when statistically controlling for sex, IQ, socioeconomic status, previous antisocial behavior, and indices of parental control. The contrasting finding, however, was that the likelihood of violent convictions was not a significant outcome after including each of these statistical controls. Of course, the study suffers from failing to measure violent content of television viewing. Also, it may have been necessary to include more participants in the study as well, given that violent convictions are relatively rare.

Conclusion

The effects of violent media have been heavily researched over the past several decades. There is now a wealth of evidence supporting the conclusion that violent video game use serves as a causal risk factor for aggressive affect, thoughts, and behavior (Anderson et al., 2010, Greitemeyer & Mügge, 2014).

The evidence for violent television and film effects is similarly overwhelmingly strong.

As our review indicates, aggressive acts differ across a wide range of severity. The bulk of research, especially experimental research, has focused on milder forms of aggression. There is much less work regarding the influence of violent media use on the more extreme forms of aggression covered in this chapter.

A central theme arising from our review is that the studies conducted on this topic do not arrive to precisely the same conclusions. Studies that tend not to detect any effects of violent media use also tend to measure the most extreme forms of aggressive behavior (e.g., group fighting, stabbings, shootings). Sample sizes appear to be a potential factor contributing to null effects in at least some of these cases. Some studies have failed to assess exposure to violent screen media, assessing total time spent rather than time on violent media.

Studies that demonstrate no relationship between violent media exposure and violent behavior also tend to include large numbers of statistical control variables, some of which are actually potential outcomes of high media violence exposure. Other control measures often tap into factors related to violent outcomes such as poor parenting, violence seen in the community, delinquent peer presence, and poor academic performance. Such factors are crucially important to parse out of the relationship between violent media use and violent outcomes. The results of these studies suggest that any bivariate relationship may be at least partially fueled by these and similar third variables. However, it is important to note that such techniques often are not pre-tested by ensuring that both violent media use and violent behavior are significantly related to each covariate. The inclusion of factors that do not meet this statistical criteria may serve to artificially deflate the relationship between violent media use and violent outcomes. In cases such as this, the variance associated between the covariate, the predictor, and the outcome, is statistically removed, even when there is no "true" relationship to be controlled. In other words, the variance in the dependent variable (violent behavior) is inappropriately attributed to the covariate, and, consequently, violent media use has less variance to "explain" the outcome (Prot & Anderson, 2013). Future research needs to do a better job of testing and reporting details of the statistical control variable.

Investigations that do report significant effects on violent behavior tend to assess more common forms of violent behavior, use more specific measures of exposure to violent media, and tend to be large-scale longitudinal studies that examine behavior over very long periods of time. This may suggest that the effects of violent media use on severe violent behavior require sustained, long-term exposure in order for such extreme forms of aggression to emerge. If this is the case, the "snapshot" method used in correlational studies may not be sufficient to detect effects of violent media use on truly violent behavior.

The subject matter discussed here has been the focus of intense debate with extreme points having been made on either side of the argument, especially within lay circles. In commenting on a murder in 2004, the lawyer Jack Thompson, stated that "We have dozens of killings in the US by children who had played these types of [violent] games. . . . These types of games are basically murder simulators. There are people being killed here almost on a daily basis" (CNN International, 2004). In contrast, the president of the Electronics Software Association, Doug Lowenstein, was cited in a 2000 interview as stating that "There is absolutely no evidence, none, that playing a violent video game leads to aggressive behavior" (Cable News Network, 2000; as cited in Anderson & Bushman, 2001). Due to the work of numerous scholars on the subject cited here, we can safely assert that the truth lies somewhere in between these extreme points of view.

A lot is already known about both the short- and long-term processes by which television, film, and video game violence exposure increases aggressive and violent behavior. The basic bio-social-cognitive models have been well-tested and validated. Nonetheless, a great deal more work is required on this topic before we fully understand all of the consequences of violent game play. For example, much more work is needed in examining such effects over long periods of time. Such work needs to include much larger samples; more precise measures of key predictor, outcome, and control variables; and a host of additional variables that have only recently begun to receive research attention. The latter category includes variables related to media violent effects on stereotypes of various outgroups, on attention deficits and impulse control problems, and on moral reasoning, beliefs, and attitudes. Longitudinal studies are often limited to a span of a few years, but this review suggests that effects on extreme forms of behavior may be best studied under much longer time periods consisting of a decade or more of observation. More work is also needed in determining the relationship between violent game play and the severity of outcomes. Findings supporting risk factor approaches to understanding aggression frequently consider the impact of an increasing number of risk factors on the likelihood of engaging in a single violent outcome (e.g., Gentile & Bushman, 2012). Much less work has been conducted on the relationship between risk factor possession and outcomes based on severity within an individual study (e.g., the number of risk factors required for highly violent outcomes to occur compared to relatively less extreme forms of violence). Without doubt, this area of study is likely to receive heavy focus by the scientific community in the next several decades.

References

Anderson, C. A., Berkowitz, L., Donnerstein, E., Huesmann, R. L., Johnson, J., Linz, D., . . . Wartella, E. (2003). The influence of media violence on youth. *Psychological Science in the Public Interest, 4*, 81–110.

Anderson, C. A., & Bushman, B. J. (2002). The effects of media violence on society. *Science, 295*, 2377–8.

Anderson, C. A., & Bushman, B. J. (2001). Effects of violent video games on aggressive behavior, aggressive cognition, aggressive affect, physiological arousal, and prosocial behavior: A meta-analytic review of the scientific literature. *Psychological Science, 12*, 353–9.

Anderson, C. A., Carnagey, N. L., Flanagan, M., Arlin, B. J., Eubanks, J., & Valentine, J. C. (2004). Violent video games: Specific effects of violent content on aggressive thoughts and behavior. *Advances in Experimental Social Psychology, 36*, 199–249.

Anderson, C. A., & DeLisi, M. (2011). Implications of global climate change for violence in developed and developing countries. In J. Forgas, A. Kruglanski, & K. Williams (Eds.), *The psychology of social conflict and aggression* (pp. 249–65). New York: Psychology Press.

Anderson, C. A., & Dill, K. E. (2000). Video games and aggressive thoughts, feelings, and behavior in the laboratory and in life. *Journal of Personality and Social Psychology, 78*, 772–90.

Anderson, C. A., Gentile, D. A., & Buckley, K. E. (2007). *Violent video game effects on children and adolescents: Theory, research, and public policy*. New York: Oxford University Press.

Anderson, C. A., & Huesmann, L. R. (2003). Human aggression: A social-cognitive view. In M. A. Hogg & J. Cooper (Eds.), *The Sage handbook of social psychology* (pp. 296–323). London: Sage Publications.

Anderson, C. A., Shibuya, A., Ihori, N., Swing, E. L., Bushman, B. J., Sakamoto, A., . . . Saleem, M. (2010). Violent video game effects on aggression, empathy, and prosocial behavior in Eastern and Western countries. *Psychological Bulletin,136*, 151–73.

Barlett, C., Branch, O., Rodeheffer, C., & Harris, R. (2009). How long do the short-term violent video game effects last? *Aggressive Behavior, 35*, 225–36.

Bartholow, B. D., Sestir, M. A., & Davis, E. (2005). Correlates and consequences of exposure to video game violence: Hostile personality, empathy, and aggressive behavior. *Personality and Social Psychology Bulletin, 31*, 1573–86.

Belsky, J., & Fearon, R. M. P. (2002). Infant-mother attachment security, contextual risk and early development: A moderational analysis. *Development and Psychopathology, 14*, 293–310.

Boxer, P., Groves, C. L., & Docherty, M. (2015). Video games do indeed influence children and adolescents' aggression, prosocial behavior, and academic performance: A clearer reading of Ferguson. *Perspectives on Psychological Science, 10*(5), 671–673.

Boxer, P., Huesmann, R. L., Bushman, B. J., O'Brien, M., & Moceri, D. (2008). The role of violent media preference in cumulative developmental risk for violence and general aggression. *Journal of Youth and Adolescence, 38*(3), 417–28.

Busching, R., Gentile, D. A., Krahé, B., Möller, I., Khoo, A., Walsh, D. A., & Anderson, C. A. (2013). Testing the reliability and validity of different measures of violent video game use in the United States, Singapore, and Germany. *Psychology of Popular Media Culture, 4*(2), 97.

Bushman, B. J., & Anderson, C. A. (2001). Is it time to pull the plug on the hostile versus instrumental aggression dichotomy? *Psychological Review, 108*, 273–9.

Bushman, B. J., & Huesmann, L. R. (2010). Aggression. In S. T. Fiske, D. T. Gilbert, & G. Lindzey (Eds.), *Handbook of social psychology* (5th ed., pp. 833–63). New York: John Wiley & Sons.

Cable News Network. (2000, May 12). *The World Today*. Atlanta, GA.

Cicchirillo, V., & Chory-Assad, R. M. (2005). Effects of affective orientation and video game play on aggressive thoughts and behaviors. *Journal of Broadcasting & Electronic Media, 49*(4), 435–49.

CNN International. (2004). Retailer pulls "murder" video game. *Cable News Network*. http://edition.cnn.com/2004/WORLD/europe/07/30/uk.manhunt.storeban/

DeLisi, M., Vaughn, M. G., Gentile, D. A., Anderson, C. A., & Shook, J. (2013). Violent video games, delinquency, and youth violence: New evidence. *Youth Violence and Juvenile Justice, 11*, 132–42.

Denniston, M. M., Swahn, M. H., Hertz, M. F., & Romero, L. M. (2011). Associations between electronic media use and involvement in violence, alcohol and drug use among United States high school students. *Western Journal of Emergency Medicine, 12*(3), 310–15.

DeWall, C. N., Anderson, C. A., & Bushman, B. J. (2011). The General Aggression Model: Theoretical extensions to violence. *Psychology of Violence, 1*, 245–58.

DuRant, R. H., Champion, H., & Wolfson, M. (2006). The relationship between watching professional wrestling on television and engaging in date fighting among high school students. *Pediatrics, 118*(2), e265–72.

Entertainment Software Association. (2014). *Essential facts about the computer and video game industry*. http://www.theesa.com/facts/pdfs/ESA_EF_2014.pdf

Eron, L. D., Huesmann, L. R. & Zelli, A. (1991), The role of parental variables in the learning of aggression. In D. Pepler & K. Rubin (Eds.), *The development and treatment of childhood aggression* (pp.169–88). Mahwah, NJ: Erlbaum.

Gentile, D. A. (2009). Pathological video-game use among youth ages 8 to 18. *Psychological Science, 20*(5), 594–602.

Gentile, D. A., & Bushman, B. J. (2012). Reassessing media violence effects using a risk and resilience approach to understanding aggression. *Psychology of Popular Media Culture, 1*(3), 138–51.

Gentile, D. A., Coyne, S., & Walsh, D. A. (2011). Media violence, physical aggression, and relational aggression in school age children: A short-term longitudinal study. *Aggressive Behavior, 37*, 193–206.

Gentile, D. A., Li, D., Khoo, A., Prot, S., & Anderson, C. A. (2014). Mediators and Moderators of long-term effects of violent video games on aggressive behavior: Practice, thinking, and action. *JAMA Pediatrics, 168*(5), 450–7.

Gentile, D. A., & Sesma, A. (2003). Developmental approaches to understanding media effects on individuals. In D. Gentile (Ed.), *Media violence and children* (pp. 87–106), Westport, CT: Praeger.

Greitemeyer, T., & Mügge, D. O. (2014). Video games do affect social outcomes: A meta-analytic review of the effects of violent and prosocial video game play. *Personality and Social Psychology Bulletin, 40*(5), 578–89.

Gunter, W. D., & Daly, K. (2012). Causal or spurious: Using propensity score matching to detangle the relationship between violent video games and violent behavior. *Computers in Human Behavior, 28*, 1348–55.

Hudziak, J. J., van Beijsterveldt, C. E. M., Bartels, M., Rietveld, M. J. H., Rettew, D. C., Derks, E. M., & Boomsma, D. I. (2003). Individual differences in aggression: Genetic analyses by age, gender, and informant in 3-, 7-, and 10-year-old Dutch twins. *Behavior Genetics, 33*, 575–89.

Huesmann, L. R., Eron, L. D., Lefkowitz, M. M., & Walder, L. O. (1984). Stability of aggression over time and generations. *Developmental Psychology, 20*(6), 1120–34.

Huesmann, L. R., Lagerspetz, K., & Eron, L. D. (1984). Intervening variables in the television violence-aggression relation: Evidence from two countries. *Developmental Psychology, 20*, 746–75.

Huesmann, L. R., Moise-Titus, J., Podolski, C., & Eron, L. D. (2003). Longitudinal relations between children's exposure to TV violence and their aggressive and violent behavior in young adulthood: 1977–1992. *Developmental Psychology, 39*(2), 201–21.

Huesmann, L. R., & Taylor, L. D. (2006). The role of the mass media in violent behavior. *Annual Review of Public Health, 27*(1), 1–23.

Johnson, J. G., Cohen, P., Smailes, E. M., Kasen, S., & Brook, J. S. (2002). Television viewing and aggressive behavior during adolescence and adulthood. *Science, 295*, 2468–71.

Konijn, E. A., Bijvank, M. N., & Bushman, B. J. (2007). I wish I were a warrior: The role of wishful identification in the effects of violent video games on aggression in adolescent boys. *Developmental Psychology, 43*(4), 1038–44.

Masten, A. S. (2001). Ordinary magic: Resilience processes in development. *American Psychologist, 56*, 227–38.

Möller, I., & Krahe, B. (2009). Exposure to violent video games and aggression in German adolescents: A longitudinal analysis. *Aggressive Behavior, 35*, 75–89.

Nisbett, R. E., & Cohen, D. (1996). *Culture of honor: The psychology of violence in the South.* Boulder, CO: Westview Press.

O'Donnell, C. R. (1995). Firearm deaths among children and youth. *American Psychologist, 50*, 771–6.

Prot, S., & Anderson, C. A. (2013). Research methods, design, and statistics in media psychology. In K. Dill (Ed.), *The Oxford handbook of media psychology* (pp. 109–36). New York: Oxford University Press.

Rideout, V. J., Foehr, U. G., & Roberts, D. F. (2010). *Generation M2: Media in the lives of 8- to 18-year-olds: A Kaiser Family Foundation study, January 2010.* Menlo Park, CA: Kaiser Family Foundation.

Robertson, L. A., McAnally, H. M., & Hancox, R. J. (2013). Childhood and adolescent television viewing and antisocial behavior in early adulthood. *Pediatrics, 131*(3), 439–46.

Schmeck, K., & Poustka, F. (2001). Temperament and disruptive behavior disorders. *Psychopathology, 34*, 159–63.

Strasburger, V. C., & Wilson, B. J. (2014). Television violence: Sixty years of research. In D. A. Gentile (Ed.), *Media violence and children* (2nd ed., pp. 135–77). Westport, CT: Praeger.

Wright, M. O., Masten, A. S., & Narayan, A. J. (2013). Resilience processes in development: Four waves of research on positive adaptation in the context of adversity. In S. Goldstein & R. B. Brooks (Eds.), *Handbook of resilience in children* (2nd ed., pp. 15–37). New York: Springer.

Ybarra, M. L., Diener-West, M., Markow, D., Leaf, P. J., Hamburger, M., & Boxer, P. (2008). Linkages between Internet other media violence with seriously violent behavior by youth. *Pediatrics, 122*(5), 929–37.

Ybarra, M. L., Huesmann, R. L., Korchmaros, J. D., & Reisner, S. L. (2014). Cross-sectional associations between violent video and computer game playing and weapon carrying in a national cohort of children. *Aggressive Behavior, 40*, 345–58.

Zwi, A. B., Krug, E. G., Mercy, J. A., & Dahlberg, L. L. (2002). World report on violence and health—Exploring Australian responses. *Australian and New Zealand Journal of Public Health, 26*(5), 405–408.

CHAPTER

19 Internet Shopping Disorder

Astrid Müller, Matthias Brand, James E. Mitchell, *and* Martina de Zwaan

Abstract

Buying disorder is defined by an extreme preoccupation with buying/shopping, by overpowering urges to buy, and by recurrent loss of control resulting in buying/shopping episodes in which the person purchases more than he or she can safely afford. The harmful spending behavior results in indebtedness, disruption of family life and personal relationships, and occasionally in unlawful behavior. Buying disorder may occur in different buying environments, including traditional offline buying in brick-and-mortar–based retailers and buying on the Internet. The online retail market offers a vast variety of shopping information, simultaneous access to many online stores, affordability, and anonymity, thereby meeting expectations for immediate reward and emotional enhancement. These aspects may contribute to the migration of traditional buying-shopping disorder into the online retail market. This chapter addresses Internet shopping disorder, focusing on empirical research and clinical experience. After a brief summary regarding buying disorder in general, the phenomenology and considerations pertaining to the etiology of Internet shopping disorder is detailed and discussed.

Keywords: Internet shopping, buying-shopping disorder, prevalence, comorbidity, etiology, treatment

Background

Shopping describes an activity in which a customer browses the available merchandise with the intention to purchase items. Browsing and purchasing may occur in different buying environments involving bricks-and-mortar–based stores, paper catalogues, TV-shopping channels, and the Internet. *E-commerce* includes the electronic trading of physical and digital goods integrating all trading steps such as online marketing, online ordering, and electronic payment (Jelassi & Enders, 2005). An increasing number of customers engage in both offline and online shopping, and some have shifted completely to online shopping. This is not surprising given the increasing online retail market. According to the US Online Retail Forecast, between 2012 and 2017, e-commerce is anticipated to increase at a compound annual growth rate of 9% (Forrester, 2017). Similarly, in Europe, online sales growth outpaces offline sales growth. For example, while in 2005 only 25% of German customers ordered consumer goods online; in 2016, about 68% of the German population aged 14 years and older regularly purchased items online (Statistica, 2018).

Appropriate online shopping is thought to be characterized by goal-directed information search, price comparisons, and efficiency. However, like conventional buying, it may become excessive under certain circumstances. This chapter reviews Internet shopping disorder, focusing on recent publications on this topic, and is also based on our clinical experience and empirical research. After a brief summary regarding buying disorder in general, the phenomenology and considerations pertaining to the etiology of Internet shopping disorder will be detailed and discussed.

Buying Disorder

Description of Buying Disorder

Buying disorder (BD) is defined by an extreme preoccupation with shopping/buying, by overpowering urges to buy and by recurrent buying episodes in which the person purchases more than he or she can safely afford, eventuating in indebtedness, disruption of family life and personal relationships, and occasionally in unlawful behavior (e.g., fraud) (McElroy, Keck, Pope, Smith, & Strakowski, 1994). The buying episodes are primarily used to satisfy emotional or identity-related needs. Hence, the purchased merchandise seldom or never gets used but instead is hidden, forgotten, hoarded, or given away. Initially, individuals with BD experience pleasure and excitement while shopping (positive reinforcement). As the disorder progresses, shopping becomes more and more a maladaptive method of coping to alleviate negative feelings, avoid self-dissatisfaction, escape from interpersonal and other conflicts, etc. (Faber & Vohs, 2004). It appears that chronic BD is mostly driven by negative reinforcement processes (Müller et al., 2012).

According to reports of treatment-seeking patients with BD, the problem is characterized by fluctuations in severity, yet by a chronic course starting in adolescence. Usually, affected individuals develop awareness of their BD problem much later, secondary to the development of negative psychosocial consequences, which contributes to the chronicity of BD.

BD must be delineated from excessive buying during episodes of mania or hypomania (McElroy et al., 1994). Furthermore, it should be differentiated from occasional innocent impulsive buying characterized by spontaneous loss of control with diminished regard for consequences, mostly driven by external cues such as commercials or retail environment, and that is not necessarily associated with high levels of psychopathology. Nevertheless, impulsive buying can take on a pathological character and turn into BD (Verplanken & Sato, 2011).

Considerations on Classification

Due to limited research, BD was not included in the fifth edition of the *Diagnostic and Statistical Manual of Mental Disorders* (DSM-5; American Psychiatric Association [APA], 2013). Given the overlap between core features of BD and other non–substance-related addictions such as gambling disorder or Internet gaming disorder, BD could be considered a behavioral addiction (Müller, Brand, Claes et al., 2019). The following DSM-5 criteria for gambling disorder (APA, 2013, p. 585) are also suitable for the description of BD:

- Persistence and recurrence of the behavior
- rritability/anxiety/sadness when cutting-down or stopping the behavior
- Loss of control and repeated unsuccessful attempts to control the behavior
- Preoccupation with the behavior
- The use of the behavior to escape or relieve a negative mood
- Deceiving others regarding the extent of the inappropriate behavior
- Jeopardizing or losing a significant relationship/job/educational or career opportunity
- Relying on others to provide money to relieve desperate financial situations caused by the behavior
- The behavior is not better explained by a manic episode

BD could also be classified as an impulse control disorder. Extreme preoccupation with shopping/buying, increasing tension before and relief following BD episodes, and repetitive failures to resist the temptation to purchase goods regardless of financial problems that makes the behavior harmful to the person or others may justify this categorization. However, the DSM-5 category "Disruptive, Impulse-Control, and Conduct Disorders" focuses not only on problems in self-control but on the violation of the rights of others (APA, 2013, p. 461). There exists some concern about the categorization of BD as an impulse control disorder given that this approach, although likely to identify patients with very severe pathological buying, may overlook those with slight or moderate forms of pathological buying.

Prevalence and Socioeconomic Aspects

The prevalence of BD is still unknown given a lack of representative studies using structured clinical interviews. A recent meta-analysis indicated a high propensity to develop BD in modern consumer societies, with point prevalence estimates of approximately 5% (Maraz, Griffiths, & Demetrovics, 2016). Representative German studies indicated that BD is an increasing problem (Hubert, Hubert, Gwozdz, Raab, & Reisch, 2014; Neuner, Raab, & Reisch, 2005). For instance, Hubert et al. (2014) investigated BD tendencies in Germany between 2010 and 2012. They compared cross-sectional samples (2010: n = 992; 2011: n = 946; 2012: n = 972) that were representative of age, gender, region, and education for the given year. The results suggested an increase of BD with rising point prevalence estimates of 6.9% in 2010, 8.9% in 2011, and 10.4% in 2012 (Hubert et al., 2014).

Previous findings are highly consistent with respect to the inverse correlation between age and BD, indicating an increased vulnerability in younger people (Maraz et al., 2016). In terms of sociodemographic variables such as marital status, education, and job situation, it appears that individuals with

BD generally are not different from those without BD (e.g., Müller, de Zwaan, Mitchell, & Zimmermann, 2016; Otero-López & Villardefrancos, 2014). In the Koran et al. study (Koran, Faber, Aboujaoude, Large, & Serpe, 2006), individuals with BD reported lower income; however, in another study BD was not related to income (Mueller et al., 2010). With regard to a possible gender effect, research has produced mixed results. In most European studies women exhibited stronger BD tendencies than men (Maraz et al., 2016; Müller, Trotzke, Mitchell, de Zwaan, & Brand, 2015). In contrast, other surveys in the United States (Koran et al., 2006) and Germany (Mueller, Mitchell, Crosby et al., 2010) did not find gender differences. More research is necessary to clarify this matter.

Psychiatric Comorbidity

Scientific data on psychiatric comorbidity refer mostly to individuals who were seeking treatment for BD. Such individuals frequently suffer from depression, anxiety disorder, binge eating disorder, and/or substance use disorders (de Zwaan, 2011). Interview data from 171 patients with BD showed that almost 90% met the lifetime criteria for an Axis I diagnosis, in particular affective (74%) and anxiety (57%) disorders (Mueller, Mitchell, Black et al., 2010). In addition, 21% reported a comorbid impulse control disorder, most commonly intermittent explosive disorder (11%).

Hoarding disorder is another comorbid mental disorder. Many individuals with BD—about 50% in treatment-seeking samples—accumulate the purchased items and experience difficulties discarding them, resulting in clutter. They meet the criteria for hoarding disorder and exhibit greater psychopathology than those without hoarding symptoms (Frost & Müller, 2014; Möllenkamp et al., 2015). Of note, according to the DSM-5, hoarding disorder can be diagnosed with and without "excessive acquisition" (APA, 2013, p. 248). The specifier "excessive acquisition" includes excessive buying of goods, acquisition of free things, and/or occasional stealing.

In clinical samples of patients with BD, 60% or more exhibit a personality disorder, most commonly avoidant, depressive, obsessive-compulsive, or borderline personality disorder (Schlosser, Black, Repertinger, & Freet, 1994). Furthermore, some patients show narcissistic and antisocial personality traits, but seldom present the full clinical picture of a narcissistic or antisocial personality disorder.

Etiology

Kellett and Bolton (2009) suggested a cognitive-behavioral model that views BD as chronic and repetitive failure in self-regulation efforts. They proposed the following four distinct stages of BD: (1) antecedents, (2) external and internal emotional triggers, (3) the act of buying, and (4) the post-purchase phase. Antecedent factors refer to early experiences and family environment, negative life events, materialistic attitudes and values, obsessional thinking style, and impulsivity. The second stage integrates internal and external triggers for BD episodes. Therein, negative affectivity, the feeling of discomfort, and negative self-appraisals are viewed as internal cues. Examples of external triggers are interaction with retail staff, the availability of credit, and marketing stimuli. In terms of the latter aspect, price promotions, odors, music, commercials, brands, and other things are considered to stimulate craving reactions. Here, the cue-reactivity paradigm that is well known from substance-related addictions can be applied in the way that individuals with BD experience an increased subjective cue reactivity to specific shopping stimuli (Starcke, Schlereth, Domass, Schöler, & Brand, 2013; Trotzke et al., 2014). The third stage—the act of buying—is characterized by mental absorption, high arousal or relief, transformation of negative mood, and by shopping in a solitary disorganized fashion. Decision-making deficits may contribute to uncontrolled buying acts (Derbyshire, Chamberlain, Odlaug, Schreiber, & Grant, 2014; Trotzke, Starcke, Pedersen, Müller, & Brand, 2015; Voth et al., 2014). In the last stage—the post-purchase state—the affected person becomes aware of the breakdown in self-regulation and experiences feelings of guilt and shame and hides the purchases. Dysfunctional cognitive schemata, low self-esteem, negative pre-buying affect, and an ignorance of negative consequences can become perpetuated through this final state; this may create the psychological internal triggers for the vicious circle of BD (Kellett & Bolton, 2009).

Neurobiological theories refer to an imbalance in serotonergic, dopaminergic, or opioid regulation. Studies in the field are still scarce. The only event-related functional magnetic resonance imaging (fMRI) study found greater nucleus accumbens activity during product presentation and a lower activation in the insula during price presentation in patients with BD compared to healthy controls (Raab, Elger, Neuner, & Weber, 2011). This study, together with neuropsychological investigations demonstrating increased specific cue-reactivity and decision-making deficits, suggests an overlap between BD and other addictive behaviors or substance use disorders (Derbyshire et al., 2014; Starcke et al., 2013; Trotzke, Starcke, Pedersen, & Brand, 2014; Trotzke, Starcke, Pedersen et al., 2015; Voth et al., 2014).

Treatment

Cognitive-behavioral therapy (CBT) has been shown to be effective in three controlled trials (Mitchell, Burgard, Faber, Crosby, & de Zwaan, 2006; Mueller et al., 2008; Müller, Arikian, de Zwaan, & Mitchell., 2013). All studies used the Compulsive Buying Scale (Faber & O'Guinn, 1992) as primary outcome variable. The intention-to-treat analyses of this outcome measure found moderate (Cohen's d = 0.56; Mueller et al., 2008) to large (d = 1.00; Müller et al., 2013) between-group effect sizes (CBT vs. waiting list). In line with Kellett and Bolton's (2009) cognitive-behavioral model, psychotherapy targets the repetitive breakdown in self-control and positive and negative reinforcement processes that result in maladaptive buying habits. The treatment consists of sessions concerning motivation to change, development of stimulus control and alternative behaviors, and cognitive restructuring as well as exposure and response prevention techniques. More disorder-specific modules address failures in money management, material values endorsement, and underlying personality traits (for a review, see Mueller, Mitchell, & Peterson, 2012). To date, literature does not yet include differential psychotherapy approaches (e.g., for patients with BD and comorbid hoarding disorder) despite the need for such specific programs.

BD has received marginal attention with respect to pharmacotherapy. To date, only a small number of controlled trials with selective serotonin reuptake inhibitors (SSRIs), along with a few open trials or case reports with opioid antagonists (naltrexone) or N-methyl-D-aspartate (NMDA) receptor antagonists (memantine), have been published (for review, see Soares, Fernandes, & Morgado, 2016).

Internet Shopping Disorder

Phenomenology and Case Example

As mentioned earlier, evidence suggests that offline BD migrates to the electronic marketplace (Chen, Tarn, & Han, 2004; LaRose, 2001; Müller, Steins-Loeber, Trotzke et al., 2019). Clinical experience shows that patients with BD increasingly engage in both shopping in brick-and-mortar–based retail stores and on the Internet, or completely shift to the e-marketplace. Duroy, Gorse, and Lejoyeux (2014) investigated the occurrence of Internet shopping disorder among 200 Parisian university students and found a prevalence rate of 16%. Generally, it seems as if Internet shopping disorder displays the same core features as conventional BD (Dittmar, Long, and Bond, 2007; Dittmar, Long, and Meek, 2004; Lyons & Henderson, 2000). Patients who compulsively purchase through the Internet describe themselves as preoccupied with shopping and buying, losing control over spending, and continuing to shop despite harmful consequences that disrupt their life (see the earlier section "Description of Buying Disorder"). The following case example illustrates the main features of Internet shopping disorder.

Despite the overlapping core features of BD offline and online, both forms differ in the retail format, in shopping cues, and in the speed of shopping and purchasing. Some patients with BD may always prefer shopping in brick-and-mortar–based stores because they appreciate the opportunity to touch merchandise and try out goods, enjoy the stimulating traditional retail environment, experience comfortable social interaction with salespersons, and receive immediate gratification. Other individuals may be particularly stimulated by specific features of the Internet that better fit their living conditions and expectancies. This subgroup may be at risk for Internet shopping disorder. We will come back to these assumptions later.

Risk Factors

FEATURES OF THE INTERNET

The online shopping environment is generally thought to provide quick information on the best economic choice and to strengthen rational consumer behavior instead of stimulating pathological buying behavior (Grewal, Iyer, & Levy., 2004; Koski, 2004). However, several features of the Internet may defeat self-control while shopping and thus may encourage BD. Shopping online is usually faster and often simpler than shopping offline and offers a vast variety of information and products. The convenience of shopping at any time of day or night from almost any place increases the risk for uncontrolled buying. As described in Kellet and Bolton's (2009) model, patients with BD prefer buying in a solitary, unobserved manner, hiding their purchases from friends and relatives. In this regard, an appeal of electronic marketplaces is that the customer is not visible, and one can keep his or her buying behavior private from others (Kukar-Kinney, Ridgway, & Monroe, 2009). The dynamic nature of the medium,

Case Example

Mary, a 35-year-old married mother of two children, suffers from frequent e-shopping. She works half-days in a nursery school and likes her job. Nevertheless, she often experiences her working days and her family life as stressful and feels exhausted and sometimes even depressed in the evening. After dinner and having put her kids to bed, she relaxes by browsing the Web; this improves her mood. She enjoys unobserved surfing through clothing online retailers. Mary becomes excited about e-mail alerts of new products; spontaneous product recommendations with nice enlarged, colored pictures of the goods; and the great body of special auctions to make attractive purchases. She starts exchanging the online offers via social network sites with her friends, seeking the best price. The evening browsing on the Internet often lasts several hours, much longer than expected. When she imagines her look in the new dress and with the fancy purse and how her friends will admire her for her style and appearance, she cannot resist the temptation to put the items in her online shopping cart and quickly click the buy button. During these moments she completely forgets her indebtedness, that she cannot afford the merchandise, and that she will conceal the purchases from her husband, regretting her behavior later on.

the use of multimedia sensory triggers (e.g., audio clips, enlarged photos), alerts of new product innovations, e-commercials, pop-ups of product recommendations, and chatrooms with salespersons or other customers may counteract rational consumer behavior by generating excitement about the products and social comparison with other customers (LaRose, 2001). Post-purchase feelings of guilt may be replaced by positive emotions triggered by substitute incentives, point programs, or free gifts. Also, free shipping and credit options may delay the consequences of inappropriate purchasing.

PERSONALITY AND USING MOTIVES

To our knowledge, only a few studies have explored psychiatric and personality factors that contribute as internal triggers to Internet shopping disorder. Most studies have originated from consumer research and examined impulse buying in convenience consumer samples but not pathological buying on the Internet.

LaRose and Eastin's (2002) survey of US students indicated that the combination of negative mood and poor self-regulation results in more online buying. Weinstein, Mezig, Mizrachi, and Lejoyeux (2015) assessed BD and anxiety in 120 habitual Internet shoppers. In this study, BD was associated with trait but not state anxiety. Hence, avoidant personality traits probably contribute to pathological online shopping.

Kukar-Kinney et al. (2009) investigated the relationship between BD tendencies and the motivation to shop and buy on the Internet in mostly female customers of an Internet women's clothing retailer. The results indicated a positive relationship between the tendency toward Internet shopping disorder and the motivations to buy unobserved, avoid social interaction while shopping and buying, and quickly experience strong positive feelings. Such using motives have already been considered important with respect to other types of Internet addiction: for example for Internet pornography use (Reid, Garos, & Carpenter, 2011), gaming (Billieux et al., 2013; Demetrovics et al., 2011; King & Delfabbro, 2014; Kuss & Griffiths, 2012a), and addictive use of social networking sites (Kuss & Griffiths, 2011).

The role of using motives and expectancies for the development and maintenance of symptoms of Internet shopping disorder was investigated by Trotzke, Starcke, Müller, and Brand (2015). In this study, the tendency toward Internet shopping disorder, symptoms of BD, and using motives was assessed in a sample of 240 female participants. Symptoms of Internet shopping disorder were examined with the short version of the Internet Addiction Test (Pawlikowski, Altstötter-Gleich, & Brand., 2013) modified for online shopping sites (s-IATshopping). The s-IATshopping consists of 12 items that are answered on a 5-point scale (1 = never to 5 = very often) resulting in sum scores ranging from 12 to 60. The s-IAT measures if people suffer from a loss of control over their Internet use and if they had tried to reduce their Internet use and failed. It also measures effects of excessive Internet use on social interactions and preoccupation with the medium. Two factors are represented by the 12 items: "loss of control/time management" and "social problems/craving" (each factor having 6 items). In the s-IATshopping, the original terms "being online" or "Internet" have been replaced by the terms "being on online shopping sites" or "Internet shopping sites" (e.g., "How often do you feel preoccupied with Internet shopping sites when off-line, or fantasize about being on online shopping sites?"). General symptoms of BD were assessed with Faber and O'Guinn's (1992) Compulsive Buying Scale (CBS). The subjects' expectancies with respect to the use of online shopping sites were measured by 14 items of the questionnaire used in

Kukar-Kinney et al.'s study (2009) and one additional item which was created specifically ("I buy rather online, because I have the chance to buy 24 hours a day"). Additionally, all subjects completed a cue-reactivity paradigm inducing subjective arousal due to confrontation with Internet shopping cues. Craving was assessed by the modified version of the Desires for Alcohol Questionnaire (Love, James, & Willner, 1998). The symptoms of Internet shopping disorder (measured by the s-IATshopping) were strongly correlated with the using motives and expectancies of using Internet shopping sites. Moreover, a structural equation model of latent level confirmed the hypothesis that the relationship between the predisposition for Internet shopping disorder (represented by the general urge to buy and arousal reactions when being confronted with shopping cues) and the symptoms of Internet shopping disorder is mediated by specific expectancies (i.e., variety, anonymity, and immediate positive feelings). In summary, the results of this study indicate that certain medium-specific aspects contribute to the symptom severity of Internet shopping disorder. This means that it is increasingly likely that someone with the predisposition for BD uses Internet shopping sites addictively if he or she has the expectancy that using shopping sites has several advantages for him or her compared to going buying offline.

In particular, the expectancy that online shopping can be done easily and independently of time and space (24/7 at any place using mobile devices), as well as the expectancy that a variety of products can been viewed and bought without having the struggle of going into several shops and that shopping can be done without face-to-face contacts (which can be shaming for some individuals) mainly contributes to the development and maintenance of Internet shopping disorder. These kinds of Internet-specific acceleration processes have already been described for the development of cybersex addiction (Brand, Snagowski, Laier, & Maderwald, 2016a). Cooper (1998) has postulated the *triple-A engine* (accessibility, affordability, and anonymity) as an accelerating factor that contributes to an overuse of Internet sex applications (e.g., pornography). We see some parallels between the triple-A engine for cybersex and accelerating factors for Internet shopping disorder. These potential common mechanisms of development and maintenance of specific types of Internet addictions should be examined in future studies.

An additional result of the study of Trotzke, Starcke, Müller, and Brand (2015) was that an overlap

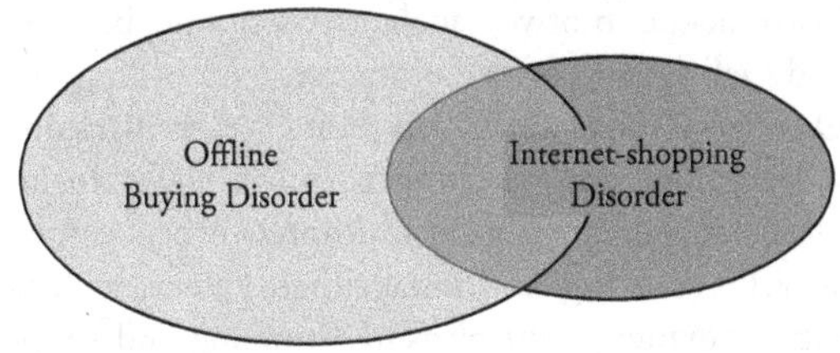

Figure 19.1 The overlap between conventional buying disorder and Internet-shopping disorder.

occurred between offline BD and Internet shopping disorder, but this overlap was only moderate. The CBS (reflecting general symptoms of BD independent of the offline-online context) and the s-IATshopping (measuring symptoms of Internet shopping disorder) were correlated with $r = .52$ in the entire sample. By using the cutoff scores for pathological buying behavior (using the CBS) or Internet shopping behavior (using the s-IATshopping), three groups were seen. First, 10% of the subjects reached the cutoff score in the CBS but not in the s-IAT, indicating that these individuals have a "traditional" offline BD but no clinically relevant signs of Internet shopping disorder. Second, 2.9% of the participants reached the cutoff score in the s-IAT solely, indicating that they have an addictive use of Internet shopping sites without symptoms of general BD, at least as measured by the CBS. Third, 3.3% of the sample reached the cutoff score in both scales, indicating that they have symptoms of both general BD and Internet shopping disorder. Although this result has to be replicated with treatment-seeking patients suffering from either offline BD or Internet shopping disorder or both, we argue that the overlap between both types of behavioral addictions is far from being exhaustive. Presumably, the phenomena of offline BD and Internet shopping disorder share some common underlying mechanisms and symptoms, but both conditions can also develop independently from each other. Future studies should consider the type and context (offline and/or online) of the addictive buying behavior (Figure 19.1).

Theoretical Models of Internet Shopping Disorder

A Social-Psychological Model of Internet Shopping Disorder

Dittmar, Long, and Bond (2007) investigated motives to buy online and found that psychological motives were distinct contributors, over and above instrumental motives such as economic benefits and efficiency of e-commerce. According to Dittmar et al. (2007), psychological motives involve "individuals' seeking to move closer to an ideal self, gain prestige, and impress other people, as well as seeking emotional enhancement, such as fun, enjoyment, and pleasure browsing and shopping, and mood regulation through seeing shopping as a leisure activity, buying to get buzz, and to improve their mood" (p. 346). In a subsequent study reported in the same publication, these investigators tested a social-psychological model of online pathological buying among students in the United Kingdom. Their findings indicated that the effect of general Internet use on Internet shopping disorder is indeed mediated by emotional and identity-related online buying motives but not by economic benefits and efficiency (Dittmar et al., 2007). Based on these results and given the strong link between materialistic values endorsement and BD, they developed a social-psychological model of Internet shopping disorder whereby the proposed link between materialistic values and online pathological buying tendencies is assumed to be mediated by psychological online buying motives, particularly by the desire for identity gain and emotional enhancement.

A Conceptual Model of Internet Shopping Disorder Based on Literature

Based on a review of the literature, Rose and Dhandayudham (2014) proposed a conceptual model that is shown in Figure 19.2. The model includes several aspects that are assumed to contribute to pathological online shopping. Most aspects were already discussed earlier, except the factor "cognitive overload." This factor pertains to the repeated stimulation and temptation potentially resulting in cognitive overload overwhelming self-control (see the earlier section "Features of the Internet"). In accordance with Muraven and Baumeister's (2000) ego depletion model, sustained resistance to temptations requires maintaining self-control efforts that, however, rely on a limited resource. Consequently, cognitive overload in one area may defeat self-control in another area resulting in a lack of willpower (i.e., a shopping spree).

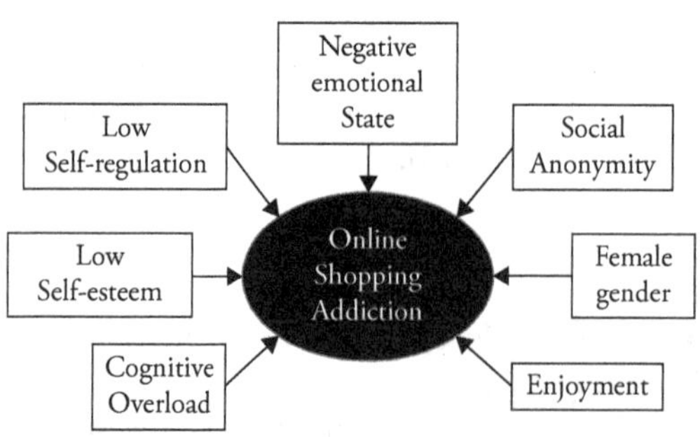

Figure 19.2 Proposed predictors for online shopping addiction based on the model of Rose and Dhandayudham (2014).

A Theoretical Model of Internet Shopping Disorder

Although most research on Internet addiction focuses on Internet gaming (Kuss, Griffiths, Karila, & Billieux, 2014), it was postulated very early in the literature on Internet addiction that other applications could also be used addictively. Young, Pistner, O'Mara, and Buchanan (1999) used the term "net compulsion" for the excessive use of online gambling, shopping, or online trading. Recently, it has been argued that, in principle, every Internet application can be used compulsively or addictively, but that the most relevant applications are gaming, gambling, social networking sites, cybersex, and shopping sites (Brand, Young, & Laier, 2014; Brand, Young Laier, Wölfling, & Potenza, 2016; Brand, Wegmann, Stark et al., 2019; Kuss & Griffiths, 2011, 2012a, 2012b; Montag et al., 2015).

Davis (2001) previously suggested that it makes sense, both clinically and scientifically, to distinguish between a generalized Internet addition and a specific type of Internet addiction. He argued that particular aspects of communication play the major role in developing a generalized Internet addiction, which is strongly related to social isolation and a lack of social support. He also argued that a generalized Internet addiction would not have developed without the medium itself. By contrast, individuals addicted to certain Internet applications, such as gaming, cybersex, or shopping sites, may have a specific predisposition toward specific activities and may also have developed an excessive or pathological behavior without or outside the Internet. Other researchers emphasize this argument by criticizing the term "addicted to the Internet" as suggesting that individuals are addicted to a delivery medium. It seems to be more appropriate to use terms like "addicted to a certain Internet application" (Starcevic, 2013). However, there are individuals who are addicted to mainly one particular Internet application, but also individuals who use a wide range of applications and lose control over their Internet use in general. This latter type of Internet addition is frequently called *generalized Internet addiction* or *generalized pathological Internet use* (Davis, 2001).

Considering Davis's (2001) theoretical arguments and recent research on psychological and neuroimaging correlates of different forms of Internet addiction, Brand et al. (2014) suggested a model of specific Internet use disorders. Although it has been argued that the different types of Internet addiction share certain core features, the main differences between a generalized and specific type of Internet addiction relate to the mechanisms of receiving positive and negative reinforcement via Internet use. Briefly, for the development of a generalized Internet addiction, psychopathological symptoms (e.g., depression, social anxiety) in combination with dysfunctional personality aspects (e.g., shyness, procrastination) and social cognitions (e.g., low perceived social support) are supposed to be the general predisposing factors. If an individual also has a dysfunctional coping style and the expectancy that the Internet provides helpful tools for avoiding negative feelings, the Internet can become a means for redirecting focus away from problems or negative mood. This represents a dysfunctional coping style and results in negative reinforcement of the predisposing factors, but also in positive reinforcement of the Internet use expectancies and the dysfunctional coping style.

For a specific type of Internet addiction to develop, Brand et al. (2014) argued that specific predispositions or vulnerabilities toward certain activities (e.g., gaming, sexual arousal) are already present, and the respective specific Internet addiction only occurs if the individual has the expectancy that certain Internet applications can be used to satisfy the specific desires. By using specific Internet applications for satisfying individual needs, gratification is experienced. This results in positive reinforcement of both the specific Internet use expectancies and also the specific predispositions and vulnerabilities. In summary, reinforcement is assumed to be a key element in processes leading to the development and maintenance of both generalized and specific Internet addiction, which is consistent with recent models on addiction and substance dependency in general (Berridge, Robinson, & Aldridge, 2009; Everitt & Robbins, 2006; Robinson & Berridge, 2000, 2008). The difference between a generalized and a specific type of Internet addiction is seen in the kinds of needs and desires that are reinforced and the main direction of reinforcement, which is a combination of positive and negative reinforcement in generalized Internet addiction and more strongly positive reinforcement in specific types of Internet addiction (although negative reinforcement of avoidance tendencies and depressive symptoms are also frequently observed in specific Internet addictions).

As pointed out earlier, the addictive or compulsive use of online shopping sites can be considered one type of specific Internet addiction (e.g., Young et al., 1999). Very recently, the aforementioned model of Brand et al. (2014) was revised and modified, resulting in a more complex model that was named Interaction of Person-Affect-Cognition-Execution (I-PACE) model of specific Internet use disorders (Brand, Young et al., 2016; Brand, Wegmann, Stark et al., 2019). This new model includes interactions between predisposing factors (e.g., neurobiological and psychological aspects), moderators (e.g., coping styles, Internet-related cognitive biases), and mediators (e.g., affective and cognitive responses to triggers) and considers their combination with executive functioning and inhibitory control. When breaking down the core elements of the I-PACE model and transferring the proposed mechanisms underlying the development and maintenance of Internet shopping disorder, we argue that predisposing factors that play a role in offline BD should also constitute person's core characteristics in making an individual vulnerable for an Internet shopping disorder. Specific temperamental features and dysfunctional personality traits, which are considered important in the context of BD and Internet shopping disorder, are high approach tendencies (Derbyshire et al., 2014; Trotzke, Starcke, Pedersen et al., 2015; Voth et al., 2014), impulsivity, neuroticism, material values, low self-esteem, and stress vulnerability (Mueller, Claes, Mitchell et al., 2010, Mueller et al., 2011; Villardefrancos & Otero-López, 2016). Moreover, psychiatric vulnerability and psychopathology (e.g., anxiety, depression) are of relevance, as in many other conditions involving addictive behaviors (de Zwaan, 2011; Mueller, Mitchell, Black et al., 2010; Müller, Steins-Loeber, Trotzke et al., 2019; Weinstein et al., 2015). Other predisposing factors are either an existent symptomatology of offline BD or a tendency toward shopping, and preferences for shopping sites. Furthermore, past research (Kukar-Kinney et al., 2009; Trotzke, Starcke, Müller, & Brand, 2015) suggested an impact of specific shopping site use expectancies

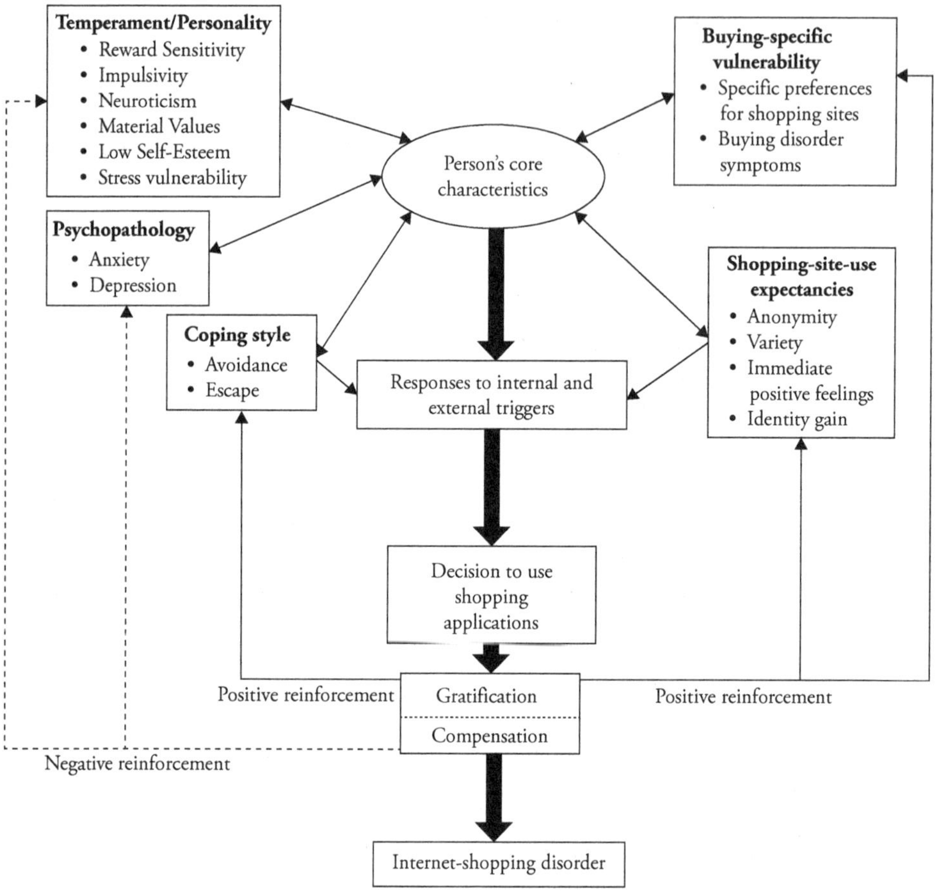

Figure 19.3 A theoretical model of internet-shopping disorder adapted from the I-PACE Model for Internet-Use Disorders.

including anonymity, variety, and the expectancy for immediate emotion regulation during browsing and shopping via the Internet (see also the earlier section "Personality and Using Motives"). As already suggested by Kellett and Bolton (2009) for conventional BD, the urge to shop and buy through the Internet can probably be triggered by internal (e.g., negative mood states, boredom, social disappointment) and external cues (e-advertisements, shopping sites). However, the combination of these predisposing factors does not necessarily result in Internet shopping disorder. It is more likely that individuals develop this specific type of Internet use disorder if they use shopping on the Internet to cope with everyday problems to avoid social conflicts, escape from reality, or to distract from negative mood (Faber & Vohs, 2004). When shopping sites are used in this situation, gratification is likely to be experienced, which results in reinforcement of both the buying-specific predispositions and the specific coping style (Brand, Wegmann, Stark et al., 2019). Expectancies about what online shopping sites can do for or help with regulating mood and experiencing pleasure are positively reinforced, while psychopathology, negative mood states, and dysfunctional personality traits are negatively reinforced (Brand, Wegmann, Stark et al., 2019). These arguments are summarized in Figure 19.3.

Conclusion and Future Directions

Although offline and online BD share core features, there is not yet a clear view on how similar or different are the phenomenology and etiology of offline BD and Internet shopping disorder. It is clinically and scientifically important to better understand how strong the relationship might be between Internet shopping disorder and the overuse of other Internet applications. Further research should address the question of whether Internet shopping disorder is a subtype of BD, a subtype of Internet addition, or both.

References

American Psychiatric Association. (2013). *Diagnostic and statistical manual of mental disorders* (5th ed.). Washington, DC: Author.

Berridge, K. C., Robinson, T. E., & Aldridge, J. W. (2009). Dissecting components of reward: "Liking," "Wanting," and Learning. *Current Opinions in Pharmacology, 9*(1), 65–73.

Billieux, J., Van Der Linden, M., Achab, S., Khazaal, Y., Paraskevopoulos, L., Zullino, D., & Thorens, G. (2013). Why do you play World of Warcraft? An in-depth exploration of self-reported motivations to play online and in-game behaviours in the virtual world of Azeroth. *Computers in Human Behavior, 29*(1), 103–109.

Brand, M., Snagowski, J., Laier, C., & Maderwald, S. (2016). Ventral striatum activity when watching preferred pornographic pictures is correlated with symptoms of internet pornography addiction. *Neuroimage, 129*, 224–32.

Brand, M., Wegmann, E., Stark, R., Müller, A., Wölfling, K., Robbins, T. & Potenza, M.N. (2019). The Interaction of Person-Affect-Cognition-Execution (I-PACE) model for addictive behaviors: Update, generalization to addictive behaviors beyond Internet-use disorders, and specification of the process character of addictive behaviors. *Neuroscience and Biobehavioral Reviews,104*, 1-10.

Brand, M., Young, K. S., & Laier, C. (2014). Prefrontal control and internet addiction: A theoretical model and review of neuropsychological and neuroimaging findings. *Frontiers in Human Neuroscience, 8*, 375.

Brand, M., Young, K. S., Laier, C., Wölfling, K., & Potenza, M. N. (2016). Integrating psychological and neurobiological considerations regarding the development and maintenance of specific internet-use disorders: An Interaction of Person-Affect-Cognition-Execution (I-PACE) model. *Neuroscience and Biobehavioral Reviews, 71*, 252–66.

Chen, K., Tarn, J. M., & Han, B. T. (2004). Internet dependency: Its impact on online behavioural patterns in e-commerce. *Human Systems Management, 23*(1), 49–58.

Cooper, A. (1998). Sexuality and the Internet: Surfing into the new millennium. *CyberPsychology & Behavior, 1*(2), 181–87.

Davis, R. A. (2001). A cognitive-behavioral model of pathological internet use. *Computers in Human Behavior, 17*(2), 187–95.

de Zwaan, M. (2011). Psychiatric comorbidity and compulsive buying. In A. Müller & J. E. Mitchell (Eds.), *Compulsive Buying. Clinical Foundations and Treatment* (pp. 87–104). New York, London: Routledge.

Demetrovics, Z., Urbán, R., Nagygyörgy, K., Farkas, J., Zilahy, D., Mervó, B., . . . E., H. (2011). Why do you play? The development of the Motives for Online Gaming Questionnaire (MOGQ). *Behavior Research Methods, 43*(3), 814–25.

Derbyshire, K. L., Chamberlain, S. R., Odlaug, B. L., Schreiber, L., & Grant, J. E. (2014). Neurocognitive functioning in compulsive buying disorder. *Annals of Clinical Psychiatry, 26*(1), 57–63.

Dittmar, H., Long, K., & Bond, R. (2007). When a better self is only a button click away: Associations between materialistic values, emotional and identity-related buying motives, and compulsive buying tendency online. *Journal of Social and Clinical Psychology, 26*(3), 334–61.

Dittmar, H., Long, K., & Meek, R. (2004). Buying on the Internet: Gender differences in on-line and conventional buying motivations. *Sex Roles, 50*(5), 423–44.

Duroy, D., Gorse, P., & Lejoyeux, M. (2014). Characteristics of online compulsive buying in Parisian students. *Addictive Behaviors, 39*(12), 1827–30.

Everitt, B. J., & Robbins, T. W. (2006). Neural systems of reinforcement for drug addiction: From actions to habits to compulsion. *Nature Neuroscience, 8*(11), 1481–89.

Faber, R. J., & O'Guinn, T. C. (1992). A clinical screener for compulsive buying. *Journal of Consumer Research, 19*(3), 459–69.

Faber, R. J., & Vohs, K. D. (2004). To buy or not to buy? Self-control and self-regulatory failure in purchase behavior. In R. F. Baumeister & K. D. Vohs (Eds.), *Self-Regulation: Research, Theory, and Applications* (pp. 517–27). New York: Guilford.

Forrester (2017, December 21). *US Online Retail Forecast. 2012 to 2017.* http://www.forrester.com/US+Online+Retail+Forecast+2012+To+2017/fulltext/-/E-RES93281?objectid=RES93281.

Frost, R. O., & Müller, A. (2014). Acquisition of possessions in hoarding disorder. In R. O. Frost & G. Steketee (Eds.), *The Oxford handbook of hoarding and acquiring* (pp. 86–99). New York: Oxford University Press.

Grewal, D., Iyer, G. R., & Levy, M. (2004). Internet retailing: Enablers, limiters and market consequences. *Journal of Business Research, 57*(7), 703–13.

Hubert, M., Hubert, M., Gwozdz, W., Raab, G., & Reisch, L. A. (2014). Compulsive buying: An increasing problem? Investigating and comparing trends in Germany and Denmark, 2010–2012. *Journal of Consumer Protection and Food Safety, 9*, 280–84.

Jelassi, T., & Enders, A. (2005). *Strategies for e-business. Creating value through electronic and mobile commerce* (pp. 4–5). London: Financial Times, Prentice Hall.

Kellett, S., & Bolton, J. V. (2009). Compulsive buying: A cognitive-behavioral model. *Clinical Psychology and Psychotherapy, 16*(2), 83–99.

King, D. L., & Delfabbro, P. H. (2014). The cognitive psychology of Internet gaming disorder. *Clinical Psychology Review, 34*(4), 298–308.

Koran, L., Faber, R., Aboujaoude, E., Large, M., & Serpe, R. (2006). Estimated prevalence of compulsive buying behavior in the United States. *The American Journal of Psychiatry, 163*(10),1806–12.

Koski, N. (2004). Impulse buying on the Internet: Encouraging and discouraging factors. *Frontiers of E-Business Research,4* (1), 23–35.

Kukar-Kinney, M., Ridgway, N. M., & Monroe, K. B. (2009). The relationship between consumers' tendencies to buy compulsively and their motivations to shop and buy on the Internet. *Journal of Retailing, 85*(3), 298–307.

Kuss, D. J., & Griffiths, M. D. (2011). Online social networking and addiction: A review of the psychological literature. *International Journal of Environmental Research and Public Health, 8*(9), 3528–52.

Kuss, D. J., & Griffiths, M. D. (2012a). Internet gaming addiction: A systematic review of empirical research. *International Journal of Mental Health and Addiction, 10*(2), 278–96.

Kuss, D. J., & Griffiths, M. D. (2012b). Internet sex addiction: A review of empirical research. *Addiction Research and Theory, 20*(2), 111–24.

Kuss, D. J., Griffiths, M. D., Karila, M., & Billieux, J. (2014). Internet addiction: A systematic review of epidemiological research for the last decade. *Current Pharmaceutical Design*, *20*(25), 4026–52.

Kuss, D. J., Louws, J., & Wiers, R. W. (2012). Online gaming addiction? Motives predict addictive play behavior in massively multiplayer online role-playing games. *Cyberpsychology, Behavior and Social Networking*, *15*(9), 480–85.

LaRose, R. (2001). On the negative effects of e-commerce: A sociocognitive exploration of unregulated on-line buying. *Journal of Computer-Mediated Communication*, *6*(3), 1-34.

LaRose, R., & Eastin, M. S. (2002). Is online buying out of control? Electronic commerce and consumer self–regulation. *Journal of Broadcasting and Electronic Media*, *46*(4), 549–64.

Love, A., James, D., & Willner, P. (1998). A comparison of two alcohol craving questionnaires. *Addiction*, *93*(7), 1091–102.

Lyons, B., & Henderson, K. (2000). *An old problem in a new marketplace: Compulsive buying on the Internet* (pp. 739–44). Melbourne: Australian and New Zealand Marketing Academy.

Maraz, A., Griffiths, M. D., & Demetrovics, Z. (2016). The prevalence of compulsive buying: A meta-analysis. *Addiction*, *111*(3), 408–19.

McElroy, S. L., Keck, P. E., Pope, H. G., Smith, J. M., & Strakowski, S. M. (1994). Compulsive buying: A report of 20 cases. *Journal of Clinical Psychiatry*, *55*(6), 242–48.

Mitchell, J. E., Burgard, M., Faber, R., Crosby, R. D., & de Zwaan, M. (2006). Cognitive behavioral therapy for compulsive buying disorder. *Behaviour Research and Therapy*, *44*(12), 1859–65.

Möllenkamp, M., de Zwaan, M., & Müller, A. (2015). Hoarding with and without excessive buying: Results of a pilot study. *Psychopathology*, *48*(1), 56–59.

Montag, C., Bey, K., Sha, P., Li, M., Chen, Y. F., Liu, W. Y., . . . Reuter, M. (2015). Is it meaningful to distinguish between generalized and specific Internet addiction? Evidence from a cross-cultural study from Germany, Sweden, Taiwan and China. *Asia Pacific Psychiatry*, *7*(1), 20–26.

Mueller, A., Claes, L., Mitchell, J. E., Wonderlich, S. A., Crosby, R. D., & de Zwaan, M. (2010). Personality prototypes in individuals with compulsive buying based on the Big Five Model. *Behaviour Research and Therapy*, *48*(9), 930–35.

Mueller, A., Mitchell, J. E., Black, D. W., Crosby, R. D., Berg, K., & de Zwaan, M. (2010). Latent profile analysis and comorbidity in a sample of individuals with compulsive buying disorder. *Psychiatry Research*, *178*(2), 348–53.

Mueller, A., Mitchell, J. E., Crosby, R. D., Gefeller, O., Faber, R. J., Martin, A., . . . de Zwaan, M. (2010). Estimated prevalence of compulsive buying in Germany and its association with sociodemographic characteristics and depressive symptoms. *Psychiatry Research*, *180*(2–3), 137–42.

Mueller, A., Mitchell, J. E., & Peterson, L. (2012). Assessment and treatment of compulsive buying. In J. E. Grant & M. N. Potenza (Eds.), *The Oxford handbook of impulse control disorders* (pp. 398–409). New York: Oxford University Press.

Mueller, A., Mitchell, J. E., Peterson, L. A., Faber, R. J., Steffen, K. J., Crosby, R. D., & Claes, L. (2011). Depression, materialism, and excessive Internet use in relation to compulsive buying. *Comprehensive Psychiatry*, *52*(4), 420–24.

Mueller, A., Mueller, U., Silbermann, A., Reinecker, H., Bleich, S., Mitchell, J. E., & de Zwaan, M. (2008). A randomized, controlled trial of group cognitive behavioral therapy for compulsive buying disorder: Posttreatment and 6-month follow-up results. *Journal of Clinical Psychiatry*, *69*(7), 1131–38.

Müller, A., Arikian, A., de Zwaan, M., & Mitchell, J. E. (2013). Cognitive behavioural group therapy versus guided self-help for compulsive buying disorder: A preliminary study. *Clinical Psychology and Psychotherapy*, *20*(1), 28–35.

Müller, A., Brand, M., Claes, L., Demetrovicz, Z., de Zwaan, M., Fernández-Aranda, F., Frost, R.O., Jimenez-Murcia, S., Lejoyeux, M., Steins-Loeber, S., Mitchell, J.E., Moulding, R., Nedeljkovic, M., Trotzke, P., Weinstein, A., & Kyrios, M. (2019). Buying-shopping disorder - is there enough evidence to support its inclusion in ICD-11? *CNS Spectrums*, *24*(4), 374–379.

Müller, A., de Zwaan, M., Mitchell, J. E., & Zimmermann, T. (2016). Pathological buying and partnership status. *Psychiatry Research*, *239*, 122–23.

Müller, A., Mitchell, J. E., Crosby, R. D., Cao, L., Claes, L., & de Zwaan, M. (2012). Mood states preceding and following compulsive buying episodes: An ecological momentary assessment study. *Psychiatry Research*, *200*(2–3), 575–80.

Müller, A., Steins-Loeber, S., Trotzke, P., Vogel, B., Georgiadou, E., & de Zwaan, M. (2019). Online shopping in treatment-seeking patients with buying-shopping disorder. *Comprehensive Psychiatry*, 94, 152120.

Müller, A., Mitchell, J. E., & de Zwaan, M. (2015). Compulsive buying. *American Journal on Addictions*, *24*(2), 132–37.

Müller, A., Trotzke, P., Mitchell, J. E., de Zwaan, M., & Brand, M. (2015). The pathological buying screener: Development and psychometric properties of a new screening instrument for the assessment of pathological buying symptoms. *PloS One*, *10*(10), e0141094.

Muraven, M., & Baumeister, R. F. (2000). Self-regulation and depletion of limited resources: Does self-control resemble a muscle? *Psychological Bulletin 126*(2), 247–59.

Neuner, M., Raab, G., & Reisch, L. (2005). Compulsive buying in maturing consumer societies: An empirical re-inquiry. *Journal of Economic Psychology*, *26*(4), 509–22.

Otero-López, J. M., & Villardefrancos, E. (2014). Prevalence, sociodemographic factors, psychological distress, and coping strategies related to compulsive buying: A cross-sectional study in Galicia, Spain. *BMC Psychiatry*, *14*, 101.

Pawlikowski, M., Altstötter-Gleich, C., & Brand, M. (2013). Validation and psychometric properties of a short version of Young's Internet Addiction Test. *Computers in Human Behavior*, *29*(3), 1212–23.

Raab, G., Elger, C., Neuner, M., & Weber, B. (2011). A neurological study of compulsive buying behavior. *Journal of Consumer Policy*, *34*, 401–13.

Reid, R. C., Garos, S., & Carpenter, B. N. (2011). Reliability, validity, and psychometric development of the hypersexual behavior inventory in an outpatient sample of men. *Sexual Addiction and Compulsivity*, *18*(1), 30–51.

Robinson, T. E., & Berridge, K. C. (2000). The psychology and neurobiology of addiction: An incentive–sensitization view. *Addiction*, *95*(Suppl 2), S9–117.

Robinson, T. E., & Berridge, K. C. (2008). The incentive sensitization theory of addiction: Some current issues. *Philosophical Transactions of the Royal Society B*, *363*(1507), 3137–46.

Rose, S., & Dhandayudham, A. (2014). Towards an understanding of Internet-based problem shopping behaviour: The concept of online shopping addiction and its proposed predictors. *Journal of Behavioral Addiction*, *3*(2), 83–89.

Schlosser, S., Black, D. W., Repertinger, S., & Freet, D. (1994). Compulsive buying. Demography, phenomenology, and comorbidity in 46 subjects. *General Hospital Psychiatry, 16*(3), 205–12.

Soares, C., Fernandes, N., & Morgado, P. (2016). A review of pharmacologic treatment for compulsive buying disorder. *CNS Drugs, 30*(4), 281-291.

Starcevic, V. (2013). Is Internet addiction a useful concept? *Australian and New Zealand Journal of Psychiatry, 47*(1), 16–19.

Starcke, K., Schlereth, B., Domass, D., Schöler, T., & Brand, M. (2013). Cue reactivity towards shopping cues in female patients. *Journal of Behavioral Addictions, 2*(1), 17–22.

Statistica. (2018, January 21). *E-Commerce in Germany.* https://www.statista.com/study/32414/e-commerce-in-germany-statista-dossier/.

Trotzke, P., Starcke, K., Müller, A., & Brand, M. (2015). Pathological buying online as a specific form of Internet addiction: A model-based experimental investigation. *PloS One, 10*(10), e0140296.

Trotzke, P., Starcke, K., Pedersen, A., & Brand, M. (2014). Cue-induced craving in pathological buying: Empirical evidence and clinical implications. *Psychosomatic Medicine, 76*(9), 694–700.

Trotzke, P., Starcke, K., Pedersen, A., Müller, A., & Brand, M. (2015). Impaired decision making under ambiguity but not under risk in individuals with pathological buying: Behavioral and psychophysiological evidence. *Psychiatry Research, 229*(1–2), 551–58.

Verplanken, B., & Sato, A. (2011). The psychology of impulsive buying: An integrative self-regulation approach. *Journal of Consumer Policy, 34*(2), 197–210.

Villardefrancos, E., & Otero-López, J. M. (2016). Compulsive buying in university students: Its prevalence and relationships with materialism, psychological distress symptoms, and subjective well-being. *Comprehensive Psychiatry, 65*, 128–35.

Voth, E. M., Claes, L., Georgiadou, E., Selle, J., Trotzke, P., Brand, M., de Zwaan, M., & Müller, A. (2014). Reactive and regulative temperament in patients with compulsive buying and non-clinical controls measured by self-report and performance-based tasks. *Comprehensive Psychiatry, 55*(7), 1505–12.

Weinstein, A., Mezig, H., Mizrachi, S., & Lejoyeux, M. (2015). A study investigating the association between compulsive buying with measures of anxiety and obsessive–compulsive behavior among Internet shoppers. *Comprehensive Psychiatry 57*, 46–50.

Young, K. S., Pistner, M., O'Mara, J., & Buchanan, J. (1999). Cyber disorders: The mental health concern for the new millennium. *Cyberpsychology and Behavior, 2*(5), 475–79.

CHAPTER

20 Technology, the Internet, and Gambling

How the Medium Can Facilitate Addiction, Adaptation, and Intervention

Howard J. Shaffer, Heather M. Gray, Sarah E. Nelson, *and* Debi A. LaPlante

Abstract

Many people worry that exposure to Internet gambling will overpower individuals' self-control, stimulate addictive behavior patterns, and provide the context to sustain addiction once it emerges. Though many researchers have attempted to evaluate this proposition, they have been limited by their methodological approaches—specifically, their use of convenience samples and self-reports of Internet gambling behavior. At the Division on Addiction, the authors collaborated with bwin.party digital entertainment to examine electronically recorded gambling data (i.e., records of actual gambling) among bwin.party subscribers. As described in this chapter, their early epidemiological studies revealed that few Internet gamblers are intemperate and that the typical Internet player gambles moderately. However, those who do use the Internet to gamble excessively often experience lasting and far-reaching harm. The authors review prevention and intervention strategies to help promote healthier Internet gambling. These cross-cutting strategies emerge from public policy, public health, corporate social responsibility, and other fields. With regard to user-initiated strategies, the authors describe what researchers have discovered about the effectiveness and reach of self-limitation and self-exclusion programs. With regard to operator-initiated strategies, they propose a series of steps leading to the development of algorithms designed to predict which Internet gamblers will require interventions to reduce gambling harm. The authors describe their approach to these steps during their work developing predictive algorithms for bwin.party. Finally, the chapter considers ethical principles that should inform the development of programs and policies designed to provide the safest possible Internet gambling experience.

Keywords: gambling, technology, Internet gambling, addiction, epidemiology, self-limitation, self-exclusion, predictive algorithms

McLuhan (1964) suggested that "The medium is the message. This is merely to say that the personal and social consequences of any medium—that is of any extension of ourselves—result from the new scale that is introduced into our affairs by each extension of ourselves, or by any new technology" (p. 7). As this book goes to press, there is ongoing debate among scholars, policymakers, the public, and others about the new scale of human activity introduced by Internet use in general and Internet gambling in particular. The overriding concern that permeates this debate is that exposure to the technological opportunities and advances that facilitate activities such as shopping, gaming, and gambling over the Internet change personal experience and social discourse. Many people suggest that these shifts and the subjective experiences associated with these changes hold the potential to overpower individuals' self-control, stimulate addictive behavior patterns, and provide the context to sustain addiction once it emerges.

The newest iteration of the *Diagnostic and Statistical Manual of Mental Disorders* from the American Psychiatric Association (i.e., DSM5: American Psychiatric Association & American Psychiatric Association DSM-5 Task Force, 2013) reflects and encourages these concerns by including Internet Gaming Addiction in an appendix, identifying it as a condition deserving of more study and suggesting that it might be a candidate for future diagnostic status. This development is part of a broader panoply of concerns about how the Internet impacts human behavior and its regulation (e.g., victimization, harrassment, bullying, sex crimes: Jones, Mitchell, & Finkelhor, 2012; McQuade, Colt, & Meyer, 2009; McQuade, Gentry, Colt, & Rogers, 2011; McQuade, Gentry, Fisk, & Rogers, 2011; Mitchell & Ybarra, 2007; Wolak, Finkelhor, & Mitchell, 2004; Ybarra, Mitchell, Wolak, & Finkelhor, 2006).

These concerns reflect a commonly observed historical pattern of apprehension often associated with the introduction of new technology (LaPlante, 2012). For example, contemporary concerns about the public health and welfare associated with using the Internet and Internet gambling are similar to those raised soon after the introduction of the printing press, telephone, radio, and television (e.g., Silver, 1979). During the 16th century, the introduction of the printing press stimulated considerable concern about its use and the subjects worthy of printing (Thompson, 2013). About a century later, one of the original references to addiction was about intemperate reading (Albanese & Shaffer, 2012). During the 1930s, some people worried about excessive radio listening and the adverse influence of jazz on the American character (Burns & PBS Online, 2014).

As these examples illustrate, new technology encourages similar concerns—some genuine and some imagined—because it tends to impact human experience in ways few can predict (Linden, 2011), and uncertainty tends to stimulate anxiety. However, Thompson reminds us that the stress associated with new technology is a double-edged sword that also can help us to grow and revise community: "Every new tool shapes the way we think, as well as what we think about. The printed word helped make our cognition linear and abstract, along with vastly enlarging our stores of knowledge. Newspapers shrank the world; then the telegraph shrank it even more dramatically. With every innovation, cultural prophets bickered over whether we were facing a technological apocalypse or a utopia" (Thompson, 2013, p. 7). If there has been any stable feature of the human condition, it has been that people tend to resist having to change. Ultimately, new uses of information technology and the psychological changes they stimulate represent both new risks and new opportunities for adaptation (McLuhan & Powers, 1989; Shapiro, 1965; Vaillant, 1977).

In this chapter, we focus our discussion on Internet gambling and some of the addiction-related health risks and benefits that might be associated with this technological medium in particular (Braverman & Shaffer, 2012; Broda et al., 2008; General Accounting Office, 2002; Gray, LaPlante, & Shaffer, 2012; LaPlante, Nelson, & Gray, 2013; LaPlante, Schumann, Labrie, & Shaffer, 2008; Nelson et al., 2008; Reilly & Smith, 2013a, 2013b; Shotton, 1991). During our consideration of technology and addiction, we review some of the work that has emerged from an ongoing collaboration between bwin.party, a large Internet gambling provider, and the Division on Addiction, a program of Cambridge Health Alliance, as it relates to risks associated with using the Internet as a medium for gambling, as well as the potential for that same technology to help to prevent, protect, and resolve excessive patterns of behavior.

Technology and the Internet

The Internet is one of the most important technological advances in history. Via its growing web of interconnected networks, the Internet has opened the door to the development of a new social system that has widespread ramifications for existing social systems. Some observers consider these technological developments as dangerous. Other observers, however, provide considerable evidence that advancing Internet technology is changing the world community for the better (Thompson, 2013). These contrasting viewpoints can be illustrated by one example, what researchers have labeled the *Internet paradox* (Kraut et al., 1998): that is, despite the Internet providing more opportunities for communication, some Internet users have reported feeling more isolated. Although newer research reveals that this effect may dissipate over time (Kraut et al., 2002), the Internet paradox—even when short-lived—reminds us about a general principle describing the overarching relationship between technology and isolation. As technology evolves, people begin to think about what technology can do for them to make things easier. Advancing technology reduces the number of people needed to complete a task; consequently, technology indirectly may encourage social isolation (Kipnis, 1991; Kraut et al., 1998).

This example illustrates that those on all sides of this discussion have the responsibility to consider both the future benefits and hazards that might become associated with this new technology. As we describe in the next section, contemporary Internet critics are providing the stimulus to develop safety features for travelers of the virtual highway—just as, for several decades now, automobile safety advocates have prompted car-makers to develop and advance new technological safety features for vehicles.

Internet Gambling: Risk and Opportunity

During the early years after the introduction of combustion engine automobiles, accidents were simply the cost of riding in a car. There were no safety belts or airbags to protect passengers. Although automobiles still present mortality and morbidity risk, deaths and injuries have been reduced. Now, there are many types of protective restraints, air bags and a host of other technologically driven safety devices (e.g., lane alert and drowsy driver warning systems, automatic braking mechanisms, backup cameras) to protect drivers from themselves and others. Few could have imagined that the very device that risked accidents someday would include technologies that could protect passengers from accidents. For the most part, these technological advances effectively protect passengers; however, it is important to remember that, under some conditions, the very devices intended to protect people can and have hurt them. For example, although unusual, airbags may cause injury to people, especially young children.

The Internet is similar to primitive automobiles in the sense that the first Internet travelers were, with few exceptions, free to navigate the sites available on the growing World Wide Web largely without restriction. However, as problems have been identified, Internet-related technology is beginning to emerge, just as it did with automobiles, to protect users. Now, for example, we have the ability to set limits on the websites that young people can visit, and biometric identification can help protect security. Nevertheless, aspects of the new technology—features and experiences with which we are unaccustomed—may facilitate excessive and risky use, particularly among early adopters of this technology. Early adopters tend to be willing to take more risks than later adopters. Furthermore, and contrary to Gladwell's popular view (2000) that early adopters of innovative technology take considerable risks, some research suggests that "early adopters act because they see the risks associated with adopting as lower than their nonadopter counterparts, partly because the risks are seen as more manageable. Risk apparently is in the eye of the beholder" (Panzano & Roth, 2006, p. 1159). Whether fueled by straightforward risk-taking or an attenuated perception of risk mixed with technology that is not yet mature, early adoption of technology provides the opportunity for personal and social problems. Furthermore, just as there are criminals and hucksters who prey on others in person, there are those who prey on others through the opportunities provided by new technology (McQuade, 2006; McQuade et al., 2009; McQuade, Gentry, Fisk, et al., 2011). The massive data breach within Target during late 2013 illustrates this duality: the same technology that allowed consumers' stolen financial data to be sold to potential thieves also permitted detection of the data breach and prompted steps to reduce further consumer harm (Krebs, 2013).

Internet Gambling: Games, Gamblers, and Gambling Involvement

As is historically common with the introduction of new technologies in general, the emergence of Internet gambling stimulated concern and predictions of trouble and tragedy. For example, many researchers initially predicted that increased access via online gambling opportunities would lead to increased prevalence of "problem gambling" (e.g., Volberg, 2000). One observer warned that, "These new technologies may provide many people with their first exposure to the world of gambling and could be argued to be more enticing than previous non-technological incarnations" (Griffiths, 1996, p. 473).

It is quite possible that certain Internet-based games are more attractive to certain people, just as certain land-based games are particularly attractive to certain people. However, as we note later, there is little evidence of a universal effect caused by specific games or specific game technology. At a different level of analysis, all gambling involves some kind of technology (e.g., craft, mechanical, technological) to deliver the game—so pitting technology against nontechnology is in some ways a straw man argument. A more useful question is to ask *what kind of technology* and *what are the impacts and effects of this technology on the human condition*? How might the Internet change the emergence, course, and recovery path associated with addiction in general and gambling-related addiction in particular?

Evidence is now available to evaluate the accuracy of some predictions about the effect of Internet gambling technology on individuals and populations. In the United Kingdom, for example, the prevalence of gambling disorder has remained relatively constant despite increased access to Internet gambling (Wardle et al., 2011). The prevalence of gambling disorders has remained relatively stable or declined slightly worldwide since the first studies during the 1970s (e.g., Kallick, Suits, Dielman, & Hybels, 1979). Despite the stability of national prevalence estimates for gambling disorders, some self-report studies (e.g., Griffiths & Barnes, 2008; Ladd & Petry, 2002; Wood & Williams, 2007) suggest higher rates of gambling-related problems among Internet gamblers compared with non-Internet gamblers. Internet gambling might be associated with higher rates of gambling problems; however, to date, these studies do not demonstrate a causal relationship between Internet gambling and gambling-related problems. Characteristics associated with both Internet gambling and elevated rates of gambling-related problems—for example, being young and male—might help account for the high rates found among Internet gamblers (Gainsbury, Russell, Hing, Wood, & Blaszczynski, 2013). Furthermore, cross-sectional surveys are point-in-time estimates that cannot reliably predict cause–effect relationships, and reliance on participant self-report hinders the ability to assess Internet gambling behavior accurately (e.g., Braverman, Tom, & Shaffer, 2014). Taken together, these methodological concerns suggest that any conclusions about Internet gambling rates, gambling problem rates among Internet gamblers, and the causal relationship between Internet gambling and gambling problems are premature (Shaffer, Peller, LaPlante, Nelson, & LaBrie, 2010).

Regarding enticement, there is little evidence that particular games or modes of gambling are universally more seductive than others so long as overall gambling involvement is considered (Halme, 2011; LaPlante, Afifi, & Shaffer, 2013; LaPlante, Nelson, et al., 2013; LaPlante, Nelson, LaBrie, & Shaffer, 2011). Research suggests instead that people who have problems with a particular form of gambling (e.g., slot machines) already are involved in other forms of gambling (Afifi, LaPlante, Taillieu, Dowd, & Shaffer, 2014; LaPlante, Afifi, & Shaffer, 2012; LaPlante, Afifi, et al., 2013; LaPlante, Nelson, et al., 2013; LaPlante et al., 2011). Thus, games that are less commonly played tend to have higher rates of problems associated with them because the people who play them are those who are most involved in gambling in general.

Epidemiologic research consistently reveals that Internet gambling participation is less prevalent than land-based forms of gambling (e.g., Wardle et al., 2011). As early adopters of a new technology, today's Internet gamblers will be different from later adopters; they might be more "serious" about gambling, calculate risk differently, or be more novelty-seeking compared with those who gamble on more common activities or adopt Internet gambling more slowly. It is not surprising, therefore, that people who report gambling on the Internet also report engaging in more forms of gambling and experiencing more gambling-related problems compared to gamblers who do not use the Internet (Gainsbury et al., 2013; Griffiths & Barnes, 2008; Ladd & Petry, 2002). As with other forms of gambling, associations between Internet gambling and elevated problems typically disappear when analyses control for the general level of gambling involvement (Afifi, LaPlante, Taillieu, Dowd, & Shaffer, 2014; LaPlante, Afifi, et al., 2013; LaPlante, Nelson, et al., 2013; LaPlante et al., 2011; Welte, Barnes, Tidwell, & Hoffman, 2009). As a more diverse population begins to engage in Internet gambling, we may expect social learning to expedite adaptation, more effective self-management and regulation, and lower levels of associated problems (LaPlante et al., 2008; LaPlante & Shaffer, 2007; Shaffer, 2005; Shaffer & Martin, 2011; Vaillant, 1977; Zinberg, 1981). As we discuss in the next section, the technology that gave rise to Internet gambling also allows researchers to evaluate this proposition.

The Public Health of Internet Gambling: Scientific Reality

A major methodological limitation plagued initial efforts to evaluate the hypothesis that Internet gambling is associated with more intense betting behavior and increased prevalence of gambling-related problems compared to traditional gambling. As we mentioned earlier, these studies tended to rely on self-reports of gambling behavior, often using associated convenience samples (Cotte & Latour, 2009; Griffiths & Barnes, 2008; Kairouz, Paradis, & Nadeau, 2012; Wood & Williams, 2007; Yani-de-Soriano, Javed, & Yousafzai, 2012). These studies tended to validate concerns about Internet gambling as being particularly dangerous.

During the past several years, at the Division on Addiction and in collaboration with bwin.party digital entertainment, we have used a different approach to evaluate the same proposition. Rather than collecting convenience samples and asking people to recall and describe their Internet gambling behavior, we have examined electronically recorded gambling data (i.e., records of actual gambling) among bwin.party subscribers. This new body of epidemiological evidence reveals that few Internet gamblers are intemperate and that the typical Internet player gambles quite moderately. For instance, one study examining patterns of fixed-odds sports betting found that the typical subscriber placed bets approximately 7 days per month (LaBrie, LaPlante, Nelson, Schumann, & Shaffer, 2007), placing only 2.5 bets per betting day, each worth €4. Further work revealed that bwin.party subscribers who played poker participated in a median of one poker session every 3 days (LaPlante, Kleschinsky, LaBrie, Nelson, & Shaffer, 2009), and those who played casino-style games bet on casino games about once every 2 weeks (LaBrie, Kaplan, LaPlante, Nelson, & Shaffer, 2008).

Other groups have examined electronically recorded betting records provided by bwin.party and other sources (Brosowski, Meyer, & Hayer, 2012) and other operators (Auer & Griffiths, 2012; Dragicevic, Tsogas, & Kudic, 2011; Fiedler, 2012a, 2012b; Gainsbury, Sadeque, Mizerski, & Blaszczynski, 2012; Gainsbury, Wood, Russell, Hing, & Blaszczynski, 2012; Siler, 2010). These studies also support the conclusion that the largest group of subscribers engages in Internet gambling in a way that is more moderate than initially predicted. Overall, despite its youth and the need for more investigation, this body of Internet gambling research seems to contradict the common conjecture that Internet gambling will create a universal public health hazard because Internet gambling offers easier access and riskier structural characteristics (e.g., speed of play, anonymity, privacy) compared with traditional land-based forms of gambling (Reilly & Smith, 2013a).

Although the current evidence suggests that Internet gambling itself does not appear to stimulate intemperate gambling at the population level, because Internet gambling is a relatively new activity, we suggest that a prudent path is to conduct an ongoing review of this matter recognizing the important contribution of temporal events. Contemporary Internet gamblers are early adopters and might not be representative of those who will follow in their footsteps. Furthermore, as with any form of gambling, we should expect a subset of Internet gamblers to gamble more intensely than the rest. Certainly, some Internet gamblers will experience gambling-related problems and be in need of assistance. We review some potential intervention strategies in the next section.

Prevention and Intervention Strategies

Prevention and intervention strategies to help promote healthier Internet gambling can arise from many sources, such as public policy, public health initiatives, corporate responsible gaming programs, awareness campaigns, and more. Although a full review of all these areas is beyond the scope of this chapter, in the following section we review strategies falling into two primary areas: (1) user-initiated strategies, such as self-limitation, and (2) operation-initiated strategies, such as predictive algorithms.

User-initiated strategies involve Internet gambling sites offering tools that allow users, on a voluntary basis, to place limits on their gambling. The most popular user-initiated strategy involve self-limitation—website features that allow users to limit the amount of money they can deposit or amount of time they can play. Self-limitation is not unique to Internet gambling. Electronic gambling machines that work with player cards also can offer self-limitation features. Research focusing on these features is mixed. Most studies find that few people take advantage of self-limitation features (e.g., ~1.2% of bwin.party subscribers, 14.6% of Svenska Spel users: Griffiths, Wood, & Parke, 2009; Nelson et al., 2008). However, this lack of use might reflect the placement and characteristics of the self-limit features as much as their inherent attractiveness to subscribers. Though no research has been done to our knowledge, it is likely that, for example, introducing self-limitation features during subscription to a gambling service would increase their use.

Even if the majority of subscribers to an Internet gambling site do not use self-limitation features, research suggests that self-limitation does have a measureable effect on gambling behavior among those who choose to use it. Studies of land-based self-limitation (i.e., electronic gambling machines) have focused on loss limits and time limits. These studies find that when gamblers are required to use these features (i.e., in laboratory experiments), they appear to be effective in reducing money spent and time played. However, as mentioned earlier, given the choice, few utilize these limit options (see Ladouceur, Blaszczynski, & Lalande, 2012, for a review of this literature). For Internet gambling, studies have examined the effect of deposit limits and time limits on gambling behavior (Auer & Griffiths, 2013; Broda et al., 2008; Nelson et al., 2008). Users of Internet self-limitation features tend to decrease their betting frequency but not the amount they wager per bet (Nelson et al., 2008). These findings suggest that these users, though they are limiting the amount of money available to spend, use this feature to help regulate their gambling involvement. Auer and Griffiths observed a different pattern: they observed that, among highly involved Internet casino gamblers with access to both monetary and time limits, monetary limits appeared to be more effective, leading to decreased theoretical loss among these gamblers (Auer & Griffiths, 2013). Different methodological choices preclude a direct comparison of these two studies, and more research is needed to identify the effects of setting monetary and time limits. Moreover, we need to interpret these findings with caution because, like studies of people seeking treatment (e.g., Berkson, 1946) in general and for gambling problems in particular, these help-seeking samples are not necessarily representative of the broader population. Another common, but more extreme, user-initiated strategy is *self-exclusion*. This tool is also available both at land-based venues and at Internet gambling sites. In some ways, the Internet allows for more strict enforcement of self-exclusion requests. Establishing a new identity under which to subscribe to a site is typically more involved and difficult than sneaking into a casino. Both self-exclusion tools are limited by the fact that gamblers can—and often do—simply access a different gambling venue. This is why self-exclusion programs ought to be considered primarily user-initiated and user-driven. Research confirms that these approaches are less about enforcement and more about providing gamblers with a straightforward way to begin the process of addressing their gambling problems. Research about land-based self-exclusion programs reliably finds that almost all of the people who use these programs are experiencing symptoms of gambling disorder, with some studies finding that almost all self-excluders qualify for the disorder (Gainsbury, 2013; Ladouceur, Jacques, Giroux, Ferland, & Leblond, 2000; Nelson, Kleschinsky, LaBrie, Kaplan, & Shaffer, 2010). This same research also finds that those who self-exclude report positive outcomes after self-exclusion, including lower levels of gambling and gambling problems and higher levels of general well-being (Ladouceur et al., 2000; Nelson et al., 2010). Less research has studied Internet self-exclusion programs. The existing work (Braverman & Shaffer, 2012; LaBrie & Shaffer, 2011) shows that those who self-exclude have higher levels of Internet gambling involvement, defined as losses, time spent gambling, and number of different forms of gambling performed. We know of no studies that have followed Internet self-excluders prospectively to identify longer term outcomes.

One important consideration for Internet gambling self-limitation and self-exclusion features is the permanency of the limit or exclusion. Again, research to date on Internet self-exclusion is scarce, but the extant research finds that, among casino self-excluders, many of those who sign up for a lifetime ban later change their minds and are frustrated by the permanency of the action (Gainsbury, 2013; Nelson et al., 2010). Current thinking about land-based programs is that these bans do not need to be permanent; however, removing oneself from a list ought to be more difficult than enrolling. By this reasoning, some programs require self-excluders to participate in exit interviews or assessments prior to reversing their ban. Similarly, at bwin.party, procedures require cooling off periods prior to changing a self-limit or self-exclusion. Subscribers who wish to reverse a self-exclusion or change a self-limit have to make the request and confirm the request days later. For both types of programs, it makes sense for barriers to be minimal for utilizing the tool but considerable for removing the limit or exclusion.

Operator-initiated strategies can take many forms, from universal deposit limits to targeted and intensive interventions with a small minority of players exhibiting the most extreme signs of a gambling disorder, to the development of algorithms that can target users based on their gambling patterns. Universal limits are sometimes problematic because this approach requires one strategy for everyone. For example, during a window of observation between 2005 and 2007, bwin.party set a single daily and monthly deposit limit for all of its subscribers, and, as we described earlier, bwin.party provided subscribers with the option to set personal limits.

Very few subscribers (i.e., less than 1%) ever reached either the corporate or the personal deposit limits (Broda et al., 2008). It is possible that subscribers controlled their deposits based on their knowledge of the limit. It is also possible that the corporate limit was set sufficiently high so that most people never approached it, whether they were experiencing gambling-related problems or not. Complicating this matter even more, subscribers who did hit the limit reduced their betting (i.e., number of bets per day) but increased the amount they wagered per bet. If bwin.party were to set the deposit limit lower, this might affect the gambling behavior of more people—in an uncertain direction. This strategy also would be indiscriminate. The amount any individual has available to wager is tied to his or her income, lifestyle, and values; the amount and meaning of these funds can vary greatly. Universal time limits offer another option; however, as with other limits, whether the time people spend engaging in gambling is harmful depends on their other obligations and values.

The flipside of these universal interventions are operator-interventions that are triggered only by a select few who undeniably demonstrate that they have a problem with gambling and that operator action is needed. In these cases, the important question is not whether the operator should intervene, but rather how. For example, the operator simply could ban these subscribers from their site. This action might effect positive change for the individual; unfortunately, it also might exacerbate gambling and any related problems. Any intervention of this kind has the potential to produce iatrogenic effects: to annoy or anger subscribers in a way that makes them increase their problematic behavior elsewhere instead of using this opportunity to address their problems. With this type of intervention, exclusion might be necessary, but operators committed to responsible gambling programs need to pair exclusion with other resources that subscribers can use to address their gambling problems—if and when they are ready to do so. Research should examine what types of interventions work and for whom among these severe cases.

Though universal interventions might target too many and intensive interventions might target too few, the holy grail of operator-initiated interventions has become the *predictive algorithm*. In brief, a predictive algorithm approach makes use of behavioral markers (i.e., information from a variety of gambling characteristics available from gambling records) to forecast potential gambling-related problems among Internet gambling subscribers. These algorithms can target subscribers according to their gambling patterns and according to *changes* in their gambling patterns, using this information to designate differing levels of potential risk. Perhaps most importantly, algorithms may provide a guide for matching responses to individuals, thus optimizing the opportunity for favorable outcomes.

For these algorithms, the devil is in the details. Some Internet gambling operators are deploying algorithms that claim to detect problematic gambling despite the absence of rigorous objective evaluation and the resulting scientific guidance that evidence provides. In some cases, there might be no evaluation and little empirical basis; in others, the evaluation and empirical foundation might exist but be kept private, thus reducing the ability of the scientific community to judge the algorithm's merit. To advance a body of science, in our work, we have been transparent about the challenges we face and the variety of methodological and procedural choices available. These challenges and choices include deciding which gambling pattern variables (i.e., potential markers) have the potential for inclusion into the algorithm, what outcomes were used to test marker relevance, how dynamic the algorithm score should be, how that score is used to determine who gets flagged, and what happens once a subscriber is flagged, among many other questions. While addressing these issues, we have been guided by the use of biomarkers in medicine, as discussed next.

Predictive Algorithms: From Biomarkers to Behavioral Markers

The predictive algorithm approach has its roots in medical biomarkers. *Biomarkers* are objectively measured and evaluated characteristics that serve as indicators of normal biologic processes, pathogenic processes, or pharmacologic responses to a therapeutic intervention (Biomarkers Definitions Working Group, 2001; Vanderstichele et al., 2008). In some cases, an underlying physiological process—which can either result from a disease state or contribute to a disease state—produces a change in measurable biological characteristics. In these cases, medical scientists can use biomarkers for early detection of problems, to diagnose diseases, to understand possible risk levels, and to target and evaluate treatments.

One of the most common examples of the use of biomarkers is the detection, diagnosis, and treatment of cancer. In the past, the identification and detection of cancer was only possible via microscopic examination of tumor tissue, long after disease onset; now, it is possible to search for active genes, their respective protein products, and other "molecular signposts" at earlier stages of cancer development (Srinivas, Kramer, & Srivastava, 2001). In other words, biomarkers can make the early detection of cancer possible. Biomarkers also are used to select and manage treatment. In the case of breast and colon cancer, biomarkers have been used to detect the *potential* for disease prior to the emergence of any cancerous cells or before cancer cells have a chance to invade adjacent tissue and establish new colonies (Hamdan, 2007). We now know that certain genes can make people particularly susceptible to certain types of cancer. For example, *BRCA1* is a type of tumor-suppressing gene that can increase risk for breast cancer from about 12% to 60%. Very few women (3–5%) who develop breast cancer have this gene, but those who do have it stand a relatively high chance of developing breast cancer. We are now able to detect this genetic mutation using a blood test, and those who have it can decide to take proactive intervention, such as double mastectomy, to prevent cancer development. The actress Angelina Jolie provides a recent, high-profile example of this approach, which is consistent with a broader trend toward more personalized and preventative medicine (Morrow, Sabatine, & de Lemos, 2008).

Just as biomarkers can provide insight into underlying biological pathology, behavioral markers can provide insight into underlying psychological or cognitive pathology. The use of behavioral markers for detection of Alzheimer's disease (AD) illustrates this relationship. Therapeutic interventions for AD are most effective during the earliest stages of the disease. However, AD begins insidiously, long before people experience symptoms or observers see signs. Consequently, researchers are searching for behavioral markers that reliably signal a form of mild cognitive impairment that often progresses to AD. For instance, a group of Spanish researchers studied a group of participants with mild cognitive impairment who later converted to AD, a group of participants with mild cognitive impairment who did not convert to AD, and cognitively healthy comparison subjects. Particular behavioral markers—including measures of delayed memory and functional activities—supplemented biomarkers to predict whether and how soon participants would develop AD (Gomar et al., 2011). These researchers concluded that developing algorithms that combine biomarkers and behavioral markers provides the best chance of identifying and treating AD during its earliest stages.

Whether researchers are working with biomarkers or behavioral markers, the three-phased process of developing predictive algorithms begins the same, often during an initial pilot study involving the measurement of candidate marker levels within two or more distinct groups (e.g., patients with AD vs. adequate comparison samples; gamblers whose behavior suggests gambling-related problems vs. adequate comparison samples; Vanderstichele et al., 2008). A marked difference between groups in marker levels suggests marker relevance (Vanderstichele et al., 2008). The second phase of marker development involves producing an operational model in the form of a tentative algorithm—for instance, using strategies involving decision trees, discriminant lines, or logistic regression models (Vanderstichele et al., 2008). During this phase, individual target markers are integrated into marker algorithms. This is important because the use of single markers often does not have sufficient accuracy for practical application (Vanderstichele et al., 2008). Integrating clinical data, such as family history and environmental factors, can further improve the accuracy of the emerging algorithm (Morrow et al., 2008). Finally, researchers should establish an estimate of the model's accuracy that is independent of the information used to build the model, often by testing the models' accuracy within an independent sample. Working in an iterative process, researchers can further refine and then test their algorithms until predictive accuracy is high enough to provide clinical utility. In the following section, we describe how we approached these steps during our work developing predictive algorithms for bwin.party.

Case Study: bwin.party Predictive Modeling

As mentioned previously, Internet gambling and the recorded bet patterns it produces provides unique opportunities to detect behavioral markers. The very technology that makes Internet gambling a potential risk allows for the study of—and intervention with—actual real-time gambling behavior.

To test a marker or algorithm, scientists need an outcome. Unfortunately, when dealing with psychological rather than physical conditions, outcomes often are difficult to come by. Though researchers now have access to real-time gambling behavior unbiased by self-report, variables derived from this behavior cannot tell us conclusively whether someone is experiencing a problem. Gambling records can inform us about "excessive" behavior but do not provide the personal context within which that behavior occurs. For example, a subscriber who loses tens of thousands of dollars gambling within a single year might not experience financial consequences, depending on his or her existing financial resources. The absence of a financial means test is an important limitation of current research efforts. No matter how complex or dynamic an algorithm, it is only as valid as the outcome, or criterion, against which it was developed. Unfortunately, the study of Internet gambling rarely provides access to diagnostic measures. Without those—or perhaps even with such data—gambling disorder remains an indeterminate construct, and the validity of measures used to identify it within this field continue to be uncertain.

Our collaboration with bwin.party has produced several proxies for gambling problems. We have used these proxies as outcomes in studies examining gambling behavior among bwin.party subscribers. The first, and in some ways least useful, proxy was membership in the group of most involved subscribers (i.e., in terms of total amount wagered or total bets or total frequency of betting) (e.g., LaBrie et al., 2007, 2008; Nelson et al., 2008). Membership in one of these "Most Involved Bettor" groups was an unsatisfactory outcome for studying gambling disorders because we did not have access to disposable income or other financial obligations and therefore had no index for the financial consequences of gambling. Among the group of subscribers who spent the most money gambling, some might have experienced little or no adverse financial consequences and others spending the same amounts might have been devastated financially. Moreover, we have no indication of the social consequences (e.g., family discord) that might be associated with these more extreme patterns of gambling.

The next set of proxies we were able to obtain, though still suffering from some limitations, was a much better surrogate for gambling problems. This set was derived from bwin.party's responsible gaming features. In different papers, we considered self-limitation, account closure for gambling-related problems, and being flagged by bwin.party as having problems as proxies for gambling-related problems (Gray et al., 2012; Nelson et al., 2008; Xuan & Shaffer, 2009). For these proxies, it was possible that some of the identified subscribers did not suffer from gambling-related problems and quite likely that others not flagged did suffer with gambling-related problems; however, it was very likely that many of those flagged were experiencing gambling problems.

Finally, we were able to survey some of bwin.party's subscribers about problems they might have with gambling. We recruited a random sample of bwin.party subscribers to complete the Brief Biosocial Gambling Screen (BBGS), a three-item screen derived from the DSM-IV criteria for pathological gambling (Gebauer, LaBrie, & Shaffer, 2010). This outcome is the most closely aligned to clinical definitions of gambling disorder, but this survey had a very low (2%) response rate. As a result, we cannot draw conclusions about bwin.party subscribers as a whole from this sample, but we can be relatively confident that those who responded positively to the BBGS items ("BBGS-positive Players") were indeed experiencing at least some level of gambling-related problems.

To begin developing an algorithm, we examined our findings from studies that used proxies and we identified variables that seemed to predict problematic gambling outcomes across proxies (e.g., Braverman, LaPlante, Nelson, & Shaffer, 2013; Braverman & Shaffer, 2012; Broda et al., 2008; Gray et al., 2012; LaBrie et al., 2008; LaBrie & Shaffer, 2011; LaPlante et al., 2009; Nelson et al., 2008; Xuan & Shaffer, 2009). Most of this work has been focused on sports betting. Through this process, we identified six potential markers of excessive Internet gambling behavior: (1) number of bets, (2) wager size, (3) multiple game involvement, (4) frequency of betting, (5) escalating pattern of bets, and (6) variability of wagers. Next, we describe these potential markers in more detail.

NUMBER OF BETS

Across proxies, subscribers who experienced problems made more bets per betting day than other players in the respective samples. For example, players who triggered bwin.party's responsible gambling interventions (i.e., RG Intervention Targets) made, on average, nine live-action sports bets per betting day. Other players in the sample made, on average, only five bets per betting day (Gray et al., 2012). Similarly, subscribers who attempted to exceed corporate deposit limits (i.e., Deposit Limit Exceeders) made many more bets than those who did not (Broda et al., 2008).

WAGER SIZE

In four separate investigations of Deposit Limit Exceeders, RG Intervention Targets, BBGS-positive Players, and subscribers who closed their accounts due to gambling-related problems (i.e., Account Closers), we have observed that players who meet criteria for potential gambling-related problems make bigger sports betting wagers than players who do not meet criteria. This was particularly the case for live-action betting. For example, the median live-action bet size among players in our population study of individuals who subscribed to bwin.party during February 2005 was €4. The comparable value for RG Intervention Targets was €12. Interestingly, we did not find that players who used bwin.party's self-limit features made larger wagers than those who did not. They tended to make smaller, but more frequent bets than other players.

GAME INVOLVEMENT

We have observed that, across all outcomes, those identified as potentially having gambling problems are more likely than others in their respective samples to engage in live-action sports betting (i.e., a more quick-cycling and instantaneous form of betting than traditional fixed odds; instead of betting on game outcomes, subscribers bet on events within games, such as who will score the next goal). More generally, across proxies, players identified by those proxies played a wider variety of games than other players. For instance, on average, players who eventually used self-limit features played 2.5 types of games, compared to an average of 2.1 games for others (Nelson et al., 2008).

FREQUENCY OF BETTING

We have defined frequency as the number of days on which a subscriber places a bet divided by the number of days on which they could have placed a bet (i.e., the duration of their subscription). Across multiple proxies for gambling-related problems, those identified by the proxies tend to gamble more frequently than their respective counterparts. This finding is consistent with the notion that excessive time spent gambling is a behavioral marker of problem and pathological gambling. Surprisingly, however, we observed that Account Closers and RG Intervention Targets have lower frequency values than their counterparts. This is likely accounted for by players with only a day or two of activity. Individuals who play only once during the duration of their subscription necessarily have the maximum possible value for frequency (i.e., 100%); furthermore, this is more likely to occur with controls than with RG Intervention Targets. When we remove subscribers with 1 day of betting activity from the dataset, RG Intervention targets have, on average, higher frequency values than their counterparts (Gray et al., 2012).

ESCALATING PATTERN OF WAGERS

The overwhelming majority of players who subscribe to bwin.party demonstrate a pattern of adaptation (LaPlante & Shaffer, 2007; Shaffer, 2005). This pattern reflects an increase in betting behavior that is followed by a decrease in play patterns as early as during the first month of play (LaPlante et al., 2008). However, adaptation is not uniformly evident among all players. For example, we discovered that, among the Most Involved Bettors, adaptation was generally slower or not apparent (LaPlante et al., 2008). This was especially true when considering live-action betting. Rather than tapering their level of involvement as they adapt to a new gambling opportunity, heavily involved bettors maintain an intense level of play over time, both during the first month of play and during the first 18 months of play. We later discovered the same phenomenon among Account Closers during their first months of play (Braverman & Shaffer, 2012); in other words, those who would go on to close their accounts for gambling-related problems increased their initial rates of play (i.e., failed to demonstrate adaptation) to a greater extent than their counterparts. This finding is consistent with diagnostic criteria for gambling disorder. In particular, according to the American Psychiatric Association (American Psychiatric Association & American Psychiatric Association DSM-5 Task Force, 2013), one criterion associated with gambling disorder involves increasing wager size over time to achieve the desired excitement previously experienced at lower levels of wagering. This process of increasing the "dose" to maintain subjective effects is known as *tolerance.*

VARIABILITY OF WAGERS

Across the array of proxies for gambling problems, we discovered a surprising trend. We observed that wager variability held just as much importance in our analyses as the other proxies. Subscribers who we could classify as having gambling problems evidenced larger day-to-day variation in the amount they wagered compared to other players who were not among the risk groups. Bet-by-bet dynamic systems analyses also showed that unpredictable wagering patterns were associated with problematic play (e.g., Braverman & Shaffer, 2012).

ALGORITHM DEVELOPMENT

To develop an algorithm based on these proxy variables, we chose one sample for development and another for validation. We ran multivariate models predicting BBGS-positive responses among our BBGS sample and then tested the resulting best models on our sample of RG Intervention Targets to ensure accuracy of the algorithm across samples. A model that included bets per day, euros per bet, frequency of wagering, variability of wager amounts, and number of different games played best distinguished subscribers who evidenced gambling problems from those who did not.

Key aspects of a predictive algorithm include how often it can generate flags and how it deals with cumulative data. The utility of the algorithm must not be time-dependent: the algorithm score needs to be valid anytime it is calculated, not just at a given time point. To create an algorithm that could flag individuals whether they had played for 1 month or 3 years, we restricted ourselves to variables that were not time-dependent. In other words, instead of a variable like "total wagered" that differs drastically depending on how long a subscriber has played, we used "average amount wagered per bet." Instead of "total bets," we used bets per day. We also chose to have the algorithm use a subscriber's cumulative betting history to generate scores. An alternative choice would have been to use only the past month or past week to generate the score. We wanted to reduce random fluctuations, so we settled on the cumulative approach.

Another aspect of algorithm development to consider is how early in the development of a gambling problem an algorithm can detect risky play patterns. During our initial developmental work identifying potential risk factors for gambling problems, we examined markers evident during the first month of play that could predict later problems (Braverman & Shaffer, 2012). Based on some of that research and work suggesting that adaptation occurs among most subscribers as early as the first week of play but is absent during that time frame for those who are among the most involved gamblers (LaBrie et al., 2007; LaPlante et al., 2008), we set our algorithm to generate its first flags after only 2 weeks of play. This empirically based decision will have to be evaluated more stringently once we have data from samples flagged by the algorithm.

The next and possibly most important decision in the predictive algorithm process is determining how to use the algorithm score. For our algorithm based mostly on sports betting behavior, the model generates a continuous score by combining the identified markers. To identify individuals in need of intervention, we created cut points above which individuals are flagged and below which they are not. How to establish that score is not at all straightforward. Selecting a higher cut point results in fewer false positives (i.e., fewer people who really do not have problems being told they might have problems) and more false negatives (i.e., more people who do have problems but do not receive flags). Alternatively, selecting a lower cut point results in more false positives and fewer false negatives. These psychometric aspects of the algorithm are referred to as specificity and sensitivity. *Specificity* refers to the proportion of players who do *not* have gambling-related problems being correctly identified as such by the algorithm. An algorithm with 100% specificity would not produce a positive result for any subscriber who does not truly have a gambling-related problem. *Sensitivity* refers to proportion of players *with* gambling-related problems who are identified by the algorithm correctly as such. An algorithm with 100% sensitivity would produce a positive result for every subscriber who has a gambling-related problem. Although it would be very easy to develop an algorithm that categorizes all subscribers as not in need of intervention—in other words, an algorithm with 100% specificity—such an algorithm would have 0% sensitivity and therefore no clinical utility.

To address these tradeoffs, we selected a tiered approach. This allows for targeted interventions that take into account varying levels of sensitivity and specificity. We identified three tiers for our algorithm approach. As Figure 20.1 illustrates, the Tier 1 cut point maximizes sensitivity, identifying approximately 80% of gamblers who are likely to develop problems associated with their gambling. Tier 2 uses a cut point that balances sensitivity and specificity, and Tier 3 identifies only those who are very likely to be experiencing problems. Each tier receives a different level of intervention targeted to the players' level of risk. We are in the process of testing different interventions within each tier to select the most effective messaging.

Once a functioning algorithm exists with selected cut points, bwin.party and other operators should consider larger issues that include ethical concerns. One important overarching concern is the balance between operator-initiated and self-initiated interventions. Operators could use algorithms to make unilateral decisions about subscribers' options, such as excluding them from future play, or they could use them as an opportunity to inform subscribers and provide them with self-initiated options. We support the latter approach for two primary reasons. First, interventions usually are more effective when the individuals to whom they are targeted experience some level of personal association and the opportunity to make decisions (e.g., Gainsbury & Blaszczynski, 2011; Wells-Parker & Williams, 2002). Second, the accuracy of any algorithm is less than 100%. As such, it would be irresponsible and potentially detrimental to force individuals to take certain actions, particularly nonreversible actions, based on data with uncertain confidence. The final sections of this chapter explore in more detail some of the limitations associated with data and the ethical challenges that confront attempts to identify and address potential health risks.

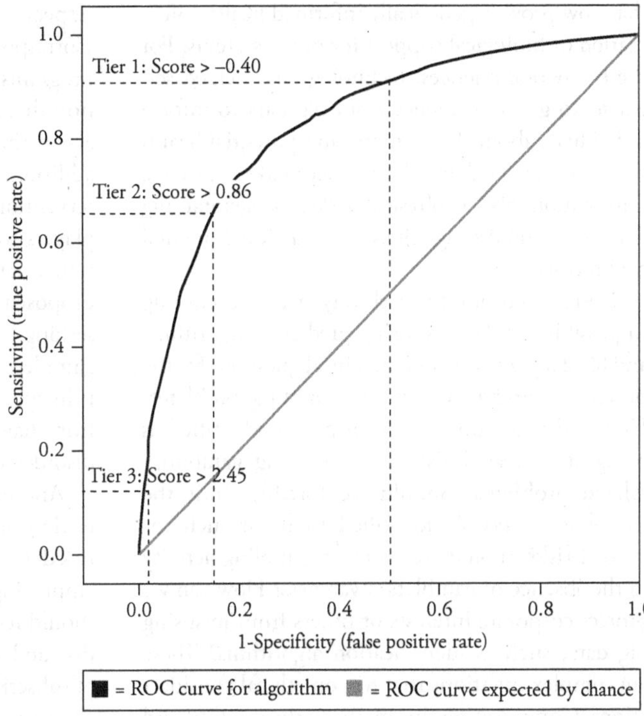

Figure 20.1 Sensitivity and specificity of bwin.party sports betting algorithm, predicting bwin.party RG Intervention Targets. (Area under curve = 0.833.)

Big Data: Considering the Signal and the Noise

Access to the bwin.party gambling records was unprecedented and opened gambling research in new and innovative ways (Shaffer et al., 2010). However, although such datasets provided new answers and a richness of information not easily matched, these and other similar datasets also have important limitations. As technology makes "big data" more widely available to researchers and the general public (e.g., the Transparency Project; http://www.thetransparencyproject.org/), one should be aware of what large datasets can and cannot provide. Nate Silver frames the discussion in this way: "We face danger whenever information growth outpaces our understanding of how to process it. The last forty years of human history imply that it can still take a long time to translate information into useful knowledge, and that if we are not careful, we may take a step back in the meantime" (Silver, 2012, p. 7). Although big data provide new opportunities to pose and answer complex questions about a vast array of phenomena, including human behavior, they also usher in new challenges and pitfalls for those who wade into the data without a map or a guide. As Nate Silver points out, when we look to big data for all of our answers, absent theory and an understanding of our own biases, we are at risk of overinterpretation and misinterpretation.

In addition, big data reflect public health principles: researchers aggregate population-level data largely in an attempt to promote the public health. For example, international teams of researchers are studying human genomes—each one consisting of a billion base pairs of DNA—to combat common human afflictions such as infections, cancer, and noncommunicable diseases. Big data projects hold the promise of yielding algorithms that, in turn, inform small data: information about individual people, collected and interpreted in the service of clinical care. Thanks to big data informing small data, for example, physicians might someday be able to identify specific genetic mutations at the root of each tumor and determine the effectiveness of potential treatments for eliminating those particular cells in different individuals.

As we already have discussed, both big data and public health strategies stimulate ethical concerns that are different from those at the level of small data or individual care. We consider these ethical concerns in the following section.

Ethical Considerations of Big Data and Predictive Modeling for Internet Gambling

As technology advances, new ethical issues confront us. Many of the end-of-life and beginning-of-life questions that currently require attention did not exist before the development of new technologies that now provide genetically informed health information or biological support for organ systems. For the behavioral sciences, technology has helped scientists to garner evidence from big data to inform individuals about their unique and potential health risks (i.e., small data). Just as biomarkers provide information about physical risks, behavioral big data are establishing clues to individual mental health risks.

Despite our ability to classify people according to possible risk factors, using predictive algorithms and big data raises important ethical questions for the prevention and treatment of gambling problems. How and when do we inform people identified as being at increased risk for developing gambling-related problems? Should we forcibly limit the gambling of people identified to be at such increased risk? Should we monitor gambling activity in the absence of gamblers' awareness? How can we protect corporate interests or others from misusing big data, such as identification algorithms? These are complex questions that rest on ethical considerations. Complicating this matter is the political and public policy context within which both the gambling and the programs intended to limit gambling-related problems exist.

There are guidelines for developing responsible gambling programs (Blaszczynski et al., 2011; Blaszczynski, Ladouceur, & Shaffer, 2004). The RENO model and the suggested general principles and minimal requirements resources provide a practical framework for building a responsible gambling initiative. However, higher level ethical principles from the life sciences provide an integrative and broader framework for these issues and can help guide gambling purveyors, consumers, and public policymakers. At a recent Harvard Medical School continuing education conference, Boyd (2013) considered ethical principles for the treatment of addiction in general. Here, we consider the four prima facie ethical principles (Beauchamp & Childress, 1989; Gillon, 1994) that can be used to guide the development of programs and policies designed to promote responsible gambling and to protect players: (1) autonomy, (2) beneficence, (3) non-maleficence, and (4) justice.

Autonomy (i.e., self-rule and the ability to make our own decisions) is a central ethical principle; in addition, we must apply this principle equally to all of those who might be affected by a policy or program (Gillon, 1994). The autonomy principle guides how institutional review boards view, for example, informed consent and confidentiality with respect to both research and treatment. Correspondingly, responsible gambling treatment programs should provide consumers with information that permits them to make informed decisions about their play and their chances of winning. In addition, the autonomy principle suggests that interventions be presented as options, permitting players to choose how to respond to their circumstance rather than be coerced. For example, some proposed self-exclusion programs require that those seeking exclusion identify themselves as a disordered gambler. This requirement violates the autonomy principle to the extent that it prevents self-excluders from having a say in whether they are considered disordered gamblers.

Another thorny issue concerns the routine collection of play pattern data for use in algorithmic risk detection and intervention programs. Operators employing risk detection algorithms often require—should require—subscribers' consent for the collection and analysis of play pattern data as a condition of subscription. One benefit of this strategy is that it allows for analysis of all subscribers' play pattern data, not just those subscribers who, for whatever reason, chose to opt-in to such a program. This circumstance avoids problems associated with self-selection. However, we must consider the possibility that embedding data tracking within the terms and conditions of subscription is inadequate for informed consent and therefore a violation of the autonomy principle.

Gillon suggests that we consider *beneficence* and *non-maleficence* together. That is, in our efforts to be helpful and to do good (i.e., beneficence), we must make every effort to avoid doing harm (i.e., non-maleficence). However, these two principles also need to be considered independently; for example, when we have no obligation of beneficence, we may still have an obligation of non-maleficence (Gillon, 1994). Specifically, as we mentioned, algorithms are not perfect. Therefore, responsible gambling programs should protect players from the limits and inaccuracies associated with algorithms. Furthermore, these programs should consider whether the intervention directly or indirectly might produce harm. For instance, algorithm-driven interventions might annoy subscribers to the point that they choose to play in less safe gambling settings. Depending on the message, interventions intended to reduce harm might stimulate adverse subjective states (e.g., anxiety). Alternatively, unscrupulous operators might create harm by intentionally misusing algorithms. For example, operators nefariously could employ a "harm reduction" program that researchers originally designed for responsibility purposes. Specifically, operators could use such a program to identify and encourage subscribers on the verge of closing their accounts or otherwise limiting their gambling—perhaps due to gambling-related problems—to deploy interventions that prevent such churn and protect potential revenues. In keeping with the spirit of this chapter, we caution that people can use the same technology to help or to hurt. Regulators, researchers, and other public health stakeholders must work with operators to ensure that they use predictive algorithms to minimize potential gambling-related harms.

We do not advocate total reliance on markers. We do encourage integrating behavioral and biological marker data with clinical judgment. For example, an elevated blood concentration of a specific protein has been identified as a biomarker for acute coronary syndrome (ACS); however, this protein also is elevated in clinical settings other than ACS. Therefore, this biomarker fails to demonstrate adequate specificity to be relied upon completely (Morrow et al., 2008). Clinical judgment and first-hand observation help fill the gap.

Justice, or fairness, is the "moral obligation to act on the basis of fair adjudication between competing claims" (Gillon, 1994, p. 185). When the resources are plentiful, it is a relatively simple task to distribute things fairly; however, when resources are scare, then it is more complicated to share resources justly. For responsible gambling programs to be moral, prevention and treatment resources should be available to all players. When these resources are not available for everyone, then the most vulnerable should receive programmatic attention. To assure fairness, we encourage algorithm users to implement tiered responsible gambling programs. For example, the system should gradually become more selective. At the beginning, everyone should have the opportunity to be screened; then, the screening resources become more focused on those identified as at-risk; finally, a responsible gambling system should target more resources for the highest risk players who face the greatest harms.

Some public health workers or policymakers might want to provide some gambling-related interventions for all players, regardless of the presence/absence of a particular gambling disorder marker, if these intercessions have demonstrated safety and efficacy. This strategy is not unlike the suggestion that everyone should be given statins to reduce inflammation regardless of elevated c-reactive proteins (Morrow et al., 2008). However, a shotgun approach will raise many ethical concerns, particularly about the potential adverse effects that such a program might stimulate among those without risk factors for gambling disorder.

Finally, Gillon reminds us that, even when we agree about the ethical principles that form the foundation of gambling treatment and prevention programs, we still might "disagree about their scope of application . . . about to what or to whom we owe these moral obligations." Furthermore, "we clearly do not owe a duty of beneficence to everyone and everything. . . . While we clearly have a prima facie obligation to avoid harming everyone, who and what count as everyone?" (1994, p. 187). There are many such ethical issues that confront marker and algorithm research for Internet gambling. For example, how should players be informed of their marker status to maximize beneficence and limit maleficence? What might players do with this information—both within the gambling setting and the community? What is the responsibility of the gambling purveyor who has identified risk to share such information with a player whether or not they have a program to prevent or alter the course of the risk?

Conclusion

Technology provokes powerful reactions when it is first introduced to society; however, history shows that, although new technologies may provoke powerful changes, they also hold the potential to self-regulate and positively influence changes. It would be premature to make a definitive statement about Internet gambling and its effects at this time. Nevertheless, key stakeholders in the field of gambling studies have learned from previous technological innovations and already are racing to minimize the potential negative impacts of this gambling medium. With more time and additional research, the full impact of the Internet on gambling and society will become clearer. With careful consideration of the risks, benefits, and ethics associated with Internet gambling, it will be possible to strive for the safest possible gambling experience in this milieu.

References

Afifi, T. O., LaPlante, D. A., Taillieu, T. L., Dowd, D., & Shaffer, H. J. (2014). Gambling involvement: Considering frequency of play and the moderating effects of gender and age. *International Journal of Mental Health and Addiction*, *12*(3), 283–294. doi:10.1007/s11469-013-9452-3

Albanese, M., & Shaffer, H. J. (2012). Addiction: The genesis and evolution of an idea and its consequences. In

H. J. Shaffer, D. A. LaPlante, & S. E. Nelson (Eds.), *The American Psychological Association's addiction syndrome handbook* (pp. 3–25). Washington, DC: American Psychological Association.

American Psychiatric Association, & American Psychiatric Association DSM-5 Task Force. (2013). *Diagnostic and statistical manual of mental disorders: DSM-5* (5th ed.). Washington, DC: American Psychiatric Association.

Auer, M., & Griffiths, M. D. (2012). Voluntary limit setting and player choice in most intense online gamblers: An empirical study of gambling behaviour. *Journal of Gambling Studies, 29*(4), 647–660.

Auer, M., & Griffiths, M. D. (2013). Voluntary limit setting and player choice in most intense online gamblers: An empirical study of gambling behaviour. *Journal of Gambling Studies, 29*(4), 647–60. doi:10.1007/s10899-012-9332-y

Beauchamp, T. L., & Childress, J. F. (1989). *Principles of biomedical ethics* (3rd ed.). New York: Oxford University Press.

Berkson, J. (1946). Limitations of the application of fourfold table analysis to hospital data. *Biometrics, 2*, 47–53.

Biomarkers Definitions Working Group. (2001). Biomarkers and surrogate endpoints: Preferred definitions and conceptual framework. *Clinical Pharmacology and Therapeutics, 69*(3), 89–95. doi:10.1067/mcp.2001.113989

Blaszczynski, A., Collins, P., Fong, D., Ladouceur, R., Nower, L., Shaffer, H. J., . . . Venisse, J. L. (2011). Responsible gambling: General principles and minimal requirements. *Journal of Gambling Studies, 27*(4), 565–73.

Blaszczynski, A., Ladouceur, R., & Shaffer, H. J. (2004). A science-based framework for responsible gambling: The Reno model. *Journal of Gambling Studies, 20*(3), 301–17.

Boyd, J. W. (2013). *Substance abuse in healthcare professionals: Ethical and legal considerations.* Paper presented at the Addiction Medicine: A Case-based Approach to Managing Addiction in Special Populations and Related Issues. Revere Hotel, Boston, MA.

Braverman, J., LaPlante, D. A., Nelson, S. E., & Shaffer, H. J. (2013). Using cross-game behavioral markers for early identification of high-risk Internet gamblers. *Psychology of Addictive Behaviors, 27*(3), 868–77. doi:10.1037/a0032818

Braverman, J., & Shaffer, H. J. (2012). How do gamblers start gambling: Identifying behavioral markers for high-risk Internet gambling. *European Journal of Public Health, 22*(2), 273–78.

Braverman, J., Tom, M., & Shaffer, H. J. (2014). Accuracy of self-reported versus actual online gambling wins and losses. *Psychological Assessment, 26*(3), 865–877.

Broda, A., Laplante, D. A., Nelson, S. E., Labrie, R. A., Bosworth, L. B., & Shaffer, H. J. (2008). Virtual harm reduction efforts for Internet gambling: Effects of deposit limits on actual Internet sports gambling behavior. *Harm Reduction Journal, 5*(1), 27.

Brosowski, T., Meyer, G., & Hayer, T. (2012). Analyses of multiple types of online gambling within one provider: An extended evaluation framework of actual online gambling behaviour. *International Gambling Studies, 12*(3), 405–19.

Burns, K., & PBS Online. (2014). *Jazz: A history of America's music: Roaring twenties.* http://www.pbs.org/jazz/time/time_roaring.htm

Cotte, J., & Latour, K. A. (2009). Blackjack in the kitchen: Understanding online versus casino gambling. *Journal of Consumer Research, 35*(5), 742–58. doi:10.1086/592945

Dragicevic, S., Tsogas, G., & Kudic, A. (2011). Analysis of casino online gambling data in relation to behavioural risk markers for high-risk gambling and player protection. *International Gambling Studies, 11*(3), 377–91. doi:10.1080/14459795.2011.629204

Fiedler, I. (2012a). Gamblers' habits: Empirical evidence on the behavior of regulars, newcomers and dropouts. *Journal of Gambling Studies, 29*(2), 289–309. doi:10.1007/s10899-012-9306-0

Fiedler, I. (2012b). The gambling habits of online poker players. *The Journal of Gambling Business and Economics.* http://ssrn.com/abstract=1908161 *or* http://dx.doi.org/10.2139/ssrn.1908161

Gainsbury, S. M. (2013). Review of self-exclusion from gambling venues as an intervention for problem gambling. *Journal of Gambling studies, 30*(2), 229–251. doi:10.1007/s10899-013

Gainsbury, S. M., & Blaszczynski, A. (2011). Online self-guided interventions for the treatment of problem gambling. *International Gambling Studies, 11*(3), 289–308. doi:10.1080/14459795.2011.617764

Gainsbury, S. M., Russell, A., Hing, N., Wood, R., & Blaszczynski, A. (2013). The impact of Internet gambling on gambling problems: A comparison of moderate-risk and problem Internet and non-Internet gamblers. *Psychology of Addictive Behaviors, 27*(4), 1092–1101. doi:10.1037/a0031475

Gainsbury, S. M., Sadeque, S., Mizerski, D., & Blaszczynski, A. (2012). Wagering in Australia: A retrospective behavioural analysis of betting patterns based on player account data. *The Journal of Gambling Business and Economics, 6*(2), 50–68.

Gainsbury, S. M., Wood, R., Russell, A., Hing, N., & Blaszczynski, A. (2012). A digital revolution: Comparison of demographic profiles, attitudes and gambling behavior of Internet and non-Internet gamblers. *Computers in Human Behavior, 28*(4), 1388–98. doi:10.1016/j.chb.2012.02.024

Gebauer, L., LaBrie, R. A., & Shaffer, H. J. (2010). Optimizing DSM IV classification accuracy: A brief bio-social screen for detecting current gambling disorders among gamblers in the general household population. *Canadian Journal of Psychiatry, 55*(2), 82–90.

General Accounting Office. (2002). *Internet gambling: An overview of the issues.* Washington, DC: Author.

Gillon, R. (1994). Medical ethics: Four principles plus attention to scope. *British Medical Journal, 309*(6948), 184.

Gladwell, M. (2000). *The tipping point: How little things can make a big difference* (1st ed.). Boston: Little, Brown.

Gomar, J. J., Bobes-Bascaran, M. T., Conejero-Goldberg, C., Davies, P., Goldberg, T. E., & the Alzheimer's Disease Neuroimaging Initiative. (2011). Utility of combinations of biomarkers, cognitive markers, and risk factors to predict conversion from mild cognitive impairment to Alzheimer disease in patients in the Alzheimer's Disease Neuroimaging Initiative. *Archives of General Psychiatry, 68*(9), 961–9. doi:10.1001/archgenpsychiatry.2011.96

Gray, H. M., LaPlante, D. A., & Shaffer, H. J. (2012). Behavioral characteristics of Internet gamblers who trigger corporate responsible gambling interventions. *Psychology of Addictive Behaviors, 26*(3), 527–35. doi:10.1037/a0028545

Griffiths, M. D. (1996). Gambling on the Internet: A brief note. *Journal of Gambling Studies, 12*, 471–3.

Griffiths, M. D., & Barnes, A. (2008). Internet gambling: An online empirical study among student gamblers. *International Journal of Mental Health and Addiction, 6*, 194–204.

Griffiths, M. D., Wood, R. T. A., & Parke, J. (2009). Social responsibility tools in online gambling: A survey of attitudes and behavior among Internet gamblers. *CyberPsychology & Behavior, 12*(4), 413–21. doi:10.1089/cpb.2009.0062

Halme, J. T. (2011). Overseas Internet poker and problem gambling in Finland 2007: A secondary data analysis of a Finnish population survey. *Nordic Studies on Alcohol and Drugs, 28*(1), 51–63.

Hamdan, M. (2007). Introduction. In *Cancer biomarkers: Analytical techniques for discovery* (pp. xvii–xxiv). Hoboken, NJ: Wiley.

Jones, L. M., Mitchell, K. J., & Finkelhor, D. (2012). Trends in youth internet victimization: Findings from three youth internet safety surveys 2000–2010. *The Journal of Adolescent Health, 50*(2), 179–86. doi:10.1016/j.jadohealth.2011.09.015

Kairouz, S., Paradis, C., & Nadeau, L. (2012). Are online gamblers more at risk than offline gamblers? *CyberPsychology, Behavior & Social Networking, 15*(3), 175–80. doi:10.1089/cyber.2011.0260

Kallick, M., Suits, D., Dielman, T., & Hybels, J. (1979). *A survey of American gambling attitudes and behavior.* Ann Arbor, MI: University of Michigan Press.

Kipnis, D. (1991). The technological perspective. *Psychological Science, 2*(2), 62–69. doi:10.1111/j.1467-9280.1991.tb00101.x

Kraut, R., Kiesler, S., Boneva, B., Cummings, J., Helgeson, V., & Crawford, A. (2002). Internet paradox revisited. *Journal of Social Issues, 58*(1), 49–74.

Kraut, R., Patterson, M., Lundmark, V., Kiesler, S., Mukophadhyay, T., & Scherlis, W. (1998). Internet paradox: A social technology that reduces social involvement and psychological well-being? *American Psychologist, 53*(9), 1017–31.

Krebs, B. (2013). Sources: Target investigating data breach. *KrebsonSecurity.* http://krebsonsecurity.com/2013/12/sources-target-investigating-data-breach/

LaBrie, R. A., Kaplan, S. A., LaPlante, D. A., Nelson, S. E., & Shaffer, H. J. (2008). Inside the virtual casino: A prospective longitudinal study of actual Internet casino gambling. *European Journal of Public Health, 18*(4), 410–6.

LaBrie, R. A., LaPlante, D. A., Nelson, S. E., Schumann, A., & Shaffer, H. J. (2007). Assessing the playing field: A prospective longitudinal study of Internet sports gambling behavior. *Journal of Gambling Studies, 23*(3), 347–62.

LaBrie, R. A., & Shaffer, H. J. (2011). Identifying behavioral markers of disordered Internet sports gambling. *Addiction Research & Theory, 19*(1), 56–65.

Ladd, G. T., & Petry, N. M. (2002). Disordered gambling among university-based medical and dental patients: A focus on Internet gambling. *Psychology of Addictive Behaviors, 16*(1), 76–9.

Ladouceur, R., Blaszczynski, A., & Lalande, D. R. (2012). Pre-commitment in gambling: A review of the empirical evidence. *International Gambling Studies, 12*(2), 215–30. doi:10.1080/14459795.2012.658078

Ladouceur, R., Jacques, C., Giroux, I., Ferland, F., & Leblond, J. (2000). Analysis of a casino's self-exclusion program. *Journal of Gambling Studies, 16*(4), 453–60.

LaPlante, D. A. (2012). Technology and its relationship to the addiction syndrome. In H. J. Shaffer, D. A. LaPlante, & S. E. Nelson (Eds.), *The APA addiction syndrome handbook: Vol. 2. Recovery, prevention, and other issues* (pp. 273–96). Washington, DC: American Psychological Association.

LaPlante, D. A., Afifi, T. O., & Shaffer, H. J. (2012). Games and gambling involvement among casino patrons. *Journal of Gambling Studies, 29*(2), 191–203. doi:10.1007/s10899-012-9307-z

LaPlante, D. A., Afifi, T. O., & Shaffer, H. J. (2013). Games and gambling involvement among casino patrons. *Journal of Gambling Studies, 29,* 191–203. doi:10.1007/s10899-012-9307-z

LaPlante, D. A., Kleschinsky, J. H., LaBrie, R. A., Nelson, S. E., & Shaffer, H. J. (2009). Sitting at the virtual poker table: A prospective epidemiological study of actual Internet poker gambling behavior. *Computers in Human Behavior, 25*(3), 711–7.

LaPlante, D. A., Nelson, S. E., & Gray, H. M. (2013). Breadth and depth involvement: Understanding Internet gambling involvement and its relationship to gambling problems. *Psychology of Addictive Behaviors, 28*(2), 396–403. doi:10.1037/a0033810

LaPlante, D. A., Nelson, S. E., LaBrie, R. A., & Shaffer, H. J. (2011). Disordered gambling, type of gambling, and gambling involvement in the British Gambling Prevalence Survey 2007. *European Journal of Public Health, 21*(4), 532–7.

LaPlante, D. A., Schumann, A., Labrie, R. A., & Shaffer, H. J. (2008). Population trends in Internet sports gambling. *Computers in Human Behavior, 24,* 2399–414.

LaPlante, D. A., & Shaffer, H. J. (2007). Understanding the influence of gambling opportunities: Expanding exposure models to include adaptation. *The American Journal of Orthopsychiatry, 77*(4), 616–23. doi:10.1037/0002-9432.77.4.616

Linden, D. J. (2011). *The compass of pleasure: How our brains make fatty foods, orgasm, exercise, marijuana, generosity, vodka, learning, and gambling feel so good.* New York: Viking.

McLuhan, M. (1964). *Understanding media: The extensions of man* (1st ed.). New York: McGraw-Hill.

McLuhan, M., & Powers, B. R. (1989). *The global village: Transformations in world life and media in the 21st century.* New York: Oxford University Press.

McQuade, S. C. (2006). *Understanding and managing cybercrime.* Boston: Pearson/Allyn and Bacon.

McQuade, S. C., Colt, J. P., & Meyer, N. B. B. (2009). *Cyber bullying: Protecting kids and adults from online bullies.* Westport, CT: Praeger.

McQuade, S. C., Gentry, S., Colt, J. P., & Rogers, M. K. (2011). *Internet addiction and online gaming.* New York: Chelsea House.

McQuade, S. C., Gentry, S., Fisk, N. W., & Rogers, M. K. (2011). *Cyberstalking and cyberbullying.* New York: Chelsea House, an Infobase Learning Company.

Mitchell, K. J., & Ybarra, M. L. (2007). Online behavior of youth who engage in self-harm provides clues for preventive intervention. *Preventive Medicine, 45*(5), 392–96. doi:10.1016/j.ypmed.2007.05.008

Morrow, D. A., Sabatine, M. S., & de Lemos, J. A. (2008). Moving toward personalized medicine. In J. A. de Lemos (Ed.), *Biomarkers in heart disease* (pp.207–288, 1st ed.). Dallas, TX: American Heart Association.

Nelson, S. E., Kleschinsky, J. H., LaBrie, R. A., Kaplan, S., & Shaffer, H. J. (2010). One decade of self-exclusion: Missouri casino self-excluders four to ten years after enrollment. *Journal of Gambling Studies, 26*(1), 129–44.

Nelson, S. E., Laplante, D. A., Peller, A. J., Schumann, A., Labrie, R. A., & Shaffer, H. J. (2008). Real limits in the virtual world: Self-limiting behavior of Internet gamblers.

Journal of Gambling Studies, 24(4), 463–77. doi:10.1007/s10899-008-9106-8

Panzano, P. C., & Roth, D. (2006). The decision to adopt evidence-based and other innovative mental health practices: Risky business? *Psychiatric Services, 57*(8), 1153–61. doi:10.1176/appi.ps.57.8.1153

Reilly, C., & Smith, N. (2013a). *Internet gambling: An emerging field of research* (pp. 1–5). Washington, DC: National Center for Responsible Gaming.

Reilly, C., & Smith, N. (2013b). *Internet gambling: An emerging field of research* (pp. 1–5). http://www.ncrg.org/resources/white-papers

Shaffer, H. J. (2005). From disabling to enabling the public interest: Natural transitions from gambling exposure to adaptation and self-regulation. *Addiction, 100*(9), 1227–30; discussion 1235.

Shaffer, H. J., & Martin, R. (2011). Disordered gambling: Etiology, trajectory, and clinical considerations. *Annual Review of Clinical Psychology, 7*(April), 483–510. doi:10.1146/annurev-clinpsy-040510-143928

Shaffer, H. J., Peller, A. J., LaPlante, D. A., Nelson, S. E., & LaBrie, R. A. (2010). Toward a paradigm shift in Internet gambling research: From opinion and self-report to actual behavior. *Addiction Research & Theory, 18*(3), 270–83.

Shapiro, D. (1965). *Neurotic styles*. New York: Basic.

Shotton, M. A. (1991). The costs and benefits of "computer addiction." *Behaviour and Information Technology, 10*(3), 219–30.

Siler, K. (2010). Social and psychological challenges of poker. *Journal of Gambling Studies, 26*(3), 401–20. doi:10.1007/s10899-009-9168-2

Silver, G. (Ed.). (1979). *The dope chronicles: 1850–1950.* San Francisco: Harper & Row.

Silver, N. (2012). *The signal and the noise: Why so many predictions fail—but some don't.* New York: Penguin.

Srinivas, P. R., Kramer, B. S., & Srivastava, S. (2001). Trends in biomarker research for cancer detection. *Lancet Oncology, 2*(11), 698–704.

Thompson, C. (2013). *Smarter than you think: How technology is changing our minds for the better.* New York: Penguin.

Vaillant, G. E. (1977). *Adaptation to life* (1st ed.). Boston: Little Brown.

Vanderstichele, H., De Meyer, G., Shapiro, F., Engelborghs, S., De Deyn, P. P., Shaw, L. M., & Trojanowski, J. Q. (2008). Alzheimer's disease biomarkers: From concept to clinical utility. In D. Galimberti & E. Scarpini (Eds.), *Biomakers for early diagnosis for Alzheimer's disease* (pp. 81–122). New York: Nova Science.

Volberg, R. A. (2000). The future of gambling in the United Kingdom: Increasing access creates more problem gamblers. *British Medical Journal, 320*(7249), 1556.

Wardle, H., Moody, A., Spence, S., Orford, J., Volberg, R., Jotangia, D., . . . Dobbie, F. (2011). *British gambling prevalence survey 2010.* London: National Centre for Social Research.

Wells-Parker, E., & Williams, M. (2002). Enhancing the effectiveness of traditional interventions with drinking drivers by adding brief individual intervention components. *Journal of Studies on Alcohol, 63*(6), 655–64.

Welte, J. W., Barnes, Grace M, Tidwell, Marie Cecile, & Hoffman, Joseph H. (2009). The association of form of gambling with problem gambling among American youth. *Psychology of Addictive Behaviors, 23*(1), 105–12. doi:10.1037/a0013536

Wolak, J., Finkelhor, D., & Mitchell, K. (2004). Internet-initiated sex crimes against minors: Implications for prevention based on findings from a national study. *The Journal of Adolescent Health, 35*(5), 424.e411–20. doi:10.1016/j.jadohealth.2004.05.006

Wood, R. T., & Williams, R. J. (2007). Problem gambling on the internet: Implications for Internet gambling policy in North America. *New Media & Society, 9*(3), 520–42. doi:10.1177/1461444807076987

Xuan, Z., & Shaffer, H. J. (2009). How do gamblers end gambling: Longitudinal analysis of Internet gambling behaviors prior to account closure due to gambling related problems. *Journal of Gambling Studies, 25*(2), 239–52. doi:10.1007/s10899-009-9118-z

Yani-de-Soriano, M., Javed, U., & Yousafzai, S. (2012). Can an industry be socially responsible if its products harm consumers? The case of online gambling. *Journal of Business Ethics, 110*(4), 481–97. doi:10.1007/s10551-012-1495-z

Ybarra, M. L., Mitchell, K. J., Wolak, J., & Finkelhor, D. (2006). Examining characteristics and associated distress related to Internet harassment: Findings from the Second Youth Internet Safety Survey. *Pediatrics, 118*(4), e1169–77. doi:10.1542/peds.2006-0815

Zinberg, N. E. (1981). High states: A beginning study. In H. J. Shaffer & M. E. Burglass (Eds.), *Classic contributions in the addictions* (pp. 241–76). New York: Brunner/Mazel.

CHAPTER

21 Digital Technologies and Sex

Internet and Smartphone Influences on Pornography Viewing and Other Sexual Behaviors

Shane W. Kraus *and* Marc N. Potenza

Abstract

The Internet has revolutionized the way in which we consume and participate in sexual activities. Digital technologies are shaping the ways in which people interact with one another romantically and sexually. This chapter reviews some of the ways in which digital technologies are potentially shaping sexual behaviors, especially those of adolescents and young adults. Evidence suggests that technologies are facilitating increasingly more sexual activities among young people and adults, yet our understanding of these remains incomplete. The Internet has made pornography highly accessible to most individuals around the world, but the effects of frequent pornography use on individuals' sexual beliefs and practices remain largely unknown. Sexting is also common among adolescents and adults, with some initial evidence finding that sexting was a partial mediator between problematic alcohol use and sexual hookups. More work on sexting behaviors is needed, particularly among vulnerable populations or groups at risk for exploitation. The wide use of smartphone applications designed to help users find casual sex partners are becoming more common, mirroring the increasing acceptability of having relationally uncommitted sex among young adults. More research is needed to investigate the influences of digital technologies on shaping the sexual practices of adolescents and emerging adults who may be spending increasingly more time online. Furthermore, more research is needed to examine both the potential benefits and risks associated with digital technologies that may facilitate sexual behaviors.

Keywords: Digital technologies, sex, pornography, smartphones, hookups, casual sex

The Internet has revolutionized the way in which people disseminate and use information. In the United States, Internet use rapidly expanded from 14% in 1995 to 87% in 2014 (Fox & Rainie, 2014). The usage of mobile cellular devices has demonstrated a similar pattern. As of 2014, an estimated 90% of American adults own a cell phone, 58% of which have Internet capabilities (Fox & Rainie, 2014). These days, people use the Internet for many purposes, including viewing of pornography (often termed "sexually explicit material"). By 2018, 95% of teenagers have access to a smartphone, and 45% reported they are online "almost constantly" (Anderson & Jiang, 2018). Approximately 78% of young adults (aged 18–24) use Snapchat and three-fourths (71%) visit social media platforms multiple times a day (Smith & Anderson, 2018). With few exceptions, Internet pornography is available to most users around the world and has become the primary means by which most individuals' access and/or share sexually explicit material (e.g., photos, web videos, erotic stories). Mobile pornography use is also increasing given the number of free and/or low-cost smartphone applications that allow users to access their preferred type of pornography while on the go and from the convenience of their private phone.

Given the rapid Internet-related technological advances that have occurred over the past two decades, societies around the world are witnessing a major behavioral shift in how people communicate with one another. Online social networking sites (e.g., Facebook, Instagram, Pinterest, Twitter, etc.) are now widely used by billions of people across the globe.

These websites allow users to build social networks and/or social relations among people who share interests, activities, and/or real-life connections. Many of these social networking sites also can be accessed from a smartphone which allows users to display their geographic location when posting or sharing status updates or photos to those listed within their social community. Given that sexual behaviors appear to be shifting as a function of recent technological advances made within the past 20 years, researchers have also started to study how geosocial networking smartphone applications (e.g., Grindr, Tinder, Bubble, OkCupid) are being used to mediate casual sex ("hookups") interactions among adolescents, men who have sex with men (MSM), and heterosexual adults. This chapter discusses some of the potential negative impacts of computer-mediated sexual behaviors among adolescents and young adults.

Internet Pornography: Sex at Your Fingertips

The Internet has transformed how people access and share pornographic material. Although definitions vary by author, pornography is typically defined as material intended to produce sexual arousal or sexual excitement in the consumer. In general, males, more so than females, report using pornography for solitary masturbation. Couples' use of pornography appears to occur less frequently; however, some couples do use pornography as a means of enhancing their sexual intimacy (Maddox, Rhoades, & Markman, 2011). Prior to the 1990s, the ease of obtaining pornography varied greatly depending on the content of the material, geographic location of the user, and laws prohibiting or restricting its sale. Recreational users of pornography often needed to visit adult bookstores, send away for materials via the postal service (i.e., getting mail delivered to the house in a "black or brown envelope"), or visit adult movie theatres. Each of these behaviors carries risks of exposing one's anonymity and private sexual practices to the public. However, beginning in the mid-1990s, Internet access began finding its way into the private homes of people, and pornography could be viewed from behind closed doors. The rapid growth of Internet pornography was most likely attributed to three significant factors: accessibility, affordability, and anonymity (Cooper, Delmonico, & Burg, 2000). In addition, the surge of Internet pornography more recently is likely attributable to the tens of thousands of websites offering free sexually explicit material (sometimes referred to as "adult-only tube sites," e.g., PornoTube, RedTube, You-Porn, Xhamster) available on the Internet (Wallace, 2011).

It is unclear how many people in the world use pornography regularly. While the exact prevalence of pornography use remains unclear, daily visits to pornographic websites are projected to be in the millions. A recent study evaluated data collected from the General Social Survey (GSS) over a 40-year period (1973–2012) and examined changes in attitudes toward pornography viewing and consumption behaviors among American young adults. Overall, they found that pornography viewing was increasing across birth generations. Specifically, 61% of young men (18–26 years old) and 36% of young women (18–26 years old) reported past year use of pornography (Price, Patterson, Regnerus, & Walley, 2016). Obtaining accurate prevalence estimates on pornography use poses a unique set of challenges for social scientists and policy lawmakers, both of whom may be interested in understanding the effects of pornography use on the sexual practices of its viewership. Data drawn from survey-based studies suggest pornography use is common among adolescents and young adults, but not completely absent from middle-aged and older adults. Although some older adults express concerns about declining sexual functioning as they age, many older adults remain sexually active (Lindau et al., 2007; Træen et al., 2018). A major limitation of the current literature is that it has focused primarily on studying the effects of pornography use among adolescents and young adults and sidestepped questions about middle-aged and older adults. Rates of pornography viewing among older men (ages 54–62 years old) have increased from 13.6% between 1973 and 1980 to 22.5% in 2008–2012, although rates for older women (54–62 years old) have remained stable (6.5%, 1973–1980 to 7.2%, 2008–2012) (Price et al., 2016). Research examining pornography use, which could include problematic pornography use, among older adults remains understudied.

Although both men and women view pornography, research suggests men are exposed to pornography at an earlier age, become more physiologically aroused when watching pornography, and are more likely to masturbate to pornography regularly (Hald, 2006; Hald & Malamuth, 2008; Kraus & Rosenberg, 2014; Morgan, 2011; Paul, 2009). As one example, one study (Sabina, Wolak, & Finkelhor, 2008) surveyed 563 college students and found that average age for first exposure to pornography for males and females was around 14 years of age. However, recent evidence suggests that age for first exposure to pornography may be on the decline for some adolescents, particularly for males, who are more likely to seek and view pornography during early adolescence (Beyens, Vandenbosch, & Eggermont, 2014; Gola, Lewczuk, &Skorko, 2016). For example, one study (Beyens et al., 2014) found that boys with an advanced pubertal stage and boys high in sensation-seeking used Internet pornography more frequently than did boys in less advanced stages of development or boys with lower levels of sensation-seeking.

Other researchers (Kraus & Rosenberg, 2014; Sinković, Štulhofer, & Božić, 2013) have found that the mean age for first exposure to Internet pornography for males was closer to 11–12 years of age. This lower age of first exposure to pornography (and presumably at an age when boys first masturbate to pornography) may be due, in part, to the increased availability of Internet access occurring in the United States and around the world. One US study found that less than half of the youth (10–17 years of age) surveyed had Internet-blocking and/or Internet-monitoring software installed on their home computers (Ybarra, Finkelhor, Mitchell, & Wolak, 2009). Currently, there exist little data on the prevalence and use of Internet-blocking and/or Internet-monitoring software programs being used on home computers to block sexually explicit materials from children and adolescents. Moreover, each year, the number of children who own a smartphone with Internet capabilities increases, and it is unknown what proportion of these children and adolescents are using their mobile devices to access pornography without their parents/guardians knowledge. As one example, a large study of Flemish teenagers (Vanden Abeele, Campbell, Eggermont, & Roe, 2014) found that 9% of teenagers viewed mobile pornography. Boys (13.9%), more so than girls (3.4%), were more likely to use their smartphone to access pornography. A recent review of 20 years of research on adolescents' pornography use found that prevalence rates vary greatly by country but, in general, adolescents' pornography users are male, sensation-seeking at a more advanced pubertal state with weak or strained family relationships (Peter & Valkenburg, 2016).

Obtaining reliable prevalence estimates of Internet pornography use and other online sexual behaviors is currently lacking in the field. Only a few studies have examined the prevalence of pornography use, with two studies assessing use in large samples of Swedish adolescents (Svedin, Åkerman, & Priebe, 2011) and US adult males (Wright, 2013). Survey data from a nationally representative study of 2,075 US adults indicated that roughly half of the participants reported lifetime pornography viewing. Among men and women with reported lifetime pornography viewing history (n = 1,461), 70% of men and 33% of women reported past-year pornography use. Among past year users of pornography, 47% of men and 16% of women reported at least monthly pornography use (Grubbs, Kraus, & Perry, 2018). Given the existing literature, researchers sometimes extrapolate prevalence estimates from studies utilizing convenience samples collected mostly from university and community members, and this process has significant limitations (e.g., selection bias; limited generalizability due to lack of cultural, sexual, and ethnic diversity; issues with sampling methods). Despite these limitations, data drawn from multiple studies (see Table 21.1) suggest that Internet pornography use is relatively more common among males than females, regardless of age, ethnicity, and country of origin. In the future, the adoption of population-based epidemiological approaches aimed at assessing the prevalence of Internet pornography and problems associated with problematic use would aid in the development and evaluation of treatment approaches for individuals requiring professional assistance.

Associations Between Mental Health Outcomes and Frequency of Pornography Use

Despite evidence suggesting that pornography use may be nonproblematic for many users and could possibly have benefits as a sexual outlet (e.g., sexual aid, educational tool used to acquire sexual health information about sexually transmitted infections), research indicates that a smaller subset of users develop difficulty moderating their use of pornography, which, in turn, is associated with negative mental health outcomes. Several studies have examined the correlates of excessive use of pornography and its associations with psychosocial and/or psychological distress (Kor et al., 2014; Kraus, Potenza, Martino, & Grant, 2015; Ross, Mansson, & Daneback, 2012). Data drawn from a US nationally representative sample of 2,075 Internet users recently found that 11% of men and 3% of women reported "feeling addicted to pornography" (Grubbs, Kraus et al., 2019). Study findings suggest that reports of more frequent pornography use are positively associated with feelings of loneliness (Yoder, Virden, & Amin, 2005), increased psycho-

Table 21.1 Proportions of adolescents and adults' reported pornography use

Sample	Authors	Country	Duration	*N*	Prevalence estimates (%)
Adults:	Baćak a & Štulhofer (2011)	Croatia	1 year	416	Female (34.2)
	Carroll et al. (2008)	United States	Weekly	813	Male (48.4), Female (3.2)
	Chi et al. (2012)	China	1 year	1,403	Male (86.2), Female (15.6)
	Gordon & Kraus (2010)	United States	Lifetime	264	Male (98.2), Female (69.3)
	Grubbs et al. (2019)	United States	1 year	1461	Male (70), Female (33)
	Hald & Malamuth (2008)	Denmark	Lifetime	688	Male (97.8), Female (79.5)
	Lam & Chan (2007)	China	Lifetime	229	Male (93)
	Morgan (2011)	United States	Six months	782	Male (78.8), Female (30.9)
	Regnerus, Gordon, & Price 2016	United States	Past week	5165	Male (46), Female (16)
	Rosser et al. (2013)	United States	90 days	1,391	Male (98.5)
	Shaughnessy et al. (2011)	Canadian	30 days	217	Male (83.3), Female (30.8)
	Sun et al. (2016)	United States	Weekly	487	Male (58.7)
	Wright (2013)	United States	1 year	14,193	Male (36)
Adolescents:	Braun-Courville & Rojas (2009)	United States	Lifetime	433	Male (85.7), Female (50.1)
	Luder et al. (2011)	Switzerland	30 days	6,054	Male (29.2), Female (1.4)
	O'Sullivan (2014)	Canadian	Lifetime	269	Male (84.4), Female (46.4)
	Ševčíková & Daneback (2014)	Czech	Lifetime	2,950	Male (61.8), Female (52.6)
	Svedin et al. (2011)	Sweden	Weekly	4,026	Male (28.6). Female (1.5)

pathology (Kor et al., 2014; Reid, Carpenter, & Lloyd, 2009; Ross et al., 2012; Twohig & Crosby, 2010), narcissism (Kasper, Short, & Milam, 2014), and impulsivity, risk-taking, and sensation-seeking (Chen et al., 2018; Wetterneck, Burgess, Short, Smith, & Cervantes, 2012).

Some evidence also indicates that higher levels of pornography use are associated with lower levels of relationship commitment, sexual satisfaction, and relational aggression among heterosexual couples (Doran & Price, 2014; Lambert, Negash, Stillman, Olmstead, & Ficham, 2012; Poulsen, Busby, & Galovan, 2013; Willoughby, Carroll, Busby, & Brown, 2016; Willoughby & Leonhardt, 2020). Specifically, both quantitative and qualitative studies posit that Internet pornography use by a partner can be problematic to romantic relationships (Ayres & Haddock, 2009; Manning, 2006), in part because it may impair healthy attachment and trust in adult pair-bond relationships (Willoughby et al., 2016). As one example, researchers (Maddox, 2011) examined associations between pornography use and relationship functioning in a random sample of 1,300 unmarried couples. They found that individuals who viewed pornography with their partner reported levels of higher dedication and sexual satisfaction than individuals who viewed pornography alone. Individuals who never viewed pornography reported the highest levels of relationship quality and lowest levels of infidelity. Another study (Doran & Price, 2014) using data on 20,000 ever-married US adults collected during 1973–2010 found males' use of pornography reduced the positive relationship between frequency of sex and happiness. Their findings also suggested that the negative relationship between pornography use and marital well-being continued to grow stronger over time, which they posited could be related to the increased accessibility to pornography occurring within the United States. However, this hypothesis awaits further research.

Among conservative Christian men, pornography use is associated with poor mental health outcome (e.g., depression, anxiety), perhaps because the behavior conflicts with individuals' intrinsic religious beliefs about moral behavior within church-abiding members (Grubbs, Sessoms, Wheeler, & Volk, 2010; Grubbs, Volk, Exline, & Pargament, 2015; Nelson, Padilla-Walker, & Carroll, 2010). For example, for some Christian men, pornography use may be ego-dystonic, thus reflected by an increase in self-reported mental health problems coupled with strong feelings of guilt and shame (Wilt, Cooper, Grubbs, Exline, & Pargament, 2016). Additional research examining the correlates of mental health, religiosity, and pornography are needed given some current gaps in understanding. More research is needed to examine the relationship between mental health outcomes and pornography use among individuals with different (i.e., non-Christian) faith perspectives, including among individuals reporting moral incongruence related to their pornography use (Grubbs, Perry, Wilt, & Reid, 2019). The existing research on mental health functioning among religious individuals has relied primarily on individuals who self-identify as Christian.

Developmental considerations regarding exposure to pornography also warrant consideration. Youth exposure may alter sexual arousal templates and lead to unrealistic expectations about dyadic sexual behaviors, and individuals have advocated for stronger legislation to help protect youth from exposure to pornography (Binford, 2018). There exist reports of pornography leading to erectile dysfunction, with self-help groups (e.g., No Fap) available for young men to cease pornography viewing (NoFap.com, 2017; Reboot Nation, 2017). Additional longitudinal studies are needed to examine these and other potential outcomes related to pornography use.

Despite the body of correlational studies examining the relationship between pornography use and negative mental health outcomes (e.g., depression, generalized anxiety), correlational research does not answer questions related to causation or explain the directionality of associations. For instance, it is unclear whether regular or even heavy pornography use may cause psychological distress, if individuals experiencing mental health problems may be more likely to have difficulty controlling their behavior because they are using pornography consumption as a means to cope with negative emotional states or stress, or if other options exist (e.g., a common feature leading to the development of psychopathology and viewing of pornography). Additional research using naturalistic longitudinal study designs would be useful in better understanding the effects and consequences of using pornography across the life span.

Pornography Use and Casual Sex

The phenomenon of having casual sex (i.e., "one-night stands" or "hookups") is not new. However, there is some evidence that hookups are becoming increasingly more deep-seated in popular culture, reflecting both evolving sexual preferences and altered social and sexual scripts (Garcia, Reiber, Massey, & Merriwether, 2012). Some data suggest that hookup behaviors (e.g., kissing, oral sex, and penetrative anal and vaginal intercourse) are becoming progressively normative among US adolescents and young adults, reflecting more accepting attitudes toward relationally uncommitted sex. Given some of the health risks associated with having unprotected sex, researchers are studying the behaviors of and reasons for having casual sex and its associated risks for adolescents and young adults. For instance, researchers (Grello, Welsh, & Harper, 2006) investigating the circumstances associated with casual sex among university students found that casual sex occurs more commonly between "friends" than strangers, and people are more likely to have one night stands when they have been drinking or using drugs. In their survey they found that men (52%), more so than women (36%) reported having engaged in casual sex. They also found that among women, but not men, casual sex was associated with depressive symptoms. Another study (Eisenberg, Ackard, Resnick, & Neumark-Sztainer, 2009) found one-fifth of sexually active adults surveyed indicated their most recent sexual partner was a casual partner (29% males, 14% females). Additionally, they found no significant associations between partner type and psychological well-being (e.g., body satisfaction, self-esteem, depressive symptoms, and suicidal ideation) as a function of partner type (i.e., casual, committed). A recent study of college-aged students found a greater proportion of men (18.6%) compared to women (7.4%) reported having had causal sex in the past 30 days. Regardless of gender, casual sex was negatively associated with well-being (e.g., self-esteem, life satisfaction) and positively correlated with psychological distress (e.g., general anxiety, social anxiety, and depression) (Bersamin et al., 2014).

Although hookup behaviors are not new, the methods for how people are finding causal sex partners are changing. People are using technology to meet others for sex, and some researchers are particularly interested in understanding what influence, if any, that pornography viewing has on young adults' sexual behaviors. Specifically, researchers are studying the associations between frequency of pornography use and engaging in risky sexual behaviors (e.g., condomless anal or vaginal sex, frequent multiple sexual partners) among adolescents, MSM, and young adults (Braithwaite, Coulson, Keddington, & Fincham, 2015; Braun-Courville & Rojas, 2009; Willoughby et al., 2014; Wright & Randall, 2012). Some researchers have proposed that pornography teaches its viewers "sexual scripts" about how to interact with other partners. According to Gagnon and Simon (2017), sexual scripts are socially constructed and influenced by societal norms and mass media in addition to one's own personal experiences, values, and preexisting attitudes. That is, sexual media potentially influence their viewers through acquisition of behavioral scripts, followed by activation and application of those scripts to everyday life (Wright, 2011). As one example, researchers (Braithwaite et al., 2015) examined the relationship between pornography use and risky sexual behavior among emerging adults in college. They found more frequent viewing of pornography was associated with a higher likelihood of hooking up and a higher number of unique hookup partners. Using both cross-sectional and longitudinal approaches that accounted for the stability of hookups over the course of an academic semester, Braithwaite and colleagues found more frequent viewing of pornography was associated with having had more previous sexual partners of all types, one-night stands, and plans to have a higher number of sexual partners in the future. They also found evidence that more permissive sexual scripts mediated the association between more frequent pornography viewing and hooking up.

Similarly, researchers (Sun, Bridges, Johnason, & Ezzell, 2016) examined the role pornography plays during dyadic sexual encounters and its associations with heterosexual men's intimacy and sexual concerns. Specifically, they found that higher levels of pornography use were associated with requests by males for their partners to perform specific sex acts commonly depicted in pornography, needing to conjure pornographic images in one's mind during sex to maintain arousal, and having concerns over one's own sexual performance and body image. Additionally, they found that higher pornography use was negatively associated with enjoying actual sex with a female partner. The authors posited that pornography provides a powerful heuristic model which could be potentially altering men's expectations and behaviors during real-life sexual encounters with female partners.

Smartphones, Sexting, and Hooking Up

Prior to the Internet, people generally met potential casual sex partners through face-to-face encounters at parties, bars, clubs, social events, etc. Today, however, people are using the Internet to find casual sex partners. Smartphone applications with customizable profiles allow users to highlight the attributes (e.g. height, weight, hair color, body type, sexual preferences, penis size, chest size, etc.) they feel are most desirable. The applications may also provide their geographic location for those interested in meeting in person for sex. In recent years, the development of smartphone applications designed to facilitate casual sex has increased as their popularity continues to rise. These smartphone applications are designed for use by non-heterosexual (e.g., Grindr, FindFred, Scruff, Skout, Hornet, etc.) and heterosexual (e.g., Tinder, Pure) individuals. Recently, researchers have started studying how these applications are being used by MSM and some of the health risks associated with meeting sex partners via the Internet (Lehmiller & Ioerger, 2014). For example, one study (Lehmiller & Ioerger, 2014) found that application users reported significantly more sexual partners and had a higher prevalence of ever having been diagnosed with a sexually transmitted infection than did non-users; however, they did not find significant differences on personality variables (e.g., erotophilia, sensation-seeking, and self-control) between users and non-users. Among college students, a recent study found that users of dating apps were more likely to have had unprotected sex with a casual sex partner the last time they engaged in sexual intercourse. Moreover, using dating apps for more than 12 months was associated with having a casual sex partner in the last sexual intercourse and with having unprotected sex with that casual partner (Choi et al., 2016).

Among a sample of young MSM who use Grindr, researchers (Winetrobe, Rice, Bauermeister, Petering, & Holloway, 2014) found 20% of the men they surveyed had unprotected anal sex with their last Grindr-met partner. Moreover, men who used Grindr for at least 1 year were more likely to report Grindr-met partners and engagement in unprotected anal intercourse, a notable risk behavior associated with the spread of HIV. Beymer et al. (2014) surveyed 7,000 MSM in Los Angeles County who used geosocial networking phone applications and found greater odds of testing positive for gonorrhea and Chlamydia compared to individuals who had met partners through in-person methods only. There were no significant differences noted for HIV or syphilis between users and non-users. A recent study found that of 686 HIV-negative Chinese MSM surveyed, 62.8% (n = 431) used geosocial networking apps (GPN) to find sexual partners. GSN apps' users as compared to non-users were younger; had an earlier age of sexual debut; and, in the past 3 months, were more likely to have used recreational drugs, more likely to have had five or more casual partners, more likely to have had group sex with males, and more likely to have had condomless anal intercourse with male steady partners (Xu et al., 2018). Among a US veteran sample, seeking sex with partners met through social media was correlated with multiple mental health concerns including depression, posttraumatic stress disorder (PTSD), insomnia, and suicidal ideation (Turban, Potenza, Hoff, Martino, & Kraus, 2016).

Currently, the use of sex-specific smartphone applications has not been studied widely among heterosexual men and women (Anzani, Di Sarno, & Prunas, 2018). The widespread use of social networking sites for sexual communication and partner seeking presents unique opportunities for the development of public health interventions intended to reduce some of the sexual risks for users (Holloway et al., 2014). Additional research is needed to better understand the psychological characteristics of app users as well as the positive sexual relationship outcomes of app use (Anzani et al., 2018).

Craigslist: Looking for that Special Casual Encounter

The use of websites such as Craigslist (a well-known classified online advertiser of jobs, housing, personals, items for sale, community activities, etc.) also appears to be another method used by individuals to post ads ("casual encounters") to find interested parties for casual sex. Results drawn from meta-analyses (Liau, Millett, & Marks, 2006) suggest that 40% of MSM have used the Internet to look for sex partners, and those who use the Internet to find sex partners are more likely to be HIV-positive than HIV-negative. Additionally, they found that MSM who used the Internet to find sex partners were more likely to have unprotected anal sex than those who did not. Overall, initial evidence suggests that, for MSM, there are a substantial percentage of men who use the Internet to find sexual partners, and these individuals are more likely to engage in unprotected sex than are men who meet their partners in person. Another study (Grov, 2012) evaluating whether MSM recruited participants from gay bars/clubs and bathhouses and off Craigslist.org, differed in behavioral and demographic characteristics. The study found that, among MSM who recently had anal sex, those on Craigslist reported the least condom use, even though 13.5% of these men were also HIV-positive. In sum, additional research is needed to examine potential risk factors associated with computer-assisted sexual behaviors, given that this method of seeking partners may continue to grow in popularity and use around the world.

Sexting and Risky Sexual Behaviors

The topic of "sexting" (defined as sending and/or receiving sexually explicit material via a cell phone) has garnered significant media attention recently. Concerned parents, policymakers, and researchers are interested in understanding the associated risks, if any, of sexting among adolescents and adults. Is sexting a gateway behavior for casual sex? A recent systematic review of 32 studies (Klettke, Hallford, & Mellor 2014) indicated that sexting is more common in adults than adolescents, and more individuals report receiving sexts than sending them. Prevalence estimates of adolescents sexting is around 10–15% (Back, Lee & Stinchfield, 2011; Klettke et al., 2014; Mitchell, Finkelhor, Jones, & Wolak, 2012; Rice et al., 2012). A recent meta-analysis of 39 studies (110,390 youth participants) found that the average prevalence estimates for sending and receiving sexts were 14.8% and 27.4%, respectively (Madigan, Ly, Rash, Van Ouytsel, & Temple, 2018). Researchers (Strassberg, McKinnon, Sustaíta, & Rullo, 2013) surveyed US high school students and found that nearly 20% of students reported they had sent a sexually explicit picture via cell phone, and, of these, over 25% indicated that they had forwarded such an image to others (a notable risk behavior which could carry legal consequences for the sender and receiver of the text).

Similar to youth, young adults are also sexting. Among adults, the prevalence of sexting is around 50% (Dir, Cyders, & Coskunpinar, 2013; Gordon-Messer, Bauermeister, Grodzinski, & Zimmerman, 2013; Klettke et al., 2014). The most common demographics associated with adult sexting include female gender, being unmarried, and LGBT identity (Dir et al., 2013; Wysocki & Childers, 2011). Demographics related to sending sexually explicit photos of oneself include white race, lesser religious service attendance, lesser education, and LGBT identity (Wysocki & Childers, 2011).

Compared to their non-sexting counterparts, those who engaged in sexting were more likely to have had recent substance abuse and engaged in high-risk sexual behaviors such as unprotected sex and sex with multiple partners in the past 3 months. Of those who engaged in sexting, roughly a third reported having sex with a new partner for the first time after sexting with that person (Benotsch, Snipes, Martin, & Bull, 2013). Similarly, researchers (Dir et al., 2013) investigating sexting behaviors among young adults found initial support for sexting as a partial mediator between problematic alcohol use and sexual hookups, and for the role of impulsivity-related features and alcohol expectancies as distal predictors in this process. Currently, additional research is needed to better understand the roles and correlates of sexting and sexual risk-taking, though it appears that these behaviors are common among both adolescent and adults.

Conclusion

This chapter reviewed some of the ways digital technologies are potentially shaping the sexual behaviors of adolescents and young adults. Internet pornography is now highly accessible to most computer users around the world. The effects of frequent pornography use on users' sexual beliefs and practices remain largely unknown. Sexting is common among adolescents and adults, with some initial evidence finding that sexting was a partial mediator between problematic alcohol use and sexual hookups. The use of smartphone applications designed to help users find casual sex partners in their geographic area is on the rise as popularity and acceptability of having relationally uncommitted sex may be increasing over time. Additional research is needed to examine the influences that digital technologies could be having on the sexual practices of adolescents and emerging adults who may be spending increasingly more time online.

Acknowledgments

This study was funded by the National Center on Addiction and Substance Abuse and grants from the National Center for Responsible Gaming (Centers of Excellence at Yale University) and supported by the Department of Psychology, University of Nevada, Las Vegas. The authors report that they have no financial conflicts of interest with respect to the content of this manuscript.

References

Anderson, M., & Jiang, J. (2018). Teens, social media & technology 2018. http://www.pewinternet.org/2018/05/31/teens-social-media-technology-2018

Anzani, A., Di Sarno, M., & Prunas, A. (2018). Using smartphone apps to find sexual partners: A review of the literature. *Sexologies, 27*(3), e61–5.

Ayres, M. M., & Haddock, S. A. (2009). Therapists' approaches in working with heterosexual couples struggling with male partners' online sexual behavior. *Sexual Addiction & Compulsivity, 16*, 55–78.

Baćak a, V., & Štulhofer, A. (2011). Masturbation among sexually active young women in Croatia: Associations with religiosity and pornography use. *International Journal of Sexual Health, 23*(4), 248–57.

Back, K. J., Lee, C. K., & Stinchfield, R. (2011). Gambling motivation and passion: A comparison study of recreational and pathological gamblers. *Journal of Gambling Studies, 27*(3), 355–70.

Benotsch, E. G., Snipes, D. J., Martin, A. M., & Bull, S. S. (2013). Sexting, substance use, and sexual risk behavior in young adults. *Journal of Adolescent Health, 52*(3), 307–13.

Bersamin, M. M., Zamboanga, B. L., Schwartz, S. J., Donnellan, M. B., Hudson, M., Weisskirch, R. S., . . . Caraway, S. J. (2014). Risky business: Is there an association between casual sex and mental health among emerging adults? *Journal of Sex Research, 51*(1), 43–51.

Beyens, I., Vandenbosch, L., & Eggermont, S. (2014). Early adolescent boys' exposure to internet pornography relationships to pubertal timing, sensation seeking, and academic performance. *Journal of Early Adolescence*, 35, 1045–1068.

Beymer, M. R., Weiss, R. E., Bolan, R. K., Rudy, E. T., Bourque, L. B., Rodriguez, J. P., & Morisky, D. E. (2014). Sex on demand: Geosocial networking phone apps and risk of sexually transmitted infections among a cross-sectional sample of men who have sex with men in Los Angeles county. *Sexually Transmitted Infections*, 90, 567–572.

Binford, W. W. (2018). Viewing pornography through a children's rights lens. *Sexual Addiction and Compulsivity, 25*, 415–444.

Braithwaite, S. R., Coulson, G., Keddington, K., & Fincham, F. D. (2015). The influence of pornography on sexual scripts and hooking up among emerging adults in college. *Archives of Sexual Behavior 44*(1), 111–23.

Braun-Courville, D. K., & Rojas, M. (2009). Exposure to sexually explicit web sites and adolescent sexual attitudes and behaviors. *Journal of Adolescent Health 45*(2), 156–62.

Carroll, J. S., Padilla-Walker, L. M., Nelson, L. J., Olson, C. D., Barry, C. M., & Madsen, S. D. (2008). Generation XXX pornography acceptance and use among emerging adults. *Journal of Adolescent Research 23*(1), 6–30.

Chen, L., Yang, Y., Su, W., Zheng, L., Ding, C., & Potenza, M. N. (2018). The relationship between sexual sensation seeking and problematic Internet pornography use: A moderated mediation model examining roles of online sexual activities and the third-person effect. *Journal of Behavioral Addictions 7*(3), 565–73.

Chi, X., Yu, L., & Winter, S. (2012). Prevalence and correlates of sexual behaviors among university students: A study in Hefei, China. *BMC Public Health, 12*(1), 972.

Choi, E. P., Wong, J. Y., Lo, H. H., Wong, W., Chio, J. H., & Fong, D. Y. (2016). The association between smartphone dating applications and college students' casual sex encounters and condom use. *Sexual & Reproductive Healthcare, 9*, 38–41.

Cooper, A., Delmonico, D. L., & Burg, R. (2000). Cybersex users, abusers, and compulsives: New findings and implications. *Sexual Addiction & Compulsivity, 7*(1–2), 5–29.

Dir, A. L., Cyders, M. A., & Coskunpinar, A. (2013). From the bar to the bed via mobile phone: A first test of the role of problematic alcohol use, sexting, and impulsivity-related traits in sexual hookups. *Computers in Human Behavior, 29*(4), 1664–70.

Doran, K., & Price, J. (2014). Pornography and marriage. *Journal of Family and Economic Issues*, 35, 489–498.

Eisenberg, M. E., Ackard, D. M., Resnick, M. D., & Neumark-Sztainer, D. (2009). Casual sex and psychological health among young adults: Is having 'friends with benefits' emotionally damaging? *Perspectives on Sexual and Reproductive Health, 41*(4), 231–7.

Fox, S., & Rainie, L. (2014). How the Internet has woven itself into American Life. Pew Research Center. Retrieved on March 12, 2014 from https://www.pewresearch.org/internet/2014/02/27/part-1-how-the-internet-has-woven-itself-into-american-life/.

Gagnon, J. H., & Simon, W. (2017). *Sexual conduct: The social sources of human sexuality*. Transaction Publishers, New York, NY.

Garcia, J. R., Reiber, C., Massey, S. G., & Merriwether, A. M. (2012). Sexual hookup culture: A review. *Review of General Psychology, 16*(2), 161.

Gola, M., Lewczuk, K., & Skorko, M. (2016). What matters: Quantity or quality of pornography use? Psychological and behavioral factors of seeking treatment for problematic pornography use. *Journal of Sexual Medicine*. 5, 815–824.

Gordon, A. K., & Kraus, S. W. (2010). Yes. Yes! Yes!!! What do Mona's moans tell us about her sexual pleasure? *Porn-Philosophy for everyone: How to think with kink* (pp. 37–51). Wiley-Blackwell, Malden, MA.

Gordon-Messer, D., Bauermeister, J. A. Grodzinski, A., & Zimmerman, M. (2013). Sexting among young adults. *Journal of Adolescent Health, 52*(3), 301–6.

Grello, C. M., Welsh, D. P., & Harper, M. S. (2006). No strings attached: The nature of casual sex in college students. *Journal of Sex Research, 43*(3), 255–67.

Grov, C. (2012). HIV risk and substance use in men who have sex with men surveyed in bathhouses, bars/clubs, and on Craigslist.org: Venue of recruitment matters. *AIDS and Behavior, 16*(4), 807–17.

Grubbs, J. B., Kraus, S. W., & Perry, S. L. (2019). Self-reported addiction to pornography in a nationally representative sample: The role of use habits, religiousness, and moral incongruence. *Journal of Behavioral Addictions*, 8, 88-93.

Grubbs, J. B., Perry, S. L., Wilt, J. A., & Reid, R. C. (2019). Pornography problems due to moral incongruence: An integrative model with a systematic review and meta-analysis. *Archives of Sexual Behavior, 48*, 397–415.

Grubbs, J. B., Sessoms, J., Wheeler, D. M., & Volk, F. (2010). The Cyber-Pornography Use Inventory: The development of a new assessment instrument. *Sexual Addiction & Compulsivity, 17*(2), 106–26.

Grubbs, J. B., Volk, F., Exline, J. J., & Pargament, K. I. (2015). Internet pornography use: Perceived addiction, psychological distress, and the validation of a brief measure. *Journal of Sex & Marital Therapy, 41*(1), 83–106.

Hald, G. M. (2006). Gender differences in pornography consumption among young heterosexual Danish adults. *Archives of Sexual Behavior, 35*(5), 577–85.

Hald, G. M., & Malamuth, N. M. (2008). Self-perceived effects of pornography consumption. *Archives of Sexual Behavior, 37*(4), 614–25.

Holloway, I. W., Dunlap, S., del Pino, H. E., Hermanstyne, K., Pulsipher, C., & Landovitz, R. J. (2014). Online social networking, sexual risk and protective behaviors: Considerations for clinicians and researchers. *Current Addiction Reports, 1*(3), 220–8.

Kasper, T. E., Short, M. B., & Milam, A. C. (2014). Narcissism and internet pornography use. *Journal of Sex & Marital Therapy, 5*, 481–486.

Klettke, B., Hallford, D. J., & Mellor, D. J. (2014). Sexting prevalence and correlates: A systematic literature review. *Clinical Psychology Review, 34*(1), 44–53.

Kor, A., Zilcha-Mano, S., Fogel, Y. A., Mikulincer, M., Reid, R. C., & Potenza, M. N. (2014). Psychometric development of the Problematic Pornography Use Scale. *Addictive larBehaviors, 39*(5), 861–68.

Kraus, S., & Rosenberg, H. (2014). The Pornography Craving Questionnaire: Psychometric properties. *Archives of Sexual Behavior, 43*(3), 451–62.

Kraus, S. W., Potenza, M. N., Martino, S., & Grant, J. E. (2015). Examining the psychometric properties of the Yale-Brown Obsessive-Compulsive Scale in a sample of compulsive pornography users. *Comprehensive Psychiatry*, 59, 117–122.

Lam, C. B., & Chan, D. K.-S. (2007). The use of cyberpornography by young men in Hong Kong: Some psychosocial correlates. *Archives of Sexual Behavior, 36*(4), 588–98.

Lambert, N. M., Negash, S., Stillman, T. F., Olmstead, S. B., & Fincham, F. D. (2012). A love that doesn't last: Pornography consumption and weakened commitment to one's romantic partner. *Journal of Social and Clinical Psychology, 31*(4), 410–38.

Lehmiller, J. J., & Ioerger, M. (2014). Social networking smartphone applications and sexual health outcomes among men who have sex with men. *PloS One, 9*(1).

Liau, A., Millett, G., & Marks, G. (2006). Meta-analytic examination of online sex-seeking and sexual risk behavior among men who have sex with men. *Sexually Transmitted Diseases, 33*(9), 576–84.

Lindau, S. T., Schumm, L. P., Laumann, E. O., Levinson, W., O'Muircheartaigh, C. A., & Waite, L. J. (2007). A study of sexuality and health among older adults in the United States. *New England Journal of Medicine, 357*(8), 762–74.

Luder, M.-T., Pittet, I., Berchtold, A., Akré, C., Michaud, P.-A., & Surís, J.-C. (2011). Associations between online pornography and sexual behavior among adolescents: Myth or reality? *Archives of Sexual Behavior, 40*(5), 1027–35.

Maddox, A. M., Rhoades, G. K., & Markman, H. J. (2011). Viewing sexually explicit materials alone or together: Associations with relationship quality. *Archives of Sexual Behavior, 40*(2), 441–8.

Madigan, S., Ly, A., Rash, C. L., Van Ouytsel, J., & Temple, J. R. (2018). Prevalence of multiple forms of sexting behavior among youth: A systematic review and meta-analysis. *JAMA Pediatrics, 172*(4), 327–35.

Manning, J. C. (2006). The impact of internet pornography on marriage and the family: A review of the research. *Sexual Addiction & Compulsivity, 13*, 131–165.

Mitchell, K. J., Finkelhor, D., Jones, L. M., & Wolak, J. (2012). Prevalence and characteristics of youth sexting: A national study. *Pediatrics, 129*(1), 13–20.

Morgan, E. M. (2011). Associations between young adults' use of sexually explicit materials and their sexual preferences, behaviors, and satisfaction. *Journal of Sex Research, 48*(6), 520–30.

Nelson, L. J., Padilla-Walker, L. M., & Carroll, J. S. (2010). 'I believe it is wrong but I still do it': A comparison of religious young men who do versus do not use pornography. *Psychology of Religion and Spirituality, 2*(3), 136.

NoFap.com. (2017). https://www.nofap.com/

O'Sullivan, L. F. (2014). Linking online sexual activities to health outcomes among teens. *New Directions for Child and Adolescent Development, 2014*(144), 37–51.

Paul, B. (2009). Predicting Internet pornography use and arousal: The role of individual difference variables. *Journal of Sex Research, 46*(4), 344–57.

Peter, J., & Valkenburg, P. M. (2016). Adolescents and pornography: A review of 20 years of research. *Journal of Sex Research, 53*(4–5), 509–31.

Poulsen, F. O., Busby, D. M., & Galovan, A. M. (2013). Pornography use: Who uses it and how it is associated with couple outcomes. *Journal of Sex Research, 50*(1), 72–83.

Price, J., Patterson, R., Regnerus, M., & Walley, J. (2016). How much more XXX is Generation X consuming? Evidence of changing attitudes and behaviors related to pornography since 1973. *Journal of Sex Research, 53*(1), 12–20.

Reboot Nation. (2017). http://www.rebootnation.org/

Reid, R. C., Carpenter, B. N., & Lloyd, T. Q. (2009). Assessing psychological symptom patterns of patients seeking help for hypersexual behavior. *Sexual and Relationship Therapy, 24*(1), 47–63.

Rice, E., Rhoades, H., Winetrobe, H., Sanchez, M., Montoya, J., Plant, A., & Kordic, T. (2012). Sexually explicit cell phone messaging associated with sexual risk among adolescents. *Pediatrics, 130*, 667–673.

Ross, M. W., Månsson, S.-A., & Daneback, K. (2012). Prevalence, severity, and correlates of problematic sexual internet use in Swedish men and women. *Archives of Sexual Behavior, 41*(2), 459–66.

Rosser, B. R. S., Smolenski, D. J., Erickson, D., Iantaffi, A., Brady, S. S., Grey, J. A., . . . Træen, B. (2013). The effects of gay sexually explicit media on the HIV risk behavior of men who have sex with men. *AIDS and Behavior, 17*(4), 1488–98.

Sabina, C., Wolak, J., & Finkelhor, D. (2008). The nature and dynamics of Internet pornography exposure for youth. *CyberPsychology & Behavior, 11*(6), 691–3.

Ševčíková, A., & Daneback, K. (2014). Online pornography use in adolescence: Age and gender differences. *European Journal of Developmental Psychology, 11*(6), 674–86.

Shaughnessy, K., Byers, E. S., & Walsh, L. (2011). Online sexual activity experience of heterosexual students: Gender similarities and differences. *Archives of Sexual Behavior, 40*(2), 419–27.

Sinković, M., Štulhofer, A., & Božić, J. (2013). Revisiting the association between pornography use and risky sexual behaviors: The role of early exposure to pornography & sexual sensation seeking. *Journal of Sex Research, 50*(7), 633–41.

Smith, A., & Anderson, M. (2018). *Social media use in 2018*. Washington, DC: Pew Internet & American Life Project.

Strassberg, D. S., McKinnon, R. K., Sustaíta, M. A., & Rullo, J. (2013). Sexting by high school students: An exploratory and descriptive study. *Archives of Sexual Behavior, 42*(1), 15–21.

Sun, C., Bridges, A., Johnason, J., & Ezzell, M. (2016). Pornography and the male sexual script: An analysis of consumption and sexual relations. *Archives of Sexual Behavior, 45*, 983–994.

Svedin, C. G., Åkerman, I., & Priebe, G. (2011). Frequent users of pornography. A population based epidemiological study of Swedish male adolescents. *Journal of Adolescence, 34*(4), 779–88.

Træen, B., Štulhofer, A., Janssen, E., Carvalheira, A. A., Hald, G. M., Lange, T., & Graham, C. (2018). Sexual activity and sexual satisfaction among older adults in four European countries. *Archives of Sexual Behavior*, 1–15.

Turban, J. L., Potenza, M. N., Hoff, R. A., Martino, S., & Kraus, S. W. (2016). Psychiatric disorders, suicidal ideation, and sexually transmitted infections among post-deployment veterans who utilize digital social media for sexual partner seeking. *Addictive Behaviors*.

Twohig, M. P., & Crosby, J. M. (2010). Acceptance and commitment therapy as a treatment for problematic internet pornography viewing. *Behavior Therapy, 41*(3), 285–95.

Vanden Abeele, M., Campbell, S. W., Eggermont, S., & Roe, K. (2014). Sexting, mobile porn use, and peer group dynamics: Boys' and girls' self-perceived popularity, need for popularity, and perceived peer pressure. *Media Psychology, 17*(1), 6–33.

Wallace, B. (2011). The geek-kings of smut. *New York Magazine*.

Wetterneck, C. T., Burgess, A. J., Short, M. B., Smith, A. H., & Cervantes, M. E. (2012). The role of sexual compulsivity, impulsivity, and experiential avoidance in Internet pornography use. *Psychological Record, 62*(1), 3.

Willoughby, B. J., Carroll, J. S., Busby, D. M., & Brown, C. C. (2016). Differences in pornography use among couples: Associations with satisfaction, stability, and relationship processes. *Archives of Sexual Behavior, 45*(1), 145–58.

Willoughby, B. J., Carroll, J. S., Nelson, L. J., & Padilla-Walker, L. M. (2014). Associations between relational sexual behaviour, pornography use, and pornography acceptance among US college students. *Culture, Health & Sexuality, 16*(9), 1052–69.

Willoughby, B. J., & Leonhardt, N. D. (2020). Behind closed doors: Individual and joint pornography use among romantic couples. *Journal of Sex Research, 57*, 77–91.

Wilt, J. A., Cooper, E. B., Grubbs, J. B., Exline, J. J., & Pargament, K. I. (2016). Associations of perceived addiction to internet pornography with religious/spiritual and psychological functioning. *Sexual Addiction & Compulsivity, 23*(2–3), 260–78.

Winetrobe, H., Rice, E., Bauermeister, J., Petering, R., & Holloway, I. W. (2014). Associations of unprotected anal intercourse with Grindr-met partners among Grindr-using young men who have sex with men in Los Angeles. *AIDS Care, 26*(10), 1303–08.

Wright, P. J. (2011). 14 Mass media effects on youth sexual behavior assessing the claim for causality.

Wright, P. J. (2013). US males and pornography, 1973–2010: Consumption, predictors, correlates. *Journal of Sex Research, 50*(1), 60–71.

Wright, P. J., & Randall, A. K. (2012). Internet pornography exposure and risky sexual behavior among adult males in the United States. *Computers in Human Behavior, 28*(4), 1410–6.

Wysocki, D. K., & Childers, C. D. (2011). 'Let my fingers do the talking': Sexting and infidelity in cyberspace. *Sexuality & Culture, 15*(3), 217–39.

Xu, J., Yu, H., Tang, W., Leuba, S. I., Zhang, J., Mao, X., . . . Shang, H. (2018). The effect of using geosocial networking apps on the HIV incidence rate among men who have sex with men: Eighteen-month prospective cohort Study in Shenyang, China. *Journal of Medical Internet Research, 20*(12), e11303.

Ybarra, M. L., Finkelhor, D., Mitchell, K. J., & Wolak, J. (2009). Associations between blocking, monitoring, and filtering software on the home computer and youth-reported unwanted exposure to sexual material online. *Child Abuse & Neglect, 33*(12), 857–69.

Yoder, V. C., Virden, T. B., III, & Amin, K. (2005). Internet pornography and loneliness: An association? *Sexual Addiction & Compulsivity, 12*(1), 19–44.

CHAPTER

22 Texting While Driving and Other Use of Digital Technology Leading to Distraction and Risk

Susan Varga *and* Federico E. Vaca

Abstract

Advances in technology have dramatically influenced and changed the world of transportation in countless way. While many improvements have been realized with the help of technology in this area, negative consequences, like distracted driving, continue to be formidable challenges to the public's safety and health. Studies have demonstrated that mobile phones, built-in navigation systems, and other in-vehicle–related entertainment/information technology (infotainment) have contributed to distracted driving, leading to increased morbidity and mortality, especially among the youth. Today, the ubiquitous use of mobile phones while driving has led to major increases of distracted driving, with some attribution to injury and fatal crashes, particularly among young drivers.

Keywords: distracted driving, accidents, secondary task, motor vehicle crash, automobiles

Technology Surge and Unintended Consequence

Advances in technology over the past 10–15 years have significantly changed the world in which we currently live. The immediacy of information sharing, access to real-time information, and ability to directly connect to one another dictates the workings of organizations globally and permeates nearly every part of the lives of individuals. The Pew Research Center's Internet & American Life Project found that cell phone ownership among adults exceeded 90% in 2013, making the cell phone the most quickly adopted consumer technology in the history of the world. Although these developments have come with great benefit to human communication, there has also been a cost to public health and safety. Some unintended consequences of these developments often include an increased sedentary lifestyle, less interpersonal interaction, and increased traffic safety threats. Studies have demonstrated that mobile phones, built-in navigation systems, and other in-vehicle–related entertainment/information technology (infotainment) have contributed to distracted driving, leading to increased morbidity and mortality, especially among the youth. In response to these challenges, counter-measures have been taken by legislators, motor vehicle companies, and private organizations to create products and prevention strategies that will enhance safety in and out of the vehicle.

The Burden of Injury in Distracted Driving

The National Highway Traffic Safety Administration (NHTSA) defines distracted driving as "anything that diverts the driver's attention from the primary tasks of navigating the vehicle and responding to critical events that takes your eyes off the road (visual distraction), your mind off the road (cognitive distraction), or your hands off the wheel (manual distraction)." NHTSA further elaborates on the definition by explaining how frequency of multitasking and the "attentional demand" of the task contribute to distraction. Each of these definitions notes that there is a secondary task or event that diverts the driver's attention away from the primary task of driving. Measuring types of distraction have involved epidemiological, observational, and simulator studies, as well as naturalistic experimental studies.

Historically, the focus of driver safety has been predominately centered on alcohol impairment and restraint use. More recently, distracted driving has emerged and has been unequivocally recognized as a widely growing impairment that can significantly undermine safety. With the growing reliance on technology and its ubiquitous presence, increasing sources of in-vehicle distraction have materialized and escalated. In 1996, Wang et al. estimated that at least 25% of motor vehicle crashes in the United States involved driver inattention, and 13% of those involved distracted drivers (Wang, Knipling, & Goodman, 1996). From the 1995–2003 National Automotive Sampling System-Crashworthiness Data System (NASS-CDS) data, Stutts et al. estimated that the overall percentage of distracted crash-involved drivers was 10.4%. This percentage was a sum of the reported and estimated events, which remained stable over that period of time (Stutts & Hunter, 2003; Stutts et al., 2005).

Driver distraction not only has significant effects on associated crash morbidity and mortality, but it also has unique characteristics in the crash profile. In 2005, Stutts et al. found that crash-involved drivers under the age of 20 and older than 70 were more likely than drivers of other ages to have been distracted at the time of their crashes.(Stutts et al., 2005) Additionally, distracted drivers were 50% more likely to have been seriously injured or killed in their crashes relative to attentive drivers. Distracted drivers were more likely than attentive drivers to have been involved in single-vehicle collision or rear-end crashes. NHTSA 2004 data demonstrated that, compared to the crashes of attentive drivers, the crashes of distracted drivers were more likely to occur during evening or nighttime hours and less likely to occur on high-speed roadways, multilane roadways, curves, and intersections. The analyses also revealed differences between collisions involving distracted drivers and those involving drivers with other forms of inattention. The majority of inattentive drivers who "looked but did not see" were angle collisions, with the vast majority of these involving turns. Comparatively, the majority of the crashes sustained by drowsy drivers were single-vehicle crashes.

A growing body of research is assessing the contribution of technology to driver distraction and associated crash risk. The 2003 NASS-CDS data reported the highest percentage of attributable source of distraction (23%) was to an outside object, person, or event, with electronic devices including cell phone use or adjusting radio, cassette, or CD accounting for 3.6% and 2.9%, respectively (Stutts & Hunter, 2003). According to the most recent NHTSA Driving Safety Summary in 2011, approximately 10% of all fatal crashes were attributable to distracted driving. Of those drivers distracted during fatal crashes, cell phones were a leading source of distraction. In 2011, 12% of all fatal distraction-affected crashes involved mobile phone use. This included talking, listening, texting, or other phone-related activities.

Populations at Risk

Driving involves heterogeneous populations acting in diverse circumstances with unique goals. An 80-year-old with cognitive slowing driving to the grocery store encounters different road challenges than a 17-year-old driving with friends through the town. Each extreme age group within the population has different vulnerabilities on the road. Additionally, men and women within the same age range find themselves responding differently to comparable road conditions. Assessing these observations gives insight into the factors that place different populations at risk on the road.

Teenage drivers have substantially higher crash risks compared to other driver age groups, and they are more likely to be involved in fatal and nonfatal crashes. The increased crash risks and frequency of this age group have been attributed to driving ability, increased risk-taking behavior, and willingness to engage in distracted driving behavior (McCartt, Hellinga, & Bratiman, 2006). On a per-mile basis, drivers aged 16–19 are overrepresented in severe crashes by a factor of 10 compared with drivers aged 40–50 (McKnight & McKnight, 2003). Even within the first few years of driving, experience-related factors largely influence the likelihood of a motor vehicle accident. The accident rate for those aged 16–18 declines almost by two-thirds, and where licensing is delayed to age 18, a similar decline in accidents occurs over the next 2 years (Twisk, Box, Shope, & Kok, 2013).

An analysis of automobile accidents rates by age of licensing and years of experience in the United Kingdom demonstrated an average decrease of 30% in the first year of driving at any age. Additionally, the effect of inexperience in novice driver accidents is evident in the fact that 16-year-old females who have built up only half the driving experience as males of the same age show a one-third higher per-mile accident rate. However, at ages where the annual mileage of the two sexes becomes similar, so does the accident rate (Williams, Preusser, Ulmer, & Weinstein, 1995). Compared with drivers aged

40–50, drivers older than age 80 are overrepresented in crashes by a factor of approximately five (Bedard, Guyatt, Stones, & Hirdes, 2002). A significant factor inflating the morbidity and mortality in older drivers is their physical frailty, which means they are more likely to die if they crash. Additionally, these drivers also tend to drive less than younger drivers, and, across all ages, those who drive less per year have a greater risk per mile driven (Langford, Methorst, & Hakamies-Blomqvist, 2006). Adjusting for these biases greatly diminishes the overrepresentation of older drivers in crashes.

Mobile Use While Driving

A Centers for Disease Control and Prevention (CDC) survey in 2011 found that more than two-thirds of US adult drivers aged 18–64 years reported talking on their cell phone while driving at least once in the past 30 days. Additionally, more than 30% of US drivers aged 18–64 years reported reading or sending text or e-mail messages while driving at least once in the past 30 days. A larger percentage of both men and women aged 25–44 years reported talking on a cell phone while driving compared with those 55–64, and a significantly larger percentage of men and women aged 18–34 reported reading or sending text or e-mail messages while driving compared with those aged 45–64 years (Naumann & Dellinger, 2013). Such findings are consistent with research showing that young drivers are more likely than experienced drivers to engage in distracting activities while driving (Poysti, Rajalin, & Summala, 2005). Additionally, these drivers are not well tuned to the effects of distraction on their driving performance, which increases their likelihood of distraction-related crashes (Horrey & Wickens, 2006; Neyens & Boyle, 2008).

Experience can be broken down into more complex driver qualities that provide protective road navigation skills. Impaired selective attention and slower information processing are associated with greater crash risk. Although young drivers perform better than older drivers on visual and motor skill tasks, they crash more frequently, which may reflect decreased hazard perception skills. In 1979, Mourant et al. demonstrated that inexperienced drivers scan the road differently than experienced drivers, which influences their steering control (Mourant & Rockwell, 1972). Studies in the 1980s and 1990s demonstrated that inexperienced drivers depend on foveal vision to guide their lateral control (Smiley, Reid, & Fraser, 1980; Summala, Nieminen, & Punto, 1996). Additionally, examination of driver eye movements showed that inexperienced drivers focus more on guiding lateral control than on hazard detection, leading to diminished hazard awareness that may increase novice drivers' crash risk (Pradhan et al., n.d.). Interestingly, simulated training can affect the pattern of eye movements and enhance hazard awareness (Pollatsek, Narayanaan, Pradhan, & Fisher, 2006). Beyond hazard awareness, other factors, such as risk-taking tendency, multitasking, and secondary tasking, contribute to the high crash rates of novice drivers (Deery & Fildes, 1999).

Driving and Secondary Tasking

Secondary tasking with mobile, in-vehicle, or other technology use accounts for additional age and gender differences in accident risk. In the 2005 NHTSA survey, there were large differences among age groups, with 10% of 16- to 24-year-olds holding phones while driving compared to 1% of drivers over age 70. Females were more likely to be holding a phone compared to males (8% vs. 5%; Glassbrenner, 2005). In the 2011 NHTSA survey, the 15- to 19-year-old group had the largest proportion of drivers (11%) involved in distraction-related fatalities, with one in five distracted by a mobile phone. Hosking et al. examined the effects of text messaging on the driving performance of young drivers in a driving simulator, with instructions to initiate text messaging with programmed scenario events. The researchers found that engaging in messaging had a negative effect on driving performance. Drivers were more likely to deviate outside the lane boundaries and less likely to respond to traffic signs. Additionally, drivers spent approximately 10% of the time looking away from the road when driving normally versus 40% when text messaging (Hosking, Young, & Regan, 2009).

In a recent landmark study published in the *New England Journal of Medicine*, Klauer et al. compared the effects of secondary tasks on driver distraction across novice and experienced drivers. This was a naturalistic study with a case-cohort randomization design using instrumented vehicles installed with accelerometers, cameras, global positioning systems, and other sensors to assess 42 newly licensed drivers and 109 adults with more driving experience. They found that engaging in a secondary task (dialing cell phone, reaching for object, eating) was associated with a significant increase in risk of crash for novice drivers. Among experienced drivers, specifically dialing a cell phone was associated with an increased crash risk (Klauer et al., 2014).

Youth, Culture, Emotion, and Technology

It is known that cell phone use increases distractibility while driving and that the youth are leading the way in using new technology. McEvoy et al. found that cell phone use was associated with a fourfold increase in crash injuries resulting in hospitalization (McEvoy, Stevenson, & Woodward, 2007). Not only does driver distraction impact young drivers differently from other age groups, but their willingness to participate in distracting activities is also higher (Ferguson, 2003). Social, emotional, behavioral, and habitual factors play a role in the willingness to engage in distracted driving. Studies show that mobile phones create additional bonding opportunities with peers (Skierkowski & Wood, 2012; Tossell et al., 2012). The Pew Internet & American Life Project found that, for teenagers, text messaging is the most popular way to communicate with their social networks, exceeding face-to-face communications, emails, and voice calls.

The Uses and Gratifications (U&G) approach focuses on social and psychological factors that consumers use when assessing their satisfaction in telecommunication. This method has been used to explain why young adults have so quickly incorporated text messaging as a form of interpersonal communication. Specifically, the idea is that consumers look to technology for gratification based on certain "needs" and "motivations." Leung et al. developed six additional gratifications that mobile technology provided compared to the offerings of traditional telephone services: "affection/sociability, relaxation/escape, immediate access, mobility, and fashion/status and coordination" (Leung & Wei, 2000). Later surveys that Grellhesl et al. conducted of college-age students found accessibility and mobility ranking highest among the gratifications listed (Grellhesl & Punyanunt-Carter, 2012). These motivations and gratifications demonstrate gain that is obtained from the use of the phones, appealing to the perceived needs of young adults.

Development and Executive Decision Making

Behavioral, structural, and functional neuroimaging (magnetic resonance imaging [MRI], magnetic resonance venography [MRV]) studies demonstrate that neural circuitry undergoes major reorganization during adolescence. For example, the prefrontal cortex (PFC) undergoes changes during this time that provide neurological foundations for the development of *executive functions*, those cognitive skills that enable the control and coordination of thoughts and behavior (Luna et al., 2001; Luna, Garver, Urban, Lazar, & Sweeney, 2004; Shallice, 1982). Additionally, performance on tasks involving inhibitory control, processing speed, working memory, decision-making, and risk-taking also continue to develop (Hooper, Luciana, Conklin, & Yarger, 2004; Luciana, Conklin, Hooper, & Yarger, 2005; Luna et al., 2004).

Structural studies demonstrate changes to the PFC in adolescence, specifically the dorsolateral (DL-PFC) and ventromedial (VL-PFC) regions. Ultimately, these changes help to improve executive functions that moderate affect and behavior. The DL-PFC is preferentially involved in executive processes and working memory, whereas the VL-PFC is involved in emotional regulation. Functional studies demonstrate an intricately developed functional link between these highly evolved structures and the limbic system during adolescence (Stuss & Alexander, 2007).

Inhibition studies evaluating impulse regulation have found that, as a whole, children and adolescents activate a larger cerebral network to perform tasks than adults. Recruited brain regions decline with age, so that only essential regions associated with task performance are activated. Luna et al. found that adolescents displayed a greater volume of activation in the DL-PFC during a response inhibition task than younger children or older adults, suggesting a greater reliance on the frontal executive network (Casey, Getz, & Galvan, 2008; Durston et al., 2002; Luna et al., 2004).

The youngest drivers begin learning to navigate the road system at a time when their neural networks are undergoing the greatest change. This physiologic reality has significant implications for the decisions young drivers make while behind the wheel. This also provides a working hypothesis for why they are more willing to engage in risk-taking behavior compared to older drivers. The manifestations of these decisions include an increased rate of mobile use while driving, decreased capacity to maneuver a vehicle, and increased rates of fatality resulting from distracted driving. Understanding this physiology and the statistics associated with it has motivated efforts to create change through education, regulation, and legislation.

Distraction and Countermeasures for Prevention

As technology has advanced, research surrounding the improvement of vehicle safety has substantially increased. The high-mounted brake light is a classic example: as research demonstrated that heightening perceptual cues signaling the slowing behavior of a vehicle impacted driver safety, the brake light became a standard requirement on all production vehicles (Mortimer, 1997). Since its institution, other automated safety features have become ubiquitous on luxury and mid-priced vehicles. Examples of crash avoidance technologies or advanced driver assistance systems (ADAS) include adaptive cruise control, forward collision warning, and blind spot monitoring. As these systems have emerged, the control of the vehicle has shifted from the driver to the system. Recent promotion of the Google Self-Driving Car using a driverless, autonomous system suggests society's interest in continuing this shift.

Current vehicle safety research includes a focus on the roles of the driver, the system, and the interplay among them. Detecting driver distraction, notifying the driver of a potential collision, and helping the driver establish safe in-vehicle behavior are of central importance. At this time, some in-vehicle systems help drivers maintain safer following distances; others solely warn them when an imminent collision looms (Dingus et al., 1997; Maltz & Shinar, 2004). Studies examining the impact of vehicle autonomy systems have yielded mixed outcomes. Muhrer et al. demonstrated the benefits of forward collision warning in combination with a braking system compared to a collision warning system alone. The braking system braked earlier and more effectively than drivers who were solely notified of the collision, thus supporting increased vehicle automation (Muhrer, Reinprecht, & Vollrath, 2012). Additional research demonstrates that some systems have impacts on driving behavior beyond their designed uses. For example, Ben-Yaacov et al. found that drivers exposed to a rear-end collision warning system maintained longer headways for at least 6 months after a short experience with the system (Ben-Yaacov, Maltz, & Shinar, 2002).

In contrast to these positive outcomes, Neubauer et al. found managing automation poses the same dangers to task engagement and alertness that externally mediated driving does, with increased distress in fatigue-prone drivers (Neubauer, Matthews, Langheim, & Saxby, 2012). Additionally, drivers sometimes adapt their behavior in ways that weaken the benefits of a safety system. Lee and Strayer (2004) write about the "usability paradox" as it relates to driving systems, noting that when an improved design of a device makes it easier to use, it creates an increased reliance on the system. When drivers become aware of the increased ease of use, they may depend on the device more frequently, thereby increasing their overall exposure to risk (Lee & Strayer, 2004). Increased comfort with a system may also lead drivers to make decisions that increase their vulnerability to adverse events. Merat et al. showed that automated driving increased the likelihood of engaging in secondary tasks, with decreased attention to the road and increased potential for deleterious effects on driver performance (Carsten, Lai, Barnard, Jamson, & Merat, 2012; Merat, Jamson, Lai, & Carsten, 2012).

Some new vehicles are being sold with in-vehicle technologies that can detect driver distraction by monitoring eye-glance directions and behavior (Dong, Hu, Uchimura, & Murayama, 2011). Other vehicles are being equipped with the ability to modify cell phone use. Some Volvo vehicles have an Intelligent Driver Information System (IDIS), which delays incoming phone calls if a driver requires greater attention to the road, such as when they are accelerating (Volvo, n.d.).

The ultimate benefit of vehicle automation will depend not only on how designers create systems, but also on how drivers adapt their behavior to the new systems and how the two work together. As Merat and Lee state,

> Designers should not assume that automation can substitute seamlessly for a human driver, nor can they assume that the driver can safely accommodate the limitations of automation. Designers, policy makers, and researchers must give careful consideration to what role the person should have in highly automated vehicles and how to support the driver if the driver is to be responsible for vehicle control. As in other domains, driving safety increasingly depends on the combined performance of the human and automation, and successful designs will depend on recognizing and supporting the new roles of the driver. (*Merat & Lee*, 2012)

Prevention Policy and Legislation

Legislation around mobile use and driving has emerged to address the crash risk that distraction poses on drivers. According to the Governor's Highway Safety Association, 12 US states (as well as the District of Columbia, Puerto Rico, Guam, and the US Virgin Islands) prohibit with primary enforcement all drivers from using handheld cell phones while driving (i.e., an officer may cite a driver for using a handheld cell phone without any other traffic offense taking place). A total of

37 states and the District of Columbia ban all cell phone use by novice drivers, but not all drivers. Currently, 41 states (as well as the District of Columbia, Puerto Rico, Guam, and the US Virgin Islands) ban text messaging for all drivers, most with primary enforcement (Governors Highway Safety Association, n.d.).

Relatively few studies have assessed the impact of legislation limiting mobile use while driving on driver behavior and fatalities. Part of the difficulty lies in the implementation and enforcement of the mobile bans, which potentially obscures outcome data. Wilson and Stimpson (2010) found that increased texting resulted in more than 16,000 estimated additional fatalities between 2001 and 2007. However, the Insurance Institute for Highway Safety's Highway Loss Data Institute (HLDI; Insurance Institute, 2011) did not observe subsequent reductions in collision claim frequency in the months after handheld cell phone laws and texting laws became effective in a number of states. In addition, Goodwin, O'Brien, and Foss (2012) found that North Carolina's restriction on teenage driver cell phone use resulted in an insignificant impact on the behavior of teenage drivers. Most recently, Lim and Chi assessed the impact of state cell phone laws on non–alcohol-related crash fatalities involving drivers under the age of 21. They found that handheld cell phone bans targeting *all* drivers reduced fatal crashes involving young drivers, but there was insufficient evidence that cell phone bans targeting *only* young drivers reduced fatal crashes (Lim & Chi, 2013).

Education and Advocacy

In response to the adverse outcomes related to distracted driving and mobile use, public and private organizations were formed to lobby and educate the public. Cell phone and insurance companies have created advocacy groups that target legislation and public awareness. Progressive auto insurance companies promote "cell phone safety" while driving and encourage their customers to practice safe cell phone behavior, consisting of not texting, waiting until the vehicle is stopped to make a call, and not talking on the phone while angry or upset (Progressive Casualty Insurance Company, n.d.). Many car insurance companies are increasing premium rates when drivers are ticketed for texting or using cell phones while driving. Since legislation is variable by state, so are the effects on the premiums.

In 2013, AT&T, Sprint, T-Mobile, and Verizon teamed up to create the first joint advertising campaign against texting while driving, titled "It Can Wait." This campaign is unprecedented, with rival companies joining together to acknowledge the risks that their products pose to safety. Beyond television and radio ads, the campaign extended into stores and communities. Perhaps this approach was a manifestation of the lessons learned from tobacco and alcohol companies, who sustained significant financial burdens when lawsuits emerged targeting the damages these products caused. Regardless, if the effects of this campaign help bring change to social norms, culture, and behavior, then the benefits to public safety will be a welcome development (CBS News, 2013). A similar media campaign has been taken up by many consumer cell phone safety advocates, most fueled by personal tragedy and loss. FocusDriven, the first national nonprofit organization created by family members who have suffered loss related to mobile distracted driving, is raising awareness and educating the public through the Internet and other media sources (FocusDriven, n.d.).

Present circumstances portend a future in which reliance on technology will continue to increase and youth will maintain the lead as a population most ready to adapt to these technological advances while remaining most vulnerable to their potential adverse effects. Furthermore, research unequivocally demonstrates the adverse effects of distracted driving on all populations. Insurance and cell phone companies alike acknowledge the distraction and crash risk that cell phone use poses while driving and have strategized to promote driving safety. Although legislation has responded to ban cell phone use in many states, implementation continues to be a challenge. Motor vehicle companies are designing and installing new technology to monitor, respond to, and counter the effects of distracted driving. In spite of numerous interventions designed to reduce distracted driving risks, cell phones continue to put individuals at risk as their use fulfills the need for human socialization and connection. Ironically, technology also has the greatest promise to alter and solve some of the problems it has created.

References

Bedard, M., Guyatt, G. H., Stones, M. J., & Hirdes, J. P. (2002). The independent contribution of driver, crash, and vehicle characteristics to driver fatalities. *Accident: Analysis and Prevention*, *34*(6), 717–27.

Ben-Yaacov, A., Maltz, M., & Shinar, D. (2002). Effects of an in-vehicle collision avoidance warning system on short- and long-term driving performance. *Human Factors*, *44*(2), 335–42.

Carsten, O., Lai, F. H., Barnard, Y., Jamson, A. H., & Merat, N. (2012). Control task substitution in semiautomated driving: Does it matter what aspects are automated? *Human Factors, 54*(5), 747–61.

Casey, B. J., Getz, S., & Galvan, A. (2008). The adolescent brain. *Developmental Review, 28*(1), 62–77.

CBS News. (2013). *Big 4 cell phone carriers to team in ads against texting-while-driving*. http://www.cbsnews.com/news/big-4-cell-phone-carriers-to-team-in-ads-against-texting-while-driving/.

Deery, H. A., & Fildes, B. N. (1999). Young novice driver subtypes: Relationship to high-risk behavior, traffic accident record, and simulator driving performance. *Human Factors, 41*(4), 628–43.

Dingus, T. A., McGehee, D. V., Manakkal, N., Jahns, S. K., Carney, C., & Hankey, J. M. (1997). Human factors field evaluation of automotive headway maintenance/collision warning devices. *Human Factors, 39*(2), 216–29.

Dong, Y. C., Hu, Z. C., Uchimura, K., & Murayama, N. (2011). Driver inattention monitoring system for intelligent vehicles: A review. *IEEE Transactions on Intelligent Transportation Systems, 12*(2), 596–614.

Durston, S., Thomas, K. M., Yang, Y. H., Ulug, A. M., Zimmerman, R. D., & Casey, B. J. (2002). A neural basis for the development of inhibitory control. *Developmental Science, 5*(4), F9–F16.

Ferguson, S. A. (2003). Other high-risk factors for young drivers: How graduated licensing does, doesn't, or could address them. *Journal of Safety Research, 34*(1), 71–7.

FocusDriven. (n.d.) http://www.focusdriven.org/

Glassbrenner, D. (2005). *Cell phone use on the roads in 2002*. National Center for Statistics and Analysis, National Highway Traffic Safety Administration. DOT HS 809 580. Washington, DC.

Goodwin, A. H., O'Brien, N. P., & Foss, R. D. (2012). Effect of North Carolina's restriction on teenage driver cell phone use two years after implementation. *Accident: Analysis and Prevention, 48*, 363–7.

Governors Highway Safety Association. (n.d.) *Distracted driving*. http://www.ghsa.org/html/stateinfo/laws/cellphone_laws.html

Grellhesl, M., & Punyanunt-Carter, N. M. (2012). Using the uses and gratifications theory to understand gratifications sought through text messaging practices of male and female undergraduate students. *Computers and Human Behavior, 28*(6), 2175–81.

Hooper, C. J., Luciana, M., Conklin, H. M., & Yarger, R. S. (2004). Adolescents' performance on the Iowa gambling task: Implications for the development of decision making and ventromedial prefrontal cortex. *Developmental Psychology, 40*(6), 1148–58.

Horrey, W. J., & Wickens, C. D. (2006). Examining the impact of cell phone conversations on driving using meta-analytic techniques. *Human Factors, 48*(1), 196–205.

Hosking, S. G., Young, K. L., & Regan, M. A. (2009). The effects of text messaging on young drivers. *Human Factors, 51*(4), 582–92.

Insurance Institute for Highway Safety and Highway Loss Data Institute. (2011). *Laws banning cellphone use while driving fail to reduce crashes, new insurance data indicate*. http://www.iihs.org/iihs/news/desktopnews/laws-banning-cellphone-use-while-driving-fail-to-reduce-crashes-new-insurance-data-indicate

Klauer, S. G., Guo, F., Simons-Morton, B. G., Ouimet, M. C., Lee, S. E., & Dingus, T. A. (2014). Distracted driving and risk of road crashes among novice and experienced drivers. *New England Journal of Medicine, 370*(1), 54–59.

Langford, J., Methorst, R., & Hakamies-Blomqvist, L. (2006). Older drivers do not have a high crash risk: A replication of low mileage bias. *Accident: Analysis and Prevention, 38*(3), 574–8.

Lee, J. D., & Strayer, D. L. (2004). Preface to the special section on driver distraction. *Human Factors, 46*(4), 583–6.

Leung, L., & Wei, R. (2000). More than just talk on the move: Uses and gratifications of the cellular phone. *Journal of Mass Communication Quarterly, 77*(2), 308–20.

Lim, S. H., & Chi, J. (2013). Are cell phone laws in the US effective in reducing fatal crashes involving young drivers? *Transport Policy, 27*, 158–63.

Luciana, M., Conklin, H. M., Hooper, C. J., & Yarger, R. S. (2005). The development of nonverbal working memory and executive control processes in adolescents. *Child Development, 76*(3), 697–712.

Luna, B., Garver, K. E., Urban, T. A., Lazar, N. A., & Sweeney, J. A. (2004). Maturation of cognitive processes from late childhood to adulthood. *Child Development, 75*(5), 1357–72.

Luna, B., Thulborn, K. R., Munoz, D. P., Merriam, E. P., Garver, K., E., Minshew, N. J., . . . Sweeney, J. A. (2001). Maturation of widely distributed brain function subserves cognitive development. *Neuroimage, 13*(5), 786–93.

Maltz, M., & Shinar, D. (2004). Imperfect in-vehicle collision avoidance warning systems can aid drivers. *Human Factors, 46*(2), 357–66.

McCartt, A. T., Hellinga, L. A., & Bratiman, K. A. (2006). Cell phones and driving: Review of research. *Traffic Injury Prevention, 7*(2), 89–106.

McEvoy, S. P., Stevenson, M. R., & Woodward, M. (2007). The contribution of passengers versus mobile phone use to motor vehicle crashes resulting in hospital attendance by the driver. *Accident: Analysis and Prevention, 39*(6), 1170–6.

McKnight, A. J., & McKnight, A. S. (2003). Young novice drivers: Careless or clueless? *Accident: Analysis and Prevention, 35*(6), 921–25.

Merat, N., Jamson, A. H., Lai, F. C., & Carsten, O. (2012). Highly Automated Driving, Secondary Task Performance, and Driver State. *Human Factors, 54*(5), 762–71.

Merat, N., & Lee, J. D. (2012). Preface to the special section on Human Factors and Automation in Vehicles: Designing highly automated vehicles with the driver in mind. *Human Factors, 54*(5), 681–6.

Mortimer, R. G. (1997). Vehicle-driver communications to reduce rear-end collisions: What makes sense and why? *Proceedings of the Human Factors and Ergonomics Society 41st Annual Meeting, 41*(2), 849–53.

Mourant, R. R., & Rockwell, T. H. (1972). Strategies of visual search by novice and experienced drivers. *Human Factors, 14*(4), 325–35.

Muhrer, E., Reinprecht, K., & Vollrath, M. (2012). Driving with a partially autonomous forward collision warning system: How do drivers react? *Human Factors, 54*(5), 698–708.

Naumann, R. B., & Dellinger, A. M. (2013). Mobile device use while driving—United States and seven European countries. *Morbidity Mortality Weekly Report, 62*(10), 177–82.

Neubauer, C., Matthews, G., Langheim, L., & Saxby, D. (2012). Fatigue and voluntary utilization of automation in simulated driving. *Human Factors, 54*(5), 734–46.

Neyens, D. M., & Boyle, L. N. (2008). The influence of driver distraction on the severity of injuries sustained by teenage drivers and their passengers. *Accident: Analysis and Prevention, 40*(1), 254–9.

Pollatsek, A., Narayanaan, V., Pradhan, A., & Fisher, D. L. (2006). Using eye movements to evaluate a PC-based risk awareness and perception training program on a driving simulator. *Human Factors, 48*(3), 447–64.

Poysti, L., Rajalin, S., & Summala, H. (2005). Factors influencing the use of cellular (mobile) phone during driving and hazards while using it. *Accident: Analysis and Prevention, 37*(1), 47–51.

Pradhan, A. K., Hammel, K. R., DeRamus, R., Pollatsek, A., Noyce, D. A., & Fisher, D. L. Using eye movements to evaluate effects of driver age on risk perception in a driving simulator. *Human Factors, 47*(4), 840–52.

Progressive Casualty Insurance Company. (n.d.) *Cell phone safety tips*. http://www.progressive.com/shop/teen-driving-cell-phone-safety/

Shallice, T. (1982). Specific impairments of planning. *Philosophical Transactions of the Royal Society of London B Biological Sciences, 298*(1089), 199–209.

Skierkowski, D., & Wood, R. M. (2012). To text or not to text? The importance of text messaging among college-aged youth. *Computers and Human Behavior, 28*(2), 744–56.

Smiley, A., Reid, L., & Fraser, M. (1980). Changes in driver steering control with learning. *Human Factors, 22*(4), 401–15.

Stuss, D. T., & Alexander, M. P. (2007). Is there a dysexecutive syndrome? *Philosophical Transactions of the Royal Society of London B Biological Sciences, 362*(1481), 901–15.

Stutts, J., Feaganes, J., Reinfurt, D., Rodgman, E. A., Hamlett, C., Gish, K., & Staplin, L. (2005). Driver's exposure to distractions in their natural driving environment. *Accident: Analysis and Prevention, 37*(6), 1093–101.

Stutts, J. C., & Hunter, W. W. (2003). Driver inattention, driver distraction and traffic crashes. *ITE Journal-Institute of Transportation Engineers, 73*(7), 34–45.

Summala, H., Nieminen, T., & Punto, M. (1996). Maintaining lane position with peripheral vision during in-vehicle tasks. *Human Factors, 38*(3), 442–51.

Tossell, C. C., Kortum, P., Shepard, C., Barg-Walkow, L. H., Rahmati, A., & Zhong, L. (2012). A longitudinal study of emoticon use in text messaging from smartphones. *Computers and Human Behavior, 28*(2), 659–63.

Twisk, D., Bos, N., Shope, J. T., & Kok, G. (2013). Changing mobility patterns and road mortality among pre-license teens in a late licensing country: An epidemiological study. *BMC Public Health, 13*, 333.

Volvo. *Intelligent Driver Information System (IDIS)*. http://www.volvocars.com/uk/pages/default.aspx

Wang, J. S., Knipling, R. R., & Goodman, M. J. (1996). The role of driver inattention in crashes; New statistics from the 1995 Crashworthiness Data System. *Association for the Advancement of Automotive Medicine, 40th Annual Proceedings*, 377–92.

Williams, A. F., Preusser, D. F., Ulmer, R. G., & Weinstein, H. B. (1995). Characteristics of fatal crashes of 16-year-old drivers: Implications for licensure policies. *Journal of Public Health Policy, 16*(3), 347–60.

Wilson, F. A., & Stimpson, J. P. (2010). Trends in fatalities from distracted driving in the United States, 1999 to 2008. *American Journal of Public Health, 100*(11), 2213–9.

CHAPTER

23 Cyberbullying, Online Addiction, and Sexting

An Overview of Online Social Risk Taking

Ruth Festl *and* Thorsten Quandt

Abstract

In public and scientific debate, the opportunities offered by digital media are often contrasted with a broad range of potential risks and harms. Negative influences are commonly anticipated for young people who have grown up with digital media in their everyday lives. This chapter systemizes different social risks faced by children, adolescents, and young adults using digital technologies. It addresses three online phenomena that arise out of or refer to social interactions with peers or adults and that are much discussed in public and current online research: cyberbullying, online addiction (with regard to social network sites and online games), and sexting. Regarding the diffusion of these phenomena, obtained rates have varied widely depending on the used definition, selected measurement instruments, and set cutoff criteria. Recently, more established instruments as well as first longitudinal studies and meta-analyses have appeared, allowing for more systematic research on social online risks. Looking at explanation patterns, individual factors such as personality features, co-occurrence with other (risky) behavior, and specific characteristics of an individual's online use were predominant in previous research; lately, aspects of social resources and social influence have become more important, emphasizing peer factors as important predictors of involvement in risky online behavior.

Keywords: online risks, cyberbullying, online addiction, sexting, adolescents, young adults

In public and scientific debate, the opportunities offered by Internet use are often contrasted with a broad range of potential dangers and harms. A negative influence is commonly anticipated for young people who have grown up with digital media in their everyday lives. However, these public concerns are often undifferentiated and oversimplified, as suggested by Livingstone and Haddon (2012):

> Children's safety gives rise to considerable public anxiety, even moral panic, over childhood freedom and innocence, an anxiety compounded by uncertainty about the power of new and complex technologies and the mass media's tendency to generalize from individual instances of harm. (p. 5)

Livingstone and Haddon have also criticized the poor and fragmented scientific evidence used to analyze the risks faced by online users. Policy decisions, in particular, should be based on more stringent findings that provide information on a person's general online behavior as well as on the potential dangers he or she may meet. However, to date, only a few studies have tried to systemize the online risks that threaten Internet users.

Livingstone, Kirwil, Ponte, and Staksrud (2014) conducted a study that overviews the general range of Internet risks faced by children and adolescents. In a large, representative sample from 25 different countries, they asked participants to indicate what things on the Internet would bother people at their age. Participants were aged between 9 and 16 years. The researchers identified four different categories of online risk (pp. 277–278).

1. Content risks with the child as recipient of mass-produced texts, images, or videos that may include pornographic or violent online content.

2. Conduct risks with the child as actor, usually within a peer context. The most common forms within this category include cyberbullying, the misuse of other users' personal information, and sexual harassment and sexting.

3. Contact risks with the child as participant in activities usually emanating from strange adults.

4. Other risks, including criminal misuse in an online context, such as receiving a virus or phishing mails as well as forms of online addiction.

Most of the online risks summarized fall into the category of content risk (55%), followed by conduct (19%) and contact risks (14%; Livingstone et al., 2014). Although content risks are the most common negative aspect of Internet use, at least in the perception of young users, this categorization also suggests that two other major risks—conduct and contact risks—arise directly out of social interaction. The prevalence of these online social risks is therefore a concern for young users who have a strong preference for social forms of Internet use. In 2015, 71% of US teenagers between 13 and 17 years of age used different social networking sites, with Facebook still being the most popular one (Lenhart, 2015). In addition, 90% of young adults between 18 and 29 years also indicated use of social media applications. The number of social media users in higher age groups is slightly lower (Perrin, 2015). User rates are equally high for another form of social digital technology use: computer games. Quandt, Festl, and Scharkow (2011) found that more than 90% of German gamers between 14 and 29 years play digital games socially, often via online platforms. Children, adolescents, and young adults, therefore, seem to be especially at risk when dealing with the negative social aspects of digital technology use.

Another negative aspect of Internet use, also classifiable as social risk, is online addiction. Livingstone et al. (2014) described this phenomenon as spending too much time online but did not find it to be very prominent in the perception of young Internet users. These (self-)perceptions notwithstanding, heavy use of social network sites (SNS) as well as social online games is widespread among young Internet users (e.g., Perrin, 2015; Quandt et al., 2011), and there are studies that point to extreme forms of use paralleled by severe psychological and social effects. These studies do not classify problematic use by the time spent online but instead by co-occurring forms of problematic behavior and corresponding perceptions. While the use of the term "addiction" in that context is still debatable (as it implies certain conceptual analogies to substance abuse), researchers are highly engaged with addiction-like forms of online behavior, especially the problematic use of online games (e.g., Festl, Scharkow, & Quandt 2013a) and social media (Griffiths, Kuss, & Demetrovics, 2014). According to this line of research, a high level of engagement with online gaming and social media does not necessarily lead to forms of problematic use, but it does seem that online addiction is a present risk for young Internet users.

This overview should not be considered all-embracing because new forms and tools for online communication and social interaction are constantly emerging, resulting in additional challenges and risks for Internet users. In this chapter, we focus on the negative aspects of social Internet use that seem to be most prominent in scientific research: cyberbullying, online addiction, sexual harassment, and sexting. These risks are often discussed in public without detailed knowledge about their prevalence or how the risks manifest themselves. We analyze these risks within the context of young Internet users.

Cyberbullying

According to Livingstone et al. (2014), cyberbullying is one of the most prevalent online risks, mentioned by both children and adolescents. A long tradition of research has investigated traditional bullying in schools starting with the pioneering work of Olweus (1979). This nondigital predecessor of cyberbullying remains one of the major social problems within schools (e.g., Gradinger, Strohmeier, & Spiel, 2009). However, within the past decade, new forms of bullying have emerged that exploit the online communication environment. This new phenomenon is usually called *cyberbullying*. Studies have confirmed a significant overlap between traditional bullying and cyberbullying (see Modecki, Minchin, Harbaugh, Guerra, & Runions, 2014). Perpetrators often use the Internet as an additional way to bully someone already known in the school context (Dehue, Bolman, & Völlink, 2008; Slonje & Smith, 2008). Despite these commonalities, some aspects of cyberbullying behavior are specifically related to the context of online communication. From a risk-taking perspective, these aspects are especially important as they can have enormous consequences for people involved in cyberbullying. The specific online characteristics of cyberbullying and the reasons behind it are discussed in the following sections.

Definition and Prevalence

Most definitions of cyberbullying are derived directly from traditional bullying research. One of the most commonly accepted concepts was provided by Smith, Mahdavi, Carvalho, Fisher & Russell (2008), who developed a definition of cyberbullying based on the traditional definition of Olweus (1994, p. 1173). They describe cyberbullying as an "aggressive, intentional act carried out by a group or individual, using electronic forms of contact, repeatedly and over time against a victim who cannot easily defend him- or herself" (p. 376). The definition draws on commonly accepted bullying criteria including "behavioral repetition" and "power imbalance." Some researchers have questioned the applicability of these traditional components in the context of an online-based behavior such as cyberbullying (e.g., Dooley, Pyzalski, & Cross, 2009). Repetitive behavior by the perpetrator may not be necessary as the harmful contents can be forwarded to other people not directly involved in first place (see Dooley et al., 2009, p. 184). The fact that cyberbullying messages can be distributed instantly to a nearly unlimited audience is one of the characteristics of online bullying that most clearly differentiate it from its traditional form (see Heirman & Walrave, 2008). One single act, therefore, can cause enormous social harm to the victimized person. However, a repeated pattern of bullying behavior is still pertinent to any analysis of the perpetration behavior.

The second criterion of bullying that needs to be discussed in light of the online communication context is the power imbalance between the perpetrator and victim. Following the enhanced possibilities of acting anonymously online (see also Heirman & Walrave, 2008), it can be assumed that the status-related differences usually observed in traditional bullying may disappear as individuals of lower physical or social standing can also perpetrate cyberbullying while hiding their real identities. In turn, not knowing the perpetrator's identity can be even more stressful for the victims because they cannot evaluate the situation correctly (Kowalski & Limber, 2007). From a psychological perspective, this uncertainty may result in an augmented perceived power imbalance between perpetrator and victim. Anonymity is not unique to cyberbullying but can also occur in the context of traditional bullying (e.g., writing an anonymous letter in the classroom). However, cyberspace, with its use of pseudonyms and fake accounts, makes it easier for the perpetrator to remain invisible. The increased power of cyberbullies can also be traced back to an enhanced exposure of victims within the online context (e.g., Heirman & Walrave, 2008; Slonje, Smith, & Frisen, 2013). The only "effective" way for a victim to hide or withdraw from cyberbullying on an SNS may be to shut down his or her account. Due to the high diffusion of private and mobile communication technologies among adolescents, bullies often have the opportunity to act online without any parental or adult control (see Heirman & Walrave, 2008; Vanden Abeele, 2016).

Investigators have used different approaches to identify specific forms of cyberbullying (see Slonje et al., 2013). Ortega-Ruiz, Elipe, Mora-Merchan, Calmaestra, and Vega (2009), for example, made a simple distinction between bullying on the Internet and bullying via mobile phones. Smith et al. (2008) also focused on the user medium and further differentiated between various applications of the Internet, such as instant messaging, pictures, and video clips. In contrast, Vandebosch and van Cleemput (2009) took a content-related approach, providing a list of direct and indirect forms of cyberbullying based on the counterparts of traditional bullying. Following this systematization, cyberbullying can be said to include various aspects of negative online social behavior: damaging another person's property; verbal and nonverbal insults made through messages, pictures, or videos; social exclusion of others (e.g., from an online group); spreading rumors about others via the Internet; forwarding personal information belonging to others; misusing other people's private property (e.g., unauthorized use of a person's account); assuming another person's identity; and other forms of public defamation (e.g., on public websites; see Vandebosch & van Cleemput, 2009, p. 1352).

There are two ways of measuring cyberbullying behavior: a behavior-based approach, as suggested by Vandebosch and van Cleemput, and a definition-based approach that measures the overall frequency of cyberbullying on different kinds of media based on a previous given definition (e.g., Smith et al., 2008). Sawyer, Bradshaw, and O'Brennan (2008) showed that a definition-based approach often underestimated traditional bullying involvement due to social desirability problems. In contrast, a behavior-based measure risks overestimating the spread of bullying because (without an explicit definition) it is not necessarily based on a common understanding and includes a list of behaviors that might not all be perceived as actual forms of bullying (see also Furlong, Sharkey, Felix, Tanigawa, & Green, 2010).

Depending in part on the approach taken, studies have yielded different prevalence rates. Most of the earlier studies referred to a definition-based measure of cyberbullying and showed comparatively low percentages of children and adolescents being involved in cyberbullying. Smith et al., for example, found that 6.6% of cybervictims were bullied on a more or less regular basis. Slonje and Smith (2008) found that only 2.5% of pupils between 12 and 20 years were cyberbullied frequently. Ybarra and Mitchell (2004) obtained a representative sample of US pupils between 10 and 17 years. They found that 12% of the sample were online aggressors, 3% were victims, and 4% had been both aggressor and victim.

Vandebosch and van Cleemput (2009) directly compared definition-based and behavior-based measures of cyberbullying involvement. Asked directly about their online bullying experiences, the pupils (between 12 and 18 years) indicated considerably lower cyberbullying rates as compared to an indirect behavioral approach: 18% admitted to cyberbullying using the definition-based approach versus 52.5% using the behavior-based approach, with the rates for victims falling at 11.1% versus 61.9%, respectively. Festl and Quandt (2014) also measured cyberbullying involvement using different behavioral criteria. Pupils who met at least one of the defined behavioral criteria (e.g., sending or receiving hurtful messages) within the past 12 months sometimes or often were considered to be involved in cyberbullying. The results revealed that 21.8% of the respondents had perpetrated cyberbullying in the previous year and that 22.5% of the respondents had been victims of cyberbullying in the same period.

These findings on the spread of cyberbullying among children and adolescents point to the importance and weight of different cyberbullying measurement approaches. A further common problem is the lack of a consistent cutoff criterion for the component of repetitive behavior. The rates of reported cyberbullying vary widely depending on whether the behavior was conducted once, twice, or several times a week, or once, twice, or several times a month, and so on. Tokunaga (2010) has synthesized results across research on cyberbullying victims and found that an average of 20–40% of young people were victims of cyberbullying. In a more recent meta-analysis considering 80 empirical studies, Modecki et al. (2014) also found variations in prevalence rates of between 5% and 32% for perpetrators (on average 16%) and between 2% and 56% for victims of cyberbullying (on average 15%). These findings confirm that future research needs to work on a commonly accepted definition of cyberbullying that can be transformed into a consensus-based measurement instrument.

Explaining Cyberbullying Involvement

Earlier studies on cyberbullying involvement have mainly focused on individual, psychologically based explanation patterns such as socio demographics or aspects of personality (see Slonje et al., 2013). Some researchers have also investigated different facets of Internet use by children and adolescents (e.g., Walrave & Heirman, 2011). In contrast, very few studies that link cyberbullying with traditional bullying research have analyzed cyberbullying from a sociostructural point of view (e.g., including peer and classroom influence). Key findings with regard to explaining cyberbullying involvement are discussed here.

Results bearing on age and gender are rather inconsistent. Some studies have found no significant age-related differences (e.g., Festl & Quandt, 2013), whereas other findings point to higher (e.g., Vandebosch & van Cleemput, 2009; Ybarra & Mitchell, 2004) or lower rates in higher age groups (e.g., Slonje & Smith, 2008). Tokunaga (2010) suggests a curvilinear relationship between a person's age and experience of cyberbullying victimization, which peaks in the middle age group. Inconsistent findings are also observed in relation to gender. Previous studies have either found no gender-related differences (e.g., Slonje & Smith, 2008; Ybarra & Mitchell, 2004) or have confirmed higher perpetration rates among male youths (e.g., Dehue et al., 2008; Walrave & Heirman, 2011). In a meta-analysis examining 122 effect sizes, Barlett and Coyne (2014) also confirmed that male adolescents were generally more likely to perpetrate cyberbullying. However, the meta-analysis also revealed that the found gender differences were moderated by the respondents' age. Specifically, female adolescents were more strongly engaged in cyberbullying during early and middle adolescence, while male perpetrators more likely acted as cyberbullies in later adolescence.

In addition, personal features such as aspects of personality, attitudes, and previous behavioral experience have been analyzed in order to explain cyberbullying involvement. Corcoran, Connolly, and O'Moore (2012), for example, showed that, in comparison to noninvolved pupils, victims of cyberbullying displayed higher levels of neuroticism. Festl and Quandt (2013) also found slight tendencies toward personality deviation among young people affected by cyberbullying. Accordingly, cyberbullies were more extroverted and less conscientious. If they had already been victimized themselves, they were also less amenable.

Positive attitudes toward cyberbullying could be identified as a risk factor associated with a higher probability of becoming a cyberbully (e.g., Festl, Scharkow, & Quandt, 2015; Festl, 2016; Walrave & Heirman, 2011). Findings moreover confirmed a high co-occurrence of traditional bullying in school and cyberbullying for both perpetration behavior and victimization experiences (e.g., Festl et al., 2015; Modecki et al., 2014). In addition, victims of cyberbullying have an increased risk of perpetrating cyberbullying and vice versa (see Festl et al., 2015; Walrave & Heirman, 2011). In the context of cyberbullying, perpetration and victimization seem to be closely connected. This suggests a smaller power imbalance than that often observed with traditional bullying (see earlier discussion; Dooley et al., 2009).

In addition to personal attributes, cyberbullying research has focused on whether Internet use in childhood and adolescence leads to different patterns of online behavior. For example, some studies have found higher Internet expertise among cyberbullies (see Walrave & Heirman, 2011; Ybarra & Mitchell, 2004). Walrave and Heirman (2011) also found that having one's own Internet access could be used as a predictor of cyberbullying. However, this finding could not be confirmed in other studies (e.g., Festl & Quandt, 2013), arguably because unrestricted access to the Internet is nearly ubiquitous, especially within older age groups of adolescents and young adults. Furthermore, studies have confirmed that children and adolescents involved in cyberbullying use the Internet more intensively (see Festl & Quandt, 2013; Walrave & Heirman, 2011), especially social forms such as instant messaging or SNS (Festl, Scharkow, & Quandt, 2013b; Festl et al., 2015; Ybarra & Mitchell, 2008). First hints on the long-term associations of social online activities and cyberbullying involvement showed that a more intensive social online use predicted a stronger engagement in cyberbullying over time (Festl & Quandt, 2016; Sticca, Ruggieri, Alsaker, & Perren, 2013). Finally, research also found a clustering regarding different forms of risky online behavior, such as a high disclosure of personal information and online contact with strangers, and cyberbullying involvement (e.g., Festl & Quandt, 2016; Kwan & Skoric, 2013; Wolak, Finkelhor, & Mitchell, 2008).

As mentioned before, only a few studies have analyzed cyberbullying involvement from the sociostructural perspective common in traditional bullying research. One reason might be the lower direct association of cyberbullying with a fixed social context; however, as already noted, cyberbullying often occurs between pupils at the same school (e.g., Smith et al., 2008). A new line of research has emerged aimed at examining social network aspects in relation to cyberbullying involvement. As an example, Festl and Quandt (2013) referred to traditional aggression and bullying research when analyzing the social position of those involved in cyberbullying. They found that pupils who had already perpetrated cyberbullying and experienced it as a victim had a more central position within the school network. Using social network analysis, Wegge, Vandebosch, and Eggermont (2014) further showed that cybervictims are often bullied by the same person both offline and online. However, the researchers could not confirm online revenge behavior for cyberbullies or cybervictims. Focusing on more direct forms of social influence, Festl et al. (2015) revealed a higher risk of becoming a perpetrator and victim of cyberbullying in school classes with a more pronounced pro-cyberbullying norm (see Festl et al., 2015).

In summary, many cyberbullying studies still are based on cross-sectional analyses, refer to a specific sample of pupils (from a few schools in a specific country) and use very different kinds of cyberbullying measures. Sociostructural analyses, in particular, need to be extended and validated on a broader empirical base.

Online Addiction

Current research on online risks for adolescents has a strong focus on addiction. Initial research into excessive online use and debate on the issue had an anecdotal basis and lacked a systematic structure. The classification systems used for medical conditions and psychological disorders, including the *International Statistical Classification of Diseases and Related Health Problems* (ICD 10; WHO, 1992) and the *Diagnostic and Statistical Manual of Mental Disorders* (DSM-IV; American Psychiatric Association, 1994) did not contain specific criteria for the new phenomenon. Internet gaming disorder (IGD) was included as a potential diagnosis in DSM-5 in 2013, as a condition that warrants further research. The 11th revision of the International Classification of diseases (adopted by the 72nd World Health Assembly of the WHO in 2019) includes "gaming disorder" (World Health Organization, 2019). It will come into effect in 2022.

Because there were no other reference points available at first, initial studies and approaches used characteristics of existing categories and symptom patterns (in particular: substance abuse, gambling, impulse control disorder) for classification and further analysis of pathological Internet use. Young (1998) was the first to identify online addiction based on empirical data. Using the criteria for pathological gambling provided in DSM-IV, she analyzed hundreds of case studies comparing problematic use with normal use to identify a new clinical disorder encompassing problematic online use or addiction. In a subsequent study (Young, 1999), she differentiated five forms of problematic Internet use: computer addiction (gaming addiction), information overload (compulsive surfing of the Internet), net compulsions (online gambling, excessive online shopping, and excessive stock trading), cybersexual addiction (addictive use of online sex sites and online pornography), and cyber-relationship addiction (compulsive involvement in relationships via the Internet). This categorization has been much discussed in the field and used as a starting point for a number of studies. It does, however, have some limitations. Some categories do not seem to constitute specific modes of Internet addiction but rather involve patterns of excessive behavior that are performed online.

Griffiths (1998) took an alternative path by proposing a general systematization of (behavioral) addiction that is applicable to diverse forms of pathological online use. He defined six addiction criteria:

- *Salience* means that the behavior has become the main activity that determines life, reasoning, and sentiment.
- *Mood modification* refers to the power of the behavior to change mood, meaning that the pathological user experiences a state of arousal or exaltation.
- *Tolerance* describes the occurrence of habituation, which reduces the (positively experienced) impact of the behavior. The consequence is an enhancement of intensity and the need to extend the behavior to obtain the desired effect.
- *Withdrawal symptoms* occur when the behavior cannot be accomplished (e.g., when there is no Internet access). These symptoms can include anything from an unpleasant state of mind, discomfort or unrest, to distinct physical effects.
- *Conflict* denotes disputes between pathological users and their environment or other activities. These conflicts can also be internalized when a pathological user is aware that his or her problematic behavior conflicts with other aims or attitudes.
- *Relapse* describes backslides into former patterns of excessive use after phases of behavioral control—often associated with a greater use or with higher intensity.

In this chapter, we refer to different kinds of social risks associated with online behavior. Young's systemization includes two forms of problematic Internet use that seem to fit into this category: computer and cyber-relationship addiction. The former refers directly to problematic use of computer games, which has been found to be especially prevalent with online games (e.g., Kuss & Griffiths, 2011). Massively multiplayer online role-playing games (MMOPRGs) form a major online gaming genre and have been the focus of much addiction research. In these games, players are closely engaged in an artificial social environment containing thousands of fellow players (see Charlton & Danforth, 2007; Wan & Chiou, 2006). Excessive use of these games can arise out of perceived social obligations, which appears to qualify online gaming as a socially based online risk. The same is true for the use of social media and, in particular, the use of SNS. If social media are considered as instruments for managing social relationships, excessive use can be assigned to the category of cyber-relationship addiction (see Young, 1999). The use of online games and SNS both show specific online characteristics and do not constitute a simple extension of an offline behavior—they are inconceivable without online communication. Excessive use of SNS is therefore not simply exaggerated relationship management via the Internet; similarly, pathological online gaming is not the same as manically playing a board game on the Internet. Online gaming and the use of SNS are widespread among children and adolescents (see Andreassen et al., 2016; Lenhart, 2015; Quandt et al., 2011).

Prevalence of Pathological Social Media Use

In the past few years, research on SNS use has intensified, especially due to the success of Facebook.

However, studies on the prevalence of pathological use have not yielded consistent results. This may be partially due to the design of previous studies. Some studies have used self-evaluation by asking users whether they feel they use SNS too often. In addition, most studies are based on specific, nonrepresentative samples (especially students). Regarding self-evaluation, up to two-thirds of SNS users indicate that they use SNS (far) too much (for an overview, see Griffiths et al., 2014, p. 125). However, the actual time spent online, especially when considered in isolation, does not seem to be an appropriate indicator of pathological use. In line with this, several studies are based on specific scales, including the Internet Addiction Scale (Young, 1998). However, rates vary greatly depending on the chosen instrument, the context of the analysis, and the thresholds selected (e.g., how many criteria have to be fulfilled in order for a user to be classified as problematic or addicted). In his study of Chinese college students, Wan (2009), for example, identified 34% of the sample as being addicted to SNS. In contrast, in a survey of Nigerian undergraduates, Alabi (2012) found that only 1.6% were addicted to Facebook. Rates lower than 10% were also identified by Marcial (2013; 4.2%) as well as Wolniczak et al. (2013; 8.6%).

Most of these previous studies refer to small, self-selected samples that focus mainly on younger female adults (see Griffiths et al., 2014; p. 131). Another problem is the lack of standard scales and cutoff criteria thereby impeding the comparison of results. Some studies have adapted general instruments such as the Internet Addiction Test (Young, 1998), whereas other researchers have used specific instruments such as the Bergen Facebook Addiction Scale (Andreassen, Torsheim, Brunborg, & Pallesen, 2012; Marcial, 2013; see Andreassen et al., 2016 for the adapted Bergen Social Media Addiction Scale). A lack of suitable standard instruments to measure addiction to SNS still remains a problem.

Explaining Pathological Social Media Use

It has been assumed that the factors influencing pathological use of SNS are part of a user's personal profile as well as his or her perceptions and strategies for successfully coping with socialization (see Turel & Serenko, 2012). Griffiths et al. (2014) point to the existence of evolutionary needs, such as relationship construction and management, as well as other basic motivations (e.g., the desire for group affiliation). Looking at personal features, age seems to be an issue as younger users seem to be particularly affected (Echeburua & de Corral, 2010). Other studies have found that certain personality characteristics, such as narcissism (La Barbera, La Paglia, & Valsavoia, 2009; Ljepava, Orr, Locke, & Ross, 2013), extroversion, and low conscientiousness (Andreassen et al., 2012; Wilson, Fornasier, & White, 2010) enhance the risk of pathologic use of SNS.

Some research also suggests that close affinity with the Internet as well as high scores in relation to other aspects of Internet addiction correlate with problematic SNS use (Andreassen et al., 2016; Kittinger, Correia, & Irons, 2012; Turel & Serenko, 2012). It is well-established that pathological forms of behavior are often paralleled by concomitant forms of problematic behavior. In line with this assumption, some studies have shown a correlation between alcoholism and pathological use of SNS (e.g., Clyton, Randall, Miller, & Oberle, 2013; Litt & Stock, 2011; Moreno, Christakis, Egan, Brockman, & Becker, 2012). However, comorbidity (Feinstein, 1970) in problematic behavior and personality disorders is still a controversial phenomenon (Aragona, 2009) as it may well be that the two concomitant forms of behavior are not distinct but based on the same latent clinical issue.

Prevalence of Pathological Game Use

An overview of the spread of pathological gaming reveals widely varying data depending on which sample or which instrument and criteria are used. Within representative surveys, the proportion of addicted players mostly falls around 1% (Festl, Scharkow, & Quandt, 2013a; Haagsma, Pieterse, & Peters, 2012; Mentzoni et al., 2011). However, among groups of adolescents and young adults, rates are slightly higher (e.g., Festl et al., 2013a; Grüsser, Thalemann, & Griffiths, 2007; Haagsma et al., 2012; Lemmens, Valkenburg, & Peter, 2009). If the focus is on online games as a specific subgroup of gamers, rates are often much higher. Analyzing users of MMORPGs, Wan and Chiou (2006), for example, classified 46% as being addicted. Charlton and Danforth (2007) have also classified 39% as addicted to online games. However, both studies are based on self-selected participants who were recruited on game-related websites that already tend to be frequented by excessive users. In contrast, Van Rooij et al. (2011) obtained a representative sample of Dutch pupils and identified a mere 1.5% as addicted to online games.

In addition, differentiation between problematic and pathological gaming often seems to be inconsistent across current research. In their meta-analytic overview, Kuss and Griffiths (2012, pp. 6–11) identified a number of different instruments for measuring gaming addiction among children and adolescents: the Pathological Video-Gaming Scale (Gentile, 2009), the modified Internet Addiction Scale (see Young, 1998), and the Game Addiction Scale (Lemmens et al., 2009). In addition, the selection of cutoff criteria for identifying problematic or addicted users varies widely. Based on the studies of Charlton and Danforth (2007), Lemmens et al. (2009) proposed a two-level approach. Users are categorized as being *problematic* if they meet more than half of the named criteria for addiction. If all of the criteria are applicable to the person, he or she is classified as being *addicted*. Studies using this classification showed that problematic use of computer games is present among a low percentage of the population (3.7%, Festl et al., 2013a; 4.1%, Mentzoni et al., 2011), and that addicted gaming behavior occurs very rarely (0.2%, according to Festl et al., 2013a; 0.6%, according to Mentzoni et al., 2011). Petry (2011), however, notes that respective criteria have to be used carefully as it seems questionable whether a classification can actually be equated with dysfunctional and clinically relevant problematic behavior.

The debate on the inclusion and use of criteria—and whether they actually reflect clinically meaningful symptoms—led to multiple proposals for measurement scales. Petry and colleagues (2014) provided an internationally comparable instrument that includes the nine gaming disorder criteria that have been derived from previous research on substance abuse and gambling. These include preoccupation, withdrawal, development of tolerance, unsuccessful attempts to stop or reduce, loss of interest in other hobbies or activities, excessive gaming despite problems, deception, escape or relief from a negative mood, and jeopardizing or losing a relationship, job, or educational or career opportunity (Petry et al., 2014, pp. 4–5). The proposition has been contested, though, as Petry and colleagues claimed this to be a "consensus" solution—an assessment regarded to be premature by a large group of researchers in the field who also criticized several base assumptions of the instrument (Griffiths et al., 2015). Alternative instruments have been proposed (Pontes & Griffiths, 2015; Pontes, Király, Demetrovics, & Griffiths, 2014) based on DSM-5 criteria, despite some more general concerns regarding the general idea of an "Internet gaming disorder" (Kuss, Griffiths, & Pontes, 2017).

The inclusion of gaming disorder in the ICD-11 seemingly settles the debate, as it includes both a definition and diagnostic criteria. Gaming disorder is defined as "a pattern of gaming behavior ('digital-gaming' or 'video-gaming') characterized by impaired control over gaming, increasing priority given to gaming over other activities to the extent that gaming takes precedence over other interests and daily activities, and continuation or escalation of gaming despite the occurrence of negative consequences" (WHO, 2019). To be diagnosed as a disorder, "the behaviour pattern must be of sufficient severity to result in significant impairment in personal, family, social, educational, occupational or other important areas of functioning and would normally have been evident for at least 12 months" (WHO, 2019). However, a large number of researchers criticized "fundamental issues" in the research on gaming disorder and therefore found the inclusion of the diagnosis in ICD-11 to be "premature" (Aarseth et al. 2017).

One major criticism is directed at the reliability of the empirical basis, which is primarily composed of nonrepresentative cross-sectional studies. Therefore, and in addition to standardized instruments and cutoff criteria, longitudinal data are needed that provide insights into the development of problematic and pathological gaming behavior over time. Gentile et al. (2011), for example, conducted a 2-year panel study on pathological use of computer games among adolescents from Singapore. They found that such behaviors were very stable over time as 84% of the respondents were consistently classified as problematic users. Van Rooij et al. (2011) also examined temporal patterns of problematic use. However, according to their results, only half of the problematic users in the survey showed analogue behavior at the second measuring point. Among a representative sample of adolescent and adult users, Scharkow, Festl, and Quandt (2014) also found that only 1% of the respondents showed constant symptoms of problematic behavior across a 2-year span. Moreover, no person exhibited an addictive behavior across all three times of measurement. According to these findings, problematic gaming seems to be selectively displayed in specific life situations. Adolescents may be particularly vulnerable to such life situations.

Explaining Pathological Game Use

To identify risk factors, one must ask what kind of gaming behavior promotes a correspondingly problematic use of computer games. Based on a representative sample, Festl et al. (2013a) found that problematic behavior is not only associated with an excessive use of digital games (see also Lemmens et al., 2009), but also with a preference for online role-playing games (MMOPRGs) and first-person shooter (FPS) games. The increased occurrence of problematic use in the context of online games, and especially online role-playing games, can be attributed to certain structural features of these games. For example, the game-inherent mechanism of positive reinforcement (Chumbley & Griffiths, 2006) as well as the multiplayer mode may strengthen not only the desire to engage in such activities but also the perceived social pressure to continue playing (see also Wan & Chiou, 2006). The cross-sectional design of most studies greatly limits inferences about causality. According to Gentile et al. (2011), adolescents who became pathological players over a period of 2 years not only used games more intensively but also identified more strongly with their avatar and visited social gaming events such as LAN-parties more often. Thus, pathological gaming behavior cannot be equated with excessive use only. Other aspects of gaming behavior, especially features that usually are implemented in online games, seem to promote pathological gaming behavior.

In addition to gaming behavior, other psychosocial risk factors can be identified. Studies show that problematic gaming behavior is positively correlated with low expectations of self-efficacy (e.g., Festl et al., 2013a; Jeong & Kim, 2010), increased aggression (Festl et al., 2013a; Grüsser et al., 2007; Lemmens et al., 2009; Mehroof & Griffiths, 2010), lower social competence (Festl et al., 2013a; Lemmens et al., 2009; Porter, Starcevic, Berle, & Fenech, 2010), and lower life satisfaction (Festl et al., 2013a; Lemmens et al., 2009; Mentzoni et al., 2011). Again, the question of causality must be raised. More complex relations have to be assumed, especially in the context of personality variables. For instance, a high level of impulsiveness was found to be not only a risk factor for pathological gaming behavior, but also to increase in the course of problematic game use (see Gentile et al., 2011, p. 322). In contrast, especially among adolescent users, Scharkow et al. (2014) found no indication that problematic gaming is systematically related to negative changes in the psychosocial lives of gamers. To sum up, conceptual specifications, more systematic research and more longitudinal data are needed to explain these partly inconsistent findings.

Sexting and Sexual Harassment

Another category of socially related online risks covers the way children and adolescents are confronted with (unwanted) sexual contact online. Initial research on sexual risk online analyzed sexual harassment by known or unknown others. Young users were seen as victims. In recent years, another phenomenon has become the predominant subject of research. *Sexting* refers to forms of online sexual contact between adolescents that are not necessarily unilateral but also can take place in the context of a romantic relationship (e.g., see Wolak & Finkelhor, 2011). However, if the respective contents are forwarded to others without permission, this clearly can be regarded an act of online sexual harassment.

Definition and Prevalence

Sexual harassment is a well-known social problem confronting people in the offline world (e.g., at school or work). It is usually defined by three different categories (Fitzgerald, Gelfand, & Drasgow, 1995): (1) gender harassment that includes verbal or visual insults of a person because of his or her gender, (2) unwanted sexual attention that involves uninvited behaviors and comments dealing with one's sexual desires with reference to another person, and (3) sexual coercion that deals with forms of physical or psychological pressure in order to evoke sexual cooperation. In general, all these components of sexual harassment can also occur in an online environment. Insults concerning a person's gender might, for example, be made actively (by rude comments in a chatroom) or passively (by gender-offensive pseudonyms; see Barak, 2005, p. 79).

Across all three forms of sexual harassment, the victim is always confronted with unwanted sexual content and behavior. However, recent research also deals with online risks that include sexual material, in most cases explicit pictures, that can also be intentionally exchanged by the involved persons (e.g., in a romantic relationship). In most studies this phenomenon is termed "sexting" (e.g., Drouin & Landgraff, 2012; Strassberg, McKinnon, Sustaita, & Rullo, 2013). Wolak and Finkelhor (2011, p. 2) describe sexting as "sexual communications with content that includes both pictures and text messages, sent using cell phones and other electronic media." However, they point to the inconsistent use of the term "sexting" in previous research and recommend an alternative term—"youth-produced sexual images"—to describe the most problematic form of the phenomenon. Analyzing an array of legally relevant cases, each including incidents with youth-produced sexual images, Wolak and Finkelhor developed a typology with two different main categories. First, aggravated incidents include criminal or abusive components: for example, when adults are involved and ask for explicit pictures of adolescents. However, peers can also create this kind of risk via sexual threats and extortion or by forwarding sexual images of others without their knowledge (see Wolak & Finkelhor, 2011). This first category aligns with the forms of sexual harassment described earlier (see Fitzgerald et al., 1995). In contrast, explorative incidents occur without these criminal or abusive elements but are produced by the young people themselves in the context of an ongoing romantic relationship or to seek attention in an intended future relationship. These pictures might not be a problem at first; however, if they are forwarded to other persons (e.g., after breaking up with the girlfriend/boyfriend), the incident can be transferred to the aggravated category and can become associated with potential harm for the involved person. Therefore, both categories of incident reflect forms of social risk.

Following Wolak and Finkelhor's (2011) suggestion, sexting should be considered as youth-produced sexual images that are forwarded via text messaging. A range of studies has explored the spread of sexting among adolescents. Temple, Paul, van den Berg, Donna Le, McElhany, and Temple (2012), for example, identified a certain proportion of adolescents between 14 and 19 years of age who had already sent a naked picture of themselves through text messaging (28%). They were also able to show that more than half of the respondents (57%) had already been asked for such a picture via the Internet. Among a high school sample, Strassberg et al. (2013) found that nearly 20% of the students had already sent a sexually explicit picture of themselves, and almost twice as many had received a corresponding image. These studies point to widespread sexting among adolescents.

However, when compared to representative data, these rates seem to be somewhat inflated. In a nationally representative study among US teens, Lenhart (2009) found that 4% of all adolescents between 12 and 17 years who owned a cell phone had sent an at least nearly nude picture or video of themselves to another person. In contrast, 15% indicated that they had already received a sexually suggestive image. In another representative study, Mitchell, Finkelhor, Jones, and Wolak (2012) obtained somewhat lower prevalence rates. According to their findings, 2.5% of respondents between 10 and 17 years had appeared in (2.1%) or created (0.4%) a sexually suggestive picture. Furthermore, 7.1% of the adolescents confirmed that they had already received a sexually suggestive picture (see Mitchell et al., 2012). Livingstone, Haddon, Görzig, and Olafsson (2011) analyzed the sending and receiving of sexual messages instead of images and videos. In a large European sample across 25 different countries, they found that 7% of children and adolescents between 11 and 16 years had been sent a sexual message on the Internet, whereas only 3% admitted to having sent one themselves. Additionally, 4% of the respondents indicated that they had been asked to talk about sex or show a private photo or video of themselves to another person on the Internet. Relying on a systematic review of six studies that used random and/or representative sample of adolescents between 10 and 19 years, Klettke, Hallford, and Mellor (2014, p. 46) found 10% "sending sexts containing sexually suggestive text or photo content" and 16% receiving sexting messages or photos.

Explaining Sexting Behavior

In general, experiences with sexting seem closely linked to increasing age. Livingstone et al. (2011), for example, found a considerably higher rate among older versus younger adolescents (see also Klettke et al., 2014; Lenhart, 2009; Temple et al., 2012). Moreover, studies generally involving older age groups (specifically young adults) also confirmed a higher occurrence of sexting (e.g., Benotsch, Snipes, Martin, & Bull, 2013; Gordon-Messer, Bauermeister, Grodzinski, & Zimmerman, 2013; Klettke et al., 2014). In addition to age differences, some studies have also identified a gender influence. Gordon-Messer et al. (2013), for example, found that young male adults were more likely to receive sexually suggestive pictures than were females. This result was also confirmed for high school students (see Strassberg et al., 2013). One reason for this gender-based difference might be that boys also ask for sexually suggestive pictures more often (see Temple et al., 2012). Walrave, Ponnet, van Ouytsel, van Gool, Heirman, and Verbeek (2015) also found that male adolescents were more willing and had more intention to send sexting messages of their own. In contrast, looking at older age groups, some studies revealed that female adults were more likely to engage in sexting (e.g., Wysocki & Childers, 2011). However, many other studies have found no gender differences (e.g., Benotsch et al., 2013; Lenhart, 2009; Temple et al., 2012; for a systematic review see also Klettke et al., 2014). In line with these results, both male and female users seem to be at the same risk of sending and receiving sexually suggestive pictures online.

Differences in sexting behavior also seem to be related to differences in adolescent cell phone use. In a nationally representative study, Lenhart (2009) found that sending sexual images of oneself was more likely among adolescents who paid the costs for their cell phones on their own (only 10% of all cell phone owners). This finding might be confused with the fact that sexting is more common in higher age groups, as parents are thought to be involved in paying cell phone costs especially among younger adolescents. In addition, not surprisingly, teenagers who send any kind of text messages have a higher probability of receiving sexual images compared to those who do not use text messaging. However, a higher risk was also found among adolescents with unlimited text messaging plans (see Lenhart, 2009). Finally, respondents who had already received sexual messages generally reported slightly stronger tendencies to leave their cell phones switched on at all times, which might reflect a higher level of perceived importance for these messages (see also Lenhart, 2009).

Many studies investigating sexting have also analyzed its relation to other variables involving sexual attitudes and behaviors. According to Temple et al.'s (2012) findings, sexting is more likely to occur among those adolescents who have already begun dating and have had sexual intercourse (see also Gordon-Messer et al., 2013). Regarding other forms of sexually risky behavior, Ferguson (2011) found a correlation between sending sexually explicit pictures and having sex without birth control in a sample of young women between 16 and 25 years. Temple et al. (2012), moreover, confirmed that female adolescents performing sexting were also more likely to engage in other forms of sexually risky behavior (e.g., to have had sex with more than one partner within the past year or to have already had sex under the influence of drugs or alcohol). This was also confirmed by Benotsch et al. (2013), who found that sexting (sending and receiving sexual suggestive messages) was predictive of having unprotected sex and multiple sex partners within the previous 3 months, even after controlling for sociodemographics, general texting behavior, and substance use. However, in a first longitudinal study among teens, Temple and Choi (2014) confirmed that even though sending a naked picture of oneself was associated with being sexually active 1 year later, active sexting behavior was not related to sexual risky behavior over time. Regarding a person's relationship status, Weisskirch and Delevi (2011) found that adolescents in a romantic relationship were more likely to send sexual images than single teenagers. This result confirms the explorative nature of sexting (see Wolak & Finkelhor, 2011), which seems to be more often used in the context of an ongoing relationship. For young adults in a relationship, the researchers confirmed a positive connection between attachment anxiety and sending a text message propositioning sexual activity. In addition to concrete sexting behavior, attachment anxiety was also associated with positive relational expectation arising out of sexting: "Those individuals high on anxiety may want to please their partners and anticipate that romantic partners will want them to provide sexually explicit images, texts, and videos" (Weisskirch & Delevi, 2011, p. 1700). In addition to the romantic partners, further studies also confirmed the relevance of peers when explaining sexting behavior. Walrave et al. (2015), for example, applied the prototype willingness model and found that the perceived social norm was the most important predictor of sexting intentions, which in turn predicted actual sexting behavior. Moreover, they revealed that the more favorably adolescents evaluate a prototype person engaging in sexting and the more they want to resemble this prototype, the more they are willing to engage in sexting behavior.

In general, studies have already provided interesting findings that may help to explain why some adolescents and young adults send or receive sexually suggestive pictures via text messaging. In addition to demographic factors and aspects of Internet and mobile phone use, such explanations relate to their general sexual behavior, facets of their personality and their social relationships. However, it should be noted that, to date, there are only very few longitudinal studies analyzing causal links between sexting and, for example, sexually risky behavior. Nevertheless, the presented results provide important insights into the nature of sexting. They indicate strongly that sexting is a significant risk for young people online, with considerable prevalence rates.

Conclusion

In this chapter, we systemized the negative social aspects faced by children, adolescents, and young adults using digital technologies. We addressed three online phenomena that arise out of or refer to social interactions with peers or adults and that are much discussed in public and, at the same time, very prominent in current online research: cyberbullying, online addiction (regarding SNS and online gaming), and sexting and sexual harassment. For each of these socially related online risks, we first examined the scientific evidence on prevalence. In general, obtained rates have varied widely depending on the definition used, the instruments selected for measurement, and how and where cutoff criteria were set. Rates for cyberbullying involvement, for example, have ranged from far below 10% (usually with definition-based measurements) to 50% and higher (usually with behavior-based measurements). Recently, some meta-analyses have appeared suggesting a moderate but still considerable involvement of young users.

The situation is not the same for the three phenomena discussed in this chapter: for pathological social media use, suitable and commonly accepted measurement instruments are still lacking, so dependable data are scarce. Gaming disorder is defined in the 11th revision of the ICD, so there is a normative reference point that will most likely be used in future studies. Current studies, applying earlier criteria and instruments, estimate gaming disorder to be a minor issue for the general population. They find it to be somewhat more common among younger players and among gamers who prefer genres typically played online.

Sexting is often considered another social online risk among adolescents and young adults. Representative studies found notable prevalence rates for sending sexually suggestive images ranging between 3% and 10%. Receiving such pictures was indicated nearly twice as often. In general, sexting can be described as a phenomenon that occurs most frequently within romantic relationships among older adolescents and younger adults.

Factors and patterns explaining these forms of risky, socially based online behaviors often refer to the individual level, especially different personality features, co-occurrence with other (risky) behavior, and specific characteristics relating to an individual's online use. Although all three phenomena are based on forms of social interaction, consideration and study of social explanation factors are still rare. In recent years, aspects of social resources and social influence have become more prominent, especially regarding research on cyberbullying and sexting behavior. These findings underline that peer factors are important determinants of involvement in risky and deviant online behavior.

Parents, teachers, and politicians are highly concerned about the online behavior of children and adolescents. Cyberbullying, online addiction, and sexting and sexual harassment are often thought to have serious consequences and a negative impact on a young user's life. Research confirms that a certain number of children and adolescents have already encountered some of these socially based online risks. According to studies, these experiences can have a negative impact on a person's life (e.g., on health issues or social relations; see, for example, Al-Dubai, Ganasegeran, Al-Shagga, Yadav, & Arokiasamy, 2013). However, most previous research is based on cross-sectional data. Therefore, it remains unclear whether certain psychosocial aspects affect or are the consequences of online risk behavior. Moreover, not all negative online experiences are automatically connected to perceived harm, at least for the youngsters concerned. Livingstone et al. (2011), for example, found that only one-quarter of those children and adolescents seeing or receiving sexually suggestive pictures felt bothered afterward. Consequences should not be underestimated, however. It seems important to focus more intensely on the people involved and to obtain more rigorous data on socially based online risks.

References

Aarseth, E., Bean, A. M., Boonen, H., Colder Carras, M., Coulson, M., Das, D., . . . Van Rooij, A. J. (2017). Scholars' open debate paper on the World Health Organization ICD-11 gaming disorder proposal. *Journal of Behavioral Addictions*, *6*(3), 267–70.

Alabi, O. F. (2012). A survey of Facebook addiction level among selected Nigerian university undergraduates. *New Media and Mass Communication*, *10*, 70–80.

Al-Dubai, S. A. R., Ganasegeran, K., Al-Shagga, M. A. M., Yadav, H., & Arokiasamy, J. T. (2013). Adverse health effects and unhealthy behaviors among medical students using Facebook. *Scientific World Journal*, *12*, 1–5.

American Psychiatric Association. (1994). *Diagnostic and statistical manual of mental disorders*. Washington, DC: Author.

Andreassen, C. S., Billieux, J., Griffiths, M. D., Kuss, D. J., Demetrovics, Z., Mazzoni, E., & Pallesen S. (2016). The relationship between addictive use of social media and video games and symptoms of psychiatric disorders: A large-scale cross-sectional study. *Psychology of Addictive Behaviors*, *30*(2), 252–62.

Andreassen, C. S., Torsheim, T., Brunborg, G. S., & Pallesen, S. (2012). Development of a Facebook Addiction Scale. *Psychological Reports, 110*(2), 501–17.

Aragona, M. (2009). The role of comorbidity in the crisis of the current psychiatric classification system. *Philosophy, Psychiatry, & Psychology, 16*(1), 1–11.

Barak, A. (2005). Sexual harassment on the Internet. *Social Science Computer Review, 23*(77), 77–92.

Barlett, C., & Coyne, S. M. (2014). Meta-analysis of sex differences in cyber-bullying behavior: The moderating role of age. *Aggressive Behavior, 40*(5), 474–88.

Benotsch, E. G., Snipes, D. J., Martin, A. M., & Bull, S. S. (2013). Sexting, substance use, and sexual risk behavior in young adults. *Journal of Adolescent Health, 52*(3), 307–13.

Charlton, J. P., & Danforth, I. D. W. (2007). Distinguishing addiction and high engagement in the context of online game playing. *Computers in Human Behavior, 23*(3), 1531–48.

Chumbley, J., & Griffiths, M. (2006). Affect and the computer game player: The effect of gender, personality, and game reinforcement structure on affective responses to computer gameplay. *CyberPsychology & Behavior, 9*(3), 308–16.

Clyton, R. B., Randall, E. O., Miller, B. K., & Oberle, C. D. (2013). Loneliness, anxiousness, and substance use as predictors of Facebook use. *Computers in Human Behavior, 29*(3), 687–93.

Corcoran, L., Connolly, I., & O'Moore, M. (2012). Cyberbullying in Irish schools: An investigation of personality and self-concept. *Irish Journal of Psychology, 33*(4), 153–65.

Dehue, F., Bolman, C., & Völlink, T. (2008). Cyberbullying: Youngsters' experiences and parental perception. *CyberPsychology & Behavior, 11*(2), 217–23.

Dooley, J. J., Pyzalski, J., & Cross, D. (2009). Cyberbullying versus face-to-face bullying: A theoretical and conceptual review. *Journal of Psychology, 217*(4), 182–88.

Drouin, M., & Landgraff, C. (2012). Texting, sexting, and attachment in college students' romantic relationships. *Computers in Human Behavior, 28*(2), 444–49.

Echeburua, E., & de Corral, P. (2010). Addiction to new technologies and to online social networking in young people: A new challenge. *Adicciones, 22*(2), 91–95.

Feinstein, A. R. (1970). The pre-therapeutic classification of co-morbidity in chronic diseases. *Journal of Chronic Diseases, 23*(7), 91–95.

Ferguson, C. J. (2011). Sexting behaviors among young Hispanic women: Incidence and association with other high-risk sexual behaviors. *Psychiatric Quarterly, 82*(3), 239–43.

Festl, R. (2016). Perpetrators on the Internet: Analyzing individual and structural explanation factors of cyberbullying in school context. *Computers in Human Behavior, 59*, 237–48.

Festl, R., & Quandt, T. (2013). Social relations and cyberbullying: The influence of individual and structural attributes on victimization and perpetration via the Internet. *Human Communication Research, 39*(1), 101–26.

Festl, R., & Quandt, T. (2014). Cyberbullying at schools: A longitudinal research project. *Diskurs Kindheits- und Jugendforschung, 1*, 109–14.

Festl, R., & Quandt, T. (2016). The role of online communication in long-term cyberbullying involvement among girls and boys. *Journal of Youth and Adolescence, 45*(9), 1931–45.

Festl, R., Scharkow, M., & Quandt, T. (2013a). Problematic computer game use among adolescents, younger and older adults. *Addiction, 108*(3), 592–99.

Festl, R., Scharkow, M., & Quandt, T. (2013b). Peer influence, internet use and cyberbullying: A comparison of different context effects among German adolescents. *Journal of Children and Media, 7*(4), 446–62.

Festl, R., Scharkow, M., & Quandt, T. (2015). The individual or the group: A multilevel analysis of cyberbullying in school classes. *Human Communication Research, 41*(4), 535–56.

Fitzgerald, L. F., Gelfand, M., & Drasgow, F. (1995). Measuring sexual harassment: Theoretical and psychometric advances. *Basic and Applied Social Psychology, 17*, 425–45. doi:10.1207/s15324834basp1704_2

Furlong, M. J., Sharkey, J. D., Felix, E., Tanigawa, D., & Green, J. G. (2010). Bullying Assessment: A call for increased precision of self-reporting procedures. In S. R. Jimerson, S. M. Swearer, & D. L. Espelage (Eds.), *Handbook of bullying in schools: An international perspective* (pp. 329–45). New York: Routledge.

Gentile, D. A., Hyekyung, C., Liau, A., Sim, T., Li, D., Fung, D., & Khoo, A. (2011). Pathological video game use among youths: A two-year longitudinal study. *Pediatrics, 127*, 319–29.

Gordon-Messer, D., Bauermeister, J. A., Grodzinski, A., & Zimmerman, M. (2013). Sexting among young adults. *Journal of Adolescent Health, 52*(3), 301–306.

Gradinger, P., Strohmeier, D., & Spiel, C. (2009). Traditional bullying and cyberbullying: Identification of risk groups for adjustment problems. *Journal of Psychology, 217*(4), 205–13.

Griffiths, M. D. (1998). Internet addiction: Does it really exist? In J. Gackenbach (Ed.), *Psychology and the Internet* (pp. 61–75). New York: Academic Press.

Griffiths, M. D., Kuss, D. J., & Demetrovics, Z. (2014). Social networking addiction: An overview of preliminary findings. In K. Rosenberg & L. Feder (Eds.), *Behavioral addictions: Criteria, evidence, and treatment* (pp. 119–41). New York: Elsevier.

Griffiths, M. D., van Rooij, A. J., Kardefelt-Winther, D., Starcevic, V., Király, O., Pallesen, S., . . . Demetrovics, Z. (2015). Working towards an international consensus on criteria for assessing internet gaming disorder: A critical commentary on Petry et al. (2014). *Addiction, 111*(1), 167–75.

Grüsser, S. M., Thalemann, R., & Griffiths, M. D. (2007). Excessive computer game playing: Evidence for addiction and aggression? *CyberPsychology & Behavior, 10*(2), 290–92.

Haagsma, M. C., Pieterse, M. E., & Peters, O. (2012). The prevalence of problematic video gamers in the Netherlands. *Cyberpsychology, Behavior, and Social Networking, 15*(3), 162–68.

Heirman, W., & Walrave, M. (2008). Assessing concerns and issues about the mediation of technology in cyberbullying. *Cyberpsychology. Journal of Psychosocial Research on Cyberspace, 2*(2), Article 1. http://cyberpsychology.eu/view.php?cisloclanku=2008111401&article=1

Jeong, E. J., & Kim, D. W. (2010). Social activities, self-efficacy, game attitudes, and game addiction. *Cyberpsychology, Behavior, and Social Networking, 14*(4), 213–21.

Kittinger, R., Correia, C. J., & Irons, J. G. (2012). Relationship between Facebook use and problematic internet use among college students. *Cyberpsychology, Behavior, and Social Networking, 15*(6), 324–27.

Klettke, B., Hallford, D. J., & Mellor, D. J. (2014). Sexting prevalence and correlates: A systematic literature review. *Clinical Psychology Review, 34*(1), 44–53.

Kowalski, R. M., & Limber, S. P. (2007). Electronic bullying among middle school students. *Journal of Adolescent Health, 41*(6), 22–30.

Kuss, J. D., & Griffiths, M. D. (2011). Internet gaming addiction: A systematic review of empirical research. *International Journal of Mental Health and Addiction, 10*(2), 278–96.

Kuss, D. J., & Griffiths, M. D. (2012). Online gaming addiction in children and adolescents: A review of empirical research. *Journal of Behavioral Addictions, 1*(1), 3–22.

Kuss, D. J., Griffiths, M. D., & Pontes, H. M. (2017). Chaos and confusion in DSM-5 diagnosis of Internet Gaming Disorder: Issues, concerns, and recommendations for clarity in the field. *Journal of Behavioral Addictions, 6*(2), 103–109.

Kwan, G. C. E., & Skoric, M. M. (2013). Facebook bullying: An extension of battles in school. *Computers in Human Behavior, 29*(1), 16–25.

La Barbera, D., La Paglia, F., & Valsavoia, R. (2009). Social network and addiction. *Studies in Health Technology and Informatics, 144*(5), 33–36.

Lemmens, J. S., Valkenburg, P. M., & Peter, J. (2009). Development and validation of a game addiction scale for adolescents. *Media Psychology, 12*(1), 77–95.

Lenhart, A. (2009, December). Teens and sexting: How and why minor teens are sending sexually suggestive nude or nearly nude images via text messaging. Pew Research Center. http://mdlbeta.oakland.k12.mi.us/os/pluginfile.php/33415/mod_resource/content/0/Resources_for_parents/Teens-and-Sexting.pdf

Lenhart, A. (2015, October). Teen, social media and technology overview 2015. Pew Research Center. file:///C:/Users/festl/Downloads/PI_TeensandTech_Update2015_0409151%20(1).pdf

Litt, D. M., & Stock, M. L. (2011). Adolescent alcohol related risk cognitions: The roles of social norms and social networking sites. *Psychology of Addictive Behaviors, 25*(4), 708–13.

Livingstone, S., & Haddon, L. (2012). Theoretical framework for children's Internet Use. In S. Livingstone, L. Haddon, & A. Görzig (Eds.), *Children, risk and safety on the Internet. Research and policy challenges in comparative perspective* (pp. 1–14). Bristol, UK: The Policy Press.

Livingstone, S., Haddon, L., Görzig, A., & Olafsson, K. (2011). *Risks and safety on the Internet: The perspective of European children. Full findings.* London: EU Kids Online.

Livingstone, S., Kirwil, L., Ponte, C., & Staksrud, E. (2014). In their own words: What bothers children online? *European Journal of Communication, 29*(3), 271–88.

Ljepava, N., Orr, R. R., Locke, S., & Ross, C. (2013). Personality and social characteristics of Facebook non-users and frequent users. *Computers in Human Behavior, 29*(4), 1602–07.

Marcial, D. E. (2013). Are you a Facebook addict? Measuring Facebook addiction in the Philippine University. *International Proceedings of Economics Development and Research, 66*, 12–15.

Mehroof, M., & Griffiths, M. D. (2010). Online gaming addiction: The role of sensation seeking, self-control, neuroticism, aggression, state anxiety, and trait anxiety. *CyberPsychology & Behavior, 13*(3), 313–16.

Mentzoni, R., Brunborg, G., Molde, H., Myrseth, H., Skouveroe, K., Hetland, J., & Pallesen, S. (2011). Problematic video game use: Estimated prevalence and associations with mental and physical health. *Cyberpsychology, Behavior, and Social Networking, 14*(10), 591–96.

Mitchell, K. J., Finkelhor, D., Jones, L. M., & Wolak, J. (2012). Prevalence and characteristics of youth sexting: A national study. *Pediatrics, 129*(1), 13–20.

Modecki, K. L., Minchin, J., Harbaugh, A. G., Guerra, N. G., & Runions, K. C. (2014). Bullying prevalence across contexts: A meta-analysis measuring cyber and traditional bullying. *Journal of Adolescent Health, 55*(5), 602–11.

Moreno, M. A., Christakis, D. A., Egan, K. G., Brockman, L. M., & Becker, T. (2012). Associations between displayed alcohol references on Facebook and problem drinking among college students. *Archives of Pediatrics and Adolescent Medicine, 166*(2), 157–63.

Olweus, D. (1979). Stability of aggressive reaction patterns in males: A review. *Psychological Bulletin 86*(4), 852–57.

Olweus, D. (1994). Annotation: Bullying at school: basic facts and effects of a school based intervention program. *Journal of Child Psychology and Psychiatry, 35*(7), 1171–90.

Ortega-Ruiz, R., Elipe, P., Mora-Merchan, J. A., Calmaestra, J., & Vega, E. (2009). The emotional impact on victims of traditional bullying and cyberbullying: A study of Spanish adolescents. *Journal of Psychology, 217*(4), 197–04.

Perrin, A. (2015, October). Social networking usage: 2005–2015. Pew Research Center. http://www.pewinternet.org/2015/10/08/2015/Social-Networking-Usage-2005-2015/

Petry, N. (2011). Commentary on van Rooij et al. (2011), "Gaming Addiction" – a psychiatric disorder or not? *Addiction, 106*(1), 213–14.

Petry, N., Rehbein, F., Gentile, D., Lemmens, J. S., Rumpf, H.-J., Mößle, T., . . . O'Brien, C. P. (2014). An international consensus for assessing internet gaming disorder using the new DSM-5 approach. *Addiction, 109*(9), 1399–06.

Pontes, H. M., & Griffiths, M. D. (2015). Measuring DSM-5 Internet gaming disorder: Development and validation of a short psychometric scale. *Computers in Human Behavior, 45*, 137–43.

Pontes, H. M., Király, O., Demetrovics, Z., & Griffiths, M. D. (2014). The conceptualization and measurement of DSM-5 Internet Gaming Disorder: The development of the IGD-20 Test. *PLoS One, 9*(10), e110137.

Porter, G., Starcevic, V., Berle, D., & Fenech, P. (2010). Recognizing problem video game use. *Australian & New Zealand Journal of Psychiatry, 44*(2), 120–28.

Quandt, T., Festl, R., & Scharkow, M. (2011). Digitales Spielen: Medienunterhaltung im Mainstream. GameStat 2011: Repräsentativbefragung zum Computer- und Konsolenspielen in Deutschland. [Digital gaming: Media entertainment at mainstream. GameStat2011: Representative survey on computer- and gaming console use in Germany] *Media Perspektiven, 9*, 414–22.

Sawyer, A. L., Bradshaw, C. P., & O'Brennan, L. M. (2008). Examining ethnic, gender, and developmental differences in the way children report being a victim of 'bullying'on self-report measures. *Journal of Adolescent Health, 43*(2), 106–14.

Scharkow, M., Festl, R., & Quandt, T. (2014). Longitudinal patterns of problematic computer game use among adolescents and adults: A two-year panel study. *Addiction, 109*(11), 1910–17.

Slonje, R., & Smith, P. K. (2008). Cyberbullying: Another main type of bullying? *Scandinavian Journal of Psychology, 49*(2), 147–54.

Slonje, R., Smith, P. K., & Frisen, A. (2013). The nature of cyberbullying, and strategies for prevention. *Computers in Human Behavior, 29*(1), 26–32.

Smith, P. K., Mahdavi, J., Carvalho, M., Fisher, S., & Russell, S. (2008). Cyberbullying: Its nature and impact in secondary school pupils. *Journal of Child Psychology and Psychiatry, 49*(4), 376–85.

Sticca, F., Ruggieri, S., Alsaker, F., & Perren, S. (2013). Longitudinal risk factors for cyberbullying in adolescence. *Journal of Community and Applied Social Psychology, 23*(1), 52–67.

Strassberg, D. S., McKinnon, R. K., Sustaita, M. A., & Rullo, J. (2013). Sexting by high school students: An exploratory and descriptive study. *Archives of Sexual Behavior, 42*(1), 15–21.

Temple, J. R., & Choi, H. J. (2014). Longitudinal association between teen sexting and sexual behavior. *Pediatrics, 134*(5), 1287–92.

Temple, J. R., Paul, J. A., van den Berg, P., Donna Le, V., McElhany, A., & Temple, B. W. (2012). Teen sexting and its association with sexual behaviors. *Archives of Pediatrics and Adolescent Medicine, 166*(9), 828–33.

Tokunaga, R. S. (2010). Following you home from school: A critical review and synthesis of research on cyberbullying victimization. *Computers in Human Behavior, 26*(3), 277–87.

Turel, O., & Serenko, A. (2012). The benefits and dangers of enjoyment with social networking websites. *European Journal of Information Systems, 21*(5), 512–28.

Vandebosch, H., & van Cleemput, K. (2009). Cyberbullying among youngsters: Profiles of bullies and victims. *New Media Society, 11*(8), 1349–71.

Vanden Abeele, M. M. P. (2016). Mobile youth culture: A conceptual development. *Mobile Media & Communication, 4*(1), 85–101.

van Rooij, A. J., Schoenmakers, T. M., Vermulst, A. A., van Den Eijnden, R. J. J., & van De Mheen, D. (2011). Online video game addiction: Identification of addicted adolescent gamers. *Addiction, 106*(1), 205–12.

Walrave, M., & Heirman, W. (2011). Cyberbullying: Predicting victimization and perpetration. *Children and Society, 25*(1), 59–72.

Walrave, M., Ponnet, K., Van Ouytsel, J., Van Gool, E., Heirman, W., & Verbeek, A. (2015). Whether or not to engage in sexting: Explaining adolescent sexting behaviour by applying the Prototype Willingness Model. *Telematics and Informatics, 32*(4), 796–08.

Wan, C. (2009, May). Gratifications and loneliness as predictors of campus-SNS Websites addiction and usage pattern among Chinese college students. Chinese University of Hong Kong. http://pg.com.cuhk.edu.hk/pgp_nm/projects/2009/Wan%20Sisi%20Candy.pdf

Wan, C. S., & Chiou, W. B. (2006). Psychological motive and online games addiction: A test of flow theory and humanistic needs theory for Taiwanese adolescents. *CyberPsychology & Behavior, 9*(3), 317–24.

Weisskirch, R. S., & Delevi, R. (2011). 'Sexting' and adult romantic attachment. *Computers in Human Behavior, 27*(5), 1697–01.

Wegge, D., Vandebosch, H., & Eggermont, S. (2014). Who bullies who online: A social network analysis of cyberbullying in a school context. *Communications, 39*(4), 415–33.

Wilson, K., Fornasier, S., & White, K. M. (2010). Psychological predictors of young adults' use of social networking sites. *Cyberpsychology, Behavior and Social Networking, 13*(2), 173–77.

Wolak, J., & Finkelhor, D. (2011, March). Sexting: A typology. Crimes Against Children Research Center. http://www.unh.edu/ccrc/pdf/CV231_Sexting%20Typology%20Bulletin_4-6-11_revised.pdf

Wolak, J., Finkelhor, D., & Mitchell, K. (2008). Is talking online to unknown people always risky? Distinguishing online interaction styles in a national sample of youth internet users. *CyberPsychology & Behavior, 11*(3), 340–43.

Wolniczak, I., Caceres-DelAguila, J. A., Palma-Ardiles, G., Arroyo, K. J., Solis-Visscher, R., Paredes-Yauri, S., . . . Bernabe-Ortiz, A. (2013). Association between Facebook dependence and poor sleep quality. A study in a sample of undergraduate students in Peru. *PLoS One, 8*(3), e59087.

World Health Organization (WHO). (1992). *ICD-10: International statistical classification of diseases and related health problems*. New York: Author.

World Health Organization (WHO). (2019). *Gaming disorder*. https://www.who.int/features/qa/gaming-disorder/en/

Wysocki, D. K., & Childers, C. D. (2011). 'Let my fingers do the talking': Sexting and infidelity in Cyberspace. *Sexuality & Culture, 15*(3), 217–39.

Ybarra, M. L., & Mitchell, K. J. (2004). Online aggressor/targets, aggressors, and targets: A comparison of associated youth characteristics. *Journal of Child Psychology and Psychiatry, 45*(7), 1308–16.

Ybarra, M. L., & Mitchell, K. J. (2008). How risky are social networking sites? A comparison of places online where youth sexual solicitation and harassment occurs. *Pediatrics, 121*(2), 350–57.

Young, K. S. (1998). Internet addiction: The emergence of a new clinical disorder. *CyberPsychology & Behavior, 1*(3), 237–44.

Young, K. S. (1999). Internet addiction: Evaluation and treatment. *Student British Medical Journal, 7*, 351–52.

PART 5

Treatment, Assessment, and Legal Considerations

Digital Technology Approaches

CHAPTER

24 Ecological Momentary Assessment and Technological Advances in Clinical Care

Isabelle Morris, Saul Shiffman, Ellen Beckjord, *and* Stuart G. Ferguson

Abstract

Ecological momentary assessment (EMA) methods provide a means by which researchers may attain highly detailed, ecologically valid, and contextually rich data on everyday experience and behavior. EMA methods are now widely used by researchers, particularly those studying health behaviors. A key reason for the popularity of EMA methods is that they allow researchers to examine both between- and within-individual differences in treatment efficacy and to explore the temporal sequences related to events of interest. Until relatively recently, EMA methods have predominately been employed as assessment and research tools. However, in recent years clinicians and researchers have begun to explore the value of real-time data collection methods as the foundation for providing tailored interventions that can respond to a patient's behaviors, moods, social context, and geographical location. This chapter discusses how EMA data can potentially be utilized to improve the delivery of health interventions. The authors conclude that while there are clearly potential benefits of utilizing real-time data collection methods for treatment delivery, considerable work remains to ensure that EMA-based interventions are appropriate, theoretically derived, and ethical in their effects on privacy and confidentiality.

Keywords: ecological momentary assessment, EMA, mHealth, eHealth, treatment

This chapter provides an introduction to *ecological momentary assessment* (EMA; Stone & Shiffman, 1994), a real-time data capture methodology used in the study of a diverse range of health behaviors. EMA enables study participants to record information about events, situations, thoughts, feelings, and behaviors in real time as they occur within participants' day-to-day lives. To date, EMA technologies have largely been employed as assessment and research tools, having demonstrated tremendous value for advancing clinical assessment through the enhancement of diagnostics by aiding the development and implementation of treatment and intervention strategies and as a means of evaluating the effects and efficacy of treatments. However, more recently, clinicians have also begun to explore the value of EMA technologies as a foundation for providing tailored interventions that respond to the patient's *real-time* behaviors, moods, social context, and geographical location.

This chapter introduces the reader to EMA and the rationale behind its use. It then outlines the various applications of EMA in health research and ultimately explores the significant potential of EMA technologies as an intervention tool to enhance clinical care.

What Is Electronic Momentary Assessment (EMA)?

EMA refers not to a single method but to a wide range of research methods, all of which share a number of key characteristics. Data collection by way of EMA is defined by the momentary or "real-time" repetitive assessment of behaviors, psychological states, or physiological responses within the environment in which they naturally occur (Shiffman, Stone,

& Hufford, 2008). While the term was first used by Stone and Shiffman (1994) only recently, synonymous research methods, such as the *experience sampling method* (Csikszentmihalyi & Larson, 1987) and self-monitoring by way of pen-and-paper diaries, have been used for much longer (Shiffman, et al., 2008). In one of the earliest accounts of the assessment of physical activity in everyday life, Hodges and colleagues reported on the use of pedometers to measure nurses' walking distances during their workday (Hodges, 1882; cited in Wilhelm, Perrez, & Pawlik, 2012). Until the 1980s, paper-and-pencil diaries were used to record cognitions, behaviors, and events such as daily reports of disease symptoms, medication intake, health behaviors, or general well-being. Recent advances in handheld technologies such as pagers, palmtop computers, and smartphones have increased the convenience of real-time data collection, allowing EMA to develop into a highly adaptable suite of research methods capable of assessing participants in an ecologically valid manner within a range of disciplinary contexts.

Typically, EMA studies sample both periodic moments in participants' day-to-day lives and targeted events of interest, often by way of surveys or diary entries administered using handheld computers such as smartphones (Shiffman et al., 2008). Sampling of periodic moments may involve "signaling" participants by way of a phone call or "beeper" multiple times per day to complete assessments on the basis of a regular or randomly selected schedule (Shiffman, 2009). Moore et al. (2013), for example, in an EMA study designed to assess the effect of substance cravings and affect on the risk of relapse, used an electronic diary to prompt participants three times daily to complete questionnaire-style assessments of their momentary affect and cravings. In doing so, the authors were able to track craving and relapse episodes over time, successfully demonstrating that participants who reported an increase in substance cravings during an early assessment were significantly more likely to report a relapse during a subsequent assessment as compared to noncraving participants.

EMA sampling can also, as previously mentioned, gather data during event-driven, targeted moments of interest. Researchers have used EMA to record all manner of event-driven phenomena including the number of cigarettes participants smoke (Ferguson & Shiffman, 2011), when medication is taken (Jónasson, Carlsen, Sødal, Jonasson, & Mowinckel, 1999), and even the occurrence of symptoms (e.g., for asthma; see MacDonell, Gibson-Scipio, Lam, Naar-King & Chen, 2012). Commonly, these two forms of assessment, prompted and event-based, are used concurrently to great effect. Finally, EMA is also commonly undertaken alongside the real-time collection of other passively sensed data using either stand-alone sensors or sensors embedded in the EMA device itself. In this manner, researchers may capture objective, clinically relevant data such as physical symptoms (e.g., heart rate or blood pressure), physical activity/inactivity, environmental conditions (e.g., one study measured electromagnetic field exposure; Bogers et al., 2013), or geospatial information (e.g., Kirchner et al., 2013).

The popularity of EMA as a research methodology has grown significantly in recent years. This is in part due to recent advances in handheld electronic technologies and the near universal accessibility of such devices (e.g., in 2013, it was estimated that there were more than 6.8 billion mobile-cellular subscriptions worldwide; International Telecommunications Union, 2013). However, EMA's appeal lies predominantly in its many advantages over other data collection techniques. The rationale behind EMA methodology has been detailed in great depth elsewhere (see Shiffman et al., 2008) so we will only touch on it briefly here. Simply put, the development of EMA methods has grown from the need for a data collection technique that is ecologically valid, free from recall-based bias, and able to intensively track behaviors and events across time.

Rationale

Ecological Validity

While laboratory-based studies afford researchers an important degree of experimental control, the interplay between contextual factors and human behavior cannot adequately be simulated, or indeed captured, in such a setting (Shiffman et al., 2008). Furthermore, phenomena demonstrated in laboratory settings may not actually occur in the "real world" (e.g., Reis & Gosling, 2010). Consequently, in order to gather data that are reliably representative, assessments must occur in the environment in which the experience or behavior occurs naturally (Shiffman et al., 2008). EMA does exactly that: assessments are completed as participants go about their day-to-day activities, and data pertaining to behaviors and experiences are recorded in the environments in which they naturally occur. For this reason, EMA methods are *ecologically valid*. That is, findings may be generalized to real-world experiences (Ferguson & Shiffman, 2011), noting of course, that any reactivity effects of participation in the study must be accounted for (Barta, Tennen, & Litt, 2012; Rowan et al., 2007). Pickering's (1991) extensive work on the topic of blood pressure monitoring serves to illustrate the importance of ecologically valid assessment methods. Pickering (1991) observed that the clinical or laboratory environment can, in some individuals, induce enough anxiety to briefly elevate blood pressure, resulting in an erroneous diagnosis of hypertension and highlighting the importance of contextual factors on participant behavior and experience. EMA methods allow researchers to observe experiences and behaviors as they change across variations in both time and context, thus ensuring a greater understanding of the antecedents and consequences of phenomena (Shiffman et al., 2008).

Momentary Assessment

Arguably the most important benefit of EMA methods is that assessments are, indeed, momentary; data are collected in real time and without the need for retrospective recall. Traditionally, self-report data are collected by way of retrospective questionnaires or interviews which require participants to recall and summarize large quantities of information after what is often a considerable time delay (e.g., "On average, how bad was your pain over the past week?") (Courvoisier, Eid, & Lischetzke, 2012; Stone, Shiffman, Schwartz, Broderick, & Hufford, 2002). Although this approach has proved to be a reliable measure of current states (Stone et al., 2002), recall of past experiences is fallible, and data gathered in this manner are prone to both random error and systematic bias (Bradburn, Rips, & Shevell, 1987; Broderick et al., 2008; Shiffman et al., 1997). In contrast, EMA focuses on current (or very recent) experiences (e.g., "At this moment, how anxious do you feel?"), thereby minimizing recall and systematic error (Heron & Smyth, 2010; Smyth & Stone, 2003).

As could be expected, discrepancies do occur between EMA- and recall-based measures of the same target phenomena (Shiffman et al., 2008). When compared to momentary approaches, recall-based measures, for example, are commonly found to overestimate the occurrence, duration, and intensity of target events (Shiffman et al., 2008; Van den Brink, Bandell-Hoekstra, & Abu-Saad, 2001). Illustrating this, Shiffman and colleagues (1997) compared smokers' memories of lapse events 12 weeks after having started a quit attempt to descriptions taken immediately after the events occurred. Recall of the context and drivers of the lapse events at the 12-week follow-up was poor, highlighting the dangers of trying to collect such information retrospectively. In another example, Garcia-Palacios et al. (2013) demonstrated that EMA methods provide a more accurate means of assessing fluctuations in self-reported chronic pain than retrospective diaries, in which patients were found to overestimate their pain levels. This research has obvious implications for the improved clinical care of individuals suffering chronic pain and other health problems that present differently within individuals rather than having a common trajectory. It is apparent that recall-based measures are, at best, inaccurate or, more troublingly, systematically biased. Thus, EMA measures, which circumvent the need for recall, hold a considerable advantage for providing more accurate data on which to base recommendations and/or clinical intervention.

Repetitive Assessment

The final defining benefit of EMA is the opportunity for intensive observation via repeated sampling of variables of interest throughout the monitoring period. Sampling patterns vary between studies; assessments may occur any number of times a day and sampling may last anywhere from 24 hours (e.g., Edmondson et al., 2013) to a year (e.g., Jamison et al., 2001). Repetitive sampling provides the researcher with numerous individual assessments that may be used to track variation in behavior, symptoms, affect, or experience across time and setting (e.g., daily fluctuations in mood), providing insight into the target phenomena's natural history. It is not surprising, therefore, that EMA methods have great potential for determining when medical interventions on target phenomena should occur and what intervention(s) should be provided. In this way, researchers may conduct causal analyses and examine questions pertaining to the antecedents and consequences of events and behaviors (Stone et al., 2007). In addition, repetitive sampling can also provide, when assessments are aggregated, scores that are representative of a participant's typical condition (i.e., average mood) while still avoiding the error and bias associated with retrospective recall (Shiffman & Stone, 1998). Put simply, repetitive sampling allows for participants' behaviors and experiences to be tracked near-continuously across time and context, thus allowing researchers insight into relationships and processes that are not adequately captured by retrospective, relatively infrequent methods of reporting.

In summary, EMA grew out of a need to improve existing data collection methods. Consequently, data collected using EMA are ecologically valid, free from random error and systematic bias, and are useful to characterize, at a high level of detail, behaviors and experiences of interest across variations in time and context.

Advancing Clinical Care Through EMA

EMA was developed as a research tool and, as such, has primarily been used in a research setting. However, recent technological advances have meant that the potential utility of EMA as an assessment tool has grown exponentially in a broad range of areas and particularly within the fields of health psychology and behavioral medicine. Broadly, the goals of clinical assessment are to develop a comprehensive understanding of the problem at hand, implement an appropriate treatment or intervention plan, and, finally, evaluate the effects and effectiveness of that treatment (Piasecki, Hufford, Solhan, & Trull, 2007). EMA has the potential to dramatically improve clinical assessment across all of these areas. There is no need, for the purposes of this chapter, to reproduce earlier reviews (see, e.g., Mehl & Conner, 2012); however, it is useful to survey the ways in which EMA methods can be used. Therefore this section explores four major applications of EMA in health research: *individual differences, temporal sequences, natural history,* and *contextual associations* and how each can contribute to improved clinical assessment and care.

Individual Differences

Possibly the simplest use of EMA is in the examination of between-individual and within-individual differences. As discussed earlier, by aggregating EMA assessments, the typical condition of an individual or group may be examined or compared. In addition, by comparing aggregated scores from different time points, changes in behavior or experience may be observed (Shiffman et al., 2008). From a health perspective, this is particularly useful for determining treatment efficacy. Mitchell et al. (2013), for instance, used EMA data on current symptoms, affect, and situation to assess the preliminary treatment efficacy of mindfulness meditation training as an intervention for attention deficit hyperactivity disorder symptoms. Mitchell and colleagues found that clinician ratings of symptomatology and executive functioning, as well as self-reported emotion dysregulation, improved in the treatment group relative to controls. Naturally, this ability to conduct "before and after" comparisons is in no way unique. However, EMA methods, as previously discussed, hold a number of advantages over traditional recall-based assessment approaches.

As EMA measures dynamic experiences in near real time it is also particularly well suited to determining treatment efficacy or individual participant responses *as they occur* (Shiffman et al., 2008). There are obvious implications here for improving clinical care: if basic aspects of assessment or monitoring can be conducted by distance, with fewer face-to-face appointments required, it could dramatically improve treatment efficiency and, in many cases, lower healthcare costs. For instance, by remotely assessing health problems that require high-frequency, long-term monitoring (e.g., diabetes, hypertension), the burden on health practitioners and patients alike could be significantly reduced by limiting clinic visits to those occasions when a problem is identified. There are several examples of EMA being used successfully to track adherence to recommended medical regimens in specific populations, such as in individuals with diabetes (e.g., Mulvaney et al., 2012).

EMA also has value in the area of so-called *telehealth*—at-home monitoring of health conditions. EMA can be used to remotely monitor postsurgical outcomes, such as pain and sleep, which can enable more ambulatory surgeries and reduce lengths of hospital stays (e.g., Costa Pombo, de Araujo, da Silva Viana, & da Costa, 2014). EMA can also be used to track symptoms among individuals with heart failure, where technology-mediated, at-home monitoring has been shown to reduce rates of hospital readmission (Cosgrove et al., 2013). This potential of EMA to enable telehealth care is made all the more significant by recent advances in handheld technologies, which mean that EMA methods are no longer restricted to simple diary entries: participants can feasibly gather assessment data in the form of video diaries, photographs, audio recordings, geographical locations (by way of geospatial positioning systems or GPS), or even physiological measures (e.g., blood glucose measures in diabetic participants). For example, individuals can report on symptoms or experiences during the day using EMA, and an EMA protocol can also integrate data that are sensed by the device being used to collect the EMA data (e.g., use the mobile device to collect data on a participant's movement) or data that are being sensed by other devices in the individual's life. This kind of sampled sensing has been used, for example, in "smart homes" that monitor use of different appliances as evidence of "normal" or "abnormal" behavior among elderly individuals who live alone (e.g., Bradford, 2013).

Temporal Sequences

The momentary and repetitive sampling that is common to all EMA methods allows researchers to capture the fine detail of the relationships that exist among experience, time, and setting (Smyth & Stone, 2003). EMA data are used to examine the temporal sequences of events: the way in which events unfold over time and context (Shiffman, 2014; Stone et al., 2007). Moreover, EMA may serve to delineate the specific antecedents and consequences of events or behaviors (Shiffman et al., 2008). This ability to capture the temporal sequences of events with a high degree of resolution has important clinical applications. Understanding the antecedents and consequences of behavior is central to the development of efficacious treatment and intervention strategies; in order to prevent a negative behavior or symptom, its causes and natural history must be understood. In the case of smoking, for example, researchers have used the analytical approach of dynamic systems modeling (traditionally used in engineering settings) to analyze EMA data in order to understand the natural history of cravings over time in relation to smoking cessation (Timms, Rivera, Collins, & Piper, 2013). These kinds of dynamic systems approaches to understanding the antecedents and consequences of smoking directly inform how and when treatment may be applied to interrupt a sequence of events that end with an undesirable outcome (e.g., smoking lapse or relapse).

EMA data have been used to categorize the situations in which smokers trying to quit may be at greater risk of relapsing back to smoking. For example, using data collected during an observational study of quitting, Shiffman and colleagues (1996) reported that the momentary risk of lapsing was greatly enhanced when a smoker was exposed to certain environmental stimuli—notably alcohol or other people smoking—and/or negative affect states. This finding is of significant importance in that it demonstrates how moment-to-moment changes in environmental factors may influence behavior. In this manner, EMA data may be used to improve understanding of behavioral antecedents and, consequently, may inform the development of optimal treatment options.

Natural History

The recording and analysis of within-individual differences over time allow researchers and clinicians to understand each individual's natural history as it relates to target phenomena (Shiffman et al., 2008). EMA offers a high resolution to the study of phenomena that have a temporal dimension (Shiffman, 2014). EMA studies have been used to reveal the individual variability of withdrawal symptoms experienced by smokers (McCarthy, Piasecki, Fiore, & Baker, 2006) and it is not surprising, therefore, that EMA has arguably become the gold standard for substance dependence research, particularly smoking addiction and cessation. The value of understanding the nature of each patient's response to target phenomena has obvious implications for clinicians. Rather than operating from a "typical" description based on means established from population studies, clinicians may measure their patient's response to a phenomenon (e.g., antecedents, behaviors, and variability in moods) as, for example, they attempt to resist smoking cues (Ferguson & Shiffman, 2009) or experience other contextual potentially high-risk events (e.g., a migraine; Houtveen & Sorbi, 2013).

Contextual Associations

Human behavior and experience are heavily influenced by social and environmental contextual factors and, thus, the generalizability of laboratory-based data is questionable (Smyth & Stone, 2003). Moreover, many health-related behaviors and experiences cannot be adequately assessed within a laboratory or clinical setting, making accurate diagnosis and treatment difficult. Many of the presenting symptoms of anxiety disorders, for example, even in patients who are significantly impaired in their day-to-day functioning, may only present under highly specific circumstances (e.g., phobic behaviors; Alpers, 2009). EMA has the ability to assess many types of behaviors, symptoms, or measures of functioning in a real-world context, allowing for the assessment of symptomatology that may be impossible to simulate in a laboratory or clinical setting. EMA is therefore able to improve the accuracy of multiples assessments as well as provide deep insights into contextual relationships that were previously unattainable. For this reason, EMA lends itself particularly well to specific aspects of substance use and substance dependence research as behavioral events such as relapse and withdrawal, which may not easily be replicated in a laboratory setting and may be highly affected by context; using EMA, these may be tracked across time and situation (Ferguson & Shiffman, 2011). Verdoux, Husky, Tournier, Sorbara, and Swandsen (2003), for example, examined the role of specific social environments on the expression of psychotic symptoms in daily life. The results suggested that, rather than social company itself, it is the dynamic changes that occur in social company that are the key driving factors behind variation in psychotic experiences. Studies such as this serve to highlight the kind of detail that is often lost in retrospective assessment: subtle person–environment interactions that are difficult to capture through retrospective recall.

In summary, while EMA is still predominantly used within a research setting, it holds considerable potential for the advancement of clinical care. EMA can be used to gain understanding of a target phenomenon, to guide the planning and implementation of treatment and intervention strategies, and even to evaluate treatment efficacy moment-by-moment. Moreover, it also has considerable potential to significantly improve access to healthcare through applications such as remote monitoring.

The Future of EMA: Combining Assessment and Intervention

We now turn to the future potential of EMA methods and associated technologies to become a significant element of not just clinical assessment but also intervention and treatment. The application of EMA technologies to treatment or intervention, whereby real-time, momentary interventions are delivered to participants as they go about their daily lives (also known as ecological momentary intervention [EMI]; Heron & Smyth, 2010) has seen a dramatic rise in popularity over the past decade. As discussed earlier, EMA technologies have already been used to implement interventions across an expansive variety of health issues such as the promotion of medication and treatment adherence (e.g., diabetes, Yoon & Kim, 2008; HIV, Moore et al., 2013), smoking cessation (e.g., Rodgers et al., 2005), the promotion of physical activity (e.g., King et al., 2008; Fukuoka et al., 2011), weight loss (e.g., Joo & Kim, 2007), reduction of anxiety (e.g., Przeworski & Newman, 2004), training of social skills (Kopelowicz, Liberman, & Zarate, 2006), and reduction of alcohol consumption (Cohn, Hunter-Reel, Hagman, & Mitchell, 2011) (for a review, see Heron & Smyth, 2010). As such, rather than provide a simple list of different clinical treatments using EMA, the following section provides a review of the potential held by EMA-based treatment and intervention before discussing the advantages and concerns associated with such techniques.

Advantages of EMA-Based Interventions

Handheld technologies have already had a significant impact on healthcare delivery and access: patients are reminded to attend appointments by way of text messages, and isolated patients may consult their healthcare professional during appointments conducted remotely over the Internet (Cohn et al., 2011). Interventions utilizing EMA technology retain all of its advantages in that it is momentary, accessible, context-sensitive, and repetitive, but EMA-based interventions also afford both the health professional and the patient a number of additional benefits. Recent technological advances, as well as the near universal availability of handheld devices such as mobile phones, have significantly improved the viability of assessment and intervention strategies utilizing such technologies (Kaplan & Stone, 2013). The (often considerable) financial burden of EMA-based research may no longer constrain intervention and study design as the majority of participants are likely to be able to provide their own equipment. Runyan et al. (2013), for instance, developed a smartphone application that was installed on university undergraduates' own mobile phones to collect momentary data about participants' use of time. Furthermore, utilizing technology that is already well known to the participant is likely to improve skill acquisition as well as make it easier for participants to incorporate new intervention behaviors, such as recording events or completing assessments, into their daily routines.

Tailored Interventions

The concept of "tailoring" intervention or treatment strategies for individual patients is not new. Intervention content is often tailored, for instance, on the basis of an individual's personal characteristics as obtained during pre-intervention interviews (Heron & Smyth, 2010). For example, Depp et al. (2010) provided individualized cognitive and behavioral interventions for participants with schizophrenia by way of text messages, the content of which was based on participants' answers to a pretrial interview as well as responses to study text messages. Alternately, the timing of an intervention may be tailored to the needs of the participant. For example, support may be provided at the request of the participant (e.g., when craving a cigarette, when feeling stressed), at times preselected by the participant (i.e., every day at 12:00 PM), or at targeted moments in which the participant believed that she would particularly need support (i.e., during typical drinking times; Heron & Smyth, 2010). However, the use of EMA technologies as a delivery platform for intervention has enormous potential beyond traditionally tailored interventions. Specifically, there is the potential to provide interventions that are tailored to the *momentary* needs of the individual (Heron & Smyth, 2010; Shiffman et al., 2008).

As previously discussed, technological advances mean that EMA methods are no longer restricted to the completion of diary entries. Similarly, interventions need not be delivered on the basis of preprogrammed schedules or self-report responses; theoretically, variables such as an individual's psychophysiological state, activity levels, context, or geographical location can all be assessed "in the moment" and then be used to guide the delivery of instantaneous, individually tailored interventions (Heron & Smyth, 2010; Patrick, Griswold, Raab, & Intille, 2008; Riley et al., 2011). Put simply, EMA has the potential to deliver interventions that evolve with the changing needs of the patient.

A recent study by Kirchner and colleagues (2013) serves to illustrate the potential of EMA as a momentary intervention provider: in a study examining the role of context on the success of smoking quit attempts, Kirchner and colleagues (2013) tracked the GPS locations of their sample, 475 adult (>18 years) smokers, throughout the first month of a quit attempt. The recorded GPS data enabled the authors to examine the success of the participants' quit attempts on a day-by-day basis, as a function of both real-time exposure to point-of-sale tobacco outlets and subjective craving to smoke. What was found was that lapsing was increasingly likely with more frequent exposure to point-of-sale tobacco. The use of geo-tagging, as demonstrated by Kirchner et al. (2013), and technologies like it, have considerable potential as a means of delivering active interventions that are based on real-world contextual information. If it is possible to identify when people will need treatment, based on momentary factors such as their geographical or situational location, then treatments can be tailored and delivered in the moment in which they will be most effective. For example, in future interventions geo-tagging could be used to identify "hotspots" in which individuals are more likely to be at risk of a targeted undesirable behavior occurring (i.e., in the case of alcohol abuse/dependence, in the vicinity of a liquor store) and to provide momentary interventions when participants move into these "high-risk" areas (i.e., a personalized SMS encouraging abstinence from alcohol). There are some risks to such an approach, however, as well as methodological and ethical implications. If one considers the example of preemptively messaging someone who approaches a geo-tagged "hotspot," there is a risk that the intervention message might cue the person to think about the risky behavior when they had been thinking about doing something else entirely, such as driving *past* rather than *to* a liquor store. Moreover, in some cases, it may be hard to delineate what exactly constitutes an "event" or target behavior. For instance, determining what exactly constitutes a "craving episode" may prove difficult. Avoiding such pitfalls may rely on the quality of the EMA data being collected (e.g., in this scenario, assessing affect and cravings in conjunction with geospatial data) to ensure that judgments made about when and how to intervene are likely to achieve the intended outcomes (see also Gustafson et al., 2011).

One intervention that has made use of this potential is the Mobylize! system (Burns et al., 2011). Mobylize! is a context-aware intervention system for depression that used a combination of EMA-reported mood and context variables with sensors embedded within a smartphone (e.g., light detection, phone usage). Machine-learning methods are then used to predict when participants were experiencing low mood and delivered a momentary intervention aimed at improving mood or supporting coping. Though continued research on this kind of preemptive approach to behavioral intervention is warranted, there is great potential for these kinds of interventions to positively impact on behavioral health disorders that may be chronic and relapsing in nature (e.g., depression, nicotine dependence, other substance dependence).

Even before the addition of EMA technology, tailoring intervention content could offer multiple advantages over generic interventions designed for a subgroup of interests (i.e., individuals with diabetes, nicotine dependence). For example, people may be more likely to attend to and thoughtfully process information if they believe it to be personally relevant. Moreover, Kreuter, Strecher, and Glassman (1999) posit that "one-size-fits-all" approaches fail to address the important role of individual differences in peoples' health-related decisions and behaviors. Indeed, tailoring the content of health messages based on participant characteristics such as motivation and self-efficacy may improve both message acceptance and willingness to change, thereby improving the likelihood of successfully enacting behavior change (Heron & Smyth, 2010).

Interventions that utilize EMA technology, however, offer additional advantages that are inherent to the methodology. For instance, changes to behavior or new, desirable habits that result from interventions delivered in a real-world setting, as opposed to a laboratory or clinic, may be more likely to be maintained. New skills and behaviors (e.g., coping strategies), despite being successfully utilized when tested in a laboratory or clinical setting, may fail to translate effectively to a real-world situation (Depp et al., 2010; Kopelowicz et al., 2006). By providing interventions within the context of the individual's day-to-day life, as opposed to during discrete periods (i.e., clinic visits), participants may have the opportunity to directly apply learned skills or behaviors to actual experiences, thereby encouraging and reinforcing behavior change (Heron & Smyth, 2010).

Another strength of combining assessment with treatment is that it may improve not only the researcher or clinician's understanding of the nature and experience of symptoms, but also the patient's. EMA methods allow the patient to actively participate in the assessment and monitoring process. Patients are able to become active partners in the therapeutic process, thereby promoting a greater understanding of symptoms and their own behavior and thus leading to improvements in patient self-efficacy, illness management, and treatment outcomes (Myin-Germeys et al., 2011). *Self-Determination Theory* (Ryan & Deci, 2000) suggests that allowing patients to gain some control over the outcome of events and to be causal agents in their own lives (or assessments and treatments), as well as providing the opportunity to interact and be connected to others, contributes to good psychological and emotional health and well-being and allows patients to experience greater motivation to engage in behavior change (Gagné & Deci, 2005; Ryan & Deci, 2000). One example of an intervention that actively promotes participant involvement is the Monitoring, Treatment, and Predication of Bipolar Episodes (MONARCA) wearable system project, a currently in-development mobile phone application that aims to provide ongoing assessment and treatment for bipolar disorder as well as encouraging and facilitating improved illness management (Puiatti, Mudda, Giordana, & Mayora, 2011). The application will require participants to complete daily assessments on mood, sleep, and medication, the results of which will provide immediate feedback to participants. The application will be used to track patient progress and help in the identification and subsequent awareness of early warning signs or symptoms of critical episodes (i.e., oncoming manic or depressive periods). Once early warning signs are identified, patient-programmable "triggers" can be used to warn participants that data collected via assessments are suggestive of an oncoming critical episode. For example, if the participant completes several entries reporting that medication has been missed, a warning may be triggered prompting the program to alert the patient, provide advice, or recommend actions to take. Future EMA designs may, ideally, make use of algorithms to identify antecedents and subsequently provide interventions without any deliberate effort on the behalf of the participant. Understanding and identifying antecedents means that illness management may be improved; rather than critical episodes seeming to occur without warning, participants and health practitioners alike would have a greater understanding of when and why events occur, improving patient self-efficacy, coping, and outcomes.

Ethical Considerations

Briefly, consideration also needs to be given to the ethical and legal issues that may arise as these technologies enable clinicians and other stakeholders to monitor patients in real time (e.g., Labrique, Kirk, Westergaard, & Merritt, 2013). While space precludes discussion of this topic here in substantial detail, potential concerns exist regarding consent, privacy, confidentiality, the potential involvement of other stakeholders such as family members, social media platforms and their owners, insurance companies, governments and employers, and the vast amount of data that can be potentially collected about individuals, and these have clinical, policy, and legislative implications (Kumar et al., 2013).

The Need for Theory-Based Interventions

To bring about effective behavior change, treatment or intervention strategies should be grounded in health behavior theory; however, this is not consistently the case, particularly in the context of real-time interventions. In a review of mobile health interventions and the health behavior models guiding them, Riley et al. (2011) concluded that current theories of health behavior were inadequate in light of the dynamic nature of modern mobile intervention strategies. Health behavior theories should be able to guide the development of complex, real-time interventions that adapt rapidly over time and in response to a variety of data; intervention content and timing should be adjusted not only at the start of an intervention but also frequently over the course of the intervention in response to assessments made or data collected during that time. Riley et al. (2011) suggest that the predominantly linear and static nature of many of the currently held theories renders them inadequate in this regard; they do not adapt to ongoing changes over the course of an intervention that may be captured using EMA methods. Furthermore, Dunton and Atienza (2008) note that the majority of current health behavior theories focus on delineating between-person differences. In contrast, theories with a focus on intra-individual variation—that is, predictors of an individual's daily and within-daily behavior—are lacking. Consequently, current theories of health behavior may be suited to tailoring intervention content and timing based on broad, pre-intervention differences, but not to tailoring an intervention to the needs of the individual as they evolve moment by moment (Riley et al., 2011). EMA offers a unique and powerful platform for improving our understanding of those mechanisms of behavior change that will be the most important to target in the development and implementation of real-time inventions designed to change behavior.

Conclusion

This chapter has provided a brief overview of both the advantages and concerns associated with implementing treatment and interventions by way of EMA methods and technologies. EMA has significant potential to provide data and technologies that may support clinicians to care for their patients. It is likely that this is a field that will undergo rapid development with the increasing ubiquity of mobile communication technologies. It is therefore of great importance that further work be done to improve our understanding of the relationships among data collection, patient involvement with the technologies, and the nature of the interventions, their monitoring, and their effectiveness. Greater attention should be given to the theoretical underpinnings of interventions that use mobile technologies to better inform their content and timing (Riley et al., 2011; see also Aronson, Marsch, & Acosta, 2013), just as consideration should be given to the ethical and legal issues that will likely arise as these technologies enable clinicians and other stakeholders to monitor patients in real time (e.g., Labrique et al., 2013).

EMA methods provide a means by which researchers may attain highly detailed, ecologically valid, and contextually rich data on everyday experience and behavior. EMA also ensures that multiple forms of psychological or physiological processes may be observed as they unfold over time, allowing researchers to conduct causal analyses and examine the antecedents and consequences of events and behavior. Applying EMA to a clinical setting has the potential to contribute significantly to the improvement of patient care, and, in some ways, it already has. Clinical assessment may be improved at multiple stages by EMA: through the enhancement of diagnostics, by aiding the development and implementation of treatment and intervention strategies, and through the evaluation of the effects and efficacy of treatments. Use of EMA in clinical care is also timely: the collection of data via EMA is in line with a healthcare system that is increasingly technology-mediated (Weinstein et al., 2013) and one in which patient-centered care is highly valued, where "patient-centered" means having a deep understanding of patients' needs, preferences, context, and outcomes, all of which may be assessed in great detail using EMA (Cosgrove et al., 2013).

While, to date, EMA technologies have largely been employed as an assessment tool within a research setting, this chapter has also provided a brief overview of EMA's growing utility as a platform for treatment and intervention. The ability of EMA technologies to provide tailored interventions that respond to patients' real-time behaviors, moods, social contexts, and geographical locations has the potential to revolutionize modern healthcare. Considerable work remains to ensure that EMA-based interventions are appropriate, theoretically derived, and ethical in their effects on privacy and confidentiality.

References

Alpers, G. W. (2009). Ambulatory assessment in panic disorder and specific phobia. *Psychological Assessment, 21*(4), 476–85. doi:10.1037/a0017489

Aronson, I. D., Marsch, L. A., & Acosta, M. C. (2013). Using findings in multimedia learning to inform technology-based behavioral health interventions. *Translational Behavioral Medicine, 3*(3), 234–43.

Barta, W., Tennen, H., & Litt, M. (2012). Measurement reactivity in diary research. In M. Mehl & T. Conner (Eds.), *Handbook of research methods for studying daily life* (pp. 108–23). New York: Guilford.

Bogers, R., Bolte, J., Houtveen, J., Lebret, E., van Strien, R., Schipper, M., . . . van Kamp, I. (2013). Design of an ecological momentary assessment study of exposure to radiofrequency electromagnetic fields and non-specific physical symptoms. *BMJ Open, 3*(8), e002933. doi:10.1136/bmjopen-2013-002933

Bradburn, N., Rips, L., & Shevell, S. (1987). Answering autobiographical questions: The impact of memory and inference on surveys. *Science, 236*, 157–61. doi:10.1126/science.3563494

Bradford, D. (2013). Detecting degeneration: Monitoring cognitive health in independent elders. *Proceedings of the Annual International Conference of the IEEE Engineering in Medicine and Biology Society, 2013*, 7029–32. doi:10.1109/embc.2013.6611176

Broderick, J. E., Schwartz, J. E., Vikingstad, G., Pribbernow, M., Grossman, S., & Stone, A. A. (2008). The accuracy of pain and fatigue items across different reporting periods. *Pain, 139*, 146–57. doi:10.1016/j.pain.2008.03.024

Burns, M. N., Begale, M., Duffecy, J., Gergle, D., Karr, C. J., Giangrande, E., & Mohr, D. C. (2011). Harnessing context sensing to develop a mobile intervention for depression. *Journal of Medical Internet Research, 13*(3), e55. doi:10.2196/jmir/1838

Cohn, A. M., Hunter-Reel, D., Hagman, B. T., & Mitchell, J. (2011). Promoting behavior change from alcohol use through mobile technology: The future of ecological momentary assessment. *Alcoholism: Clinical and Experimental Research, 35*(12), 2209–15. doi:10.1111/j.1530–0277.2011.01571.x.

Cosgrove, D. M., Fisher, M., Gabow, P., Gottlieb, G., Halvorson, G. C., James, B. C.... Toussaint, J. S. (2013). Ten strategies to lower costs, improve quality, and engage patients: The view from leading health system CEOs. *Health Affairs (Millwood), 32*(2), 321–27. doi:10.1377/hlthaff.2012.1074

Costa Pombo, N. G., de Araujo, P. J., da Silva Viana, J. M., & da Costa, M. D. (2014). Evaluation of a ubiquitous and interoperable computerised system for remote monitoring of ambulatory post-operative pain: A randomised controlled trial. *Technological Health Care, 22*(1), 63–75. doi:10.3233/thc-130774

Courvoisier, D. S., Eid, M., & Lischetzke, T. (2012). Compliance to a cell phone-based ecological momentary assessment study: The effect of time and personality characteristics. *Psychological Assessment, 24*(3), 713–20. doi:10.1037/a0026733

Csikszentmihalyi, M., & Larson, R. (1987). Validity and reliability of the experience-sampling method. *Journal of Nervous and Mental Disease, 175*(9), 526–36. doi:10.1097/00005053-198709000-00004

Depp, C. A., Mausbach, B., Granholm, E., Cardenas, V., Ben-Zeev, D., Patterson, T. L.,... Jeste, D. V. (2010). Mobile interventions for severe mental illness: Design and preliminary data from three approaches. *Journal of Nervous and Mental Disease, 198*(10), 715–21. doi:10.1097/NMD.0b013e3181f49ea3

Dunton, G. F., & Atienza, A. A. (2008). The need for time-intensive information in healthful eating and physical activity research: A timely topic. *Journal of the American Dietetic Association, 109*, 30–5. doi:10.1016/j.jada.2008.10.019

Edmondson, D., Shaffer, J. A., Chaplin, W. F., Burg, M. M., Stone, A. A., & Schwartz, J. E. (2013). Trait anxiety and anger measured by ecological momentary assessment and their correspondence with traditional trait questionnaires. *Journal of Research in Personality, 47*(6), 843–52. doi:10.1016/j.jrp.2013.08.005.

Ferguson, S. G., & Shiffman, S. (2009). Cue-induced cravings for cigarettes. *Current Cardiovascular Risk Reports, 3*, 385–90. doi:10.1007/s12170-009-0057-0

Ferguson, S. G., & Shiffman, S. (2011). Using the methods of ecological momentary assessment in substance dependence research—smoking cessation as a case study. *Substance Use & Misuse, 46*, 87–95. doi:10.3109/10826084.2011.521399

Fukuoka, Y., Komatsu, J., Suarez, L., Vittinghoff, E., Haskell, W., Noorishad, T., & Pham, K. (2011). The mPED randomized controlled clinical trial: Applying mobile persuasive technologies to increase physical activity in sedentary women protocol. *BMC Public Health, 11*, 933–40. http://www.biomedcentral.com/1471–2458/11/933

Gagné, M., & Deci, E. L. (2005). Self-determination theory and work motivation. *Journal of Organizational Behavior, 26*, 331–62. doi:10.1002/job.322

Garcia-Palacios, A., Herrero, R., Belmonte, M. A., Castilla, D., Guixeres, J., Molinari, G.,... Botella, C. (2013). Ecological momentary assessment for chronic pain in fibromyalgia using a smartphone: A randomized crossover study. *European Journal of Pain, 18*(6):862–72. doi: 10.1002/j.1532–2149.2013.00425.x.1016/j.jrp.2013.08.005

Gustafson, D. H., Shaw, B. R., Isham, A., Baker, T., Boyle, M. G., & Levy, M. (2011). Explicating an evidence-based, theoretically informed, mobile technology-based system to improve outcomes for people in recovery for alcohol dependence. *Substance Use and Misuse, 46*(1), 96–111. doi:10.3109/10826084.2011.521413

Heron, K. E., & Smyth, J. M. (2010). Ecological momentary interventions: Incorporating mobile technology into psychosocial and health behaviour treatments. *British Journal of Health Psychology, 15*(1), 1–39. doi:10.1348/135910709x466063

Houtveen, J. H., & Sorbi, M. J. (2013). Prodromal functioning of migraine patients relative to their interictal state—an ecological momentary assessment study. *PloS One, 8*(8), e72827. doi:10.1371/journal.pone.0072827

International Telecommunications Union. (2013). *Information and communications technology statistics.* http://www.itu.int/en/ITU-D/Statistics/Pages/stat/default.aspx

Jamison, R. N., Raymond, S. A., Levine, J. G., Slawsby, E. A., Nedeljkovic, S. S., & Katz, N. P. (2001). Electronic diaries for monitoring chronic pain: One-year validation study. *Pain, 91*, 277–78. doi:10.1016/s0304-3959(00)00450–4

Jonasson, G., Carlsen, K. H., Sodal, A., Jonasson, C., & Mowinckel, P. (1999). Patient compliance in a clinical trial with inhaled budesonide in children with mild asthma. *European Respiratory Journal, 14*, 150–54.

Joo, N., & Kim, B. (2007). Mobile phone short message service messaging for behaviour modification in a community-based weight control programme in Korea. *Journal of Telemedicine and Telecare, 13*, 416–20.

Kaplan, R. M., & Stone, A. A. (2013). Bringing the laboratory and clinic to the community: Mobile technologies for health promotion and disease prevention. *Annual Review of Psychology, 64*, 471–98. doi:10.1146/annurev-psych-113011–143736

King, A. C., Ahn, D. K., Oliveira, B. M., Atienza, A. A., Castro, C. M., & Gardner, C. (2008). Promoting physical activity through hand-held computer technology. *American Journal of Preventive Medicine, 34*, 138–42.

Kirchner, T. R., Cantrell, J., Anesetti-Rothermel, A., Ganz, O., Vallone, D. M., & Abrams, D. B. (2013). Geospatial exposure to point-of-sale tobacco: Real-time craving and smoking-cessation outcomes. *American Journal of Preventive Medicine, 45*(4), 379–85. doi:10.1016/j.amepre.2013.05.016

Kopelowicz, A., Liberman, R. P., & Zarate, R. (2006). Recent advances in social skills training for schizophrenia. *Schizophrenia Bulletin, 32*, S12–23. doi:10.1093/schbul/sbl023

Kreuter, M. W., Strecher, V. J., & Glassman, B. (1999). One size does not fit all: The case for tailoring print materials. *Annals of Behavioural Medicine, 21*(4), 276–83. http://www.ncbi.nlm.nih.gov/pubmed/10721433

Kumar, S., Nilsen, W. J., Abernethy, A., Atienza, A., Patrick, K., Pavel, M.,... Swendeman, D. (2013). Mobile health technology evaluation: The mhealth evidence workshop. *American Journal of Preventative Medicine, 45*(2), 228–36. doi:10.1016/j.amepre.2013.03.017

Labrique, A. B., Kirk, G. D., Westergaard, R. P., & Merritt, M. W. (2013). Ethical issues in mHealth research involving persons living with HIV/AIDS and substance abuse. *AIDS Research and Treatment, 2013*, Article ID 189645, doi:10.1155/2013/189645

MacDonell, K., Gibson-Scipio, W., Lam, P., Naar-King, S., & Chen, X. (2012). Text messaging to measure asthma medication use and symptoms in urban African American emerging adults: A feasibility study. *Journal of Asthma, 49*(10), 1092–96. doi:10.3109/02770903.2012.733993

McCarthy, D. E., Piasecki, T. M., Fiore, M. C., & Baker, T. B. (2006). Life before and after quitting smoking: An electronic diary study. *Journal of Abnormal Psychology, 115*, 454–66. doi:10.1037/0021-843X.115.3.454

Mehl, M. R., & Conner, T. S. (Eds.). (2012). *Handbook of research methods for studying daily life*. New York: Guilford.

Mitchell, J. T., McIntyre, E. M., English, J. S., Dennis, M. F., Beckham, J. C., & Kollins, S. H. (2013). A pilot trial of mindfulness meditation training for ADHD in adulthood: Impact on core symptoms, executive functioning, and emotion dysregulation. *Journal of Attention Disorders, 21*(13):1105–20.

Moore, T. M., Seavey, A., Ritter, K., McNulty, J. K., Gordon, K. C., & Stuart, G. L. (2013). Ecological momentary assessment of the effects of craving and affect on risk for relapse during substance abuse treatment. *Psychology of Addictive Behaviour, 28*(2):619–24.

Mulvaney, S. A., Rothman, R. L., Dietrich, M. S., Wallston, K. A., Grove, E., Elasy, T. A., & Johnson, K. B. (2012). Using mobile phones to measure adolescent diabetes adherence. *Health Psychology, 31*(1), 43–50. doi:10.1037/a0025543

Myin-Germeys, I., Birchwood, M., & Kwapil, T. (2011). From environment to therapy in psychosis: A real-world momentary assessment approach. *Schizophrenia Bulletin, 37*, 244–7. doi:10.1093/schbul/sbq164

Patrick, K., Griswold, W. G., Raab, F., Intille, S. S. (2008). Health and the mobile phone. *American Journal of Preventive Medicine, 35*(2), 177–81. doi:10.1016/j.amepre.2008.05.001

Piasecki, T. M., Hufford, M. R., Solhan, M., & Trull, T. J. (2007). Assessing clients in their natural environments with electronic diaries: Rationale, benefits, limitations, and barriers. *Psychological Assessment, 19*(1), 25–43. doi:10.1037/1040–3590.19.1.25

Pickering, T. G. (1991). Clinical applications of ambulatory blood pressure monitoring: The white coat syndrome. *Clinical and Investigative Medicine, 14*, 212–7.

Przeworski, A., & Newman, M. G. (2004). Palmtop computer-assisted group therapy for social phobia. *Journal of Clinical Psychology, 60*, 179–88. doi:10.1002/jclp.10246

Puiatti, A., Mudda, S., Giordano, S., & Mayora, O. (2011, August 30–September 3). *Smartphone-centred wearable sensors network for monitoring patients with bipolar disorder.* Paper presented at the 33rd Annual International Conference of the IEEE EMBS. doi:10.1109/IEMBS.2011.6090613

Reis, H. T., & Gosling, S. D. (2010). Social psychological methods outside the laboratory. In S. T. Fiske, D. T. Gilbert, & G. Lindzey (Eds.), *Handbook of social psychology* (5th ed., pp. 82–114). New York: Wiley.

Riley, W. T., Rivera, D. E., Atienza, A. A., Nilsen, W., Allison, S. M., & Mermelstein, R. (2011). Health behavior models in the age of mobile interventions: Are our theories up to the task? *Translational Behavioral Medicine, 1*(1), 53–71. doi:10.1007/s13142-011-0021-7

Rodgers, A., Corbett, T., Bramley, D., Riddell, T., Wills, M., Lin, R. B., & Jones, M. (2005). Do u smoke after txt? Results of a randomised trial of smoking cessation using mobile phone text messaging. *Tobacco Control, 14*, 255–61. doi:10.1136/tc.2005.011577

Rowan, P. J., Cofta-Woerpel, L., Mazas, C. A., Vidrine, J. I., Reitzel, L. R., Cinciripini, P. M., & Wetter, D. W. (2007). Evaluating reactivity to ecological momentary assessment during smoking cessation. *Experimental and Clinical Psychopharmacology, 15*, 382–9. doi:10.1037/1064–1297.15.4.382

Runyan, J., Steenbergh, T., Bainbridge, C., Daugherty, D., Oke, L., & Fry, B. (2013). A smartphone ecological momentary assessment/intervention "app" for collecting real-time data and promoting self-awareness. *Plos One,* 8(8), e71325. doi:10.1371/journal.pone.0071325

Ryan, R. M., & Deci, E. L. (2000). Self-determination theory and the facilitation of intrinsic motivation, social development, and well-being. *American Psychologist, 55*, 68–78. doi:10.1037110003-066X.55.1.68

Shiffman, S. (2009). How many cigarettes did you smoke? Assessing cigarette consumption by global report, time-line follow-back, and ecological momentary assessment, *Health Psychology, 28*(5), 519–26. doi:10.1037/a0015197

Shiffman, S. (2014). Conceptualizing analyses of ecological momentary assessment data. *Nicotine Tobacco Research, 16*(Suppl 2): S76–87. doi:10.1093/ntr/ntt195

Shiffman, S., Hufford, M., Hickcox, M., Paty, J. A., Gnys, M., & Kassel., J. D. (1997). Remember that? A comparison of real-time versus retrospective recall in smoking lapses. *Journal of Consulting and Clinical Psychology, 65*(2), 292–300. doi:10.1037/0022-006X.65.2.292.a

Shiffman, S., Paty, J. A., Gnys, M., Kassel, J. A., & Hickcox, M. (1996). First lapses to smoking: Within-subjects analysis of real-time reports. *Journal of Consulting and Clinical Psychology, 64*(2), 366–79. doi:10.1037/0022-006X.64.2.366

Shiffman, S., & Stone, A. A. (1998). Introduction to the special section: Ecological momentary assessment in health psychology. *Health Psychology, 17*(1), 3–5. doi:10.1037/h0092706

Shiffman, S., Stone, A. A., & Hufford, M. R. (2008). Ecological momentary assessment. *Annual Review of Clinical Psychology, 4*, 1–32. doi:10.1146/annurev.clinpsy.3.022806.091415

Smyth, J. M., & Stone, A. A. (2003). Ecological momentary assessment research in behavioural medicine. *Journal of Happiness Studies, 4*, 35–52. doi:10.1023/A:1023657221954

Stone, A. A., & Shiffman, S. (1994). Ecological momentary assessment (EMA) in behavioral medicine. *Annals of Behavioral Medicine, 16*(3), 199–202.

Stone, A. A., Shiffman, S., Atienza, A. A., & Nebeling, L. (2007). Historical roots and rationale of ecological momentary assessment (EMA). In A. Stone, S. Shiffman, & A. Atienza (Eds.), *The science of real-time data capture: Self-reports in health research.*

Stone, A. A., Shiffman, S., Schwartz, J. E., Broderick, J. E., & Hufford, M. R. (2002). Patient non-compliance with paper diaries. *British Medical Journal, 324*, 1193–4. doi:10.1136/bmj.324.7347.1193

Timms, K. P., Rivera, D. E., Collins, L. M., & Piper, M. E. (2013). A dynamical systems approach to understand self-regulation in smoking cessation behavior change. *Nicotine & Tobacco Research, 16*(Suppl 2):S159–68. doi:10.1093/ntr/ntt149

Van den Brink, M., Bandell-Hoekstra, E., & Abu-Sadd, H. (2001). The occurrence of recall bias in pediatric headache: A comparison of questionnaire and diary data. *Headache, 41*, 11–20. doi:10.1046/j.1526–4610.2001.111006011.x

Verdoux, H., Husky, M., Tournier, M., Sorbara, F., & Swendsen, J. D. (2003). Social environments and daily life occurrence of psychotic symptoms: An experience sampling test in a non-clinical population. *Social Psychiatry and Psychiatric Epidemiology, 38*, 654–61. doi:10.1007/s00127-003-0702-8

Weinstein, R. S., Lopez, A. M., Joseph, B. A., Erps, K. A., Holcomb, M., Barker, G. P., & Krupinski, E. A. (2013). Telemedicine, telehealth, and mobile health applications that work: Opportunities and barriers. *American Journal of Medicine, 127*(3), 183–7. doi:10.1016/j.amjmed.2013.09.032

Wilhelm, P., Perrez, M., & Pawlik, K. (2012). Conducting research in daily life: A historical review. In M. R. Mehl & T. S. Conner (Eds.), *Handbook of research methods for studying daily life* (pp. 62–88). New York: Guilford.

Yoon, K., & Kim, H. (2008). A short message service by cellular phone in type 2 diabetic patients for 12 months. *Diabetes Research and Clinical Practice, 79*, 256–61.

CHAPTER

25 Virtual Reality Training in Job Interviewing for People with Mental Health Disorders or Disabilities

Morris D. Bell *and* Matthew J. Smith

Abstract

Job interviewing is often the first big hurdle for people seeking employment and may be especially difficult for someone with a psychiatric disorder or disability. Performing well in a job interview often requires coping with the emotional demands of the interaction and having the necessary social skills to establish rapport with the interviewer in order to present oneself in a favorable way. Virtual Reality Job Interview Training (VR-JIT) was created specifically for people with severe and persistent mental illness (SPMI) and other potential employment handicaps (e.g., physical disability, felony convictions, first job) to help them overcome their fears, learn the necessary skills, and develop self-confidence to do well during a job interview. The chapter begins by reviewing vocational rehabilitation services for individuals with SPMI, explains the scientific foundations of the VR-JIT training program, describes the special features of the online tool, and presents research findings on its acceptability and efficacy among individuals with SPMI and other disabilities. The authors observed that trainees largely adhered to VR-JIT and could master the skills and earn excellent scores by the end of training. VR-JIT had a moderate to large effect on improving job interview skills in live role-play interviews and increasing self-confidence for job interviews. Moreover, 6-month follow-up survey results suggest that VR-JIT increased access to employment or other competitive volunteer positions as well as reduced the number of weeks to obtaining their employment goal

Keywords: virtual reality, job interview training, social skills training, vocational rehabilitation, serious and persistent mental illness

Job interviewing is often the first big hurdle for people seeking employment. It is frequently an anxiety-provoking experience but may be especially difficult for someone with a psychiatric disorder or disability. Performing well in a job interview often requires coping with the emotional demands of the interaction and having the necessary social skills to establish rapport with the interviewer and to present oneself in a favorable way. Virtual Reality Job Interview Training (VR-JIT) is the focus of this chapter and was created specifically for people with severe and persistent mental illness (SPMI) and other potential employment handicaps (e.g., physical disability, felony convictions, first job) to help them overcome their fears, learn the necessary skills, and develop self-confidence to do well during a job interview. The chapter begins by reviewing vocational rehabilitation services for individuals with SPMI, explains the scientific foundations of the VR-JIT training program, describes the special features of the online tool, and presents research findings on its acceptability and efficacy among individuals with SPMI and other disabilities.

Why Focus on Work?

Improving vocational rehabilitation services has become a national priority for promoting recovery for individuals with SPMI (i.e., schizophrenia, other psychotic disorders, mood disorders, and posttraumatic stress disorder [PTSD]). Competitive employment rates for individuals with SPMI are approximately 10–20% (Brekke, Levin, Wolkon, Sobel, & Slade, 1993; Marwaha & Johnson, 2004; Marwaha et al., 2007) yet more than 75% of individuals with SPMI prefer returning to some kind of productive activity (Becker, 2002). When these individuals attempt to return to work, they often lack access to appropriate work activity, which leads to further discouragement. Unemployment is a primary source of morbidity, and costs associated with SPMI exceed US$6 billion per year (Rice & Miller, 1998). Obtaining work, on the other hand, is associated with improvement in symptoms and self-esteem (Bell, Lysaker, & Milstein, 1996; Bond, Resnick et al., 2001; Mueser et al., 1997). Moreover, stigma associated with unemployment may be lessened when individuals with SPMI return to work (US Department of Health and Human Services, 2003) by helping to reintegrate people into their community, a key objective of the Americans with Disabilities Act. The President's New Freedom Commission on Mental Health Report, *Achieving the Promise,* reinforced that the goal of the mental health system is to help people with mental illnesses in "living, working, learning, and participating fully in the community" (US Department of Health and Human Services, 2003), and, to meet that goal, recovery-oriented mental health systems emphasize vocational services.

A leading approach to providing this vocational service has been *supported employment* (SE). Derived from procedures in the field of developmental disabilities, SE includes integration with clinical settings, rapid job development and coaching, psychosocial supports, negotiating reasonable accommodations with employers, and benefits counseling. A series of articles in the journal *Psychiatric Services,* dedicated to evidence-based psychiatry, included SE as an evidence-based practice (Bond, Becker et al., 2001). Research on SE has repeatedly demonstrated that it is more effective at improving competitive work outcomes than other models of vocational rehabilitation for SPMI, with more than 15 randomized controlled trials of "high fidelity" supporting SE programs (Bond, Dietzen, McGrew, & Miller, 1995; Bond, Drake, & Becker, 2008; Cook et al., 2005). Reports from the Employment Intervention Demonstration Project (EIDP), an evaluation of SE programs for people with SPMI located in eight sites nationwide in the United States, strongly suggested that at least part-time employment in competitive work is possible for individuals with SPMI (Cook et al., 2005). Most of these jobs were low-skilled and part-time yet integrated at or above minimum wage. After the first 6 months, 30–40% were employed at any one time. Of the various jobs obtained, 18% were full-time (Mueser et al., 2004). Individual Placement and Support (IPS) is a standardized version of SE which is now available in a toolkit from the Substance Abuse and Mental Health Service Administration (SAMHSA) (Bond, Becker et al., 2001). This toolkit explains the principles of IPS, provides training modules to staff, and has a fidelity rating instrument to determine degree of successful implementation.

Individuals with SPMI using SE services still face substantial obstacles to finding appropriate work. As noted, almost half of individuals with SPMI receiving SE services do not obtain work even after 2 years of services, and, for the half who do, it takes on average 6 months until they obtain their first jobs (Bond et al., 2008). One of the obstacles to successful job attainment is the requirement in many situations for the applicant to have a standard job interview. Even in situations in which the vocational specialist may have "carved out" a possible position for their client, the client will still need to meet with the hiring manager and will face many of the same questions that would occur in a standard interview. An informal poll of vocational specialists at a national rehabilitation conference indicated that at least half of their clients participated in standard job interviews, and, in almost all cases, their clients had to meet with the potential employer ahead of time to answer questions about their suitability for the job. Very often even these informal interviews led to unfavorable outcomes.

Vocational specialists know that they need to prepare their clients for job interviews, whether the client is receiving supported employment or involved in less-intensive vocational services such as job clubs or employment counseling. Usually, vocational specialists will role-play the interview with clients because this method creates an opportunity to help the client get comfortable with the situation and gives the vocational specialist the chance to give corrective feedback. Indeed, role-playing is one of the best ways to expose a person to an interpersonal stressor and to teach interpersonal skills. However, there are multiple limitations to these live role-plays. They are limited by the skillfulness of the role-play trainer and the amount of time that can be devoted to repeating the role-plays. Additionally, feedback may not be systematic, there is usually no transcript or video of the role-play for review, there is usually no scoring or examination of good or poor responses, and many clients may feel embarrassed and awkward doing live role-plays. It was for these reasons that Dr. Morris Bell decided to develop a computer-based virtual reality (VR) job interview training program that would provide immersion into a realistic simulated job interview.

Scientific Foundation for Job Interview Role-Play Training

Cognitive Impairment and Behavioral Learning Approaches

A growing body of evidence identified cognitive impairments as a primary source of functional loss and disability in schizophrenia and related disorders (Green, 1996). Cognitive impairments are common, often precede illness onset, and may be linked to core neurobiological substrates of the disorder. The relationship between cognition and work outcomes has also been amply demonstrated. For example, cognitive impairment is associated with lower levels of employment in cross-sectional comparisons of employed versus unemployed individuals with SPMI (Meltzer, 1999; Meltzer & McGurk, 1999), retrospective studies of SPMI individuals with good versus poor vocational outcome (Bellack, Gold, & Buchanan, 1999), prospective studies of SPMI individuals (McGurk & Mueser, 2003a; Mueser, 2002b), and studies of individuals with SPMI receiving vocational rehabilitation (Bell, Bryson, & Wexler, 2003; Bryson, Bell, Kaplan, & Greig, 1998; Gold, Goldberg, McNary, Dixon, & Lehman, 2002b; Lysaker, Bell, Zito, & Bioty, 1995), including individuals receiving SE (Bryson et al., 1998; Gold, Goldberg, McNary, Dixon, & Lehman 2002a; McGurk & Mueser, 2003a, 2003b, 2006a, 2006b; Mueser, 2002a, 2002b). In summary, despite differences in methods across studies, a consistent pattern emerges from this literature showing that better cognitive functioning predicts better work outcomes (Evans et al., 2003; McGurk & Mueser, 2004).

Recently, social cognition has emerged as an important area for investigation, particularly in understanding social dysfunction related to mental illness. Social cognition includes such abilities as emotion recognition, theory of mind, cognitive and emotional empathy, and social attribution bias. While these aspects of mental life may be dependent on neurocognition, they appear to have explanatory power of their own (Couture, Penn, & Roberts, 2006; Green et al., 2008; Pinkham & Penn, 2006). For example, in one study, social cognition measures explained vocational outcomes independent of neurocognition, and there is evidence that social cognition plays an important role in deficits of social skills (Bell, Fiszdon, Greig, & Wexler, 2010; Mueser et al., 1996) and are related to overall community functioning (Smith et al., 2012, 2014c).

Efforts to remediate neurocognitive impairments have gained increased attention, with several meta-analyses generally supporting their efficacy (Fiszdon & Reddy, 2012; Kurtz, Moberg, Gur, & Gur, 2001; McGurk, Twamley, Sitzer, McHugo, & Mueser, 2007; Twamley, Jeste, & Bellack, 2003; Wykes, Huddy, Cellard, McGurk, &N Czobor, 2011). These methods rely principally on drill and repeat practice to increase performance without relying on "top-down" instruction because such instruction is less effective due to cognitive impairments in verbal memory, processing speed, and executive function. Behavioral learning approaches such as errorless learning, shaping, and social modeling are often recommended as ways to change behavior despite cognitive limitations (Liberman, 2009). The simulated role-plays in VR-JIT take advantage of these behavioral learning principles using implicit learning through repetition of role-plays to improve performance, shaping behavior through feedback and reward, and scaffolding difficulty to optimize challenge while reducing error and discouragement. The approach also takes advantage of other important basic principles from the behavioral treatment literature related to exposure therapy and social skills training.

Exposure and Fear Reduction

One of the first concrete achievements in behavior therapy was the development of systematic desensitization to reduce anxiety to feared stimuli (Wolpe, 1973). Exposure therapy has been used for a variety of disorders including phobias, panic disorder, obsessive-compulsive disorder, and PTSD. In recent years, VR software has become a useful tool for bringing life-like experiences into the clinic to help veterans with combat-related PTSD and for phobias such as fear of heights and flying (Krijn, Emmelkamp, Olafsson, & Biemond, 2004; Rizzo, Reger, Gahm, Difede, & Rothbaum, 2009). For most people, a job interview is a highly anxiety-provoking situation. VR-simulated role-play allows exposure to the feared stimulus in a safe environment in which the trainee may exercise maximum control. Following the principles of exposure therapy, repeated role-plays allow the trainee to gradually experience less fear and gain an increasing sense of mastery. By having multiple levels of stress exposure, the trainee may practice at a lower level of challenge and then increase the difficulty level once mastery has been achieved at the lower level. This follows the principle of gradually exposing people to a hierarchy of feared stimuli in conventional behavioral treatments for anxiety disorders. In this way, the trainee may eventually develop the confidence and skill to deal with even very difficult interview situations.

Social Skills Training

Social skills training is aimed at improving social competence across a range of different areas, such as the quality of social relationships, job performance, or interacting with healthcare professionals, and it is widely accepted as an evidence-based practice (Bellack, Mueser, Gingerich, & Agresta, 2013; Liberman, DeRisi, & Mueser, 1989). Skills training involves teaching complex social skills by breaking them down into smaller steps and practicing the skills in role plays and in community settings, which has been shown to improve social functioning and social support across multiple studies (Dilk & Bond, 1996; Heinssen, Liberman, & Kopelowicz, 2000; Kurtz & Mueser, 2008; Mueser, Wallace, & Liberman, 1995; Wallace, 1998). While such training is effective, it requires professionals who must be trained to adequate levels of fidelity to effectively implement the intervention. It is most often administered in a group format, which further limits the frequency and intensity of the training. These limitations are not present when the social skills can be practiced using VR tools. While there are some advantages to live role-play, such as being able to receive feedback about tone of voice or nonverbal behaviors, VR-JIT, as will be described later, allows for highly personalized role-plays with precise feedback and coaching and may be repeated as often as the consumer wants without fear of embarrassment.

Description of the Special Features of Virtual Reality Job Interview Training

Innovative Virtual Reality Technology

The development of this technology began when Dr. Bell observed a demonstration of one of SIMmersion's (www.simmersion.com) VR tools that trained US military chaplains to perform suicide screenings. SIMmersion has created interactive training software for the Department of Defense, the Federal Bureau of Investigations, the National Institute on Alcohol Abuse and Alcoholism, and others using proprietary software that allows trainees to influence the behavior of the simulated character. Dr. Bell was impressed by the compelling VR created by the SIMmersion software and thought that it could help individuals with SPMI be more successful in job interviews. Through the National Institute of Mental Health (NIMH) Small Business Innovation Research (SBIR) grant awarded to SIMmersion, with Dr. Bell as scientific proponent and advisor, this idea became a reality.

SIMmersion Technology

SIMmersion simulations combine video, voice recognition, and *nonbranching logic* (described later) to create an interactive environment that allows trainees to encounter complex social cues and realistic interpersonal exchanges. Another key distinguishing feature of SIMmersion simulations is that trainees experience a sense of "presence" that allows them to become immersed in the training and creates real-world experience. This helps trainees build skills, clarify concepts, and increase retention. SIMmersion's simulations provide superior training because they impact the trainee in three ways: didactic e-learning, role-play practice, and extensive feedback on the practice.

To make the simulation as life-like as possible, an actor, in the role of "Molly Porter," a Human Resource Hiring Manager, was video recorded. This video was separated into thousands of response clips that are played at appropriate times during the simulated conversation. Trainees have face-to-face conversations with Molly using a microphone to participate in the interactive environment and react to complex social cues.

In VR-JIT, the trainee interviews with Molly for a job at a new department store (e.g., Target) that will be opening soon. There are eight possible jobs, including cashier, customer service, inventory, security, grounds and facilities, janitor, food service, and stock clerk. Throughout the interview, the trainee responds to questions regarding work history, needs, and skills. Molly appears to have memory, with her behavior guided by an advanced "emotional model." For example, if a trainee responds inappropriately to several questions, Molly may become dismissive, but if the trainee continually answers appropriately, Molly becomes friendly and encouraging. Trainee questions and statements include a wide variety of natural choices, which allow trainees to answer Molly's questions both appropriately and inappropriately. Based on the trainee's statement, the software selects a reply for Molly. Selection is based on three factors: (1) the version of Molly's personality selected at the start of the session (friendly, business-like, or serious), (2) the entire history of the conversation, and (3) Molly's evolving relationship with the trainee or emotional state, driven by trainee statements. Each of these factors is used to compute conditional probabilities associated with each possible reply, and one is selected. Molly stays true to her character version and the emotional state created during the role-play, and thus she behaves somewhat differently each time the system is used.

For trainees, the goal is to get the job. To help them achieve this goal, they receive three layers of feedback. The first layer is from an on-screen coach who provides nonverbal cues (e.g., smiling, applauding, or showing thumbs down) regarding the trainee's choice of statements. The second layer is an interactive, color-coded transcript available during and after the conversation that explains what Molly was looking for in a response and what was right (green font) or wrong (red font) about each trainee response. This transcript also lets the trainee replay individual exchanges, sections of dialogue, or the entire conversation. The third layer is summative feedback at the conclusion of the conversation on what was accomplished or where trainees need additional improvement on each of eight learning objectives (i.e., Be Honest, Be Dependable, Display Teamwork, Be Positive, Ask for Thursdays Off, Showing Interest in the Position, Be Professional, Make a Good Impression). In addition, VR-JIT contains an interactive e-learning component that provides trainees with information they need to practice to develop job interview skills and provides insight into the eight learning objectives.

The technology includes several key features to address the needs of individuals with SPMI or other disabilities. *Speech recognition* allows trainees to practice speaking prescripted positive responses to difficult questions in a pressure-free environment. Then, in a "real" interview, he or she can use the rehearsed answers practiced within the simulation. Although these answers are not "memorized," they get incorporated into the trainees' interviews through implicit learning. Trainees can also try out inappropriate statements to learn how the interviewer will respond.

Another key feature is the "online" job application. Completing a job application takes time and practice. Trainees *complete an employment application* that includes questions about their employment history, skills, and contact information. This "online" procedure is based on applications currently in use by employers such as Target and Home Depot. This practice prepares trainees to accurately complete such applications. Additionally, information in the application about schooling, previous employment, and military service are used to populate the list of questions that Molly may ask during the interview.

The simulation also allows the trainee *to indicate "yes" or "no"* to the following characteristics: mental illness, substance abuse, felony conviction, autism, first job, spinal cord injury, other visible disability, and other hidden disability (e.g., attention deficit hyperactivity disorder [ADHD]). Each of these characteristics is used to adapt the training to the specific backgrounds of the trainee, which creates an individualized interview experience.

Prior to the virtual interview, trainees are instructed that *they must negotiate* Thursday afternoons off because they have a standing clinical appointment. To make such a request in a respectful way at the right time is challenging for many trainees but is the sort of issue that commonly occurs. This challenge was built into the dialogue because it brings up psychological issues that can overwhelm people who are trying to return to work but know that their recovery requires continued support.

Finally, VR-JIT provides trainees with the option to *disclose their psychiatric disability* at any time throughout the interview. This option helps trainees learn when it may (or may not) be advisable to disclose and how to request accommodations. When disclosure occurs, Molly will explain that her company complies with the American with Disabilities Act and will make reasonable accommodations. She may ask what accommodations may be necessary. Such options are unique to this software and provide trainees an opportunity to decide whether disclosure makes sense for them and if so, to learn an effective way to do it. However, VR-JIT does not advocate for trainees to disclose and only provides the opportunity to learn an effective method to do so.

Nonbranching Logic

This technology allows trainees to do and say what they want, when they want, within the confines of a safe simulation using conditional probabilities that go beyond the branching logic of a "choose your own adventure." Molly has memory, emotion, and a personality; this variability encourages repeated practice and makes the exchanges with Molly seem like a real conversation. This feature provides hours of self-paced training in a safe and judgment-free environment.

Scoring

At the end of each role-play, along with the summative feedback described earlier, trainees receive scores for each of the eight learning objectives with a perfect score totaling 100. If a trainee gets 90 or better, he or she is informed: "You got the job! You made a great impression on Molly and she decided to offer you the job. Congratulations!"

Research Findings for Virtual Reality Job Interview Training

Feasibility and Tolerability Study

SIMmersion and Dr. Bell developed the prototype of VR-JIT through a NIMH SBIR Phase 1 grant that also supported testing its feasibility and tolerability with a representative sample of individuals with SPMI in vocational rehabilitation. Participants had a strong positive response to the prototype and reported it was easy to use, an enjoyable experience, and realistic and helpful. Almost all described the virtual interview as anxiety-provoking but that the anxiety lessened as they became more skilled. They saw the benefit of its special features and believed that they could learn the skills being taught through this method. Participants were enthusiastic about using the final product when it became available (Bell & Weinstein, 2011).

SBIR-Phase 2

Based on Phase 1 acceptability and potential, SIMmersion and Dr. Bell were awarded SBIR Phase2 funding to finalize VR-JIT by adding the extensive e-learning materials and the "online job application" component and building out a comprehensive, flexible, and individualized job interview simulation that includes detailed scoring and feedback. The final product also uses scaffolding across three levels of difficulty in Molly's personality from easy (i.e., Friendly) to medium (i.e., Businesslike) to hard (i.e., Serious). At the most difficult level, Molly may be dismissive, accusatory, and even ask illegal questions. Learning to manage such questions and to win Molly over is challenging but possible. As described earlier, this dialogue is individualized so that Molly can be very challenging by asking precisely those questions that may make the trainee most uncomfortable, such as, "I see there are gaps in your work history; can you explain them?" By reviewing the interview transcripts, the trainee learns about what Molly was exploring in her question and how she understood your response. On the next role-play, the trainee can benefit from this information if the same question arises. However, a strong advantage of this tool is that each interview is different, and, while some questions will be repeated, there will always be new challenges. This allows trainees to generalize their understanding of interview questions so that they can be prepared for the unexpected.

SBIR Efficacy Studies

SIMmersion and Dr. Bell partnered with Drs. Michael Fleming and Matthew Smith and their team at Northwestern University to finalize VR-JIT and evaluate whether it enhanced job interview skills and increased self-reported self-confidence in interviewing ability. Thus, we compared VR-JIT trainees with a wait-list control group on scores from two pre- and two post-training job interview role-plays and on scores from a self-report of their self-confidence in job interviewing.

Methods

We conducted randomized controlled trials in five community-dwelling cohorts of individuals with various disabilities. Three cohorts were supported by SBIR Phase 2 funding, while the Department of Psychiatry and Behavioral Sciences at Northwestern University supported the recruitment of two additional cohorts. We first report on the SBIR Phase 2 cohorts that included (1) individuals with SPMI (83.8% with a mood disorder; 16.2% with schizophrenia; n = 37), (2) veteran outpatients with PTSD (and 84.8% with a co-occurring mood disorders; n = 33), and (3) young adults with autism spectrum disorders (n = 26; Smith et al., 2014a., 2014b, 2015d). Participants (n = 96) were randomized at a ratio of 2 (VR-JIT) to 1(control) so that 64 were in the VR-JIT group and 32 in the wait-list control group.

Results

VR-JIT Trainees (n = 64) showed excellent adherence to the intervention with 55 of 64 participants (86%) completing 8 or more hours of training and the remaining 9 trainees completing 5–7 hours. There were some dips in performance as the participants transitioned to more difficult levels of "Molly." However, the learning curve (Figure 25.1) shows that most participants made rapid gains in skill acquisition, with 87% obtaining a score of 100 at the hardest level at least once by the end of training.

Training Experience

At the end of training, participants reported high satisfaction on the Training Experience

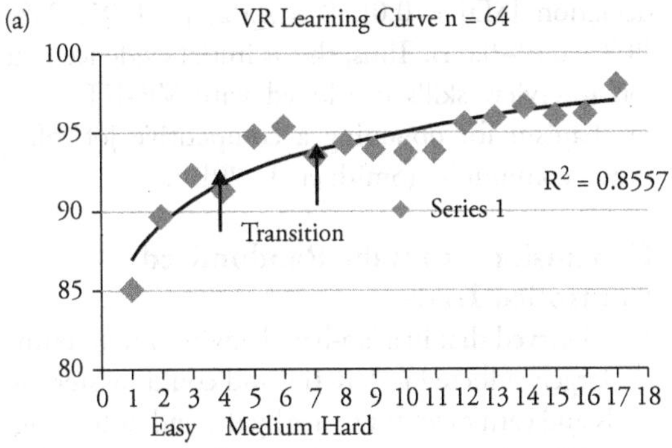

Figure 25.1 Virtual reality (VR) learning curve (n = 64).

Questionnaire (TEQ; Likert Scale of 1–7; higher is better, Table 25.1).

Role-Play Interview Improvement

ANCOVA was performed with post-treatment role-play scores as the dependent variable, treatment group and diagnostic group as fixed factors, and pre-treatment role-play scores as the covariate. This analysis showed a significant treatment condition effect for VR-JIT (F (1,89) = 1 2.8, p<0.001). There was very little improvement for controls (Cohen's d = 0.05) and a moderate improvement for VR-JIT trainees (Cohen's d = 0.52). Two items in the VR-JIT group had large improvement effect sizes: sharing things positively and sounding honest (both Cohen's d >0.70) (Smith et al., 2014a, 2014b, 2015d). Differences by diagnostic group were not significant (p = 0.64), suggesting that VR-JIT trainees with a range of disabilities may acquire new skills when given the proper training.

Improvement in Self-Reported Confidence

ANCOVA with post-test self-reported job interview confidence as the dependent variable and pre-test self-report confidence as the covariate showed a significant VR-JIT effect (F (1,87) = 12.18, p <0.001). Controls showed a small improvement (Cohen's d = 0.36) while VR-JIT trainees showed a large improvement (Cohen's d = 1.04). Item frequencies revealed that 46.8% of VR-JIT trainees described themselves before training as being (moderately, very, or extremely) comfortable with job interviewing, while those rates improved to 79.2% after training (Smith et al., 2014a, 2014b, 2015d). Again, differences by diagnostic group were not significant (p = 0.50).

Table 25.1 Mean score on Training Experience Questionnaire (TEQ)

TEQ Items	
Ease of use	5.9 (1.0)
Enjoyable	6.1 (1.2)
Helpful	6.3 (1.2)
Instilled confidence	6.1 (1.3)
Prepared for interviews	6.1 (1.0)

Employment Outcomes in SPMI

Although there was no follow-up planned to determine whether VR-JIT improved employment outcomes, subsequent funding from the Department of Psychiatry and Behavioral Sciences at Northwestern University facilitated the collection of a brief employment outcome survey from participants 6 months after post-test evaluation. Seventy-four of 96 (77%) participants completed a survey of their employment status and their opinion about VR-JIT's helpfulness. Given that individuals with SPMI and veteran cohorts were both chronically ill, we evaluated their outcomes independently from the young adults with autism spectrum disorders. We found that 25% of controls and 51% of VR-JIT trainees received a job offer, which was significant after adjusting for covariates. Moreover, the likelihood that trainees received a job offer increased for each completed VR-JIT training interview (odds ratio [OR]: 1.41, 95% confidence interval [CI]: 1.02–1.95, p <0.05), and a greater number of completed VR-JIT interviews was associated with fewer weeks until a job offer was received (B = −3.679, SE = 1.37, p <0.05) (Smith et al., 2015a).

Employment Outcomes in Autism

Given that young adults with autism spectrum disorders have better functional outcomes if they work or volunteer (Henninger & Taylor, 2013; Taylor, 2009), we evaluated if VR-JIT was associated with obtaining a competitive job or volunteer position. We observed that 53.3% of VR-JIT trainees obtained a job or volunteer position by 6-month follow-up while only 25% of controls obtained a position (p = 0.09), which was significant after adjusting for covariates (p < 0.05). Moreover, we observed that interview role-play performance improvement between pre- and post-test was associated with completing more interviews during the follow-up period (r = 0.55, p <0.05) (Smith et al., 2015b).

Additional Efficacy Studies

We evaluated VR-JIT in two additional randomized controlled trials of individuals with schizophrenia

(n = 32) or a history of substance use disorders (n = 24). We observed (via ANCOVA) that VR-JIT trainees with schizophrenia significantly improved their job interviewing skills ($F(1,29) = 15.0$, $p < 0.001$; Cohen's d = 0.92) compared to controls, who appeared to regress to the mean (Cohen's d = −0.42). VR-JIT trainees with schizophrenia had a higher rate of obtaining job offers compared to controls (47.8% vs. 14.3%, $p = 0.055$). Similar to the SPMI cohort, we observed that completing more virtual interviews in the schizophrenia cohort was also related with spending fewer weeks searching for employment ($r = -0.63$, $p < 0.001$) and improving one's confidence ($r = 0.46$, $p < 0.05$) (Smith et al., 2015c).

Among the individuals with a substance use disorder, we observed a moderate improvement in role-play performance among VR-JIT trainees compared to controls (Cohen's d = 52). However, this improvement did not attain statistical significance ($F(1,22) = 1.8$, $p = 0.097$). Moreover, we observed that VR-JIT trainees were more likely than controls to obtain a competitive position (78.6% vs. 44.4%, $p < 0.05$). Similar to prior studies, we observed that using VR-JIT was correlated with spending fewer weeks searching for a job ($r = -0.36$, $p < 0.05$) (Smith et al., 2016).

Across all five of our cohorts, we asked the VR-JIT trainees during the 6-month follow-up about their training experience, and, of the trainees who completed the survey (n = 83), 91.5% agreed or strongly agreed that "Looking back, my job interview training was helpful to me"; 89.2% agreed or strongly agreed that "I think it gave me more confidence to go on a job interview"; 90.4% agreed or strongly agreed that "I feel better prepared for interviews"; and 78.3% agreed or strongly agreed "I think refreshing my training skills with the intervention will help me get a job in the future."

Job Interview Skills as a Mechanism for Employment

Although common sense tells us that doing well on the interview helps individuals obtain employment, there are little data to support this relationship. Our data provided the opportunity to evaluate whether interviewing skills were a mechanism for employment via enhancement by VR-JIT. As displayed in Figure 25.2, we observed a significant mediation where the number of virtual interviews completed by n = 79 trainees predicted post-test interview skills, which then predicted receiving a job offer by 6 months (product of coefficients = 0.02, standard deviation [SD] = 0.01, $\beta = 0.02$, $p < 0.05$; 95% PCI = 0.01–0.04). Thus, this is initial evidence that job interview skills developed with VR-JIT are a mechanism for obtaining a competitive job offer in the community (Smith et al., 2017).

Conclusions from the Randomized Controlled Trials

We observed that in a lab-based environment, trainees largely adhered to VR-JIT and could master the skills and earn excellent scores by the end of training. VR-JIT had a moderate to large effect on improving job interview skills in live role-play interviews and increasing self-confidence for job interviews across all five cohorts. Moreover, 6-month follow-up survey results suggest that VR-JIT increased access to employment or other competitive volunteer positions as well as reduced the number of weeks to obtaining this access. Last, we observed that skills enhanced with VR-JIT may be a mechanism for community employment.

What Comes Next?

As of this writing, there are eight scientific papers on the efficacy of VR-JIT that were published in peer-reviewed journals (Smith et al., 2014a, 2014b, 2015a, 2015b, 2015c, 2015d, 2016, 2017). The papers related to the autism spectrum disorder and veteran subsamples were picked up by the public press; stories about the research appeared on the NBC Today Show, Fox News, CNN, and WGN Nightly News; and a lengthy video interview and story appeared in the online *Wall Street Journal*. Other coverage included the *Chicago Tribune*, Everyday Health with Sanjay Gupta, Autism Speaks, Reuters, *Calgary Journal*, and *The Business Standard*. Headlines stated: "FBI Training Software Repurposed to Help Autistic Adults Get Jobs," and "Adults with Autism Get Help from Human Simulator to Navigate Job Interviews." This display of public interest in VR-JIT was not so much about the science but rather the common-sense appeal of a VR job interview training system and its potential societal impact on the lives of people with disabilities.

As of this writing, three research proposals have been funded to continue the evaluation of VR-JIT. First, the National Institute of Mental Health (NIMH) funded an evaluation of the effectiveness and initial implementation of VR-JIT to determine if the intervention can be delivered in everyday rehabilitation practice to individuals with SPMI in a cost-effective manner (R01 MH110524, PI:

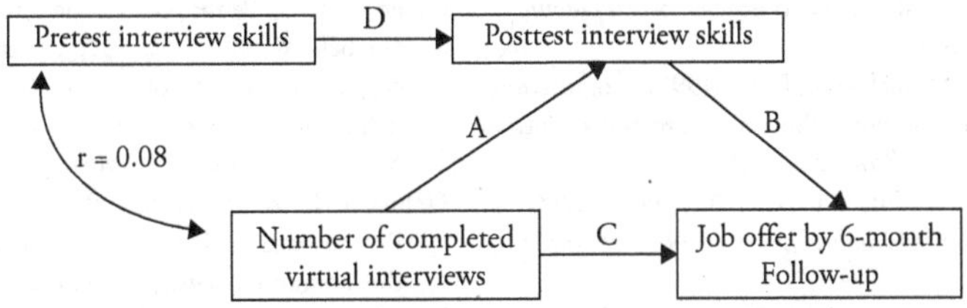

Figure 25.2 Interview skills as a mechanism of obtaining a job offer after virtual reality job interview training. The number of completed virtual interviews were related to post-test interview skills (Path A: B = 2.66, p <.01 (standard deviation [SD] = .85, β = .20, 95% PCI = .08 to .33)); in turn post-test interview skills were related to obtaining a job offer (Path B: B = .01, p <.05 (SD = .01, β = .28, 95% PCI = .01 to .53); and completed virtual interviews were related to obtaining a job offer (Path C: B = .09, p <.05 (SD = .05, β = .30, 95% PCI = .01 to .54). We evaluated if post-test interview skills mediated the relationship between the number of completed virtual interviews and obtaining the job offer to determine if interview skills are a mechanism of employment. Our analysis determined that when accounting for pretest interview skills as a covariate, Path C becomes nonsignificant (B = .07, p >.10 (SD = .05, β =.23, 95% PCI = .06 to .49).

M. Smith). Second, NIMH funded a study to modify VR-JIT for transition-age youth on the autism spectrum, which includes a preliminary evaluation of delivering the modified VR-JIT to students in a high school setting (R34 MH111531, PI: M. Smith). The third proposal was funded by the Kessler Foundation (https://kesslerfoundation.org/) to evaluate the effectiveness and implementation of VR-JIT for 1,000 high school students with disabilities receiving federally mandated transition services (PI: M. Smith).

Additionally, VR-JIT has gone through a feasibility assessment by the Veterans Administration (VA) Division of Veterans Benefits and is currently in field trials in four states to be used with veterans with service-connected disabilities in the VA's vocational rehabilitation program. It is also being used in multiple other programs including an Easter Seals program to reintegrate ex-offenders back into the community and a psychosocial clubhouse that offers SE to individuals with SPMI. VR-JIT has also been implemented by multiple academic (e.g., Marywood University, Conestoga College, the University of Idaho, Mercyhurst University), healthcare (the Mayo Clinic, Rady Children's Hospital), community, and government organizations. SAMSHA has posted VR-JIT on its list of evidence-based programs and practices. Individual users have also been able to obtain access to VR-JIT online at https://jobinterviewtraining.net.

VR-JIT is a sophisticated use of VR software to solve a very specific training problem: learning the skills and developing the self-confidence for job interviews. However, it also serves as an example of the broad potential of VR simulations for other kinds of social skills training for which role-playing could be a part. In the future, additional features to enhance VR-JIT could allow feedback on tone of voice, posture, and facial expressions. This emotion monitoring is currently under development at the Massachusetts Institute of Technology (MIT) Media Lab. For example, MIT students used emotion recognition software and feedback to improve their job interviewing skills. Independent ratings of digital recordings of the students before and after training showed substantial improvement in their eye contact, posture, tone of voice, and other nonverbal features that are important for job interviews (Hoque, Courgeon, Martin, Mutlu, & Picard, 2013).

Learning theory is the scientific foundation for rehabilitation services of this kind. New methods that teach skills more effectively have the potential to improve rehabilitation outcomes. VR and other technological teaching innovations hold significant promise for helping people with disabilities learn new skills or recover lost skills so that they can live better and more integrated lives within their own communities.

References

Becker, D. (2002). *Supported employment toolkit.* Lebanon, NH: Psychiatric Research Center.

Bell, M., Bryson, G., & Wexler, B. E. (2003). Cognitive remediation of working memory deficits: Durability of training effects in severely impaired and less severely impaired schizophrenia. *Acta Psychiatrica Scandinavica 108*(2), 101–9.

Bell, M. D., Fiszdon, J. M., Greig, T. C., & Wexler, B. E. (2010). Social attribution test—multiple choice (SAT-MC) in schizophrenia: Comparison with community sample and relationship to neurocognitive, social cognitive and symptom measures. *Schizophrenia research, 122*(1), 164–71.

Bell, M. D., Lysaker, P. H., & Milstein, R. M. (1996). Clinical benefits of paid work activity in schizophrenia. *Schizophrenia Bulletin, 22*(1), 51–67.

Bell, M. D., & Weinstein, A. (2011). Simulated job interview skill training for people with psychiatric disability: Feasibility and tolerability of virtual reality training. *Schizophrenia Bulletin, 37*(suppl_2), S91–7.

Bellack, A. S., Gold, J. M., & Buchanan, R. W. (1999). Cognitive rehabilitation for schizophrenia: Problems, prospects, and strategies. *Schizophrenia Bulletin, 25*(2), 257.

Bellack, A. S., Mueser, K. T., Gingerich, S., & Agresta, J. (2013). *Social skills training for schizophrenia: A step-by-step guide.* New York: Guilford.

Bond, G. R., Becker, D. R., Drake, R. E., Rapp, C. A., Meisler, N., Lehman, A. F., . . . Blyler, C. R. (2001). Implementing supported employment as an evidence-based practice. *Psychiatric Services, 52*(3), 313–22.

Bond, G. R., Dietzen, L. L., McGrew, J. H., & Miller, L. D. (1995). Accelerating entry into supported employment for persons with severe psychiatric disabilities. *Rehabilitation Psychology, 40*(2), 75–94.

Bond, G. R., Drake, R. E., & Becker, D. R. (2008). An update on randomized controlled trials of evidence-based supported employment. *Psychiatric Rehabilitation Journal, 31*(4), 280.

Bond, G. R., Resnick, S. G., Drake, R. E., Xie, H., McHugo, G. J., & Bebout, R. R. (2001). Does competitive employment improve nonvocational outcomes for people with severe mental illness? *Journal of Consulting and Clinical Psychology, 69*(3), 489–501.

Brekke, J. S., Levin, S., Wolkon, G. H., Sobel, E., & Slade, E. (1993). Psychosocial Functioning and Subjective Experience in Schizophrenia. *Schizophrenia Bulletin, 19*(3), 599–608.

Bryson, G., Bell, M. D., Kaplan, E., & Greig, T. (1998). The functional consequences of memory impairments on initial work performance in people with schizophrenia. *Journal of Nervous and Mental Disease, 186*(10), 610–5.

Cook, J. A., Leff, H., Blyler, & C. R., et al. (2005). Results of a multisite randomized trial of supported employment interventions for individuals with severe mental illness. *Archives of General Psychiatry, 62*(5), 505–12.

Couture, S. M., Penn, D. L., & Roberts, D. L. (2006). The functional significance of social cognition in schizophrenia: A review. *Schizophrenia Bulletin, 32*(suppl_1), S44–63.

Dilk, M. N., & Bond, G. R. (1996). Meta-analytic evaluation of skills training research for individuals with severe mental illness. *Journal of Consulting and Clinical Psychology, 64*(6), 1337.

Evans, J. D., Heaton, R. K., Paulsen, J. S., Palmer, B. W., Patterson, T., & Jeste, D. V. (2003). The relationship of neuropsychological abilities to specific domains of functional capacity in older schizophrenia patients. *Biological Psychiatry, 53*(5), 422–30.

Fiszdon, J. M., & Reddy, L. F. (2012). Review of social cognitive treatments for psychosis. *Clinical Psychology Review, 32*(8), 724–40.

Gold, J. M., Goldberg, R. W., McNary, S. W., Dixon, L. B., & Lehman, A. F. (2002a). Cognitive correlates of job tenure among patients with severe mental illness. *American Journal of Psychiatry, 159*, 1395–402.

Gold, J. M., Goldberg, R. W., McNary, S. W., Dixon, L. B., & Lehman, A. F. (2002b). Cognitive correlates of job tenure among patients with severe mental illness. *American Journal of Psychiatry, 159*(8), 1395–402.

Green, M. F. (1996). What are the functional consequences of neurocognitive deficits in schizophrenia? *The American Journal of Psychiatry, 153*(3), 321.

Green, M. F., Penn, D. L., Bentall, R., Carpenter, W. T., Gaebel, W., Gur, R. C., . . . Heinssen, R. (2008). Social cognition in schizophrenia: An NIMH workshop on definitions, assessment, and research opportunities. *Schizophrenia Bulletin, 34*(6), 1211–20.

Heinssen, R. K., Liberman, R. P., & Kopelowicz, A. (2000). Psychosocial skills training for schizophrenia: Lessons from the laboratory. *Schizophrenia Bulletin, 26*(1), 21.

Henninger, N. A., & Taylor, J. L. (2013). Outcomes in adults with autism spectrum disorders: A historical perspective. *Autism, 17*(1), 103–16.

Hoque, M. E., Courgeon, M., Martin, J.-C., Mutlu, B., & Picard, R. W. (2013). MACH: My automated conversation coach. *Proceedings of the 2013 ACM International Joint Conference on Pervasive and Ubiquitous Computing*, 697–706.

Krijn, M., Emmelkamp, P. M., Olafsson, R. P., & Biemond, R. (2004). Virtual reality exposure therapy of anxiety disorders: A review. *Clinical Psychology Review, 24*(3), 259–81.

Kurtz, M. M., Moberg, P. J., Gur, R. C., & Gur, R. E. (2001). Approaches to cognitive remediation of neuropsychological deficits in schizophrenia: A review and meta-analysis. *Neuropsychology Review, 11*(4), 197–210.

Kurtz, M. M., & Mueser, K. T. (2008). *A meta-analysis of controlled research on social skills training for schizophrenia.* Washington, DC: American Psychological Association.

Liberman, R. P. (2009). *Recovery from disability: Manual of psychiatric rehabilitation.* Arlington, VA: American Psychiatric Publishing.

Liberman, R. P., DeRisi, W. J., & Mueser, K. T. (1989). *Social skills training for psychiatric patients.* Pergamon.

Lysaker, P. H., Bell, M. D., Zito, W. S., & Bioty, S. M. (1995). Social skills at work: Deficits and predictors of improvement in schizophrenia. *Journal of Nervous and Mental Disease, 183*(11), 688–92.

Marwaha, S., & Johnson, S. (2004). Schizophrenia and employment. *Social Psychiatry and Psychiatric Epidemiology, 39*(5), 337–49.

Marwaha, S., Johnson, S., Bebbington, P., Stafford, M., Angermeyer, M. C., Brugha, T., . . . Toumi, M. (2007). Rates and correlates of employment in people with schizophrenia in the UK, France and Germany. *British Journal of Psychiatry, 191*(1), 30–7.

McGurk, S. R., & Mueser, K. T. (2003a). Cognitive functioning and employment in severe mental illness. *Journal of Nervous and Mental Disease, 191*(12), 789–98.

McGurk, S. R., & Mueser, K. T. (2003b). Cognitive functioning and employment in severe mental illness. *Journal of Nervous and Mental Disease, 191*, 789–98.

McGurk, S. R., & Mueser, K. T. (2004). Cognitive functioning, symptoms, and work in supported employment: A review and heuristic model. *Schizophrenia Research, 70*(2), 147–73.

McGurk, S. R., & Mueser, K. T. (2006a). Cognitive and clinical predictors of work outcomes in clients with schizophrenia receiving supported employment services: 4-year follow-up. *Administration and Policy in Mental Health and Mental Health Services Research, 33*(5), 598–606.

McGurk, S. R., & Mueser, K. T. (2006b). Cognitive and clinical predictors of work outcomes in clients with schizophrenia receiving supported employment services: 4-year follow-up. *Administration and Policy in Mental Health and Mental Health Services Research, 33*, 598–606.

McGurk, S. R., Twamley, E. W., Sitzer, D. I., McHugo, G. J., & Mueser, K. T. (2007). A meta-analysis of cognitive remediation in schizophrenia. *American Journal of Psychiatry, 164*(12), 1791–802.

Meltzer, H. Y. (1999). Outcome in schizophrenia: Beyond symptom reduction. *Journal of Clinical Psychiatry, 60*(Suppl 3), 3–8.

Meltzer, H. Y., & McGurk, S. R. (1999). The effects of clozapine, risperidone, and olanzapine on cognitive function in schizophrenia. *Schizophrenia Bulletin, 25*(2), 233–56.

Mueser, K. T. (2002a). Cognitive impairment, symptoms, social functioning, and vocational rehabilitation in schizophrenia. In H. Kashima, I. R. H. Falloon, M. Mizuno, & M. Asai (Eds.), *Comprehensive treatment of schizophrenia: Linking neurobehavioral findings to psychosocial approaches* (pp. 344–51). Tokyo: Springer-Verlag.

Mueser, K. T. (2002b). Cognitive impairment, symptoms, social functioning, and vocational rehabilitation in schizophrenia. In H. Kashima, I. R. H. Falloon, M. Mizuno, & M. Asai (Eds.), *Comprehensive treatment of schizophrenia: Linking neurobehavioral findings to psychosocial approaches* (pp. 344–51). Tokyo: Springer-Verlag.

Mueser, K. T., Becker, D. R., Torrey, W. C., Xie, H., Bond, G. R., Drake, R. E., & Dain, B. J. (1997). Work and nonvocational domains of functioning in persons with severe mental illness: A longitudinal analysis. *Journal of Nervous and Mental Disease, 185*(7), 419–26.

Mueser, K. T., Clark, R. E., Haines, M., Drake, R. E., McHugo, G. J., Bond, G. R., . . . Swain, K. (2004). The Hartford study of supported employment for persons with severe mental illness. *Journal of Consulting and Clinical Psychology, 72*(3), 479.

Mueser, K. T., Doonan, R., Penn, D. L., Blanchard, J. J., Bellack, A. S., Nishith, P., & DeLeon, J. (1996). Emotion recognition and social competence in chronic schizophrenia. *Journal of Abnormal Psychology, 105*(2), 271.

Mueser, K. T., Wallace, C. J., & Liberman, R. P. (1995). New developments in social skills training. *Behaviour Change, 12*(1), 31–40.

Pinkham, A. E., & Penn, D. L. (2006). Neurocognitive and social cognitive predictors of interpersonal skill in schizophrenia. *Psychiatry Research, 143*(2), 167–78.

Rice, D. P., & Miller, L. S. (1998). Health economics and cost implications of anxiety and other mental disorders in the United States. *British Journal of Psychiatry*.

Rizzo, A., Reger, G., Gahm, G., Difede, J., & Rothbaum, B. O. (2009). *Virtual reality exposure therapy for combat-related PTSD, Post-traumatic stress disorder*. In P. J. Shiromani, T. M. Keane, & J. E. LeDoux (Eds.), *Post-traumatic stress disorder: Basic science and clinical practice* (pp. 375–399). New York: Humana.

Smith, M. J., Bell, M. D., Wright, M. A., Humm, L. B., Olsen, D., & Fleming, M. F. (2016). Virtual reality job interview training and 6-month employment outcomes for individuals with substance use disorders seeking employment. *Journal of Vocational Rehabilitation, 44*(3), 323–32.

Smith, M. J., Fleming, M. F., Wright, M. A., Jordan, N., Humm, L. B., Olsen, D., & Bell, M. D. (2015a). Job offers to individuals with severe mental illness after participation in virtual reality job interview training. *Psychiatric Services, 66*(11), 1173–9.

Smith, M. J., Fleming, M. F., Wright, M. A., Losh, M., Humm, L. B., Olsen, D., & Bell, M. D. (2015b). Brief report: Vocational outcomes for young adults with autism spectrum disorders at six months after virtual reality job interview training. *Journal of Autism and Developmental Disorders, 45*(10), 3364–9.

Smith, M. J., Fleming, M. F., Wright, M. A., Roberts, A. G., Humm, L. B., Olsen, D., & Bell, M. D. (2015c). Virtual reality job interview training and 6-month employment outcomes for individuals with schizophrenia seeking employment. *Schizophrenia Research, 166*(1–3), 86–91.

Smith, M. J., Ginger, E. J., Wright, K., Wright, M. A., Taylor, J. L., Humm, L. B., . . . Fleming, M. F. (2014a). Virtual reality job interview training in adults with autism spectrum disorder. *Journal of Autism and Developmental Disorders, 44*(10), 2450–63.

Smith, M. J., Ginger, E. J., Wright, M., Wright, K., Boteler Humm, L., Olsen, D., . . . Fleming, M. F. (2014b). Virtual reality job interview training for individuals with psychiatric disabilities. *Journal of Nervous and Mental Disease, 202*(9), 659–67.

Smith, M. J., Horan, W. P., Cobia, D. J., Karpouzian, T. M., Fox, J. M., Reilly, J. L., & Breiter, H. C. (2014c). Performance-based empathy mediates the influence of working memory on social competence in schizophrenia. *Schizophrenia Bulletin, 40*(4), 824–34.

Smith, M. J., Horan, W. P., Karpouzian, T. M., Abram, S. V., Cobia, D. J., & Csernansky, J. G. (2012). Self-reported empathy deficits are uniquely associated with poor functioning in schizophrenia. *Schizophrenia Research, 137*(1–3), 196–202.

Smith, M. J., Humm, L. B., Fleming, M. F., Jordan, N., Wright, M. A., Ginger, E. J., . . . Bell, M. D. (2015d). Virtual reality job interview training for veterans with posttraumatic stress disorder. *Journal of Vocational Rehabilitation, 42*(3), 271–9.

Smith, M. J., Smith, J. D., Fleming, M. F., Jordan, N., Brown, C. H., Humm, L., . . . Bell, M. D. (2017). Mechanism of action for obtaining job offers with virtual reality job interview training. *Psychiatric Services, 68*(7), 747–50.

Taylor, J. L. (2009). The transition out of high school and into adulthood for individuals with autism and for their families. *International Review of Research in Mental Retardation, 38*, 1–32.

Twamley, E. W., Jeste, D. V., & Bellack, A. S. (2003). A review of cognitive training in schizophrenia. *Schizophrenia Bulletin, 29*(2), 359.

US Department of Health and Human Services. (2003). *Achieving the promise: Transforming mental health care in America*. Final Report. Rockville, MD: Author.

Wallace, C. J. (1998). Social skills training in psychiatric rehabilitation: Recent findings. *International Review of Psychiatry, 10*(1), 9–19.

Wolpe, J. (1973). *The practice of behavior therapy*. Pergamon.

Wykes, T., Huddy, V., Cellard, C., McGurk, S. R., & Czobor, P. (2011). A meta-analysis of cognitive remediation for schizophrenia: Methodology and effect sizes. *American Journal of Psychiatry, 168*(5), 472–85.

CHAPTER

26 The Promise and Problem of E-Assessment

Michael D. Franzen *and* Matthew J. L. Page

Abstract

There has been an explosion in the development of electronic methods for psychological assessment. These include use of handheld devices, desktop computers, and platform-based Internet methods. This development has occurred separately in the commercial environment and in the research environment. This development of new methods presents great promise to improve the accuracy, ecological validity, and range of constructs in psychological assessment. However there are also many problems involved in the development of these electronic methods, including the need to train clinicians in their use, the need to develop safeguards for privacy, and the need to develop methods to ensure the integrity of the data collected. This chapter outlines some of the main considerations in moving forward.

Keywords: psychological assessment, electronic test administration, ecological momentary assessment, real-time data collection, assessment

Electronic assessment or *e-assessment* refers to the use of both electronic devices (e.g., mobile devices) and the use of electronic media (e.g., the Internet) to conduct psychological assessment. It is not a matter of *if* e-assessment will come to augment or supplant traditional psychological assessment, but rather *how* mental health professionals will adjust to it. The reality is that e-assessment methods are already occurring. The forces behind this change derive from social, demographic, economic, and political influences. The advent of personal computers, handheld electronic "smart" devices, and wired and wireless technologies have had significant impact on our social structure and life. Smart phones, smart automobiles, and even smart homes are becoming ubiquitous, and psychological assessment is interfacing with these developments as a participant in our culture. As a larger proportion of our populace has grown up with these devices already integrated into daily life, new technology seems less like science fiction and more like second nature. Younger patients and clinicians in particular expect and want to use psychological assessment methods congruent with other aspects of their electronic lives. Moreover, the federal government is mandating changes in healthcare delivery that will rely on electronic methods. The use of electronic assessment is expected to increase efficiency, help reduce overall costs, and increase accuracy in data collection and interpretation.

Traditional psychological assessment involves the measurement of cognitions, emotional states, or behaviors. Conventionally, psychological assessment is conducted by having an examiner interact with and observe a patient. For cognitive assessment, the psychologist may pose certain problems such as asking which designs are similar (visual-spatial perception) or how two words are alike (verbal abstraction skills). For emotional assessment, the psychologist may ask whether a patient has experienced certain subjective states such as depressed mood. For behavioral assessment, the psychologist may observe the patient and measure the frequency or duration of a target behavior. In each case, the psychologist is making a decision about an observation and recording it, typically using paper and pencil. In e-assessment, the patient interacts with an electronic device such as a desktop computer or handheld device, which then records the relevant data to be reviewed and interpreted later by the psychologist.

It is attendant on today's researchers and clinicians to understand the positive and negative issues involved in e-assessment and to use this understanding to harness and direct the development and use of electronic means of psychological assessment. Rather than allowing the development of these methods to proceed aimlessly, government and regulatory agencies are developing policies and guidelines to systematize the application of electronic methods. Assessment professionals, and especially those specializing in the development of assessment methods, should be active participants in these endeavors. Mental health practitioners are now engulfed in electronic advances in their professional activities whether they are research, consultation, therapy, or assessment. Most of the focus has been on the development of methods for interventions and in telehealth applications or in research applications. This chapter focuses on psychological assessment.

For some providers, increasing incorporation of technology may evoke anxiety. A growing reliance on laptops, tablets, webcams, mobile phones, and other innovative devices will cost money and require training, which seems counterintuitive to the seeming promise of increased efficiency with the advent of these technologies. Providers who rely on face-to-face talk therapy and paper-and-pencil data collection, particularly those who are not "tech-savvy," may worry about their skills becoming obsolete, Moreover, the technology wave carries a host of ethical concerns. New guidelines are needed to handle issues like patient confidentiality, data storage, and psychometric properties of electronic instruments, particularly as psychological services transition further away from professional supervision and into the homes of patients.

Regardless of these concerns, it is clear that the high-tech movement is sweeping the mental health field, ready or not. In light of these changes, continuing discussion is warranted, both to establish best practices for electronic mental health practice and to allay the fears of traditionalists. Among scientific attention to assessment in research contexts, little has been written about electronic assessment methods, or *e-assessment*, in the provider's office, despite new electronic scoring and even administration options for the most popular assessment tools. Although the public's popularity and familiarity with handheld devices have encouraged publishers to create assessment tools on tablets and laptops, data collection via the Internet is less novel and still underutilized. Researchers have also established methods for electronic, naturalistic data collection in real-time using *ecological momentary assessment* (EMA; Shiffman, Stone, & Hufford, 2008; Stone & Shiffman, 1994). In spite of these options, transitioning these devices from research into practice has been slow (Piasecki, Hufford, Solhan, & Trull, 2007).

Regardless of whether an individual practitioner decides to embrace the new technology, it is clear that changes have already occurred. We cannot predict the future, but we can envision that it will be very different from the present. By initiating and maintaining this discussion, the mental health community can better control the direction and outcome.

In this chapter, we describe current practices in e-assessment, consider its benefits and drawbacks, and offer suggestions for structures and strictures to allow ethically and scientifically responsible development of e-assessment. chapter is not meant as a comprehensive or exhaustive treatment of the topic. Instead, in presenting an overview of the developing technologies, their advantages, and relevant concerns, we aim to encourage a continuing discussion of best practices in e-assessment. Whether the reader is leery of these new technologies or eager to incorporate them in practice, all mental health providers should be mindful of the rapidly expanding e-assessment trend and how to best address ethical concerns during its implementation.

The Many Facets of E-Assessment

We are well aware that a variety of professionals may be involved in the development and use of psychological assessment. However, in some jurisdictions access to and professional use of psychological assessment instruments may be limited to individuals who are licensed to practice psychology. Therefore when our comments are germane to the professional practice of psychology we will use the term "psychologist" rather than the more inclusive but unwieldy terms "mental health professional" or "assessment professional."

Just as there are a variety of traditional psychological assessment techniques and conceptualizations, so, too, are there a multitude of activities and concepts in e-assessment. For the purposes of this chapter, we consider e-assessment as existing in a matrix of overarching concepts. E-assessment can include the use of electronic scoring after traditional administration and the use of automated report writing after traditional administration. For example, currently, a psychologist can purchase either a scoring program for the Minnesota Multiphasic Personality Inventory-2 (MMPI-2; Butcher, Dahlstrom, Graham, Tellegen, & Kaemmer, 1989), in which several pages of profiles are generated after raw scores are entered or may elect to have the software generate an automated narrative report that can be used to write a more detailed and nuanced evaluation report. Another approach would involve the use of electronic media to administer the test, such as having a patient complete tasks on-screen in the clinician's office. This approach would also include either score or report generation. E-assessment might also allow the assessment to be conducted in the office under the direct supervision of the practitioner or in a remote setting with the patient and possible additional staff. In the latter case, the clinician may be in simultaneous electronic communication with the patient, or the results may be communicated to the clinician's office for later review and interpretation. Grosch, Gottlieb, and Cullum (2011) describe another model of e-assessment in which a provider and patient are in two different locations and communication occurs via electronic means. This model may be seen to be similar to the current models of telepsychology under development in which psychotherapy is conducted via teleconferencing.

E-assessment might also differ regarding the constructs targeted. These can include subjective patient ratings, symptom checklists, or observed behaviors, which can all provide useful information for traditional emotional, behavioral, and personality constructs. Some e-assessment tools collect more concrete data, such as blood pressure and medication consumption, sometimes even without the user being aware of the data collection. Cognitive constructs such as memory or visual-spatial processing might be fruitfully addressed using electronic methods. Yet another variant of e-assessment is in the use of virtual reality to conduct naturalistic assessment. Luxton (2014) has presented initial concepts in the use of virtual reality, although this discussion focuses on therapeutic interventions provided in a virtual reality environment. Initial applications of this technology have targeted the treatment of posttraumatic stress disorder (PTSD; Reger et al., 2011), although development of assessment models using virtual reality are easily imagined as well.

E-assessment can be divided into two basic categories: *standardized psychological assessment* using electronic methods, and *electronic monitoring* of mood states or discrete behaviors. In the first category, psychological assessment of traditional psychological constructs such as personality or cognitive skill could be completed using electronic stimuli and scoring. In the second category, electronic methods are used to help obtain individual data regarding the occurrence of behaviors such as angry statements or cigarette use. Both of these categories can be further subdivided into *local storage* or *immediate electronic transmission* of the data. The assessment of memory could be conducted using an instrument provided through software loaded onto a computer located in a professional's office or on a tablet connected to a central administration and scoring program located in the cloud. Assessing the occurrence of discrete behaviors or mood states could be conducted on a device the subject uses. In this case, information may be retained by the device and then copied into an electronic file in the professional's office, transmitted instantaneously to the professional, or sent to a central file located on a remote server and accessed by the professional at a later time. Although there are opportunities for breaches of confidentiality in all of these instances, there would seem to be a higher potential for breaches when storage is located outside of the provider's office. There is also greater control over the standardization of the test administration when it is conducted in the office. Conversely, there may be greater relation to the targeted constructs for the assessments conducted in the open environment, presumably when the mental health professional is not present.

There are already multiple examples of electronic methods of assessment in which test administration and scoring occur in the professional's office using a local storage method. Some popular neuropsychological tests such as the Wisconsin Card Sorting Test (Heaton, Chelune, Talley, Kay, & Curtiss, 1993), a measure of abstract visual problem solving and concept formation, are available either in standard administration form or electronic administration form. Other tests, such as the Iowa Gambling Task (Bechara, Damasio, Damasio, & Anderson, 1994), which is designed to measure executive functioning and problem solving in a more emotionally laden context, are available only in electronic form. Many personality and behavioral questionnaires such as the MMPI-2 (Butcher et al., 1989), Personality Assessment Inventory (PAI; Morey, 2007), and Behavior Rating Inventory of Executive Function (BRIEF; Gioia, Isquith, Guy, & Kenworthy, 2000) are available as paper-and-pencil administration with either hand scoring or computer scoring, or alternatively using computerized administration.

Test publishers are moving to a model that involves administration and scoring over the Internet, with storage of the data in a remote server controlled by the test publisher. Pearson publishers is marketing two basic methods of e-assessment that they call Q-global and Q-interactive. Q-global involves the clinician administering a test and then entering the data into a web-based scoring and interpretation system. Q-interactive involves administering the test on an electronic device and accessing it through a web-based system. In both cases, the patient information and test scores are stored remotely. Psychological Assessment Resources, Inc. (PAR) is marketing PARiConnect, which allows the clinician the option to enter raw test data and obtain scoring and interpretation, administer tests electronically in the office with immediate scoring and interpretation, or administer assessment to patients electronically without the patient and clinicians in the same physical space but instead connected electronically. Here again the patient information is stored remotely under the control of the test publisher.

Although there are multiple electronic methods available and more in development, not all tests are available in electronic forms, and test users have not necessarily seemed eager to adopt electronic methods. Rabin et al. (2014) surveyed clinical neuropsychologists and found that very few neuropsychologists used electronic assessment methods when those methods were available. These practices will surely change in the near future as publishers place greater emphasis on electronic administration and scoring options.

Potential Benefits of E-Assessment

Potential benefits of e-assessment are varied. The existence of electronic versions may increase availability and accessibility of test materials and may allow for greater accuracy in administration and scoring. Electronic versions of tests may allow for the collection of more sophisticated data, such as reaction time and variability indices. For example, the Conners Continuous Performance Test not only calculates average reaction times but also calculates the standard deviation of those reaction times overall as well as the reaction times in specific time periods during the assessment or as a function of other variables, such as the interstimulus interval. There may be greater compliance with assessment conducted in ecological or naturalistic settings and improvements in test development. When the assessment is conducted by an electronic device recording data instead of requiring the subject to record the information, the task demands on the subject are lessened, thus reducing the chance that the subject may fail to record relevant data. Although specific benefits will vary test to test, these potential advantages, accompanied with constant and innovative improvements in technology, paint an exciting picture for the future of e-assessment.

With increasing societal savviness, comfort, and reliance on day-to-day technology, one of the most obvious benefits of e-assessment is the potential for easier access to assessment methods using the Internet and cell phones. Latest estimates suggest that roughly 85% of Americans access the Internet and 90% use cell phones (Smith, 2014; Zickuhr, 2013). Given this accessibility, many psychologists and other mental health professionals have been incorporating online collection of psychological assessment data. Doing so may save on costs and on time, allowing the clinician to gather referential psychological information before the patient even walks through the door (Luxton, Pruitt, & Osenbach, 2014). Patients may even be able to receive immediate feedback about their responses for appropriate variables. Additionally, because it does not require the presence of a professional, e-assessment provides the opportunity for individuals in remote or rural settings to be assessed. Cell phones and tablets allow for even more venues for access to assessment materials in the form of "apps," many of which are available to users for a small fee or may even be free. Although many of these apps are in line with a self-help approach to psychology, clinicians may find it useful to recommend and incorporate these apps. Doing so may be useful both for collecting data in assessment services and for keeping therapy patients engaged in their treatment between sessions.

The use of electronic assessment methods may improve the accuracy and validity of data. Of particular note is the improvement in validity when using real-time collection methods such as EMA, compared to traditional self-report methods. Asking patients to reflect on their current symptoms and previous history through interview and rating scales is an inherent and common part of clinical practice and relatively simple to conduct (Moskowitz & Young, 2006). However, many authors have argued that self-report methods, particularly those relying on retrospective reports, have questionable validity.

Recall or response bias, whether intentional or unintentional, often influences self-report. Some have argued that the office setting and presence of professionals create demand characteristics that may lead both patients to present a false image to their provider and providers to elicit information in a way that conforms to a former hypothesis (Kanter, Kohlenberg, & Loftus, 2002; Orne, 1962; Rosenthal, 2002). Even the most honest patients may be vulnerable to bias in their memory of previous events and symptoms (Tversky & Marsh, 2000). Jones and Johnston (2011) also argue that individuals tend to report rounded figures when making estimates of symptoms and behaviors. Furthermore, self-report rating scales require a certain level of effort that may be too burdensome for patients lacking adequate cognitive capacity (Piasecki et al., 2007). EMA and other e-assessment methods may allow reporters to overcome at least some of these biases when data are collected in their natural environment, without the influence of a professional's presence or the cognitive burden of generating accurate recollections and estimations (Piasecki et al., 2007; Shiffman & Stone, 1998).

EMA may be particularly helpful for variables that are difficult to estimate otherwise. For example, researchers have explored electronic diaries for a variety of applications, including alcohol consumption (Piasecki et al., 2014), social interactions (Janicki, Kamarck, Shiffman, & Gwaltney, 2006), and mood states (Trull et al., 2008). Recording accurate data about these variables through traditional interviews with patients can be difficult given the complexity and instability of many behaviors and mood states. E-assessment may also allow for more sophisticated collection of biological data. A variety of cell phone "apps" have been developed in recent years that use creative methods to collect such data. Users are able to press their fingers to a phone's camera to track heart rate and to estimate the length of sleep cycles and disturbances by having their phone detect motion and noise on their mattress during sleep. Sleep-related apps may even log useful statistics such as sleep duration and efficiency, estimated sleep quality, and audio-recordings of noises during the night (Tsukayama, 2014). A plethora of other health apps are available to monitor other variables such as diet, cigarette use, and exercise. Many of these apps require minimal direct input from the user, thus reducing cognitive burden. Some technology experts argue that America will see a rise in the use of wearable monitoring devices in the next several decades that will encourage regular evaluation of biological markers and will make these data even more accessible to providers (Anderson, 2014). For providers such as neuropsychologists, attempting to identify cognitive deficits related to health behaviors and for therapists targeting improvements in these activities, these methods may be highly appealing.

E-assessment can also be useful in evaluating time-related variables that would be otherwise difficult or cumbersome to measure. A number of computerized cognitive or neuropsychological tasks, such as the Conners Continuous Performance Test (Conners, 2004), utilize electronic measures of response speed to stimuli occurring every few seconds for several minutes. These tasks serve as a valuable tool in evaluating sustained attention, impulsivity, and arousal (Ballard, 2001). As variability in response time becomes a more frequent parameter of clinical interest, e-assessment devices could allow accurate and immediate calculation of such variables (Johnson et al., 2007). E-assessment is particularly useful for variables that change often and require frequent data collection to capture accurately, such as mood, attention, pain, and fatigue (Affleck, Zautra, Tennen, & Armeli, 1999). In the naturalistic environment, e-assessment may also be a useful way to evaluate antecedents and consequences of behaviors by tracking the time at which they occur.

Of course, completion of assessment records in naturalistic settings has been available for decades, at least in nonelectronic forms. Completing thought records and tracking behaviors through paper methods are common components of cognitive-behavioral therapy. Neuropsychologists may also rely on sending patients home with rating scales and open-ended measures. However, patients often have suboptimal adherence and commitment to these assessment measures. In contrast, EMA methods tend to have a high level of compliance compared to written methods, and adherence may even be facilitated by electronic reminders such as alarms and email (Jones et al., 2012; Piasecki et al., 2007). Compliance itself may be a useful variable to evaluate through e-assessment by comparing the number of completed assessments to the number of electronic prompts (Shiffman, 2009).

When there is e-assessment of variables for which interpretation is based on normative information, those data can be transmitted to a central server location where it is added to the normative base. Future results can be compared to an up-to-date and ever-improving database. Frequently, assessment data are interpreted by calculating the relation of the subject's scores to a large group of data from other individuals. The raw scores are translated to standard scores, which indicate how far above or below the normative average the subject's scores fall. These normative translations are based on a sample collected at a given point in time prior to the publication of the test. The use of the multiple remote assessment devices can continually add to the normative sample, increasing the stability of the normative transformations and their interpretations as well as keeping the normative comparisons more accurate and contemporary. The gradual change in distributions of cognitive variables, as part of what is known as the *Flynn effect*, can be accounted for more readily (Flynn, 2009). Currently, it can take 4–5 years to obtain a sufficient sample to construct a normative base and another 2–3 years before the instrument is published. That instrument can remain on the market for decades, but its accuracy may decline with each successive year. The original Wechsler intelligence scales were used for nearly four decades before they were re-normed (Wechsler, 1981). The MMPI has only been re-normed once in its long and venerable history (Butcher et al., 1989).

Possible difficulties with this rolling normative approach include the need for increased oversight to maintain the integrity of the data. Currently, when tests are normed, the test publisher will contract with a clinician or researcher to collect and transmit the information to the publisher. The professional is responsible for ascertaining the individual's characteristics (age, gender, health, diagnosis). When these data are collected remotely outside the presence of the professional, alternate methods will be needed to monitor the quality of the data, such as making sure it is the patient or subject who is actually providing the data to the device. The use of electronic administration of longer performance measures of memory or intellectual function could take place in the professional's office where such oversight would be possible. This would be less true in those instances in which assessment of attention or brief measures of memory take place outside the clinician's office.

E-assessment also facilitates the use of alternate forms. For example, the second edition of the Conners Continuous Performance Test (Conners, 2004) is capable of virtually infinite alternate forms because the choice of the target letter presented on the computer screen and the time interval between stimuli presentations varies around certain parameters (order of stimulus items, inter-stimulus interval, presentation duration). It would also be possible to construct alternate forms of verbal memory tests using lists of words that are equated for frequency and typicality of usage in the English language, perhaps even while controlling for demographic variables. Each time the test is administered, the program could generate an alternate form.

Of course there are current limitations to the development of a broader array of tests for different target skills and sensory modalities. The most highly developed electronic modality is visual presentation and response or entering data using keystrokes or a mouse. Greater development of touchpad technology as well as voice recognition technology will allow greater variability in item administration and response. Many current electronic visual memory tests involve administration of visual stimuli followed by multiple-choice recognition procedures. Using a stylus and draw pad, or finger and touchpad, will allow the test taker to draw the visual stimuli, mirroring traditional tests of visual memory. The response could then be scored by a professional or other personnel, or conceivably by the program itself. Verbal memory tests could involve auditory and/or visual presentation of word lists or passages, with examinees responding either by clicking on a multiple-choice alternative, typing in the word, or speaking into the device's microphone.

These e-assessment ideas may soon be realized and published. A number of innovative assessment measures have become available in recent years using administration methods with technological enhancements. The latest versions of the Wechsler Adult Intelligence Scale (WAIS-IV; Wechsler, 2008), the Wechsler Intelligence Scale for Children (WISC-V; Wechsler, 2014), and the Wechsler Memory Scale (WMS-IV; Wechsler, 2009) can now be administered through Pearson's Q-interactive service, offering new administration features that are made possible using tablets and the Internet. The benefits of these methods include immediate scoring of subtests, automatic audio-recording during administration for later review, and automated components of administration such as scoring, timing, and displaying stimuli. These changes are touted to improve speed, accuracy, and reliability in administration by reducing demands on the examiner.

Electronic devices also allow for the possibility of adaptive testing, adjusting the assessment protocol dynamically based on the examinee's performance on initial items or measures (Bauer et al., 2012). For example, Chorpita and Nakamura (2008) argue that dynamic means of diagnostic structured interviewing, using a Bayesian algorithm to guide examiners to determine which questions to ask to assess diagnostic criteria efficiently, can significantly reduce error rates and even lower administration time by as much as 99%. It is easy to conceive of a computer program that could direct examiners in their evaluation of diagnostic criteria using evidence-based algorithms for a host of disorders. Similarly, there are multiple versions of adaptive educational testing, including the Graduate Management Admission Test (GMAT) and the Graduate Record Examination (GRE). In fact, many psychological tests of ability already have rudimentary adaptive protocols in which there are rules for establishing basals and ceilings. Electronically administered tests will allow even greater adaptive capacity as the next item can be automatically determined by performance on the most recent item.

As publishers continue to integrate technology into assessment materials, more creative improvements in administration are conceivable (Bauer et al., 2012). There is the potential that by allowing electronic devices to monitor aspects of the assessment protocol, the examiner may ultimately gain greater control over the testing environment and may obtain more accurate and thorough psychological data to interpret.

Potential Drawbacks of E-Assessment

There are numerous complications related to the implementation of e-assessment, but these drawbacks can also be conceptualized as challenges to be met. Broadly, many mental health professionals, and especially psychologists who spend a considerable percentage of their time in assessment activities, are concerned about what technology will mean to the fundamentals of their practice. Some practitioners may also be concerned that e-assessment will obviate the need for the professional in the assessment process. At least with current technology, qualitative data collection and automated scoring may be limited, and some fear that observational data will be underutilized. Others are apprehensive about patient engagement with technologically advanced methods, particularly for certain demographic groups. Training of providers in e-assessment is also a concern, as most clinicians practicing today were trained before these methods were available, and graduate programs are not currently required to incorporate e-assessment into their curriculum. There are significant concerns regarding safeguarding the integrity of tests and guarding the privacy of the patient when e-assessment is used. Finally, the transformation of paper-and-pencil tasks to electronic versions requires careful consideration as they may not be equivalent to the original versions. Let us examine these concerns individually.

For many providers, a major concern about e-assessment relates to fundamental changes in the assessment process and what it might mean for interpretation. Neuropsychological assessment provides a potential example. Neuropsychological assessment involves the measurement of cognitive and emotional/behavioral variables in the context of brain–behavior relations. Although academic assessment shares procedures, such as tests of intelligence, personality assessment, and measures of emotional state, neuropsychological assessment generally involves the evaluation of subjects with known or suspected central nervous dysfunction, such as closed head injury or seizure disorder. The interpretation of neuropsychological assessment is conducted in the context of knowledge about brain structure and function. Interacting with a patient during an evaluative interview and throughout neuropsychological testing provides a wealth of information that extends much further than the numerical values the patient scores on tests and rating scales. Supporters of Edith Kaplan's Boston Process Approach (Kaplan, 1988, 1990) might argue that information collected via observations of behaviors and qualitative aspects of performance is more important than the quantitative test results (Bauer & Bowers, 2013).

Some assessment experts may argue that with greater reliance on electronic and automated testing procedures, qualitative components of the evaluation process may fall through the cracks (Bauer et al., 2012). These concerns are particularly relevant for assessments conducted outside the professional's presence (Luxton et al., 2014). Allowing a computer to have more input in test interpretation may reduce the amount of valuable observational data available to the clinician, potentially resulting in an incomplete conceptualization of the patient. However, this distinction between qualitative and quantitative data is not a clear line of demarcation. The issue is whether e-assessment can capture aspects of the process in which the subject engages (qualitative) as well as the eventual score (quantitative).

E-assessment methods need not be reductive, and some researchers and clinicians even argue that enhanced technological testing procedures may provide more data about qualitative processes. For example, Davis et al. (2011) created a digital version of the classic Clock Drawing Test in which software records precise pen strokes and the time it takes the patient to create them. This program essentially provides the professional with a video recording of the drawing, allowing for more careful observation and better interpretation of process variables such as latency, planning, and commission errors. Similar electronic applications to other visual construction tasks are certainly feasible. Ultimately, it will be important for mental health professionals to continue examining test performance thoroughly, integrating behavioral observations and context, as e-assessment continues to develop.

Although technological components of assessment may be exciting to some users, not all patients will be comfortable using electronic methods and may become less engaged, which in turn could compromise the reliability and validity of the assessment. In fact, individuals who are older, less educated, and poorer are less likely to use the Internet, and some ethnic minority groups are less likely to use cell phones (Luxton et al., 2014; Smith, 2014; Zickuhr, 2013). Conversely, given the popularity of Internet and cell phone use among some groups (e.g., children/adolescents), these individuals may be more engaged when incorporating electronic methods (Jackson, von Eye, Fitzgerald, Witt, & Zhao, 2011). As electronic methods for everyday tasks become more integrated across the sociodemographic spectrum, insufficient familiarity or discomfort with technology will likely become a shrinking concern. However, as with traditional assessment methods, the patient's ability to engage with the type of materials and administration format used needs to be considered in choosing an assessment approach.

Furthermore, it is important not to assume that demographic factors like age are always a barrier to technological savviness. Even 20 years ago, computerized methods were being used to assess elderly patients, who rated the devices as easy to use (Cutler et al., 1993; Ritchie et al., 1993). Moreover, even among demographic groups who are less likely to use technology, a majority of these groups report that they use the Internet and cell phones (Smith, 2014; Zickuhr, 2013). Instead of assuming that individuals from these groups, such as elderly patients, will be less comfortable with electronic methods, the clinician should assess the patient's familiarity and comfort with technological methods regardless of age, just as the clinician would assess language proficiency. Consequentially, it may also be important for clinicians to retain traditional assessment methods for those times when they seem better suited to individuals. It is similarly important for researchers and test developers to investigate these factors when constructing normative samples.

Another concern is that the growing availability of e-assessment resources may make it more likely that inadequately trained or supervised individuals may use or misuse technological methods. It will be important not only to provide training to qualified practitioners, but also to ensure that use of e-assessment is restricted to qualified and trained individuals. Traditionally, regulatory bodies have licensed practice at very broad levels and have left the oversight of specific professional activities to the individually constituted professional boards of examiners. For example, states license the general practice of psychology, but individual practitioners are expected to practice within the scope of their training and experience. There are fairly well defined standards regarding psychotherapy and traditional assessment. It will be necessary to determine if or the extent to which practice in e-assessment should require additional distinct training and regulatory control.

Electronic transmission and storage of clinical data pose challenges for compliance with the standards of the Health Insurance Portability and Accountability Act (HIPAA) (Luxton et al., 2014). It is an important ethical dictate and legal requirement that mental health professionals protect patient privacy. The use of e-assessment needs to follow these requirements, and providers will have to work along with test publishing companies to meet this mandate (Bauer et al., 2012). Medical identity theft and breach of protected health information pose a major threat to Americans, and risks of these crimes should be considered carefully when relying on e-assessment methods. Concerns regarding device encryption, remote transmission of data, location of data storage, and how long data are stored all warrant consideration. If e-assessment results are stored within general healthcare records, there may be greater availability of assessment results to other professionals, making it possible for providers without the needed background knowledge to interpret results, perhaps incorrectly (Myrvik et al., 2014). There will need to be safeguards implemented to restrict access to assessment data to those professionals with adequate training and experience, just as there are currently safeguards regarding who can purchase psychological assessment measures. At the minimum, tests should contain posted warnings regarding the qualifications of the intended user and a statement that use for other than what the test was designed for may result in misinterpretation. The use of electronic methods of transmission and storage of data may also be complicated by Internet connection difficulties or equipment malfunction. Most mental health professionals do not possess the technical knowledge and skills to remediate these difficulties and instead rely on information technicians, such as computer support staff. In the case of e-assessment, even these technicians need to follow the professional and ethical standards of mental health providers.

Remote electronic data collection raises a host of other concerns. When assessment is conducted outside of a professional's office, there is an inherent risk that someone other than the patient is completing the assessment (Naglieri et al., 2004). Bauer et al. (2012) recommend that test developers incorporate procedures to verify that the user is indeed the target patient. Additionally, when test materials leave the confines of the practitioner's office, there arises an inherent risk for breach of test security (Luxton et al., 2014). For example, if patients are asked to complete an assessment tool from their home computer using the Internet, they will be able to save a "screenshot" or picture of the screen with a simple keystroke when completing the measure. Having measures available on the Internet allows individuals to learn and distribute methods for responding to items in order to create a desired profile or outcome (Naglieri et al., 2004). Other individuals may also be present at the time of the assessment or may later gain access to information shared electronically. Finally, staff may not be available to answer questions that arise concerning items on self-report measures (Myrvik et al., 2014). Clinicians would also be unable to intervene should patients have emotional and potentially self-injurious reactions to the assessment process. At the very least, patients should be well-informed of these inherent risks before administration of remote e-assessment.

Professional organizations have addressed concerns about e-assessment and computerized test administration. For example, in a joint statement from the American Academy of Clinical Neuropsychology and the National Academy of Neuropsychology, Bauer et al. (2012) stressed that "even when a traditional examiner-administered test is programmed for computer administration, it becomes a new and different test." Almost any change in administration has the potential to affect the quality of the data, and the psychometric properties of some measures may improve or decline when administered electronically. When data collection is remote, patients may react and present differently in the face of a computer or cell phone screen than they would in person, and they may be subject to unpredictable environmental distractions (Luxton et al., 2014). It is vital to recognize that transitioning from a paper-and-pencil or interview format to an e-assessment method may require a new normative comparison sample. For example, the Tower of London–Drexel University (Culberston & Zillmer, 2005) records the time it takes the subject to initiate a response on each item and tallies these times to obtain a summary score. The result is influenced by not only the subject's performance, but also by how long it takes the examiner to respond. Having an electronic version of this task eliminates the response time of the examiner, which when summed over 10 items may reduce the score and artificially result in more patients exhibiting faster performance when compared to the slower scores in the traditional method of administration. Consequentially, the professional may be more likely to incorrectly interpret the performance as impulsive.

Although such concerns merit attention, the literature does offer a number of instances in which electronic versions of assessment tools were found to be comparable to their traditional counterparts. Stolwyk, Lee, McKay, and Ponsford (2013) found that paper and computerized versions of the Austin Maze, a spatial memory task, had a number of comparable properties. Similarly, Clionsky and Clionsky (2014) reported that the iPad version and the paper-and-pencil version of the Memory Orientation Screening Test (Clionsky & Clionsky, 2010) are psychometrically equivalent. O'Halloran et al. (2008) examined the traditional and computerized versions of a sizeable neuropsychological test battery in a sample of schizophrenic patients and also generally found equivalence, with one exception: the computerized version exhibited better temporal reliability. Even if paper and computer versions of tests are ultimately found to be equivalent, development of electronic test versions warrants investigation into psychometric equivalence across populations of interest. The presence or absence of psychometric equivalence is an empirical question, the answer for which should not be assumed in either direction.

Although EMA may expand the type and accuracy of data that can be collected, it is important to recognize that the act of assessment through electronic means may alter the variable that is measured. For example, if e-assessment allows for more frequent measurement of a certain behavior, increased awareness on behalf of the patient may trigger change in the variable (Affleck et al., 1999). Of course, this type of reactivity may be present in traditional assessment methods as well, and reactivity may actually be beneficial to the patient if a treatment goal is to alter the assessed behavior. However, reactivity needs to be addressed carefully in the research, development, and clinical application of e-assessment methods, given the increase in utilization of these methods. It will be important for test developers to consider ways to reduce reactivity. For example, reactivity may be minimized when using e-assessment methods that do not reveal data to the patient at the time of collection (Affleck et al., 1999) or when data collection is automated.

Ease in access to e-assessment tools also raises concerns about the qualification of their users. Access to the e-assessment instruments could presumably be conducted via downloads from "app stores." Some of these require limited access, and the prevailing standard is to have the purchasing individual read and electronically sign an End Users Licensing Agreement (EULA). Undoubtedly the reader has already clicked the EULA when downloading other apps and software purchased via the Internet. There is presumably no other verification of appropriate authorization, and it is likely that most users simply click without reading the EULA. For access to electronic psychological assessment methods, some other mechanism is obviously necessary to verify that the user is authorized to use the instrument by virtue of training, credentials, and license. Currently, test publishers require documentation of the credentials of the test user before test materials can be purchased. A similar system needs to be in place for electronic purchases. Possible solutions include already available technology such as thumbprint identification or retinal scans. Many pharmacies already use thumb print technology to access prescriptions to controlled substances. Furthermore, there needs to be a method that allows the licensed professional to monitor the use of the assessment procedures and interpretation of results. However, the recent history of the use of apps suggests that early solutions regarding test security may be insufficient, and this issue warrants continued attention.

In addition to all of these broad concerns, each different form of e-assessment will have its own challenges. For example, Grosch et al. (2011) point out that implementation of teleconference for assessment, or what the authors term "teleneuropsychology," will raise different issues about informed consent and privacy, such as who may be present in either of the remote locations during the assessment and disclosure to the patient that absolute privacy guarantees may not be possible. This type of e-assessment will require high-quality transmission methods and backup equipment in case of temporary technical failure. Only those assessment methods and instruments that have been shown to be reliable and valid in the teleconferencing setting should be used. Some initial data have been gathered supporting the use of some dementia assessment instruments in teleneuropsychology (Cullum, Weiner, Gehrmann, & Hynan, 2006; Hildebrand, Chow, Williams, Nelson, & Wass, 2004), but this is obviously only the beginning. It is clear that there are various ethical and practical factors to consider when designing and practicing with each specific e-assessment tool.

Future Directions

Compared to the fast rate at which technology is advancing the field of psychological assessment, practitioners seem apprehensive to embrace these changes (Bauer et al., 2012; Naglieri et al., 2004; Piasecki et al., 2007). Their hesitation is potentially telling of important considerations that have yet to be thoroughly addressed. As we have discussed, a number of technical, ethical, and practical concerns are associated with the various forms for e-assessment, and some more so than others. It is also possible that new concerns may arise as e-assessment is implemented and developed. Therefore, it is important that individual practitioners and professional organizations actively participate in the oversight of this movement. Although some guidelines have been offered by governing organizations and task forces (American Psychological Association [APA], 2013; Bauer et al., 2012; Naglieri et al., 2004), publication and implementation of specific policies for e-assessment have been relatively slow. For example, the American Psychological Association has issued broad guidelines for the conduct of Internet-based psychological assessment (APA, 2013). Although the guidelines underline the responsibility of the individual clinician in using such measures, they do not offer specific practices. What is needed is a set of specific standards to guide psychologists and other practitioners who wish to utilize e-assessment and remain within ethical and professional mores. Establishment of these recommendations for specific practices in e-assessment, particularly regarding the risks and drawbacks, may be what is needed to make providers feel more comfortable in making electronic adaptations.

In developing standards for e-assessment, it is extremely important that electronic assessment methods are considered in the context of developing standards and requirements of electronic medical records (EMR). The implementation of EMR is required by the federal government as part of the effort to reduce medical error, reduce the cost of healthcare, and provide portability of information. This is of particular relevance given the Health Information Technology for Economic and Clinical Health Act, requiring most clinicians to implement EMR (HITECH Act, 2009). Psychological assessment is an important part of healthcare. Typically, under most state laws, the storage of psychological assessment records is the responsibility of the individual psychologist or practitioner conducting the assessment. Many clinicians have responded to this responsibility by keeping reports from the evaluation in the general medical record and raw test scores and protocols in a separate file that the professional or service maintains. If assessment is conducted and the results are stored electronically, it is attendant upon the practitioner to maintain the integrity of the tests and ensure that some mechanism is created to protect against others who might be privy to the general healthcare records gaining access to original test materials. This could be more easily accomplished in a solitary practice, but might be problematic in a multispecialty practice that utilizes a single general electronic healthcare records system or when working within institutional settings. There is not clear agreement regarding the inclusion of standardized test scores in narrative reports. However there is fairly general consensus regarding access to raw scores and test stimuli.

Little has been written in the literature about electronic storage of e-assessment records in EMR databases. Steinfeld and Keyes (2011) discuss some of the important aspects of integrating psychological information into EMR systems but do not address the issue of psychological assessment record storage. Barak (2003, 2004; Barak & Buchanan, 2004) has written about the application of electronic assessment methods primarily for vocational counseling. Here of course there are different concerns from those involved with cognitive testing, but some of the same issues may be relevant, and the differences underline the need for broad-based guidelines as each type of assessment may have its own integrity and ethical issues. Smith et al. (2011) discuss the use of Internet-based assessment in the context of a collaborative assessment framework, but this does not contain standardized instruments, such as intellectual assessment and neuropsychological measures that are more appropriately used under the control of a licensed psychologist. Baker and Bufka (2011) discuss telehealth applications of interventions, and although the use of electronic psychological assessment might fall under some of these same considerations, e-assessment needs to develop with consideration of the factors which differentiate it from teleheath interventions.

Grosch et al. (2011) note that there are few resources or guidelines available to the clinician conducting neuropsychological assessment in the context of Internet use, a point similarly applicable to e-assessment in general. Rather, e-assessment technology seems to be outpacing the profession's capacity to control it. Clearly, there is a need for the development of more specific guidelines and suggestions for best practices. We hope that the information presented in this chapter highlights the need to develop these specifics, building off of what guiding principles are already available (e.g., APA, 2013; Bauer et al., 2012). After reviewing the potential benefits and complications associated with e-assessment, we close the chapter with a few recommendations.

First, mental health providers should educate themselves regarding use of e-assessment. Even if an individual clinician decides not to use e-assessment in his or her own practice, other professionals will do so. Optimal care for many patients will require communication with these other professionals, which will necessitate familiarity with e-assessment. As well as educating themselves, providers should participate in the development of professional, legal, and clinical standards for the use of e-assessment.

Second, professional organizations (e.g., American Psychiatric Association, American Psychological Association, National Academy of Neuropsychology) should develop organized and systematic oversight and specific recommendations for the use of e-assessment, with test developers and publishers also involved in these efforts. In addition to promulgating standards in the form of best practices recommendations, professional organizations need to develop educational materials (e.g., continuing education) to assist the clinician in acquiring the knowledge and skills needed for sound implementation. Training programs need to be involved at two levels.

One is in the development and evaluation of e-assessment instruments and applications. Another is in the integration of e-assessment into training curricula. Each of these stakeholders (clinicians, test publishers, professional organizations, regulatory bodies) brings a different perspective to the discussion. The stakeholders all share a common broad goal: namely, development and use of accurate, sound, culturally sensitive assessment instruments which can be used safely and ethically. However, because they have somewhat different goals and perspectives, each will make an idiosyncratic contribution to the process.

Finally, for all of these e-assessment methods, issues of billing and coding need to be addressed. Regardless of any supporting research regarding the scientific validity and clinical utility of e-assessment, it will not be widely adopted unless providers are able to ethically and legally bill for the services provided. This will require extensive work at the regulatory and legislative level.

It may at first appear that traditional psychological assessment of emotional and behavioral constructs using checklists would be the main activity for the arena of e-assessment. However, e-assessment of performance and cognitive constructs is also possible and is, in fact, already extant for many of the constructs of attention, problem solving, and memory. We predict that future developments will include the use of voice-activated assessment for language and verbal memory assessment, use of drawing programs for construction tasks or visual memory tasks, and the use of virtual reality for more complex behavioral tasks. Clearly this is just the beginning. The activity of academics and researchers who are usually at the forefront of new ideas has been piqued. The publishing companies see a potential for profit and are pursuing it. The individual practitioner may be intrigued by the "coolness" factor, may be motivated by the potential ease and economy, or may simply see it as a way to practice more consistently with other aspects of his or her lifestyle. Regardless, much of psychological assessment is already becoming electronically based, whether we are ready or not. To paraphrase Ornette Coleman, the future is now.

References

Affleck, G., Zautra, A., Tennen, H., & Armeli, S. (1999). Multilevel daily process designs for consulting and clinical psychology: A preface for the perplexed. *Journal of Consulting and Clinical Psychology, 6*, 746–54. doi:10.1037/0022-006X.67.5.746

American Psychological Association (APA). (2013, July 31). *Guidelines for the practice of telepsychology.* http://www.apapracticecentral.org/ce/guidelines/telepsychology-guidelines.pdf

Anderson, J. (2014, May 14). *The internet of things will thrive by 2025.* Pew Research Internet Project. http://www.pewinternet.org/files/2014/05/PIP_Internet-of-things_0514142.pdf

Baker, D. C., & Bufka, L. F. (2011). Preparing for the telehealth world: Navigating legal, regulatory, reimbursement, and ethical issues in an electronic age. *Professional Psychology: Research and Practice, 42*, 405–11. doi:10.1037/a0025037

Ballard, J. C. (2001). Assessing attention: Comparison of response-inhibition and traditional continuous performance tests. *Journal of Clinical and Experimental Neuropsychology, 23*, 331–50. doi:10.1076/jcen.23.3.331.1188

Barak, A. (2003). Ethical and professional issues in career assessment on the Internet. *Journal of Career Assessment, 11*, 3–21. doi:10.1177/106907202237457

Barak, A. (2004). Psychological applications on the internet: A discipline on the threshold of a new millennium. *Applied & Preventive Psychology, 8*(1999), 231–45. doi:10.1016/S0962-1849(05)80038–1

Barak, A., & Buchanan, T. (2004). Internet-based psychological testing and assessment. In R. Kraus, J. S. Zack, & G. Stricker (Eds.), *Online counseling: A handbook for mental health professionals* (pp. 217–39). New York: Elsevier Science.

Bauer, R. M., & Bowers, D. (2013). Intellectual antecedents to the Boston process approach. In L. Ashendorf, R. Swenson, & D. Libon (Eds.), *The Boston process approach to neuropsychological assessment: A practitioner's guide* (pp. 23–38). New York: Oxford University Press.

Bauer, R. M., Iverson, G. L., Cernich, A. N., Binder, L. M., Ruff, R. M., & Naugle, R. I. (2012). Computerized neuropsychological assessment devices: Joint position paper of the American Academy of Clinical Neuropsychology and the National Academy of Neuropsychology. *Archives of Clinical Neuropsychology, 27*, 362–73. doi:10.1080/13854046.2012.663001

Bechara, A., Damasio, A. R., Damasio, H., & Anderson, S. W. (1994). Insensitivity to future consequences following damage to human prefrontal cortex. *Cognition, 50*(1–3), 7–15. doi:10.1016/0010–0277(94)90018–3

Butcher, J. N., Dahlstrom, W. G., Graham, J. R., Tellegen, A., & Kaemmer, B. (1989). *The Minnesota Multiphasic Personality Inventory-2 (MMPI-2): Manual for administration and scoring.* Minneapolis: University of Minnesota Press.

Chorpita, B. F., & Nakamura, B. J. (2008). Dynamic structure in diagnostic structured interviewing: A comparative test of accuracy and efficiency. *Journal of Psychopathology and Behavioral Assessment, 30*, 52–60. doi:10.1007/s10862-007-9075-8

Clionsky, M., & Clionsky, E. (2014). Psychometric equivalence of a paper-based and computerized (iPad) version of the Memory Orientation Screening Test (MOST). *The Clinical Neuropsychologist, 28*, 747–55. doi:10.1080/13854046.2014.913686

Clionsky, M. I., & Clionsky, E. (2010). Development and validation of the Memory Orientation Screening Test (MOST): A better screening test for dementia. *American Journal of Alzheimer's Disease and Other Dementias, 25*, 650–6. doi:10.1177/1533317510386216

Conners, K. C. (2004). *Conners Continuous Performance Test (CPT II). Version 5 for Windows. Technical guide and software manual.* North Tonawanda, NY: Multi-Health Systems.

Culberston, W. C., & Zillmer, E. A. (2005). *Tower of London-Drexel University technical manual* (2nd ed.). North Tonawanda, NY: Multi-Health Systems.

Cullum, C. M., Weiner, M. F., Gehrmann, H. R., & Hynan, L. S. (2006). Feasibility of telecognitive assessment in dementia. *Assessment, 13*, 385–90. doi:10.1177/1073191106289065

Cutler, N. R., Shrotriya, R. C., Sramek, J. J., Veroff, A. E., Seifert, R. D., Reich, L. A., & Hironaka, D. Y. (1993). The use of the Computerized Neuropsychological Test Battery (CNTB) in an efficacy and safety trial of BMY 21,502 in Alzheimer's disease. *Annals of the New York Academy of Sciences, 695*, 332–6. doi:10.1111/j.1749–6632.1993.tb23079.x

Davis, R., Penney, D. L., Pittman, D., Libon, D. J., Swenson, R., & Kaplan, E. (2011). *The Digital Clock Drawing Test (dCDT)—I: Development of a new computerized quantitative system.* Abstract presented at the 39th annual meeting of the International Neuropsychological Society, Boston, MA.

Flynn, J. R. (2009). *Beyond intelligence: Beyond the Flynn effect.* Cambridge: Cambridge University Press.

Gioia, G. A., Isquith, P. K., Guy, S., & Kenworthy, L. (2000). *BRIEF: Behavior Rating Inventory of Executive Function.* Odessa, FL: Psychological Assessment Resources. doi:10.1076/chin.8.4.249.13513

Grosch, M. C., Gottlieb, M. C., & Cullum, C. M. (2011). Initial practice recommendations for teleneuropsychology. *Clinical Neuropsychologist, 25*, 1119–33. doi:10.1080/13854046.2011.609840

Health Information Technology for Economic and Clinical Health (HITECH) Act6, Title XIII of Division A and Title IV of Division B of the American Recovery and Reinvestment Act of 2009 (ARRA), Pub. L. No. 111-5, 123 Stat. 226 (Feb. 17, 2009).

Heaton, R. K., Chelune, G. J., Talley, J. L., Kay, G. G., & Curtiss, G. (1993). *Wisconsin Card Sorting Test manual: Revised and expanded.* Odessa, FL: Psychological Assessment Resources.

Hildebrand, R., Chow, H., Williams, C., Nelson, M., & Wass, P. (2004). Feasibility of neuropsychological testing of older adults via videoconference: Implications for assessing the capacity for independent living. *Journal of Telemedicine and Telecare, 10*, 130–34. doi:10.1258/135763304323070751

Jackson, L. A., von Eye, A., Fitzgerald, H. E., Witt, E. A., & Zhao, Y. (2011). Internet use, videogame playing and cell phone use as predictors of children's body mass index (BMI), body weight, academic performance, and social and overall self-esteem. *Computers in Human Behavior, 27*, 599–604. doi:10.1016/j.chb.2010.10.019

Janicki, D. L., Kamarck, T. W., Shiffman, S., & Gwaltney, C. J. (2006). Application of ecological momentary assessment to the study of marital adjustment and social interactions during daily life. *Journal of Family Psychology, 20*, 168–72. doi:10.1037/0893–3200.20.1.168

Johnson, K. A., Kelly, S. P., Bellgrove, M. A., Barry, E., Cox, M., Gill, M., & Robertson, I. H. (2007). Response variability in Attention Deficit Hyperactivity Disorder: Evidence for neuropsychological heterogeneity. *Neuropsychologia, 45*, 630–8. doi:10.1016/j.neuropsychologia.2006.03.034

Jones, M., & Johnston, D. (2011). Understanding phenomena in the real world: The case for real time data collection in health services research. *Journal of Health Services Research & Policy, 16*, 172–6. doi:10.1258/jhsrp.2010.010016

Jones, M., O'Connor, D., Schwartz, J., Johnston, D., French, D., & de Bruin, M. (2012). Opportunities and challenges in real time data capture: Methods in Health Psychology Symposium II. *European Health Psychologist, 14*(4), 93–9.

Kanter, J. W., Kohlenberg, R. J., & Loftus, E. F. (2002). Demand characteristics, treatment rationales, and cognitive therapy for depression. *Prevention & Treatment, 5*, Article 41. doi:10.1037/1522–3736.5.1.541c

Kaplan, E. (1988). A process approach to neuropsychological assessment. In T. Boll, & B. K. Bryant (Eds.), *Clinical neuropsychology and brain function: Research, measurement, and practice* (pp. 129–67). Washington, DC: American Psychological Association.

Kaplan, E. (1990). The process approach to neuropsychological assessment of psychiatric patients. *Journal of Neuropsychiatry and the Clinical Neurosciences, 2*, 72–87.

Luxton, D. D. (2014). Artificial intelligence in psychological practice: Current and future applications and implications. *Professional Psychology: Research and Practice, 45*, 332–9. doi:10.1037/a0034559

Luxton, D. D., Pruitt, L. D., & Osenbach, J. E. (2014). Best practice for remote psychological assessment via telehealth technologies. *Professional Psychology: Research and Practice, 24*, 27–35. doi:10.1037/a0034547

Morey, L. C. (2007). *The Personality Assessment Inventory manual.* Lutz, FL: Psychological Assessment Resources.

Moskowitz, D. S., & Young, S. N. (2006). Ecological momentary assessment: What it is and why it is a method of the future in clinical psychopharmacology. *Journal of Psychiatry & Neuroscience, 31*, 13–20.

Myrvik, M. P., Beverung, L. M., Panepinto, J. A., Igler, E. C., Englebert, N., & Bingen, K. M. (2014). Integration of electronic patient-reported outcomes (ePROs) into pediatric clinic settings across hematology/oncology/bone marrow transplant. *Clinical Practice in Pediatric Psychology, 2*, 39–49. doi:10.1037/cpp0000052

Naglieri, J. A., Drasgow, F., Schmidt, M., Handler, L., Prifitera, A., Margolis, A., & Velasquez, R. (2004). Psychological testing on the Internet: New problems, old issue. *The American Psychologist, 59*, 150–62. doi:10.1037/0003-066X.59.3.150

O'Halloran, J. P., Kemp, A. S., Gooch, K. N., Harvey, P. D., Palmer, B. W., Reist, C., & Schneider, L. S. (2008). Psychometric comparison of computerized and standard administration of the neurocognitive assessment instruments selected by the CATIE and MATRICS consortia among patients with schizophrenia. *Schizophrenia Research, 106*, 33–41. doi:10.1016/j.schres.2007.11.015

Orne, M. T. (1962). On the social psychology of the psychological experiment: With particular reference to demand characteristics and their implications. *American Psychologist, 17*, 776–83. doi:10.1037/h0043424

Piasecki, T. M., Cooper, M. L., Wood, P. K., Sher, K. J., Shiffman, S., & Heath, A. C. (2014). Dispositional drinking motives: Associations with appraised alcohol effects and alcohol consumption in an ecological momentary assessment investigation. *Psychological Assessment, 26*, 363–9. doi:10.1037/a0035153

Piasecki, T. M., Hufford, M. R., Solhan, M., & Trull, T. J. (2007). Assessing clients in their natural environments with electronic diaries: Rationale, benefits, limitations, and barriers. *Psychological Assessment, 19*, 25–43. doi:10.1037/1040–3590.19.1.25

Rabin, L. A., Spadaccini, A. T., Brodale, D. L., Grant, K. S., Elbulok-Charcape, M. M., & Barr, W. B. (2014). Utilization rates of computerized tests and test batteries among clinical neuropsychologists in the United States and Canada. *Professional Psychology: Research and Practice, 45*, 368–77. doi:10.1037/a00379987

Reger, G. M., Holloway, K. M., Candy, C., Rothbaum, B. O., Difede, J., Rizzo, A. A., & Gahm, G. A. (2011). Effectiveness of virtual reality exposure therapy for active duty soldiers in a military mental health clinic. *Journal of Traumatic Stress, 24*, 93–6. doi:10.1002/jts.20574

Ritchie, K., Allard, M., Huppert, F. A., Nargeot, C., Pinek, B., & Ledesert, B. (1993). Computerized cognitive examination of the elderly (ECO): The development of a neuropsychological examination for clinic and population use. *International Journal of Geriatric Psychiatry, 8*(11), 899–914. doi:10.1002/gps.930081104

Rosenthal, R. (2002). Experimenter and clinician effects in scientific inquiry and clinical practice. *Prevention & Treatment, 5*, Article 38. doi:10.1037/1522-3736.5.1.538c

Shiffman, S. (2009). Ecological momentary assessment (EMA) in studies of substance use. *Psychological Assessment, 21*, 486–97. doi:10.1037/a0017074

Shiffman, S., & Stone, A. A. (1998). Introduction to the special section: Ecological momentary assessment in health psychology. *Health Psychology, 17*(1), 3–5. doi:10.1037/h0092706

Shiffman, S., Stone, A. A., & Hufford, M. R. (2008). Ecological momentary assessment. *Annual Review of Clinical Psychology, 4*, 1–32. doi:10.1146/annurev.clinpsy.3.022806.091415

Smith, A. (2014, January 6). *African Americans and technology use: A demographic portrait.* Pew Research Internet Project. http://www.pewinternet.org/files/2014/01/African-Americans-and-Technology-Use.pdf

Smith, R. E., Fagan, C., Wilson, N. L., Chen, J., Corona, M., Nguyen, H., . . . Shoda, Y. (2011). Internet-based approaches to collaborative therapeutic assessment: New opportunities for professional psychologists. *Professional Psychology: Research and Practice, 42*, 494–504. doi:10.1037/a0025392

Steinfeld, B. I., & Keyes, J. A. (2011). Electronic medical records in a multidisciplinary health care setting: A clinical perspective. *Professional Psychology: Research and Practice, 42*, 426–32. doi:10.1037/a0025674

Stolwyk, R. J., Lee, S., McKay, A., & Ponsford, J. L. (2013). Exploring what the Austin maze measures: A comparison across conventional and computer versions. *Brain Impairment, 14*, 243–52. doi:10.1017/BrImp.2013.23

Stone, A. A., & Shiffman, S. (1994). Ecological momentary assessment (EMA) in behavioral medicine. *Annals of Behavioral Medicine, 16*, 199–02.

Trull, T. J., Solhan, M. B., Tragesser, S. L., Jahng, S., Wood, P. K., Piasecki, T. M., & Watson, D. (2008). Affective instability: Measuring a core feature of borderline personality disorder with ecological momentary assessment. *Journal of Abnormal Psychology, 117*, 647–61. doi:10.1037/a0012532

Tsukayama, H. (2014, September 22). *Sleep-tracking apps: Can they really help you rest easy?* The Washington Post. http://www.washingtonpost.com/blogs/the-switch/wp/2014/09/22/sleep-tracking-apps-can-they-really-help-you-rest-easy/

Tversky, B., & Marsh, E. J. (2000). Biased retellings of events yield biased memories. *Cognitive Psychology, 40*, 1–38. doi:10.1006/cogp.1999.0720

Wechsler, D. (1981). *Wechsler adult intelligence scale-revised.* San Antonio, TX: Psychological Corporation.

Wechsler, D. (2008). *Wechsler adult intelligence scale* (4th ed.). Bloomington, MN: Pearson.

Wechsler, D. (2009). *Wechsler memory scale* (4th ed.). Bloomington, MN: Pearson.

Wechsler, D. (2014). *Wechsler intelligence scale for children* (5th ed.). Bloomington, MN: Pearson.

Zickuhr, K. (2013, September 25). *Who's not online and why.* Pew Research Internet Project. http://www.pewinternet.org/files/old-media//Files/Reports/2013/PIP_Offline%20adults_092513_PDF.pdf

CHAPTER

27 Telemental Health

Mitigating the Practitioner's Risk

Pietro J. Lynn, Esq

Abstract

The Internet and advances in technology are substantially increasing our ability to communicate. Those remote audio and video communications technologies offer mental healthcare professionals with the opportunity to clinically engage with patients outside of the traditional office setting. However, with those opportunities come new challenges. Clinicians interested in utilizing remote communications technology to treat patients, *telemental health*, should carefully consider new legal exposures inherent in treating patients outside the office before incorporating telemental health into their practices. Telemental health raises new issues for mental healthcare professionals in the context of malpractice claims, personal jurisdiction, informed consent, licensing, and compliance with the Health Insurance Portability and Accountability Act (HIPAA). This chapter identifies the new and sometimes subtle problematic issues associated with telemental health, exploring the nature of the risks to the telemental health clinician and discussing a practical approach to minimizing the exposures.

Keywords: telemental health, licensure, malpractice, risk mitigation, jurisdiction

The emergence of new technologies in communications and information sharing presents an opportunity for mental health professionals to provide services to their patients more efficiently and conveniently. Digital communication by email, text message, video conferencing, or other Internet-based software using voice and/or images has dramatically broadened the mechanisms by which information may be shared between the mental health professional and the patient. At the same time, the costs associated with those technologies have diminished, making them widely available. We live in a time when virtually everyone with a computer or handheld device and access to a wireless network can engage in video conferencing and other forms of digital communication. Accordingly, there is a far greater opportunity for mental health professionals to assess or treat patients outside the physical presence of the professional or to practice *telemental health*.

Most patients are accustomed to using electronic communications, such as email and text messages or some variation of video conferencing, to exchange information with family, friends, schools, government, or business associates. It is foreseeable that patients will expect and even demand to use such technologies to communicate with mental health providers. It is equally reasonable to anticipate that patients will include treatment information in their electronic communications and will expect similarly substantive responses from the clinician. Those professional communications, depending on content, can often be considered the provision of professional services. Clinicians must be careful when they decide to practice telemental health as its obvious benefits create equally significant legal risks and exposures.

Likewise, entrepreneurial clinicians may wish to operate websites that dispense mental health diagnoses or advice based on interactive technologies and sophisticated software. Website-based treatment is becoming an increasingly popular and potentially lucrative form of mental healthcare that will likely expand in the future. Nonetheless, to the extent that they are also platforms for the provision of telemental health services, the risks identified in this chapter should be equally concerning.

The goal of this chapter is to identify some of telemental health's most significant risks and to propose strategies to mitigate them. It is important for clinicians to understand what constitutes telemental health treatment, its potential limitations and differences in comparison to traditional treatment, and the impact of those limitations/differences on the clinician's liability exposure to licensing authorities, governmental agencies, and patients. Only when clinicians are aware of the risks can they take necessary steps to mitigate them through thoughtful and proactive planning and practices.

What Is Telemental Health?

There are numerous state statutes that establish a definition of telemental health. Although the definitions vary somewhat by jurisdiction, those differences seem to be minor. In general, telemental health is characterized by the provision of mental health services remotely, where the patient is not in the presence of the mental health professional at the time that assessment, treatment, or other mental health services are rendered. The American Psychiatric Association states that telemedicine "typically refers to the use of telecommunications technology to assist in the practice of medicine" (Recupero & Fisher, 2014, p. 1). Similarly, the American Psychological Association adopted a broadly useful definition that can be applied as a general guide. It considers "telepsychology" (telemental health for psychologists) to be "the provision of psychological services using telecommunications technologies" (Joint Task Force for the Development of Telepsychology Guidelines for Psychologists, 2013, p. 792). "Telecommunications technologies" are defined as "the preparation, transmission, communication, or related processing of information by electrical, electromagnetic, electromechanical, electro-optical, or electronic means" (2013, p.792).

When professionals provide mental health services, whether in person or remotely, the communication is subject to legal and professional standards for licensed providers. When the professional engages in telemental health, it raises additional concerns, particularly those created by providing treatment across state lines. Other concerns include obtaining appropriate informed consent, complying with the requirements of the Health Insurance Portability and Accountability Act (HIPAA), and broadening exposure to malpractice and licensing risks. If the professional relationship does not qualify as a mental health service, all of those risks largely vanish. The obvious conclusion is that, when appropriate and feasible, risk can be mitigated by limiting website-based services or distance professional communications to services that fall outside the defined parameters of mental healthcare.

One method for accomplishing that goal is to restrict the scope of teleservices to "coaching." *Coaching* is a consultative service and hence is not subject to the strict regulations and liability exposures inherent in the provision of mental health services. With some exceptions, states generally do not require registration or a license to sell coaching or consulting services in person or at a distance (Hart, Blattner, & Leipsic, 2001). The distinction may be difficult to discern, although it is a meaningful and potentially important one.

Few published legal cases raise and discuss the difference between coaching and therapy. Authors in both fields have described potential distinctions, although there are so many variations in psychotherapeutic approaches and coaching that a solid rationale is needed to establish a particular service as falling within one or the other category. Meneghello (2013) notes that therapy "usually involves healing issues from the past, sometimes traumatic or unresolved childhood issues" (p. 39). According to a survey of mental health therapists, the therapist "discerns and treats" psychopathology through "behavioral, cognitive, or analytic intervention" (Hart et al., 2001, p. 230).

Coaching services are neither retrospective nor based on treating personal psychological issues. Rather, they tend to be "prospective, focusing on goals, untapped potential, and critical success factors in a whole person who seeks to maximize his or her fulfillment in life and work" (Hart et al., 2001, p. 230). A life coach would not engage in an inquiry into past traumas and relationships in order to develop a plan to treat some identified psychological condition. Instead, the coach develops plans for success and offers behaviors to maximize the client's potential to achieve articulated goals.

The best practice for coaches is to design services that clearly avoid the criteria defining mental health treatment and to formally establish strict parameters for professional interactions with the client and then maintain the discipline necessary to work only within the established parameters. Again, if it isn't telemental health, the provider's risk is substantially diminished.

What Are the Differences/Limitations Inherent in Telemental Health?

If professionals are willing to incorporate telemental health as a component of their practices, it is important to understand the inherent limitations of the media to be utilized in the context of treatment. Traditional clinical care is provided with the patient in the professional's presence. Observation of the patient is often considered an important component in the exercise of professional judgment. The clinician relies on visual and verbal cues, like voice tone, facial expressions, body language, and other indicators of the patient's emotional state. It is often believed that those nonverbal cues enhance judgments about the patient's diagnosis and treatment.

Additionally, when the patient is present in the clinician's office, the clinician will have a measure of control over external factors that could impact the patient's presentation. That is not the case for telemental health services. For example, it could be important for the telemental health provider to know if someone is present when the patient is communicating to the provider and, if so, the identity of that person. It is foreseeable that the patient may not always provide accurate information about who is present, even if asked by the clinician. The clinician will have limited or no means to independently verify whether the patient has been truthful, which could have a profound impact on a patient's presentation and thereby affect the clinician's conclusions. Hence, drawing professional judgments can become more challenging with telemental health.

Furthermore, the patient's ability to convey information accurately through the selected medium may impact the content or quality of communications. If a patient has difficulties using the technology and struggles to communicate, or has anxiety around the technology, it may be hard to discern the impact or distorting influence on the patient's overall presentation. Likewise, the clinician may have difficulties with the medium that distract and interfere with assessment and treatment. (It is critical to risk mitigation that the telemental health professional thoroughly understand the operations and relative strengths and weaknesses of the technology used with patients. The professional should also make sure that the patient is sufficiently fluent in operating the technology to support effective treatment.)

It may also be challenging to determine what, if any, impact there is on the patient's presentation or the clinician's interpretation because of the inherent limitations of the technology itself. The quality of video conferencing or audio communications can be limited by Internet connections or cell phone coverage. Interrupted calls or video connections almost certainly complicate the treatment in ways that the clinician would never experience in an office settling. Although this factor seems less significant with the trend toward increasingly better connectivity, the issue must be considered by the professional and identified as a risk inherent in remote treatment.

Malpractice in the Context of Telemental Health

Patients can sue clinicians in civil court whom they allege have committed malpractice. *Malpractice* is generally established when the professional breaches the standard of care for the profession and that breach causes some legally identifiable harm.

There is very little guidance regarding telehealth malpractice, mostly because the issue is still emerging. "Case law is understandably underdeveloped on the issue of telehealth malpractice, with the majority of cases only addressing claims against physicians prescribing medication over the Internet" (Schumacher, 2015, p. 427). Issues that the courts will need to address include jurisdiction and choice of law, including the standard of care which will apply and whether or not there is a different standard of care applicable to telehealth as opposed to direct treatment.

In a malpractice action, the provider is generally held to the established standard of care in the state where he or she treated the patient. If the service is Internet-based or provided remotely, it becomes less clear which state's standards for mental health services will be applied to determine if malpractice has occurred. Likewise, the courts must decide if the standard of care is different for telemental health than for traditional mental health services.

Currently, the American Psychiatric Association's stated position is that "standards of ethics, practice guidelines, and other policies apply to telepsychiatry, just like in-person care" (Hilty, n.d.). The Guidelines for the Practice of Telepsychology, however, suggest that there may indeed be or should be a different standard of care. It is recommended that the psychologist "take particular care to evaluate and assess the appropriateness of utilizing these technologies prior to engaging in, and throughout the duration of, telepsychology practice to determine if the modality of service is appropriate, efficacious and safe" (Joint Task Force, 2013, p. 10). The Guidelines for the Practice of Telepsychology also instructs the practitioner to consult the "burgeoning research in telepsychology" to determine whether it is appropriate and, if so, how best to treat the patient remotely (p. 10). Psychologists are expected to consider the client's "particular needs, the multicultural and ethical issues that may arise" and to review "the most appropriate medium . . . or best options available for the service delivery" (p. 10). Telemental health professionals who do not consult the literature or consider the patient's specific circumstances in planning and delivering care do so at their own peril.

Although there are no reported cases establishing the standard of care as a matter of law in tele*mental* health malpractice claims, there is a growing body of decisions in the area of tele*health* malpractice claims (i.e., relating to the provision of medical treatment by electronic means). In *Marsingill v. O'Malley* (2006), the Alaska Supreme Court considered a case in which a surgical patient, Marsingill, called her surgeon during the night because of ongoing symptoms. The surgeon correctly advised the patient that he could not evaluate her over the phone but that, if she felt badly enough to call him at night, she should go to the emergency room for treatment. The doctor explained that Marsingill would likely undergo unpleasant treatment at the emergency room. He did not explain the full scope of the possible danger facing Marsingill if she failed to seek emergency care and did not make a firm treatment recommendation. Marsingill suffered brain injury and partial paralysis because she did not receive timely treatment of a serious condition.

A jury ultimately decided that the surgeon did not breach the standard of care. However, the evidence at trial focused on the appropriate phone communications to be made when a patient calls with the same symptoms, as distinct from the communications to be made during an examination. The surgeon's testifying expert indicated that it was inappropriate to alarm patients during a call, that there were a number of benign conditions that could have been diagnosed based on the information Marsingill provided, and that the surgeon had stated that he could not diagnose her over the phone. This testimony served as the basis for arguing that the surgeon acted properly even though he did not warn Marsingill that she could be suffering from a very serious condition.

Marsingill is instructive because it supports a different standard of care for phone calls than for in-person treatment and suggests a lower standard of care for emergency phone calls. There is less information available via telephone than during a face-to-face encounter and, thus, presumably, likely diminished accuracy in diagnosis. *Marsingill* is very helpful for the sporadic user of distance treatment. If the call is an isolated and singular event, like an emergency, there is likely to be a low standard of care. If telecommunications are a normal part of the patient–mental healthcare professional relationship, however, the *Marsingill* approach likely will not apply. When the clinician uses technology frequently, it is expected that attempting to apply a lower standard of care based on inadequate available data by virtue of the technology will not suffice, but rather that the provider will be held to a standard resembling or paralleling that applied to more traditional or face-to-face procedures with patients. (The *Marsingill* case supports the contention that often the safest response to the emergency call for care is to tell the patient to report to the emergency room.)

There are several common-sense solutions to the potential legal problems associated with telemental healthcare. The practitioner must (1) restrict the use of telemental health services unless it will be part of the services regularly provided, (2) establish a thoughtful protocol to reduce risk in relation to the extent electronic media will be incorporated into his or her practice, and (3) obtain informed consent in a manner that alerts the patient to the limitations of telemental healthcare and protects the provider from claims that may be unique to distance treatment.

Restricting the use of telemental health services in the context of more traditional face-to- face treatment may be a challenge. Patients may demand an opportunity to engage in distance treatment when unable to meet with the provider. They may also seek communications about their condition through electronic media outside of regular treatment appointments. Telemental health practitioners must be intentional and thoughtful about the circumstances in which they will engage in communications with the patient that constitute treatment. Only then can the risk mitigation process begin.

If preferred or indicated, the risk may be mitigated by clear communications that there will be no provision of telemental health services and that the patient may not make contact for any purposes other than for scheduling in person office appointments. If there is an emergency, the clinician may explain to the patient that an appointment can be made or the patient can seek emergency care from a hospital. The provider can explain his or her concerns around the shortcomings of telemental health and, based on that rationale, decline to engage in it.

Alternatively, the clinician may define the circumstances under which telemental health services will be provided. When those communications may occur and what media are acceptable should be an explicit component of that discussion. Each telemental health medium has its advantages and disadvantages. How those varying options are to be selected and integrated into a practice should be a considered decision. Text messages and emails seem to be especially limiting to a clinician attempting to understand the totality of the patient's presentation. Practitioners should ask themselves if the convenience and popularity of those media are worth the risk of mistaken professional conclusions. In contrast to text messages and emails, more complete clinical information will typically be presented either through video conferencing or telephone communications. At least those media provide the clinician with tone, inflection, and elements of demeanor, and, in the case of video conferencing, facial expressions. As discussed earlier, although potential shortcomings remain with remote services, such as the impact of additional unknown persons in the room with the patient or the occurrence of technology or Internet problems (e.g., insufficient image resolution, media failure), they nonetheless appear to be a good alternative to traditional treatment.

When the clinician establishes protocols for telemental health with patients, the procedures should be in writing and specifically identify the electronic communications that the patient may use with the professional and vice versa. The clinician should also explain the reasons for the protocols and fully explicate the limitations of the medium for diagnosis and treatment.

The clinician should also be sure to consider patient expectations for responsiveness. Many providers have smartphones that can receive calls, emails, and text messages at almost any location. When policies are ambiguous or insufficiently explained, the use of certain telemental health media may create extreme expectations for promptness in replying. An established and explicit telemental health timeliness protocol can avoid a situation in which a delay in responding, which purportedly caused harm, might otherwise appear to be unreasonable and provide a potential basis for a successful malpractice claim. More generally, to manage risk, the telemental health professional should address expectations for responding and other such potential questions or issues explicitly and at the outset of the relationship in a formal, written document. For example, the document should cover the *mutual* understanding between the patient and the provider about timeliness of responses. However, clinicians must understand that once a mutual expectation is established, they must comply with its terms. If the agreement indicates responses within 24 hours, that is a promise that must be met. If clinicians cannot meet their own standards, it will be difficult to establish adherence to the standard of care in the event of malpractice litigation. One viable alternative is an explicit agreement with patients that they use electronic communications at their own risk, with no response expected.

Furthermore, it can be helpful to identify alternative methods of seeking emergency care for the patient and to include these arrangements in the written document. The telemental health agreement should direct the patient to an emergency room or other viable facility or service if emergency care is required and the provider does not respond in a timely manner. The patient should be asked to sign the document demonstrating that he or she understands and accepts the risks inherent in telemental health services. This document should be separate and distinct from any informed consent document and maintained in the patient file. It is sensible to update the document with the patient as circumstances change or on a routine basis (e.g., after 6 months) as a prophylactic measure to reduce malpractice exposure.

It is also useful to the telemental health clinician to establish protocols for use of the media to provide mental health services. There should be explicit rules for when, how, and what media will be used. For example, a clinician might establish a rule that only emergencies will warrant the use of electronic communications and then only by email. Email has the benefit of being a written communication, one that is easily saved should some later dispute arise with the patient.

Providers should also contact their malpractice insurance carriers to ensure that telemental health services are covered by their policy. Although most telemental health services are likely to be covered for in-state practice, they are not necessarily covered for interstate practice (DeAngelis, 2012).

Informed Consent for Telemental Health

Informed consent is a necessary part of any mental health provider (MHP)–patient relationship. At the outset, a legally recognized MHP–patient relationship can be established over the Internet. In the case of psychiatrists, for example, "when the service provided falls within the broad category of medicine, and is provided under an express, or implied, agreement between the Internet physician and the user patient, and the service in some manner contributes to the user's medical care, directly or indirectly, the necessary elements exist to establish a legally recognized physician-patient relationship" (Blum, 2003, p. 439). This analysis is equally applicable to any mental health professional providing services over the Internet that fall within the category of mental health treatment. Therefore, the provision of services requires informed consent. "Informed consent is crucial to protect patients from unauthorized and unforeseen uses of their medical information. Any telemedicine interaction, accordingly, requires informed consent not only because medical information might be obtained, transmitted or stored during the telemedicine consultation, but also because patients are engaging in a specific medical procedure" (Spielberg, 1999, pp. 287–289).

In general, ethical standards that apply to mental health services also apply to telemental health services (DeAngelis, 2012). As telehealth gains popularity, however, experts have begun developing guidelines specifically for professionals providing services via the Internet. The American Counseling Association Code of Ethics (2014) includes a section titled "Distance Counseling, Technology, and Social Media." Section H.2.a discusses informed consent and disclosure, stating that, in addition to the "usual and customary protocol of informed consent between counselor and client for face-to-face counseling" (p. 17), informed consent for telemental health services invokes new issues, such as a provider's distance counseling credentials, physical location of practice, risks and benefits of engaging in use of distance counseling and/or technology, possibility of technology failure and alternate methods of service delivery, anticipated response time, and potential denial of insurance benefits.

Similarly, the Guidelines for the Practice of Telepsychology (Joint Task Force, 2013) state, "Psychologists strive to obtain and document informed consent that specifically addresses the unique concerns related to the telepsychology services they provide. When doing so, psychologists are cognizant of the applicable laws and regulations, as well as organizational requirements that govern informed consent in this area" (p. 12). Ultimately, informed consent must specifically address unique hurdles raised in the telemental health arena.

Most states do not require additional informed consent before a telemental health encounter over and above what is required for an in-person encounter. However, according to Thomas and Capistran (2017), 20 states and the District of Columbia require a physician to obtain additional informed consent before a telemedicine encounter (p. 10). As these authors further note (2016), nine states and the District of Columbia require a psychologist to obtain additional patient informed consent (p. 2). In 2015, AB 809 in California revised the informed consent requirements relating to licensed healthcare providers, including psychologists and counselors, delivering health care services via telehealth by permitting consent to be provided orally or in writing and deleting the requirement that the healthcare provider who obtains consent be at the originating site where the patient is physically located (Medical Board of California, n.d.).

Similarly, Kentucky regulations (201 Ky. Admin. Regs. 26:310) require informed consent, in writing, that covers the specifics of telepsychology:

> A credential holder using telehealth to deliver psychological services or who practices telepsychology shall, upon initial contact with the client.... Inform the client in writing about:
>
> (a) The limitations of using technology in the provision of telepsychology;
> (b) Potential risks to confidentiality of information due to technology in the provision of telepsychology;
> (c) Potential risks of disruption in the use of telepsychology;
> (d) When and how the credential holder will respond to routine electronic messages;
> (e) In what circumstances the credential holder will use alternative communications for emergency purposes;
> (f) Who else may have access to client communications with the credential holder;
> (g) How communications can be directed to a specific credential holder;
> (h) How the credential holder stores electronic communications from the client; and
> (i) The reporting of clients required by 201 KAR 26:145, Section 7.

The Kentucky statutory standard establishes a helpful guide for telemental health providers outside of that state. Informed consent should be contained in a robust document that explores the variety of issues raised in this chapter. The document should serve as the basis for a detailed conversation with the patient about each of the statutory issues. The conversation should culminate with the patient endorsing that he or she understands and agrees to telemental health treatment, as distinct from traditional treatment.

Licensing Issues

Sometimes the telemental healthcare professional may know that the patient is in a jurisdiction outside the state(s) where the clinician is licensed. The licensing issues are easily understood because the professional knows where he or she is working. At other times, the clinician may not know where the patient is located and has no way of knowing without asking. Furthermore, the patient may not be honest with the clinician when asked. Email, text messages, phone calls, or video conferencing will not ordinarily identify the patient's location for the clinician. This can be a problem because providing services outside of the state of licensure may lead to discipline or even criminal charges.

Professional licensure is granted state by state, and thus the provision of telemental services across state lines inevitably raises licensing questions (unless the provider is licensed across the states in question). Many states' laws do not address telemental health, but all states have addressed the issue of cross-border licensing. The question remains how to apply existing regulations to the practice of telemental health across state lines.

Few cases explore this issue. One that does is a 2014 Pennsylvania case involving the Pennsylvania psychology licensing board's attempt to stop a psychologist who was not licensed in Pennsylvania from delivering psychological services to patients who resided in Pennsylvania (*Abraham v. Bureau of Prof'l & Occupational Affairs, State Bd. of Psychology*, 2014). In that case, Dr. Abraham listed a Pennsylvania address as his business location and listed a telephone number with a Pennsylvania area code but was only licensed to practice psychology in Israel, not in Pennsylvania. From his location in Israel, he provided counseling services to clients in Pennsylvania using the phone and Skype. The State Board of Psychology imposed a civil penalty and ordered Dr. Abraham to cease and desist from holding himself out as a psychologist in Pennsylvania until he obtained a license in the state. Dr. Abraham appealed, and a Pennsylvania Court affirmed the Board's order that a license was needed, even though Dr. Abraham claimed to be treating patients in Israel. It was unclear what significance the Court placed on Dr. Abraham listing a Pennsylvania business address on his website. Nonetheless, the court relied heavily on the fact that the patients were located in Pennsylvania in finding a licensing violation. It is probably fair to assume that the most important factor was the location of the *patient* as opposed to the provider.

The approach in the *Abraham* case is supported by states with specific licensing guidelines for the use of telemental health. Those states require professionals to be licensed in the state in which the patient is receiving services (Medical Board of California, n.d.; 201 Ky. Admin. Regs. 26:310). As noted in the context of medical care: "Seemingly unable to relinquish traditional concepts, a physician is considered by too many jurisdictions as practicing medicine in the state where the *patient* is located (termed the originating site), which is the fundamental contributor to the licensure barrier, as the provision of medical care by [telemedicine] is still caught by the originating site's licensure state law requirements" (Siegal, 2012, p. 14). A Vermont statute (26 V.S.A. § 3018) indicates that professionals who provide telepractice services to persons in Vermont are deemed to be practicing in Vermont and must be licensed by the Board; yet Vermont licensed psychologists who provide telepractice services to clients outside of Vermont nonetheless remain under the jurisdiction of the Board. In summary, considering these types of decisions, statutes, and regulations, it seems prudent for the telemental health professional to assume it is necessary to be licensed in the state where the provider is located *and* the state where the patient is receiving care.

Most states have guest licensure provisions that allow a professional licensed in another state to provide services for a brief period of time (usually ranging from 10 to 30 days in a given calendar year) under specified conditions. In many instances, a provider has to file a formal application for temporary licensure and receive official approval, and it should not be assumed that one can practice temporarily in another state if the length of that activity is restricted. Furthermore, some states have adopted some special-purpose licensure, "allowing practitioners to obtain a limited license for the delivery of specific health services under particular circumstances, which can be regarded as suitable for the [telemedicine] care" (Siegal, 2012, p. 15). Some states issue licenses via reciprocity; that is, these states will issue a license to an applicant with a valid, unrestricted license to practice medicine in another state if the other state's requirements for licensure are substantially equivalent.

Although obtaining a short-term or limited license or even a full license in the state where the patient is located is a potential solution to the problem, it is not always a complete solution. If the patient moves to a state where the professional is not licensed, the risks are again present. The danger is further compounded if the patient does not inform or misinforms the telemental health professional about his or her location. It is doubtful that ignorance will be a defense to charges that there has been unlicensed treatment. A licensing authority could effectively argue that a professional engaging in telemental health has a duty to control the location of services because of licensing laws. If the patient moves to a jurisdiction where the provider is unlicensed, with or without informing the clinician, a licensing board could easily contend that the professional bears all of the risk of violating state laws.

It may be challenging for professionals to limit treatment to jurisdictions in which they are licensed. The best solutions may come from the technology and media used for telemental health services or merely from common-sense precautions. One obvious way to determine if the patient is in a location where the provider has a license is to ask the patient to pan the room with a video camera before every treatment session. If the room is one that the clinician knows is in the patient's home, the risk is mitigated. Consultants may also work with the provider to supply technology that will identify the location of the patient at the time of treatment (although the provider needs to inform the patient about the capacity to do so and probably should include this capability in the consent form). The technology needed to determine someone's location is already widely available for cell phones. Again, a careful, thoughtful approach to the practice of telemental health can limit the exposures.

Personal Jurisdiction

It is often important for telemental healthcare providers to not only consider where they are practicing so that licensing requirements are met, but also where they are engaging in their professional activities for purposes of personal jurisdiction. That is, the clinician may wish to ask him- or herself: Where can I be sued in my telemental health practice? What laws will govern claims against me? There are obvious disadvantages to litigating a case outside the state in which the professional works. Each state has different laws, juror attitudes, and judicial approaches to discovery. Defending telemental health practices in far-flung, potentially hostile jurisdictions can be a significant inconvenience and disadvantage. The telemental healthcare professional may inadvertently create the basis for claims in distant states or even foreign countries by virtue of distance treatment.

A person may be subject to suit in a forum state where he or she has established "minimum contacts" (*Internat. Shoe Co. v. Washington*, 1945, p. 319). To establish minimum contacts the person must have "purposefully avail[ed]" himself of the "privileges and benefits of conducting activities within the forum" (*World-Wide Volkswagen Corp. v. Woodson*, 1980, p. 297). It is clear that when a patient travels out of state for treatment with a healthcare provider there is no minimum contact with the patient's home state (e.g., see *Ghanem v. Kay*, 1984; *Walters v. St. Elizabeth Hosp. Med. Ctr.*, 1982). Under those facts, the patient can only sue the clinician where the patient was treated.

What constitutes purposeful availment becomes complicated in the context of Internet contacts. The law seems clear that if the patient finds the provider online, so long as all the treatment is in the provider's state, there is no jurisdiction in the patient's state of residence (*Paterno v. Laser Spine Inst.*, 2014). However, there may be jurisdiction over the telemental health provider in all locations where he or she uses "electronic and telephonic means to project themselves into [a state] to conduct business transactions" (p. 372). Passive websites do not confer jurisdiction in all states where the website can be accessed. Websites that are interactive for commercial transactions may confer personal jurisdiction in any state where the website is used (*Halas v. Dick's Sporting Goods*, 2013).

Applied to telemental health, it seems clear from the personal jurisdiction cases that if the professional provides services through electronic or telephonic means to patients, he or she must be prepared to defend those professional services in any state (and potentially any country) where the patient is located at that time. Once jurisdiction is established, the courts in those states may use their laws to determine the outcome of the case.

There is no way to eliminate the possibility of lawsuits in jurisdictions outside of the state in which the clinician works. Patients can initiate suit at any time in any place. The courts then must sort out which cases may go forward and which ones are improperly filed for lack of personal jurisdiction. Nonetheless, there are methods which may limit that risk of litigation outside of the clinician's home state. For example, the clinician can use a telemental health agreement that includes a choice of venue and a choice of law provision to be signed at treatment onset—an agreement as to where the provider can be sued and the law that will govern any claims.

The choice of venue clause should be prominent within the document and explicitly state that any litigation between the patient and the provider must be filed within the provider's home state. Likewise, the choice of law provision should identify the state law that will govern any claims arising from the treatment relationship. Although there is some danger that a trial court in another state could find the provisions invalid for public policy reasons, such clauses are often enforced by the courts in other contexts. The inclusion of the choice of law and venue language provides additional certainty to the practice of telemental health by likely limiting the places where the practitioner can be sued and the laws that will be applied to the litigation.

HIPAA Compliance

HIPAA (1996) created privacy rules for "covered entities." Under HIPAA, health and mental health providers are considered covered entities and must comply with the privacy provisions. The right to privacy extends to all "individually identifiable health information" held or transmitted by a covered entity in any form of media, whether electronic, paper, or oral. That information is known as protected health information (PHI). HIPAA compliance can be challenging for the telemental health provider.

Where a mental healthcare professional violates HIPAA privacy provisions, there is exposure to both civil and criminal penalties. The Department of Health and Human Services may impose civil money penalties for each individual act constituting failure to comply with a privacy rule (42 U.S.C. § 1320d-05). The penalties range from $100 per violation to $1,000, depending on the covered entity's culpability. More concerning for the practitioner is the potential criminal exposure for violations of HIPAA's privacy rules. A person who knowingly obtains or discloses PHI in violation of HIPAA faces a fine of $50,000 per violation, with a cap of $1.5 million, and up to 1 year's imprisonment (42 U.S.C. § 1320d-06).

The penalties under HIPAA require careful consideration of the potential pitfalls of telemental health privacy protections. It is obvious that delivering mental health services using technology that lacks adequate security creates substantial exposures. Whether the professional utilizes Skype, email, or text messaging, there is a foreseeable danger that other persons will be able to access the PHI without the patient's consent. That potential has generated conversation about how best to mitigate the risk and ensure HIPAA compliance while still embracing the advantages of distance treatment.

The first step in complying with HIPAA is a careful analysis of the technology being considered for service delivery. The professional should evaluate the likelihood and potential impact of the risk in connection with the electronic PHI (e-PHI). Efforts must be made to implement appropriate security measures to address the risks identified in the risk analysis. The process by which the risk was determined, the security measures adopted, and the reasons for those measures all should be documented to demonstrate the provider's intent and efforts to protect the e-PHI in the event of a breach.

To appropriately evaluate the use of technology in the delivery of telemental health for privacy purposes, the clinician should consult with experts to determine the level of security provided by any software platform. For example, if a clinician wishes to utilize Skype or some other common video conferencing software to conduct therapy, the professional will need to make a technical inquiry to determine if the encryption capability makes that software sufficiently secure so that there is no significant risk of unauthorized persons accessing the therapy materials or records. Likewise, text messages or emails may be available on servers to unauthorized persons, like employers who regularly monitor employee emails. Wireless Internet networks utilized to facilitate telemental health may not be entirely secure. Attention must be paid to network security. In short, the covered entity, the telemental health professional, must analyze the stream of communication of e-PHI from start to finish. Obviously, clinicians who fail to perform the detailed inquiry need to determine how effectively the technology they use protects privacy are engaging in risky professional behaviors that could easily result in fines and licensing action.

Conclusion

Telemental health is an intriguing and potentially attractive option for many mental healthcare providers. It is more convenient for patients and clinicians. Services can be provided and treatment received almost anywhere. There is the lucrative possibility of software-driven, web-based assessment and treatment. However, the obvious benefits are accompanied by some not so obvious risks. The telemental health practitioner must carefully consider those risks and implement sound mitigation strategies.

References and Legal Citations

Abraham v. Bureau of Prof'l & Occupational Affairs, State Bd. of Psychology, No. 64 C.D. 2014, 2014 WL 3893352 (Pa. Commw. Ct. Aug. 11, 2014).

American Counseling Association. (2014). ACA Code of ethics. http://www.counseling.org/resources/aca-code-of-ethics.pdf.

American Psychiatric Association Council on Psychiatry & Law. (2014). Resource document on telepsychiatry and related technologies in clinical psychiatry. *American Psychiatric Association Resource Documents.* https://www.psychiatry.org/psychiatrists/search-directories-databases/library-and-archive/resource-documents

Blum, J. D. (2003). Internet medicine and the evolving legal status of the physician-patient relationship. *Journal of Legal Medicine, 24*, 413–55.

DeAngelis, T. (2012). Practicing distance therapy, legally and ethically. *Monitor on Psychology, 43*(3), 52.

Ghanem v. Kay, 624 F. Supp. 23 (D.C.C. 1984).

Halas v. Dick's Sporting Goods, 964 N.Y.S. 2d 808 (N.Y. App. Div. 2013)

Hart, V., Blattner, J., & Leipsic, S. (2001). Coaching versus therapy: A perspective. *Consulting Psychology Journal: Practice and Research, 53*(4), 229–37. doi:10.1037//1061–4087.53.4.229

Hilty, D. (n.d.) Standard of care and state based regulations. American Psychiatric Association Telepsychiatry Toolkit. https://www.psychiatry.org/psychiatrists/practice/telepsychiatry/standard-of-care-state-based-regulations

Internat. Shoe Co. v. Washington, 326 U.S. 310 (1945).

Joint Task Force for the Development of Telepsychology Guidelines for Psychologists. (2013). Guidelines for the practice of telepsychology. *American Psychologist, 68*(9): 791–800. doi:10.1037/a0035001

Marsingill v. O'Malley, 128 P.3d 151 (Alaska 2006).

Medical Board of California. (n.d.) Practicing medicine through telehealth technology. http://www.mbc.ca.gov/Licensees/Telehealth.aspx

Meneghello, K. (2013). Life coaching: Four things you didn't know. *Oregon State Bar Bulletin, 73*, 38–9.

Paterno v. Laser Spine Inst., 23 N.E.3d 988 (N.Y. 2014).

Schumacher, A. (2015). Telehealth: Current barriers, potential progress. *Ohio State Law Journal, 76*, 409–39.

Siegal, G. (2012). Enabling globalization of health care in the information technology era: Telemedicine and the medical World Wide Web. *Virginia Journal of Law and Technology, 17*, 1–34.

Spielberg, A. R. (1999). Online without a net: Physician-patient communication by electronic mail. *American Journal of Law & Medicine, 25*, 267–95.

Thomas, L., & Capistran, G. (2017). State telemedicine gaps analysis: Physician practice standards & licensure. *American Telemedicine Association.* http://www.americantelemed.org/docs/default-source/policy/2016_50-state-telehealth-gaps-analysis-md-physician-practices-licensure.pdf?sfvrsn=2.

Walters v. St. Elizabeth Hosp. Med. Ctr., 543 F. Supp. 559 (W.D. Pa. 1982).

World-Wide Volkswagen Corp. v. Woodson, 444 U.S. 286 (1980).

PART 6

Applications of Digital Technology to Promote Psychological Welfare and Health in Special Groups

CHAPTER

28 Mobile Applications to Help Women Achieve Better Behavioral Health in the Postpartum Period

Dawn W. Foster *and* Ariadna Forray

Abstract

Various theoretical perspectives have informed intervention and program development in postpartum health, including the transtheoretical model, the health belief model, and cognitive and social processes. Mobile technology has been used in recent years to address and promote postpartum health. Mobile technologies utilizing theoretically grounded interventions can be harnessed to improve postpartum behavioral health by decreasing two major barriers to treatment in this population: avoidance of pharmacotherapy and convenient treatment delivery. Specifically, mobile technologies in the postpartum period can tailor messages to user characteristics (e.g. age, number of children, history of depression); link the user with others for increased social support; provide convenient, cost-effective, evidence-based treatment to large populations regardless of location; and provide the ability to send time-sensitive communications to devices. Current interventions for postpartum women include a mobile application for depression that promotes social connectedness and text messaging to promote smoking cessation in perinatal women. Mobile technologies represent a rich medium by which to deliver and facilitate personalized interventions for a variety of health behaviors in postpartum women.

Keywords: postpartum, text messaging, depression, pregnancy, smoking cessation

Background

Many health problems associated with the peri- and postnatal time period can be prevented with adequate and timely medical care or intervention (McCarthy & Maine, 1992; Thaddeus & Maine, 1994). Mobile technology has been used in recent years to combat maternal and child health problems and to promote postpartum health (Cormick et al., 2012; Noordam, Kuepper, Stekelenburg, & Milen, 2011). Additional efforts to understand underlying mechanisms and develop empirically validated and theory-based interventions and programs for postpartum health are warranted.

This chapter begins by presenting various theoretical perspectives that have informed intervention and program development in postpartum health. The chapter then presents existing mobile interventions that have been applied for promoting postpartum health. Implications and future avenues for research are then discussed.

Transtheoretical Model

One of the long-used theoretical frameworks is the *transtheoretical model* (TTM). The TTM is a model of behavior change that has been widely disseminated and helps to elucidate and facilitate change across a broad spectrum of health behaviors (Prochaska & Velicer, 1997). The TTM describes both processes and stages of change. Stages of change represent a continuum of events leading to change in behavior (precontemplation, contemplation, preparation, action, and maintenance). Stages of change also facilitate differentiation of the target population in a way that assists the tailoring of intervention content to specific needs. Precontemplators often do not recognize a need to change or lack awareness that change is possible. As an example, a pregnant woman who smokes cigarettes and is not thinking about quitting, or does not view her smoking as a problem, would be categorized as a precontemplator. Contemplators are also not actively making a change; however, they are beginning to think about doing so. Here, a pregnant woman who smokes but is considering quitting soon would be categorized as a contemplator. The preparation stage is categorized by intentions to make a change or having attempted behavior change in the past year. A pregnant woman who intends to stop smoking or tried to quit recently would be classified as being in the preparation stage. The action stage includes individuals who have made or are currently making a change in their behavior. A pregnant woman who is actively reducing or stopping cigarette use would be classified as being in the action stage. Beyond the action stage is the maintenance stage. Here, individuals have been abstinent for more than 6 months (not smoking for at least 6 months). For some behaviors, including many addictive behaviors, it is also important to consider *relapse*, as change does not often occur in linear fashion. During relapse, the individual may regress to an earlier stage (smoking a cigarette after having abstained for a year). When this happens, the individual is encouraged to rebuild motivation to change the behavior.

In addition to stages of change, the TTM also proposes processes of change. These provide a framework for understanding mechanisms hypothesized to mediate change. Processes of change are comprised of cognitive and behavioral mechanisms and include social liberation, consciousness raising, environmental reevaluation, dramatic relief, self-liberation, self-reevaluation, counterconditioning stimulus control, reinforcement management, and helping relationships. As pregnant and postpartum women move across the continuum of stages toward better health practices and away from risky behaviors, a consistent pattern of utilization of processes has been demonstrated. Importantly, processes of change provide both strategies and methods for intervention delivery and determinants of behavioral change, which facilitate the generation of meaningful program objectives.

As a general example, a TTM-based mobile intervention for smoking cessation during pregnancy might target women in the precontemplation or contemplation stage: those who have not yet quit smoking. The mobile intervention might employ text messages as a strategy to promote health during the peri- and postnatal time. Examples of message content might include highlighting the woman's ability to control situations and triggers of the problem behavior (stimulus control), encouraging appraisal of values with respect to managing the problem behavior (self-reevaluation), considering how the behavior may affect her or her baby's health (environmental reevaluation), and suggesting that the woman reward herself for making positive changes (reinforcement management).

The TTM is sensitive to early indications of change by examining and building on constructs related to decision-making and self-efficacy. The model has much clinical utility. It has been applied as a means for tailoring intervention approaches to readiness to change, has demonstrated efficacy as a diagnostic tool and as an intervention for risky behaviors, and has been applied as a framework for studying and promoting peri- and postpartum health (Aveyard et al., 2006; Fahrenwald & Walker, 2003; Hacker, Brown, Cabral, & Dodds, 2005; Horowitz, 2003; Huang, Wu, Huang, Chien, & Guo, 2013; Lawrence, Aveyard, Evans, & Cheng, 2003; Ruggiero, Tsoh, Everett, Fava, & Guise, 2000; Slade, Laxton-Kane, & Spiby, 2006). Thus, the TTM has much clinical utility in encouraging behavior change and can be readily applied using mobile and web-based technology to increase progression along the stage of change continuum.

Health Belief Model

The health belief model (HBM) is a widely used theory in health behavior research and proposes that beliefs about health problems, perceptions of the benefits of action and barriers to action, and self-efficacy impact health behaviors (Baghianimoghadam, Zolghadar, Moghadam, Darayi, & Jozy, 2012; Stout, 1997; Zweig, LeFevre, Kruse, 1988). HBM constructs include perceived severity, which refers to the subjective assessment of a health problem or behavior and its potential consequences. For example, a pregnant woman perceiving that drinking alcohol or smoking cigarettes is very harmful to her and her baby's health may not be likely to use those substances. Furthermore, perceived susceptibility is described by the HBM as the subjective assessment of one's risk for developing a particular problem. Here, a pregnant woman who perceives herself and her baby as vulnerable to health problems might be more motivated to avoid risky behaviors or to engage in healthy behaviors compared to a pregnant woman who does not perceive herself or her baby as vulnerable. Perceived seriousness and perceived susceptibility are powerful in prompting individuals to adopt healthy behaviors or avoid risky behaviors (Chen, Fox, Cantrell, Stockdale, & Kagawa-Singer, 2007; Chen, Lee, Chou, Kuo, & Hsu, 2007; Iriyama, Nakahara, Jimba, Ichikawa, & Wakai, 2007). This has been demonstrated in risky sexual behaviors (Iriyama et al., 2007), getting vaccinations (Chen, Fox et al., 2007), and other health behaviors (Brown, Ottney, & Nguyen, 2011; Daddario, 2007; Kloeblen & Batish, 1999; Sharifirad et al., 2013). Furthermore, perceptions of benefits of a certain health behaviors (e.g., believing that eating healthy foods will be beneficial to oneself and one's baby) influence the likelihood of taking action to protect health, as do perceptions about barriers and whether obstacles exist with respect to behavior change. The HBM further posits that cues to action (or triggers that prompt health behaviors) are also important in promoting health, and these could include, for example, having fresh fruit on the coffee table rather than candy, as a cue to eat in a healthy fashion. Cues can range in intensity and can be related to perceived susceptibility, seriousness, benefits, and barriers. Self-efficacy is included in the HBM and refers to the perception of one's competence to successfully perform a behavior or successfully refrain from engaging in a risky behavior. Theory-based strategies to prevent adverse health outcomes around pregnancy have evolved and range from contraceptive behaviors (Baghianimoghadam et al., 2012; Brown et al., 2011; Hall, 2012; Hester & Macrina, 1985), labor and delivery (Baghianimoghadam et al., 2012), breastfeeding (Sweeney & Gulino, 1987), prenatal care (Stout, 1997; Zweig et al., 1988), and prevention of low birth weight (Ekhtiari, Majlessi, Foroushani, & Shakibazadeh, 2014). Furthermore, the HBM and the TTM have some common features, including the identification of self-efficacy as an important factor in health promotion. Self-efficacy is important from a motivational standpoint as postpartum or pregnant women with high self-efficacy are encouraged to tackle challenging tasks and engage in behavior change (de Vries & Backbier, 1994; Gao, Sun, & Chan, 2014; Kaiser, Razurel, & Jeannot, 2013).

An HBM-based mobile intervention might, for example, include content that highlights risks and benefits of specific behaviors as well as ways for overcoming barriers or obstacles. A woman with a newborn may know that physical activity is a healthy behavior; however, she may perceive barriers to exercising ("I need sleep more than I need to go to the gym," or "I don't have the energy to exercise when my baby is sleeping," etc.). A mobile intervention that, for example, provides helpful tips for enjoyable ways of engaging in physical activity may provide important benefits. Messages sent by text or via a smartphone application might suggest postpartum exercise classes suitable for new moms at nearby health clubs or yoga studios. Theoretically based content such as this may be expected to build self-efficacy, address barriers, and encourage behavior change to promote postpartum health.

Other Theoretical Perspectives

Social Processes

Social connections and social support are critical to the mental health of new mothers. A lack of effective social skills and social support networks has been suggested as predictive of relapsing into substance use and risky behaviors (Abroms, Windsor, & Simons-Morton, 2008; Charlton, 1990; Rogers & King, 2013), and it is a widely held perspective that social support from friends and family can facilitate healthy behaviors (Chassin, Presson, Sherman, McLaughlin, & Gioia, 1985). Moreover, research supports the perspective that connectedness can boost favorable outcomes in various domains including depressive symptomatology, substance abuse, and suicide ideation (Seil, Desai, & Smith, 2014).

Cognitive Processes

Social-cognitive models of health behavior change have been applied in theory-based interventions (Abroms et al., 2008; An et al., 2008) and have been used to promote postpartum health (Mesters, Gijsbers, Bartholomew, Knottnerus, & Van Schayack, 2013). There is interest in and research on the role of automatic processes in all psychological domains, including social-cognitive processes (Bargh, Schwader, Hailey, Dyer, & Boothby, 2012). There are two broad categories of behavior: *reflective processes*, which are goal-directed and flexible, and *automatic processes*, which occur without thought or awareness (Strack & Deutsch, 2004). Interventions that target automatic processes to change health-related behaviors are important, and there is an opportunity to implement these on a large scale using mobile technologies.

One approach that has gained traction in promoting healthy behaviors is the use of *cognitive bias modification* (CBM) to change impulsive or automatic processes that may underlie health risk behaviors (Marteau, Hollands, & Fletcher, 2012). CBM has been used as a treatment for a wide range of disorders including anxiety and addictive disorders. Impulsive processes (e.g., attentional bias for a substance) may predominate when executive control is compromised (Wiers, Gladwin, Hofmann, Salemink, & Ridderinkhof, 2013). Postpartum women often experience significant sleep disturbance (Insana, Williams, & Montgomery-Downs 2013), and sleep deprivation may diminish executive function and lead an individual to rely more on automatic processes (Gohar et al., 2009). Thus, this type of intervention is particularly well-suited for postpartum women. Using mobile technologies to change automatic processes associated with unhealthy behaviors among pregnant and postpartum women may enhance efforts to promote health, and, when coupled with efforts to increase stage of change, promote readiness to change, increase self-efficacy, and reinforce healthy behaviors.

Mobile Phones for Health Promotion

Modern technology-based programs that use contemporary methods of delivery, such as phone-based interventions, are often attractive to mothers and soon-to-be mothers, and capable of delivering interventions at a high standard of consistency. Some of the main benefits of using mobile phones among postpartum women is the decrease of two major barriers to treatment: avoidance of the use of medications and convenience of treatment delivery. Treatment delivery in the immediate postpartum period is challenging due to high parenting demands and multiple treatment barriers (e.g., time, childcare, transportation, etc.). These demands may also increase the risk of perinatal women developing a mood disorder or relapsing to unhealthy behaviors, such as smoking.

Important characteristics of media such as mobile devices include the promotion of interaction between mothers and also between mothers and the programs. Interactive technology has demonstrated utility as a health promotion and education tool. Phone-assisted data collection may be linked with web-based platforms for flexible and quick data collection and may be relatively inexpensive. Principles for effective phone-based programs include varied and comprehensive teaching methods, sufficient dose, appropriate timing, positive relationships, theory-driven qualities, socioculturally relevance, and outcome evaluations (Katz et al., 2011; Lund, Rasch et al., 2014). For example, programs that provide and reinforce educational materials can increase knowledge and solidify it through interesting and interactive challenges or quizzes. Furthermore, relevance, including cultural or geographic relevance, may increase interest, applicability, and acceptability of a given program within a particular population. Phone-based interactive programs permit tailoring of messages to specific user characteristics (ethnicity, stage of change, etc.), which is often an important element of contemporary programs (Lichtenstein, 1997). Web-based programs may have multiple research, contextual, and logistical advantages over other delivery channels, including the ability to integrate the data collection and intervention components, thereby facilitating continuous monitoring of both process and outcome evaluation measures. Additionally, phone and web interfacing programs may ensure fidelity and completeness and ensure consistency across delivery environments.

The use of mobile phones in intervention delivery affords additional advantages in that mobile phones are relatively ubiquitous and transportable. Their use has grown considerably since they were first introduced in the 1980s, and advances in technology continue to make new functions available. Many researchers use emerging technologies such as mobile phones due to their enhanced versatility, declining cost, and rapid increase in utilization. Health services around the globe use mobile phones to support health, including self-management of chronic disorders (Gammon et al., 2005; Tasker, Gibson, Franklin, Gregor, & Greene, 2007) and improving medication adherence (Puccio et al., 2006).

Existing Mobile Applications

Assessment and Prevention

Mobile phones have been applied in the assessment and measurement of health and related outcomes among pregnant and post-partum women. Qualitative studies have utilized focus groups to better understand access to mobile phones, experience with receiving and sending text messages, and perceived benefits of using mobile phones for health promotion (Jennings, Ong'ech, Simiyu, Sirengo, & Kassaye, 2013). Interviews conducted via mobile phone have been used and results showed that mobile phones are generally acceptable and feasible in the collection of maternal and child health data (van Heerden, Norris, Tollman, Richter, & Rotheram-Borus, 2013). Other phone assessments among the pregnant population include a psychosocial assessment for perinatal depression (Cardone, Kim, Gordon, Gordon, & Silver 2006), which encourages dynamic and interactive phone exchanges between the health professional and the patient. This method for reaching patients at risk for perinatal depression has demonstrated excellent clinical utility, and the majority of women were readily engaged. Programs such as this may improve expectancies and efficacy related to healthcare and access, which may in turn improve outcomes related to seeking and adhering to antenatal and postnatal care.

Regarding prevention of adverse health outcomes, one program that targets maternal and child health is called Text4baby and is designed to send educational messages to pregnant and postpartum women. The goal of Text4baby is to promote healthy behaviors and prevent risky behaviors during the sensitive peri- and postpartum period. Messages were refined via focus groups at community centers located in six cities across the nation and were tailored to women with low health literacy (Whittaker et al., 2012). One of the challenges found with the low health literacy population is the potential for sharing cell phones, which may pose some difficulty with participants not receiving messages and having special privacy concerns (Poorman, Gazmararian, Elon, & Parker, 2014). Prevention efforts (e.g., "Wired Mothers," a cluster-randomized controlled trial to encourage use of antenatal care; Lund, Nielsen et al., 2014) targeting this population have demonstrated trends toward improved quality of care, with more women attending antenatal care following receipt of reminder text messages. Additionally, prevention efforts have included community-based phone programs to complement gaps in clinical services for HIV prevention efforts (Jennings et al., 2013), and these efforts may improve readiness to engage in antenatal and postnatal care uptake and retention. Taken together, efforts with respect to prevention of adverse health outcomes during and after pregnancy have shown some benefit with respect to promoting postpartum health.

Intervention

Mobile phones are increasingly being utilized in health systems because there is great potential to overcome barriers relating to access to healthcare, convenience, and adherence to prescribed regimens. Existing research has implemented and evaluated interventions delivered via mobile phones to promote health during pregnancy and the postpartum period. Mobile phone interventions have been employed to encourage antenatal care attendance and adherence in low-income settings (Lund, Rasch et al., 2014) and have been found to contribute to improved health of mother and child. Mobile phone interventions have further been used to evaluate levels of satisfaction of antenatal care, anxiety levels, and pregnancy outcomes in the context of a randomized controlled trial (Jareethum et al., 2008). Findings from this research show that women who received the intervention had higher levels of satisfaction regarding antenatal care services and also had lower anxiety levels during the antenatal period relative to pregnant women who did not receive the intervention (Jareethum et al., 2008).

In a recent randomized controlled trial, 497 pregnant women were randomized to receive Text4baby only (control condition) or Text4baby and Quit4baby, an interactive and intensive text messaging smoking cessation program. The 7-day point prevalence of abstinence in women receiving the Quit4baby intervention was significantly greater at 1 and 3 months compared to the control group: 28.80% versus 15.79% at 1 month (p <0.01) and 35.20% versus 22.67% at 3 months (p <0.01), respectively (Abroms, Johnson et al., 2017). These findings indicate that an intensive smoking cessation text messaging program may help female smokers quit smoking during pregnancy.

Current Efforts

Many interventions currently being implemented or tested target health behaviors and illustrate how mobile phones utilize the different theories related to health behavior change. For the purposes of this chapter, we focus on four such interventions that exemplify several unique ways in which health behavior change for perinatal women is being implemented utilizing mobile technology. *SmokefreeMOM* is a mobile text messaging service designed for pregnant women in the United States to help them quit smoking. This program provides around-the-clock encouragement, advice, and tips to help pregnant women and mothers quit smoking and remain abstinent. The program is flexible and meets women at various levels of stage of change, with the option of receiving messages about quitting smoking, cutting down on smoking, or health risks of smoking (National Cancer Institute, 2014). In an acceptability and feasibility trial it was found to be more favorably rated than the control text message quitline referral condition in its helpfulness at 3-month follow-up (P <.01) and in its frequency of messaging at 3-month follow-up (P <.01) (Abroms, Chiang, Macherelli, Leavitt, & Montgomery, 2017). Further study is needed to evaluate whether this readily available free resource can promote cessation in pregnant smokers.

Few interventions have been developed to target social connectedness on a community-wide level. *Momba Depression* is a smartphone application currently under study (NCT01816945, clinicaltrials.gov) that promotes community-wide maternal mental health through an application platform based on promoting social connectedness, maternal–fetal and maternal–infant attachment, and social support. The application contains a token-based economy and reward system grounded in principles of behavioral economics. Mothers in their third trimester of pregnancy are provided with a smartphone, Internet connectivity, access to the Momba application, and training on how to use it. Applications such as this may promote connections between mother and baby, foster a sense of community, build social support, increase knowledge about motherhood, and highlight availability of and access to local resources, all of which may be important to the mental health of postpartum women.

An expansion of the Momba platform is currently being tested to deliver financial incentives to increase abstinence from smoking in the postpartum period (NCT02237898; clinicaltrials.gov). The *Momba Smoking* application consists of financial incentives delivered via a smartphone and a carbon monoxide sensor designed to interface wirelessly with a smartphone to measure breath carbon monoxide. This intervention utilizes one of the most effective interventions for short-term smoking cessation—*contingency management*—to decrease smoking in pregnant and postpartum women (Higgins et al., 2010; Washio et al., 2011) and reduces the burden of implementing such an intervention among postpartum women. As real-world, community settings may be accessed through the use of smartphone technology, this intervention has the potential to expand the use of evidence-based treatments.

The authors are currently piloting a smartphone application called PARIS, a perinatal attentional retraining intervention for smoking. This application uses a CBM intervention—attentional retraining using a visual probe task—delivered via mobile phones to prevent relapse to smoking in postpartum women. This intervention is similar to one used in a study recently published for social anxiety (Enock, Hofmann, & McNally, 2014) and targets both smoking- and stress-related cues. Consistent with a classical conditioning paradigm, attentional bias in addictive behaviors may result from repeated pairings between the rewarding effects of drugs and substance-related cues (Field & Cox, 2008; Franken, 2003; Robinson & Berridge, 1993). This may result in substance-related cues capturing and holding the attention of users (attentional bias) and eliciting substance-seeking behaviors (Franken, 2003; Robinson & Berridge, 1993). Attentional bias to smoking cues remains elevated in former smokers (Field & Cox, 2008; Franken, 2003; Robinson & Berridge, 1993), particularly in naturalistic settings and under conditions of stress. Postpartum women often experience significant stress (Paul, Downs, Schaefer, Beiler, & Weisman, 2013). Stress may be a major driver of relapse in postpartum women (Letourneau et al., 2007; Park et al., 2009) and is associated with an attentional bias toward emotionally negative information (MacLeod, Rutherford, Campbell, Ebsworthy, & Holker, 2002). Targeting automatic processes to reduce attentional bias toward smoking and stress cues may be protective against relapse to smoking. One of the main benefits of this smartphone intervention is that it may facilitate the delivery of a behavioral intervention in higher doses. The number of training sessions has been associated with the degree of reduction in attentional bias (Hakamata et al., 2010). This intervention also has the potential to overcome two major barriers to treatment in this patient population: avoidance of the use of medication and the burden of treatment attendance at a time when parenting demands are high.

Future Directions

Many phone interventions utilize short message service (SMS), otherwise known as text messages. SMS is a powerful communication medium (particularly in young adults) and can be sent from the Internet or from another mobile phone to one or multiple mobile devices. Thus, SMS-based interventions utilize an inexpensive and important medium of communication. The majority of published mobile phone interventions are text-message based, with relatively few utilizing applications developed specifically for smartphones (Fanning, Mullen, & McAuley, 2012). However, it is important for researchers to consider the growing population of smartphone users. A multinational survey of 4,000 participants from 21 countries suggested that 53% of mobile phone users were able to access multimedia services including data services, email, and websites (Urban, 2007). Contextually, smartphone applications, or "apps," may provide a rich and entertaining educational forum. Furthermore, the use of a nonhuman (computerized) medium facilitates confidential and personalized management of progress pertaining to sensitive and socially stigmatized issues such as smoking or drinking behaviors.

Immediate demographics intake and stage-matching offers individualized attention based on the specific needs of each person, a task that would be difficult to manage in a group setting. Moreover, information may be easily updated and expanded since programs may reside on a single server, and curricula may potentially be accessed by anyone at any location worldwide as long as their device has Internet connectivity. It is important to note that, as with any intervention component that requires few human resources, smartphone apps may not be appropriate replacements for counselors or healthcare providers. Apps cannot supervise behavioral and experiential activities performed by individuals during intervention processes. Thus, programs should be designed to do what they can and should not be intended to assume the role of counselor.

Theoretically grounded interventions that recognize the potential of mobile technologies may provide researchers with an effective tool for promoting health. Behavioral scientists have described the potential that mobile devices have in facilitating the understanding of multiple health behaviors including alcohol use (Collins, Kashdan, &Gollnisch, 2003; Irvine et al., 2012; Suffoletto, Calabria, Ross, Callaway, & Yealy, 2012), and meta-analyses demonstrate support for mobile technology efficacy in influencing smoking cessation (Whittaker et al., 2009). In this chapter, we described how novel mobile interventions are being tested and used in different ways to improve postpartum behavioral health. The ability to tailor messages to user characteristics (e.g., age, stage of pregnancy), the cost-effective deliverability and scalability to large populations regardless of location, and the ability to send time-sensitive communications to devices are among the possible benefits of mobile phone–based interventions, and importantly, there is an ability to link the user with others for increased social support. As such, mobile devices including mobile phones and smartphones represent a rich medium by which to deliver and facilitate confidential and personalized management of progress pertaining to sensitive or socially stigmatized issues during and after pregnancy.

References

Abroms, L. C., Chiang, S., Macherelli, L., Leavitt, L., & Montgomery, M. (2017). Assessing the National Cancer Institute's SmokefreeMOM text-messaging program for pregnant smokers: Pilot randomized trial. *Journal of Medical Internet Research, 19*(10), e333.

Abroms, L. C., Johnson, P. R., Leavitt, L. E., Cleary, S. D., Bushar, J., Brandon, T. H., & Chiang, S. C. (2017). A randomized trial of text messaging for smoking cessation in pregnant women. *American Journal of Preventive Medicine, 53*(6), 781–90.

Abroms, L. C., Windsor, R., & Simons-Morton, B. (2008). Getting young adults to quit smoking: A formative evaluation of the X-Pack Program. *Nicotine and Tobacco Research, 10*(1), 27–33.

An, L. C., Bluhm, J. H., Foldes, S. S., Alesci, N. L., Klatt, C. M., Center, B. A., . . . Manley, M. W. (2008). A randomized trial of a pay-for-performance program targeting clinician referral to a state tobacco quitline. *Archives of Internal Medicine, 168*(18), 1993–9.

Aveyard, P., Lawrence, T., Cheng, K. K., Griffin, C., Croghan, E., & Johnson, C. (2006). A randomized controlled trial of smoking cessation for pregnant women to test the effect of a transtheoretical model-based intervention on movement in stage and interaction with baseline stage. *British Journal of Health Psychology, 11*(Pt 2), 263–78.

Baghianimoghadam, M. H., Zolghadar, R., Moghadam, B. B., Darayi, M., & Jozy, F. (2012). Related factors to choose normal vaginal delivery by mothers based on Health Belief Model. *Journal of Education and Health Promotion, 1*, 17.

Bargh, J. A., Schwader, K. L., Hailey, S. E., Dyer, R. L., & Boothby, E. J. (2012). Automaticity in social-cognitive processes. *Trends in Cognitive Sciences, 16*(12), 593–605.

Brown, W., Ottney, A., & Nguyen, S. (2011). Breaking the barrier: The Health Belief Model and patient perceptions regarding contraception. *Contraception, 83*(5), 453–8.

Cardone, I. A., Kim, J. J., Gordon, T. E., Gordon, S. M., & Silver, R. K. (2006). Psychosocial assessment by phone for high-scoring patients taking the Edinburgh Postnatal Depression Scale: Communication pathways and strategies. *Archives of Women's Mental Health, 9*(2), 87–94.

Charlton, A. (1990). [Social and personal obstacles in the fight against smoking at group and at individual level]. *Hygie, 9*(2), 16–20.

Chassin, L., Presson, C., Sherman, S. J., McLaughlin, L., & Gioia, D. (1985). Psychosocial correlates of adolescent smokeless tobacco use. *Addictive Behaviors, 10*(4), 431–5.

Chen, C. M., Lee, P. H., Chou, Y. H., Kuo, S. F., & Hsu, Y. H. (2007). Avoidance of environmental tobacco smoke among pregnant Taiwanese women: Knowledge, self-efficacy, and behavior. *Journal of Women's Health (Larchmt), 16*(6), 869–78.

Chen, J. Y., Fox, S. A., Cantrell, C. H., Stockdale, S. E., & Kagawa-Singer, M. (2007). Health disparities and prevention: Racial/ethnic barriers to flu vaccinations. *Journal of Community Health, 32*(1), 5–20.

Collins, R. L., Kashdan, T. B., & Gollnisch, G. (2003). The feasibility of using cellular phones to collect ecological momentary assessment data: Application to alcohol consumption. *Experiments in Clinical Psychopharmacology, 11*(1), 73–8.

Cormick, G., Kim, N. A., Rodgers, A., Gibbons, L., Buekens, P. M., Belizan, J. M., & Althabe, F. (2012). Interest of pregnant women in the use of SMS (short message service) text messages for the improvement of perinatal and postnatal care. *Reproductive Health, 9*, 9.

Daddario, D. K. (2007). A review of the use of the health belief model for weight management. *Medsurg Nursing, 16*(6), 363–6.

de Vries, H., & Backbier, E. (1994). Self-efficacy as an important determinant of quitting among pregnant women who smoke: The phi-pattern. *Preventive Medicine, 23*(2), 167–74.

Ekhtiari, Y. S., Majlessi, F., Foroushani, A. R., & Shakibazadeh, E. (2014). Effect of a self-care educational program based on the Health Belief Model on reducing low birth weight among pregnant Iranian women. *International Journal of Preventive Medicine, 5*(1), 76–82.

Enock, P. M., Hofmann, S. G., & McNally, R. J. (2014). Attention bias modification training via smartphone to reduce social anxiety: A randomized, controlled multi-session experiment. *Cognitive Therapy and Research, 38*, 200–16.

Fahrenwald, N. L., & Walker, S. N. (2003). Application of the Transtheoretical Model of behavior change to the physical activity behavior of WIC mothers. *Public Health Nursing, 20*(4), 307–17.

Fanning, J., Mullen, S. P., & McAuley, E. (2012). Increasing physical activity with mobile devices: A meta-analysis. *Journal of Medical Internet Research, 14*(6), e161.

Field, M., & Cox, W. M. (2008). Attentional bias in addictive behaviors: A review of its development, causes, and consequences. *Drug and Alcohol Dependence, 97*(1–2), 1–20.

Franken, I. H. (2003). Drug craving and addiction: Integrating psychological and neuropsychopharmacological approaches. *Progress in Neuropsychopharmacological and Biological Psychiatry, 27*(4), 563–79.

Gammon, D., Arsand, E., Walseth, O. A., Andersson, N., Jenssen, M., & Taylor, T. (2005). Parent-child interaction using a mobile and wireless system for blood glucose monitoring. *Journal of Medical Internet Research, 7*(5), e57.

Gao, L. L., Sun, K., & Chan, S. W. (2014). Social support and parenting self-efficacy among Chinese women in the perinatal period. *Midwifery, 30*(5), 532–8.

Gohar, A., Adams, A., Gertner, E., Sackett-Lundeen, L., Heitz, R., Engle, R., . . . Bijwadia, J. (2009). Working memory capacity is decreased in sleep-deprived internal medicine residents. *Journal of Clinical Sleep Medicine, 5*(3), 191–7.

Hacker, K., Brown, E., Cabral, H., & Dodds, D. (2005). Applying a transtheoretical behavioral change model to HIV/STD and pregnancy prevention in adolescent clinics. *Journal of Adolescent Health, 37*(3 Suppl), S80–93.

Hakamata, Y., Lissek, S., Bar-Haim, Y., Britton, J. C., Fox, N. A., Leibenluft, E., . . . Pine, D. S. (2010). Attention bias modification treatment: A meta-analysis toward the establishment of novel treatment for anxiety. *Biological Psychiatry, 68*(11), 982–90.

Hall, K. S. (2012). The Health Belief Model can guide modern contraceptive behavior research and practice. *Journal of Midwifery and Women's Health, 57*(1), 74–81.

Hester, N. R., & Macrina, D. M. (1985). The health belief model and the contraceptive behavior of college women: Implications for health education. *Journal of the American College of Health, 33*(6), 245–52.

Higgins, S. T., Bernstein, I. M., Washio, Y., Heil, S. H., Badger, G. J., Skelly, J. M., . . . Solomon, L. J. (2010). Effects of smoking cessation with voucher-based contingency management on birth outcomes. *Addiction, 105*(11), 2023–30.

Horowitz, S. M. (2003). Applying the transtheoretical model to pregnancy and STD prevention: A review of the literature. *American Journal of Health Promotion, 17*(5), 304–28.

Huang, C. M., Wu, H. L., Huang, S. H., Chien, L. Y., & Guo, J. L. (2013). Transtheoretical model-based passive smoking prevention programme among pregnant women and mothers of young children. *European Journal of Public Health, 23*(5), 777–82.

Insana, S. P., Williams, K. B., & Montgomery-Downs, H. E. (2013). Sleep disturbance and neurobehavioral performance among postpartum women. *Sleep, 36*(1), 73–81.

Iriyama, S., Nakahara, S., Jimba, M., Ichikawa, M., & Wakai, S. (2007). AIDS health beliefs and intention for sexual abstinence among male adolescent students in Kathmandu, Nepal: A test of perceived severity and susceptibility. *Public Health, 121*(1), 64–72.

Irvine, L., Falconer, D. W., Jones, C., Ricketts, I. W., Williams, B., & Crombie, I. K. (2012). Can text messages reach the parts other process measures cannot reach: An evaluation of a behavior change intervention delivered by mobile phone? *PLoS One, 7*(12), e52621.

Jareethum, R., Titapant, V., Chantra, T., Sommai, V., Chuenwattana, P., & Jirawan, C. (2008). Satisfaction of healthy pregnant women receiving short message service via mobile phone for prenatal support: A randomized controlled trial. *Journal of the Medical Association of Thailand, 91*(4), 458–63.

Jennings, L., Ong'ech, J., Simiyu, R., Sirengo, M., & Kassaye, S. (2013). Exploring the use of mobile phone technology for the enhancement of the prevention of mother-to-child transmission of HIV program in Nyanza, Kenya: A qualitative study. *BMC Public Health, 13*, 1131.

Kaiser, B., Razurel, C., & Jeannot, E. (2013). Impact of health beliefs, social support and self-efficacy on physical activity and dietary habits during the post-partum period after gestational diabetes mellitus: Study protocol. *BMC Pregnancy and Childbirth, 13*, 133.

Katz, K. S., Rodan, M., Milligan, R., Tan, S., Courtney, L., Gantz, M., . . . Subramanian, S. (2011). Efficacy of a randomized cell phone-based counseling intervention in postponing subsequent pregnancy among teen mothers. *Maternal and Child Health Journal, 15*(Suppl 1), S42–53.

Kloeblen, A. S., & Batish, S. S. (1999). Understanding the intention to permanently follow a high folate diet among a sample of low-income pregnant women according to the Health Belief Model. *Health and Education Research, 14*(3), 327–38.

Lawrence, T., Aveyard, P., Evans, O., & Cheng, K. K. (2003). A cluster randomised controlled trial of smoking cessation in pregnant women comparing interventions based on the transtheoretical (stages of change) model to standard care. *Tobacco Control, 12*(2), 168–77.

Letourneau, A. R., Sonja, B., Mazure, C. M., O'Malley, S. S., James, D., & Colson, E. R. (2007). Timing and predictors of postpartum return to smoking in a group of inner-city women: An exploratory pilot study. *Birth, 34*(3), 245–52.

Lichtenstein, E. (1997). Behavioral research contributions and needs in cancer prevention and control: Tobacco use prevention and cessation. *Preventive Medicine, 26*(5 Pt 2), S57–63.

Lund, S., Nielsen, B. B., Hemed, M., Boas, I. M., Said, A., Said, K., . . . Rasch, V. (2014). Mobile phones improve antenatal care attendance in Zanzibar: A cluster randomized controlled trial. *BMC Pregnancy and Childbirth, 14*, 29.

Lund, S., Rasch, V., Hemed, M., Boas, I. M., Said, A., Said, K., . . . Nielsen, B. B. (2014). Mobile phone intervention reduces perinatal mortality in Zanzibar: Secondary outcomes of a cluster randomized controlled trial. *JMIR mHealth and uHealth, 2*(1), e15.

MacLeod, C., Rutherford, E., Campbell, L., Ebsworthy, G., & Holker, L. (2002). Selective attention and emotional vulnerability: Assessing the causal basis of their association through the experimental manipulation of attentional bias. *Journal of Abnormal Psychology, 111*(1), 107–23.

Marteau, T. M., Hollands, G. J., & Fletcher, P. C. (2012). Changing human behavior to prevent disease: The importance of targeting automatic processes. *Science, 337*(6101), 1492–5.

McCarthy, J., & Maine, D. (1992). A framework for analyzing the determinants of maternal mortality. *Studies in Family Planning, 23*(1), 23–33.

Mesters, I., Gijsbers, B., Bartholomew, K., Knottnerus, J. A., & Van Schayck, O. C. (2013). Social cognitive changes resulting from an effective breastfeeding education program. *Breastfeeding Medicine, 8*(1), 23–30.

National Cancer Institute, T. C. R. B. (2014). http://women.smokefree.gov/smokefreemom.aspx

Noordam, A. C., Kuepper, B. M., Stekelenburg, J., & Milen, A. (2011). Improvement of maternal health services through the use of mobile phones. *Tropical Medicine and International Health, 16*(5), 622–6.

Park, E. R., Chang, Y., Quinn, V., Regan, S., Cohen, L., Viguera, A., . . . Rigotti, N. (2009). The association of depressive, anxiety, and stress symptoms and postpartum relapse to smoking: A longitudinal study. *Nicotine and Tobacco Research, 11*(6), 707–14.

Paul, I. M., Downs, D. S., Schaefer, E. W., Beiler, J. S., & Weisman, C. S. (2013). Postpartum anxiety and maternal-infant health outcomes. *Pediatrics, 131*(4), e1218–24.

Poorman, E., Gazmararian, J., Elon, L., & Parker, R. (2014). Is health literacy related to health behaviors and cell phone usage patterns among the text4baby target population? *Archives of Public Health, 72*(1), 13.

Prochaska, J. O., & Velicer, W. F. (1997). The transtheoretical model of health behavior change. *American Journal of Health Promotion, 12*(1), 38–48.

Puccio, J. A., Belzer, M., Olson, J., Martinez, M., Salata, C., Tucker, D., & Tanaka, D. (2006). The use of cell phone reminder calls for assisting HIV-infected adolescents and young adults to adhere to highly active antiretroviral therapy: A pilot study. *AIDS Patient Care and STDS, 20*(6), 438–44.

Robinson, T. E., & Berridge, K. C. (1993). The neural basis of drug craving: An incentive-sensitization theory of addiction. *Brain Research Reviews, 18*(3), 247–91.

Rogers, E. R., & King, S. R. (2013). Intervention based on social cognitive theory: Evaluating adolescents' knowledge of OTC pain medications. *Journal of the American Pharmacological Association,* 53(1), 30–8.

Ruggiero, L., Tsoh, J. Y., Everett, K., Fava, J. L., & Guise, B. J. (2000). The transtheoretical model of smoking: Comparison of pregnant and nonpregnant smokers. *Addictive Behaviors, 25*(2), 239–51.

Seil, K. S., Desai, M. M., & Smith, M. V. (2014). Sexual orientation, adult connectedness, substance use, and mental health outcomes among adolescents: Findings from the 2009 New York City Youth Risk Behavior Survey. *American Journal of Public Health, 104*(10), 1950–6.

Sharifirad, G. R., Tol, A., Mohebi, S., Matlabi, M., Shahnazi, H., & Shahsiah, M. (2013). The effectiveness of nutrition education program based on health belief model compared with traditional training. *Journal of Education and Health Promotion, 2,* 15.

Slade, P., Laxton-Kane, M., & Spiby, H. (2006). Smoking in pregnancy: The role of the transtheoretical model and the mother's attachment to the fetus. *Addictive Behaviors, 31*(5), 743–57.

Stout, A. E. (1997). Prenatal care for low-income women and the health belief model: A new beginning. *Journal of Community Health Nursing, 14*(3), 169–80.

Strack, F., & Deutsch, R. (2004). Reflective and impulsive determinants of social behavior. *Personality and Social Psychology Review, 8*(3), 220–47.

Suffoletto, B., Calabria, J., Ross, A., Callaway, C., & Yealy, D. M. (2012). A mobile phone text message program to measure oral antibiotic use and provide feedback on adherence to patients discharged from the emergency department. *Academy of Emergency Medicine, 19*(8), 949–58.

Sweeney, M. A., & Gulino, C. (1987). The health belief model as an explanation for breast-feeding practices in a Hispanic population. *ANS Advances in Nursing Science, 9*(4), 35–50.

Tasker, A. P., Gibson, L., Franklin, V., Gregor, P., & Greene, S. (2007). What is the frequency of symptomatic mild hypoglycemia in type 1 diabetes in the young? Assessment by novel mobile phone technology and computer-based interviewing. *Pediatric Diabetes, 8*(1), 15–20.

Thaddeus, S., & Maine, D. (1994). Too far to walk: Maternal mortality in context. *Social Science and Medicine, 38*(8), 1091–10.

Urban, A. (2007). Mobile television: Is it just a hype or a real consumer need? *Observatorio Journal, 3,* 45–58.

van Heerden, A., Norris, S., Tollman, S., Richter, L., & Rotheram-Borus, M. J. (2013). Collecting maternal health information from HIV-positive pregnant women using mobile phone-assisted face-to-face interviews in Southern Africa. *Journal of Medical Internet Research, 15*(6), e116.

Washio, Y., Higgins, S. T., Heil, S. H., Badger, G. J., Skelly, J., Bernstein, I. M., . . . Hanson, J. D. (2011). Examining maternal weight gain during contingency-management treatment for smoking cessation among pregnant women. *Drug and Alcohol Dependence, 114*(1), 73–6.

Whittaker, R., Borland, R., Bullen, C., Lin, R. B., McRobbie, H., & Rodgers, A. (2009). Mobile phone-based interventions for smoking cessation. *Cochrane Database of Systematic Reviews, 4,* CD006611.

Whittaker, R., Matoff-Stepp, S., Meehan, J., Kendrick, J., Jordan, E., Stange, P., . . . Rhee, K. (2012). Text4baby: Development and implementation of a national text messaging health information service. *American Journal of Public Health, 102*(12), 2207–13.

Wiers, R. W., Gladwin, T. E., Hofmann, W., Salemink, E., & Ridderinkhof, K. R. (2013). Cognitive bias modification and cognitive control training in addiction and related psychopathology: Mechanisms, clinical perspectives, and ways forward. *Clinical Psychological Science, 1*(2), 192–212.

Zweig, S., LeFevre, M., & Kruse, J. (1988). The health belief model and attendance for prenatal care. *Family Practice Research Journal, 8*(1), 32–41.

CHAPTER

29 Use of Digital Technology to Provide or Enhance the Delivery of Interventions for Adolescents

Deepa R. Camenga *and* Grace E. Kong

Abstract

Adolescence is a critical period for the onset of mental health disorders, yet only about one-third of affected adolescents receive mental healthcare. Barriers to such care include poor access, stigma, and the lack of availability of proper resources to identify and treat mental health disease. Thus, the delivery of mental health services via new technologies may help mitigate some of these barriers. Digital technology–based interventions show promise for the treatment of various mental health conditions in adolescents. This chapter provides an overview of computer- and Internet-based therapeutic programs, texting programs using mobile phones, and serious games as they apply to a variety of conditions including depression/anxiety, eating disorders, and tobacco smoking, as well as mental healthcare utilization. The unique needs of adolescents are discussed in relation to the scaling of digital technologies and future directions for technology-enhanced mental healthcare.

Keywords: computer, online, mobile phone, mental health, adolescent

Introduction

Mental healthcare services worldwide are faced with a pressing need to identify novel methods to engage adolescents. Adolescence is a critical period for the onset of mental health disorders. A review found that 1 out of 4 adolescents meet lifetime criteria for a *Diagnostic and Statistical Manual of Mental Disorders* (DSM) mental disorder (Costello, Mustillo, Keller, & Angold, 2004). In that study, anxiety disorders represented the most common condition (31.9%), followed by behavioral disorders (19.1%), mood disorders (14.3%), and substance-use disorders (11.4%), with approximately 40% of those with one class of disorder also meeting criteria for another class of lifetime disorder (Merikangas et al., 2010).

Despite the prevalence of mental health disorders in this age group, only about one-third of adolescents receive mental healthcare (Merikangas et al., 2011). Barriers to mental healthcare include poor access, stigma, and the lack of availability of proper resources to identify and treat mental health disease (Renton et al., 2014). The delivery of mental health services via new technologies may help mitigate some of these barriers. Adolescents, in particular, are especially appropriate for this platform of care as they have already embraced a variety of digital technologies for entertainment, socializing, and education. According to the Pew Research Institute, 93% of adolescents have access to a computer at home, 78% own a cell phone, and 75% send text messages on their phones (Madden, Lenhart, Duggan, Cortesi, & Gasser, 2013). As a result of the strong penetration of technology use among adolescents, an increasing number of mental health interventions have begun to utilize digital technologies.

Although a majority of digital interventions are delivered via computer-based online modules, there are a small number of interventions that utilize mobile phone or gaming applications. Text messages and mobile applications ("apps") have the potential to enhance clinical care at many stages of treatment, from treatment engagement to supporting treatment gains and facilitating adherence and follow-up (Price et al., 2013). As compared to desktop applications, mobile phones have the added benefit of being able to provide real-time feedback in real-world contexts as they are generally carried on the user. Mobile phone apps also have the ability to provide more complex functionality than text messaging alone (Price et al., 2013). For example, apps have the added capability of using geo-location services, app-based homework guides, and more developed educational curricula (Price et al., 2013). Additionally, video games are also emerging as a modality to help treat mental health conditions. In particular, "serious" video games, or video games that use computer-based entertainment technology to teach, train, or change behavior, are being developed to help treat certain mental health conditions (Burns, Webb, Durkin, & Hickie, 2010).

This chapter provides an overview of initiatives described in the published scientific literature through 2014 that utilize digital technology to improve mental health in adolescents aged 13–17 years. Modalities such as computer/Internet-based therapeutic programs, texting programs, and video games will be discussed as they apply to a variety of conditions including depression, anxiety, and smoking cessation, as well as mental healthcare utilization. Additionally, the unique needs of adolescents will be discussed in relation to the scaling of digital technologies for mental health and future directions for digital technologies for mental health.

Depression and Anxiety

A variety of digital technologies are utilized to enhance the treatment of adolescent depression and anxiety. Overall, evidence to date suggests that computer-based technologies may have positive effects on depression and anxiety in adolescents (National Collaborating Centre for Mental Health, 2014). Although many technology-based interventions focus on young adults and adults, only a few focus entirely on adolescents aged 13–17 years. This section provides an overview of interventions that focus on the treatment of depression and/or anxiety in adolescents.

Computer-Based Interventions

Computer-based interventions that target anxiety and depression in adolescents are most frequently based on cognitive-behavioral therapy (CBT). CBT explores the relationship between thoughts, behaviors, and emotions and seems to be particularly amenable to a computerized delivery method as it is highly structured and knowledge-based (National Collaborating Centre for Mental Health, 2014). CBT has proved effective for the treatment of anxiety disorders in children and young people (James et al., 2013; Reynolds et al., 2012) and also may be effective for the treatment of depression in adolescents (Spirito, Esposito-Smythers, Wolff, & Uhl, 2011). A meta-analysis of computerized CBT intervention for young people found that, compared to control conditions, computerized CBT had a medium effect on self-rated depression and anxiety, a large effect on clinician-rated depression severity, and small effect on preventing relapse (National Collaborating Centre for Mental Health, 2014).

Project CATCH-IT (Competent Adulthood Transition with Cognitive-behavioral, Humanistic and Interpersonal Training) is an online depression-treatment program that delivered CBT and interpersonal psychotherapy based on a community-resiliency concept model. The program is delivered within primary care settings and consists of 14 sessions, 15 to 20 minutes in length, that use reading materials and skills-building exercises (Van Voorhees et al., 2007). Studies of Project CATCH-IT have focused on how primary care engagement in combination with the online program affects depression outcomes. For example, a randomized controlled trial (RCT) of 84 adolescents and young adults aged 14–21 years sought to determine how physician-delivered brief advice (BA) versus motivational interviewing (MI) could enhance participation outcomes in Project CATCH-IT (Hoek et al., 2011). The adolescents were included if they were at risk for depression (having depressed mood, anhedonia, and/or irritability for "at least a few days in last 2 weeks") (Hoek et al., 2011) and randomized to either physician MI + Project CATCH-IT or BA + Project CATCH-IT. Both groups experienced decreases in depressive symptoms; however, at 6-month follow-up, the MI group demonstrated significantly fewer depressive episodes and reported less hopelessness as compared with the BA group (Hoek et al., 2011). An evaluation of outcomes at 1-year post intervention similarly found decreases in depressive symptoms in both groups; however, fewer adolescents randomized to MI reported a depressive episode (Saulsberry et al., 2013).

MoodGYM also utilizes CBT to target depression and anxiety in adolescents through five sessions that contain interactive modules, quizzes, and homework. Several studies evaluated the efficacy of MoodGYM in young adults (Calear, 2009; Ellis, 2013; Sethi, 2010), and this program was also tested in secondary schools with general samples of adolescents who were not at elevated risk for developing depression (Calear, Christensen, Mackinnon, Griffiths, & O'Kearney, 2009). An RCT comparing MoodGYM and a usual high school health curriculum in a general sample of 157 adolescent girls found that MoodGYM resulted in a faster decline in depressive symptoms; however, adherence to the five-session module was low (O'Kearney, Kang, Christensen, & Griffiths, 2009). Similarly, a cluster RCT of 30 Australian secondary schools (*N* = 1,477) randomized a population-based sample of students aged 12–17 years to MoodGYM or a wait-list control. The study found that at 6-month follow-up, participants in the intervention condition had significantly lower levels of anxiety and males had fewer symptoms of depression (Calear et al., 2009).

Last, a Dutch-based program, *Grip op je dip online (Master Your Mood Online)* is an online group CBT-based program aimed at 16- to 25-year-olds. This program uses moderated group chat sessions delivered in six sessions. Participants also complete online homework and exercises. A study of 244 16- to 25-year-olds with Center for Epidemiological Studies Depression Scale scores between 10 and 45 found that, compared to wait-list control, participants in Master Your Mood had a greater decrease in depressive symptoms (van der Zanden, Kramer, Gerrits, & Cuijpers, 2012). Given the popularity of social networking among adolescents, there is a possibility that future studies may evaluate unmoderated peer online networks as a treatment modality for anxiety and depression.

Several computerized CBT interventions also target anxiety, including *ThinkFeelDo, BRAVE for Teenagers*, and *CoolTeens. ThinkFeelDo* is a CD-ROM–based computerized CBT program for anxiety and depression. The intervention consists of six modules that use quizzes, exercises, and video clips with narrators to guide participants through the sessions. Unlike previously described interventions, this computerized CBT intervention requires a trained facilitator to guide the participants through the computerized program and to encourage reflection on the materials (Stallard, Richardson, Velleman, & Attwood, 2011). A pilot RCT of the program was conducted with 20 adolescents aged 11–16 years with an anxiety disorder or depression. This pilot study showed that, compared to the wait-list control, ThinkFeelDo resulted in improvements in measurements of depression but not anxiety (Stallard et al., 2011). BRAVE for Teenagers-ONLINE is an online CBT-based anxiety treatment program used to treat social phobia, generalized anxiety disorder, separation anxiety, and specific phobia in adolescents aged 13–17 years. The program consists of 10 weekly sessions with 5–6 parent sessions. The sessions utilize reading materials, questions and answers, games and quizzes, and weekly email contact with a therapist to review homework and session activities. An RCT of 115 12- to 18-year-olds randomized to either BRAVE for Teenagers-ONLINE with minimal therapist support, face-to-face counseling, or wait-list control found that online delivery of CBT was equally efficacious as clinic-based, face-to-face therapy (Spence et al., 2011). CoolTeens is another computerized CBT program delivered via CD-ROM (rather than online) that targets anxiety. This program involves a small level of therapist involvement via weekly phone calls (Cunningham et al., 2009; Wuthrich et al., 2012). A small RCT of 43 14- to 17-year-olds with a diagnosis of anxiety found adolescents randomized to the CoolTeens condition, compared to those in the wait-list control group, were more likely to have significant reductions in the total number of anxiety disorders, the average severity for all disorders, and the severity of the primary anxiety disorder (Wuthrich et al., 2012).

Mobile Phone–Based Applications: Texting and Apps

Overall, mobile phone–based interventions are fewer and less developed than computerized interventions; however, there is growing interest in the use of this platform for mental health treatment. *MEMO* is a CBT-based mobile phone–based depression intervention aimed at preventing the onset of depressive symptoms in general populations of adolescents (rather than in treatment-seeking samples). The intervention delivers up to two messages per day for up to 9 weeks, and the messages contain a mixture of texts, video messages, and animated cartoons (Whittaker et al., 2012). The intervention was found to have reasonable adherence and satisfaction among New Zealand students aged 13–17 years (Whittaker et al., 2012). An RCT of 855 adolescents randomized to MEMO or an attention-matched control condition of text messages focusing on healthy eating, responsible environmental practices, and cyberbullying is ongoing.

The *Mobile Tracking Young People's Experiences* (mobiletype) app allows adolescents with mild or moderate symptoms of depression to self-monitor depressive symptoms, stress, coping strategies, daily activities, eating, sleeping, exercise patterns, and alcohol and cannabis use. The data are then uploaded to a report which is accessed by the primary care provider and is used to help determine appropriate treatment approaches and management plans. An RCT of 163 14- to 24-year-olds identified by their primary care physician as having mild to moderate symptoms of depression found that the mobiletype's self-monitoring increased emotional self-awareness; however, there were no differences with respect to changes in depressive symptoms as compared to the attention-matched control group which kept a daily log of activities (Reid et al., 2011). The application has also been found to assist primary care doctors with diagnosis, medication management, and referrals (Reid et al., 2013).

Serious Video Games

Serious video games are also emerging as a modality for the treatment of depression and are a subtype of computerized interventions as they are delivered via computer but use interactive gaming components. *SPARX* (Smart, Positive, Active, Realistic, X-factor thoughts) is a CD-ROM-based serious game used for the treatment of depression among adolescents, and it is based on the interactive fantasy game The Journey (Merry, Stasiak, Shepherd, Frampton, Fleming, & Lucassen , 2012). SPARX utilizes avatars to allow users to undertake challenges in a fantasy world in order to practice CBT skills. Participants in SPARX completed the seven modules of the game over 4–7 weeks and were prompted to speak with their referring physician if they were not improving. A randomized controlled noninferiority trial of 187 adolescents with mild to moderate depression comparing SPARX and treatment as usual (assessment by a general practitioner with referral to face-to-face therapy as necessary) showed that SPARX was noninferior to treatment as usual in reducing depressive symptoms and demonstrated a mean reduction on the Children's Depression Rating Scale-Revised of 9.05 for SPARX and 7.45 for treatment as usual (Merry et al., 2012).

Other Mental Health Conditions

A small number of studies have explored the application of digital technologies to a variety of other mental health conditions such as phobia and eating disorders. For example, a small study of children and adolescents aged 8–17 years demonstrated that a single 2.5-hour session of computer-delivered spider exposure therapy reduced self-rated and researcher-rated fear of spiders (Muris, Merckelbach, Holdrinet, & Sijsenaar, 1998). Another study evaluated a computer-based program for posttraumatic stress disorder (PTSD). The program provided online access to educational materials for children and parents, and this material aimed at normalizing and relieving trauma reactions. Using a self-help approach that incorporated cognitive and resiliency theory, the website contained sections that promoted strategies such as relaxation, coping statements, problem-solving, increasing pleasant events, identifying personal strengths, and reflection on the traumatic event (Cox, Kenardy, & Hendrikz, 2010). An RCT of 85 children and adolescents aged 7–16 years in the website access or a control group after hospitalization for an unintentional injury showed that only 56.3% of participants randomized to the website reported using it during the study. At 6-month follow-up, children and adolescents randomized to the website reported a decrease in anxiety symptoms, while those in the control reported an increase in symptoms. However, an intention-to-treat analysis found that these differences in anxiety symptoms were not significant.

Several studies have also evaluated the use of digital technology for the prevention of eating disorders in adolescents. Specifically, studies have evaluated the use of computer-based CBT and online therapy (Bruning Brown, Winzelberg, Abascal, & Taylor, 2004; Jones et al., 2008; Pretorius et al., 2009) for the prevention of eating disorders. The program, *StudentBODIES*, is based on cognitive-behavioral body image interventions and consists of an 8-week psychoeducational intervention. Participants have the ability to post on a group discussion forum, which is monitored by research assistants supervised by a licensed psychologist. An RCT of 157 high school girls without suspicion for an existing eating disorder were recruited to a wait-list control group or StudentBODIES in combination with an Internet-delivered parent education intervention. The parent education component consisted of a self-directed 4-week program that provided psychoeducation around supporting healthy body image in adolescents. Adolescents in the StudentBODIES intervention group reported fewer eating-disordered symptoms compared to the control group post-treatment; however, differences did not persist at the 3-month follow-up (Beintner, Jacobi, & Taylor, 2012).

Substance Use

Another large area for potential development of digital technologies is for adolescent substance use. Given the stigma and legal implications of underage substance use, technology-aided implementations offer promise for reducing stigma and increasing engagement, access, and retention in services (National Collaborating Centre for Mental Health, 2014). Overall, the most diverse and developed area of digital technology–based interventions is in smoking cessation; however, there are several computer-based interventions that target other types of substance use in adolescents. This section focuses technology-based interventions for adolescent substance use broadly with the following section specifically focusing on smoking cessation.

Although a meta-analysis found a small overall effect size for computer-delivered treatments for alcohol and tobacco (Cohen d 0.2; p <0.001), a majority included interventions focused on young adults and adults (Rooke, Thorsteinsson, Karpin, Copeland, & Allsop, 2010). However, a handful of interventions specifically target adolescents in school, clinical, and community settings. For example, a computer-based alcohol prevention intervention provided 10 sessions via CD-ROM to teach adolescents skills necessary to avoid alcohol. The modules covered topics such as goal-setting, coping, peer pressure, refusal skills, self-efficacy, problem-solving, decision-making, effective communication, and time management. An RCT included 514 urban adolescents (mean age 11.5 years) recruited from after-school community programs who were randomized to the computerized program and a parent intervention consisting of a 30-minute educational session or a control group. The results showed that adolescents in the intervention group reported less monthly alcohol use than control youths at posttest and at 1- and 2-year follow-up assessments (Schinke, Schwinn, Di Noia, & Cole, 2004). Additionally, marijuana and cigarette use was also reduced among the intervention group. Another computer-based program combined the Dutch-based Obrebro Prevention Program and a computerized intervention. The Obrebro Prevention program is designed to provide parents with education about how to communicate clear rules about underage alcohol use and maintain a zero-tolerance position toward youth drinking (Koutakis, Stattin, & Kerr, 2008). This intervention was combined with four student-led digital (computer-based) educational sessions aimed at forming healthy attitudes toward alcohol use and developing refusal skills. A cluster randomized trial of 3,490 students (mean 12.68 years) from 19 high schools in the Netherlands found that the combination of the Orebro Prevention Project and the student-led digital intervention resulted in reduced likelihood of heavy drinking at a 10-month follow-up, but not at a 22-month follow-up (Koning et al., 2009). Another computerized intervention sought to provide gender-specific drug prevention intervention to adolescent girls. The intervention, *RealTeens*, provided nine computer sessions on a variety of topics, including goal-setting, decision-making, coping, self-esteem, assertion, communication, media influences, peer pressure, and drug facts. A study of 236 Canadian adolescent girls in seventh through ninth grade (mean age 14 years) recruited via a youth-oriented website and randomized to RealTeens versus a control condition (no intervention) found that girls participating in the intervention reported lower levels of self-reported past-30-day alcohol, marijuana, poly-drug, and total substance use at 6-month follow-up (Schwinn, Schinke, & Di Noia, 2010). Another gender-specific prevention program also targeted adolescent girls but simultaneously involved mothers to strengthen the quality of girls' relationships with their mothers and increase the ability to resist substance use (Fang & Schinke, 2013). The program consisted of nine interactive modules that encouraged adolescents and mothers to participate in skill demonstrations, guided rehearsal, and immediate feedback. An RCT of 108 Asian American adolescent girls aged 10–14 years and their mothers randomized to the intervention or control group (no intervention) found that intervention-arm girls reported fewer episodes of alcohol drinking, marijuana use, and misuse of prescription drugs at 2-year follow-up (Fang & Schinke, 2013).

Several studies have also evaluated the effect of computerized normative feedback on substance use. *SafERTeens* is a computerized brief intervention that is delivered to adolescents presenting to the emergency room with medical or injury-related concerns (Walton et al., 2010). The computerized brief intervention is interactive, based on MI, and has components that focus on goal-setting and personalized feedback for alcohol, violence, and weapon carriage. Additionally, there are exercises that focus on the potential benefits of staying away from drinking and fighting, five tailored role plays (e.g., anger management, conflict resolution, alcohol refusals, not drinking and driving), and information about referral. An RCT of 726 adolescents aged 14–18 years presenting to the emergency department with a past-year history of alcohol use and aggression examined the brief computer intervention, the same intervention with a counselor present, or a control group (self-help brochure). At 6-month follow-up, participants in the computer intervention and therapist intervention both showed self-reported reductions in alcohol consequences (computer, −29.1%; therapist, −32.2%; control, −17.7) (Walton et al., 2010). However, differences did not persist at the 12-month follow-up (Cunningham et al., 2012). Another computer-delivered normative feedback program was designed to be delivered in middle schools. The "Your Decisions Count: Alcohol, Tobacco and Other Drugs" program for middle schools is based on the Transtheoretical Model and is an Internet-based, computerized tailored intervention program (Evers et al., 2012). The intervention consists of three separate interactions with the computer program a month apart. An RCT of 1,590 students in 22 middle schools examined the computer program and control condition (pre- and post-intervention surveys only). The study results showed that the computer program yielded significant reductions in the percentage of "ever-users" of alcohol, tobacco, marijuana, and other drugs at a 3-month follow-up (Evers et al., 2012).

Smoking Cessation

Many new developments have progressed in the area of adolescent smoking cessation (see reviews by Hutton et al., 2011; Park & Drake, 2014). The Internet-supported interventions are categorized into Internet-based interventions, other online activities (e.g., blogs, support groups), and computer programs without Internet components (Barak, Klein, & Proudfoot, 2009).

Internet-Based Interventions

Internet-based interventions utilize a variety of theoretical models to promote smoking cessation. *NOT Plus* (Mermelstein & Turner, 2006) enhanced the delivery of the American Lung Association's Not on Tobacco (NOT; Dino et al., 2001; Horn, Dino, Kalsekar, & Mody, 2005) program using an Internet-based platform. The NOT Plus program is an adolescent smoking cessation program delivered in school and community settings and utilizes the Social Cognitive Theory. An RCT of 351 adolescent smokers in the standard NOT condition (n = 170) and the NOT Plus condition (which included Internet access) (n = 181) showed that the self-reported abstinence in the past 7 days for both groups did not significantly differ at the end of treatment (NOT: 4.7%; NOT Plus: 12:2%, p = .06), but the quit rates in the NOT Plus (13.8%) was higher than the standard NOT condition (0.6%, p <.05) at the 3-month follow-up assessment. *Stomp Out Smoke* (SOS; Patten et al., 2006), based on Social Learning Theory, Health Communication, and Decision Making Theories, is an Internet-based intervention designed to be completed in the home. The SOS program consists of interactive quizzes, email interactions with a quit coach, a private journaling function that allows adolescents to keep records of their personal quit strategies, a quit plan, and a list of supporters, as well as an art gallery in which to post artwork. An RCT comparing SOS versus BA in a medical setting (consisting of four MI- and CBT-based face-to-face sessions) found that the 30-day point-prevalence, biochemically confirmed smoking abstinence rates for BA and SOS at weeks 24 (BA: 12%, SOS: 6%) and 36 (BA: 13%, SOS: 6%) did not significantly differ.

Internet-Assisted Instruction (IAI) is a 4-week Internet-based smoking cessation intervention that provides a variety of resources for smoking cessation. In addition to information on health effects of smoking, adolescents were provided with (1) education about auricular acupressure for smoking cessation, (2) opportunities to interact with professional assistance on smoking cessation via email, (3) opportunities to interact with other adolescents on a discussion forum to share their experiences of smoking cessation efforts, and (4) a personalized quit plan based on information collected via an online questionnaire (also see Chen, Yeh, & Chao, 2006). This intervention was combined with auricular acupressure among adolescent smokers in Taiwan (Chen et al., 2006). Auricular acupressure is thought to improve smoking cessation efforts through reducing cigarette craving and altering sense of taste, which may make cigarette smoke less appealing. Using a quasi-experimental design, 77 high school smokers were assigned to either 4 weeks of an auricular acupressure and Internet-based smoking cessation intervention or auricular acupressure only. Adolescents were instructed to stimulate five auricular points for at least 1 minute, 3–5 minutes per day for 4 weeks. The results showed that the quit rates based on serum cotinine level (<100 ng/mL) were higher in the intervention group with an IAI component (15.78%) than the auricular acupressure only group (2.56%).

The *Consider This* program (Buller et al., 2008) is an Internet-based program based on social cognitive theory and has 73 online activities, which are organized into six modules and focus on building positive expectancies and self-efficacy to quit smoking. The contents are individually tailored based on the changes in smoking status or susceptibility to smoke status from the previous session. Middle school students (grades 6–9) in Australia (n = 2,077) and the

United States (n = 1,234) were randomized to *Consider This* or the control condition (i.e., received standard health education). The results from the Australian sample indicated that students who reported smoking a whole cigarette in the past 30 days in the intervention group were more likely to report not smoking in the past 30 days, relative to those in the control group, at the end of the school year. However, the treatment effect was not found in the American sample.

Smoking Zine is an Internet-based smoking prevention and cessation intervention that has been evaluated in high-school students in 14 schools in Toronto (Norman, Maley, Li, & Skinner, 2008) and among American Indian adolescents attending a summer camp in South Dakota (Bowen, Henderson, Harvill, & Buchwald, 2012). Smoking Zine focuses on increasing self-efficacy through assessments, quizzes, and tailored feedback in five stages. The theoretical framework underlying the intervention are based on the Theory of Reasoned Action/Planned Behavior (Montaño, Kasprzyk, & Taplin, 1997), the Transtheoretical Model of behavioral change (Prochaska, Redding, & Evers, 1997), and Social Cognitive Theories (Bandura, 1986).

In an RCT, 9th to 11th graders (n = 1,402; 15% smokers) in 81 classes in the Toronto area were randomized to receive Smoking Zine or the control condition (Norman, Maley, Li & Skinner). In this trial, Smoking Zine was accompanied by an offline component, which included paper journals of one's own assessment scores from the online assessments and a 10-minute single group session that included MI to motivate students to be smoke-free using tailored assessment scores and journal entries in a single 1-hour classroom session. Tailored emails encouraging students to stay abstinent and to use the Smoking Zine website were sent for 6 months. The control condition included activities that require a similar level of engagement as the treatment group but focused on climate change instead of tobacco. The results showed that the smoking cessation outcome rates at the 3-month and 6-month follow-up assessments did not differ between the conditions; however, smokers reported a decrease in their intentions to smoke and increased their resistance to smoke at 6-month follow-up. Additionally, nonsmokers in the treatment group were less likely than nonsmokers in the control group to engage in heavy smoking during the treatment period.

The second evaluation of the Smoking Zine included a cultural modification of the intervention through feedback from American Indian youth (Bowen et al., 2012). The changes included culturally relevant context such as a summer powwow and images relevant to American Indian youth. American Indian adolescents attending a summer camp were randomized to access Smoking Zine during their 1-hour of computer time during the 6 weeks of camp (n = 64) or to the control condition (n = 49) that did not have access to Smoking Zine during this time. The results showed that the nonsmoking status (self-reported never smoking even a part of a cigarette) did not change from baseline to follow-up: 85% of the intervention group and 83% of the control group were nonsmokers at baseline, and 83% of the intervention group and 80% of the control group were nonsmokers at 1-month follow-up.

Other Online Activities (Blogs, Support Groups)

Breathing Room is an Internet-based, "virtual world" chat room program in which adolescents can have real-time discussions with a trained smoking-cessation counselor who uses MI strategies, as well as with virtual peers though the use of avatars (animated figures) (Woodruff, Edwards, Conway, & Elliott, 2001). *Breathing Room* also allows avatars to navigate various locations, such as a shopping mall which contains billboards and storefront advertisements with anti-smoking themes. The virtual counselor covers session topics focused on assessing readiness to quit, discussing the benefits and costs of quitting, identifying barriers to quitting, increasing self-efficacy, developing a quitting plan, and managing lapses. Adolescent smokers participate in seven 1-hour interventions for a 2-month period using a designated computer at school before or after school hours or during lunch times. Two studies evaluated the efficacy of *Breathing Room.* The pilot study recruited 26 high school adolescents who reported smoking at least once in the past month (Woodruff, Edwards, Conway, & Elliott, 2001). The results showed self-reported past-week abstinence of 22% at the end of treatment and 33% at the 1-month follow-up. A second trial randomized adolescent smokers to Breathing Room (n = 77) or an assessment-only condition (n = 59). At the end of treatment, the abstinence rate of the intervention group was higher than the control group (35% vs. 22%), but they did not differ at 1-year follow-up (Woodruff, Conway, Edwards, Elliott, & Crittenden, 2007).

Computer Programs Without an Internet Component

A Smoking Prevention Interactive Experience (ASPIRE; Prokhorov et al., 2008), based on the Social Cognitive Theory and the Transtheoretical

Model of Change, is an adolescent smoking prevention and cessation intervention delivered on a CD-ROM in the classrooms. The curriculum consists of five weekly sessions in one school semester and two booster sessions in the following semester, and each session is about 30 minutes long. The program has eight educational tracks that use animations, video clips, and interactive activities. Each session assesses smoking status and stage of smoking acquisition or cessation, and activities are tailored to the specific stage and designed to move adolescents through the stages toward smoking cessation for smokers and reduce the likelihood of initiation among nonsmokers. An RCT examined ASPIRE compared to the National Cancer Institute's *Clearing the Air* self-help booklet (Prokhorov et al., 2008). Students from 16 high schools in the greater Houston area were randomized to ASPIRE (n = 610) or the control condition (n = 550). Of the 1,160 participants, 62 were smokers at baseline. The results showed that at 18-month follow-up, smoking initiation rates determined by self-reported smoking were lower in the ASPIRE condition (1.9% vs. 5.8%); however, smoking cessation rates in the two groups did not differ.

Pathways to Change (PTC; Redding et al., 1999; Velicer & Prochaska, 1999; Velicer et al., 1993) is an interactive computer-based smoking prevention and cessation intervention based on the Transtheoretical Model of Change. PTC uses appealing video clips to offer tailored advice and encouragement based on the readiness to change (i.e., not initiate smoking for nonsmokers and quitting for smokers). PTC (10 minutes long) was administered as part of an adolescent smoking cessation intervention in a routine medical care setting along with a brief counseling session (10 minutes long) and up to two 10-minute in-person or telephone booster sessions (Hollis et al., 2005). This combined intervention was called *Teen Reach* (Research Approaches to Cancer in a Health Maintenance Organization). Smoking and nonsmoking adolescents receiving routine medical care were randomized and up to two 10-minute in-person or telephone booster sessions (Hollis et al., 2005). The efficacy of Teen Reach was examined through randomizing smoking and nonsmoking adolescents to either Teen Reach (n = 1,254) or a control intervention (n = 1,272) (Hollis et al., 2005). The control condition received 5 minutes of advice on healthy eating. The results showed that the participants in Teen Reach, relative to the control condition, were more likely to self-report past-30 day abstinence at 1-year follow-up (77.2% vs. 72.8%) and at 2-year follow-up (72.8% vs. 68.6%). Treatment effects were stronger for smokers at baseline compared to nonsmokers.

The *Computerized Adolescent Smoking Cessation Program* (CASCP; Fritz, Hardin, Gore, & Bram, 2008) adapted the contents of the NOT program into a computerized intervention. The CASCP consisted of four 30-minute sessions: the first two modules focus on increasing motivation to quit by providing information on the gains of quitting, and the third and fourth modules focus on increasing self-efficacy. The CASCP included the use of video and audio clips and animated figures. A total of 121 adolescent smokers were recruited from high schools and randomized to receive CASCP (n = 61) or no intervention (n = 60) (Fritz, Hardin, Gore, & Bram, 2008). At the end of treatment, 14% of the intervention and 5% of the control condition self-reported quitting; at 1-month follow-up, the quit rate in the intervention condition was 23% and no information on the control condition was provided.

Summary

There is growing interest in the application of digital technologies to adolescent mental health interventions. A variety of digital technologies have been utilized to improve the treatment of anxiety, depression, and substance use disorders including nicotine dependence; however, fewer applications have been developed to target other common mental health conditions. Overall, Internet- and computer-based formats are popular, and many digitize educational curricula and self-monitoring tools. Text messaging is also emerging as a modality for the treatment of depression and smoking cessation, although it is far less well studied than computer-based interventions.

Initial findings suggest that computer-delivered interventions for adolescent depression, anxiety, and substance use have promising results. Data support the use of computer-delivered modalities for smoking cessation, and a few have tested interventions targeting alcohol use; however, other common co-occurring drugs such as marijuana and tobacco are also addressed. The interventions also target a variety of populations from both school-based and clinical populations, and a few studies have developed gender-specific or culturally tailored interventions. Future research is needed to determine how to improve on the existing findings and continue to determine how to best disseminate these digital technology-based interventions.

Scaling Technology-Based Interventions for Mental Healthcare in Adolescents

Although there are many promising interventions that utilize digital technology to improve mental health outcomes, traditionally few interventions are scaled to a level where there is measurable impact on public health (DeAngelis, 2010). Several considerations have been described when scaling digital technologies for mental health, including data security and confidentiality, having an accessible mental healthcare workforce to support users of digital technologies, and having an appropriate technologic infrastructure to support e-health. Within this framework, adolescents have unique needs that should be considered when disseminating and scaling technologies for mental health. First and foremost is the issue of data security and privacy. Adolescents need enhanced education about the need to keep protected health information confidential, and this is especially true when they are utilizing technologies such as mobile phone applications and texting in real-world contexts. Additionally, as parents often pay for their adolescents' computers, mobile phones, and Internet access, there needs to be enhanced discussion with parents about the need to respect the privacy of their adolescents' health information on digital platforms, even though the adolescents may not own the device by which the information is being communicated. Even if digital technologies are employed, face-to-face professional assistance still needs to be available to adolescents as none of the digital tools takes the place of intensive, higher level care. Additionally, adolescents have unique needs when navigating the mental healthcare system; namely, they may need to seek confidential mental healthcare without the direct supervision of their parents. Ideally, as adolescents age, they should be increasingly encouraged to independently manage their own healthcare. Digital technologies, such as text messaging and mobile apps, may also help encourage adolescents to independently manage appointments and other aspects of their healthcare.

Future Directions

It seems that digital technology–based mental health interventions are accepted by adolescents; however, some studies have shown that long-term engagement may be low. Therefore, future interventions will need to focus on enhancing functionality to keep adolescents engaged with the self-directed interventions. When considering the application of digital technologies for conditions with potential safety risks such as depression, future interventions may necessitate the development of real-time monitoring through moderators, sophisticated text recognition software, or direct involvement of clinicians. Overall, digital technologies should strive to provide increasingly tailored support. Digital technologies are unlikely to replace face-to-face therapies, especially among those adolescents with more severe mental health disorders; however, digital technologies may augment existing therapies for adolescents. Future research is needed to determine how to best integrate this promising therapeutic modality into adolescent mental healthcare.

References

Bandura, A. (1986). *Social foundations of thought and action: A social cognitive theory*. Englewood Cliffs, NJ: Prentice Hall.

Barak, A., Klein, B., & Proudfoot, J. G. (2009). Defining internet-supported therapeutic interventions. *Annals of Behavioral Medicine, 38*(1), 4–17. doi:10.1007/s12160-009-9130-7

Beintner, I., Jacobi, C., & Taylor, C. B. (2012). Effects of an Internet-based prevention programme for eating disorders in the USA and Germany: A meta-analytic review. *European Eating Disorders Review, 20*(1), 1–8. doi:10.1002/erv.1130

Bowen, D. J., Henderson, P. N., Harvill, J., & Buchwald, D. (2012). Short-term effects of a smoking prevention website in American Indian youth. *Journal of Medical Internet Research, 14*(3), e81. doi:10.2196/jmir.1682

Bruning Brown, J., Winzelberg, A. J., Abascal, L. B., & Taylor, C. B. (2004). An evaluation of an Internet-delivered eating disorder prevention program for adolescents and their parents. *Journal of Adolescent Health, 35*(4), 290–6. doi:10.1016/j.jadohealth.2003.10.010

Buller, D. B., Borland, R., Woodall, W. G., Hall, J. R., Hines, J. M., Burris-Woodall, P., . . . Saba, L. (2008). Randomized trials on consider this, a tailored, internet-delivered smoking prevention program for adolescents. *Health Education & Behavior, 35*(2), 260–81. doi:10.1177/1090198106288982

Burns, J. M., Webb, M., Durkin, L. A., & Hickie, I. B. (2010). Reach out central: A serious game designed to engage young men to improve mental health and wellbeing. *Medical Journal of Australia, 192*(SUPPL. 11), S27–30.

Calear, A. L., Christensen, H., Mackinnon, A., Griffiths, K. M., & O'Kearney, R. (2009). The YouthMood project: A cluster randomized controlled trial of an online cognitive behavioral program with adolescents. *Journal of Consulting and Clinical Psychology, 77*(6), 1021–32.

Chen, H. H., Yeh, M. L., & Chao, Y. H. (2006). Comparing effects of auricular acupressure with and without an internet-assisted program on smoking cessation and self-efficacy of adolescents. *The Journal of Alternative and Complementary Medicine, 12*(2), 147–52. doi:10.1089/acm.2006.12.147

Costello E. J., Mustillo, S., Keller G., & Angold A. (2004). Prevalence of psychiatric disorders in childhood and adolescence. In B. L. Levin, K. D. Hennessy, & J. Petrila (Eds.), *Mental health services: A public health perspective* (pp. 111–28). Oxford, UK: Oxford University Press.

Cox, C. M., Kenardy, J. A., & Hendrikz, J. K. (2010). A randomized controlled trial of a web-based early intervention for children and their parents following unintentional injury.

Journal of Pediatric Psychology, 35(6), 581–92. doi:10.1093/jpepsy/jsp095

Cunningham, M. J., Wuthrich, V. M., Rapee, R. M., Lyneham, H. J., Schniering, C. A., & Hudson, J. L. (2009). The Cool Teens CD-ROM for anxiety disorders in adolescents: A pilot case series. *European Child and Adolescent Psychiatry, 18*(2), 125–9. doi:10.1007/s00787-008-0703-y

Cunningham, R. M., Chermack, S. T., Zimmerman, M. A., Shope, J. T., Bingham, C. R., Blow, F. C., & Walton, M. A. (2012). Brief motivational interviewing intervention for peer violence and alcohol use in teens: One-year follow-up. *Pediatrics, 129*(6), 1083–90. doi:10.1542/peds.2011–3419

DeAngelis, T. (2010). Getting research into the Real World. *Monitor on Psychology.* http://www.apa.org/monitor/2010/11/dissemination.aspx

Dino, G. A., Horn, K. A., Goldcamp, J., Maniar, S. D., Fernandes, A., & Massey, C. J. (2001). Statewide demonstration of not on tobacco: A gender-sensitive teen smoking cessation program. *Journal of School Nursing, 17*(2), 90–7.

Evers, K. E., Paiva, A. L., Johnson, J. L., Cummins, C. O., Prochaska, J. O., Prochaska, J. M., . . . Gökbayrak, N. S. (2012). Results of a transtheoretical model-based alcohol, tobacco and other drug intervention in middle schools. *Addictive Behaviors, 37*(9), 1009–18. doi:10.1016/j.addbeh.2012.04.008

Fang, L., & Schinke, S. P. (2013). Two-year outcomes of a randomized, family-based substance use prevention trial for Asian American adolescent girls. *Psychology of Addictive Behaviors, 27*(3), 788–98. doi:10.1037/a0030925

Fritz, D. J., Hardin, S. B., Gore, P. A., Jr., & Bram, D. (2008). A computerized smoking cessation intervention for high school smokers. *Pediatric Nursing, 34*(1), 13–7.

Hoek, W., Marko, M., Fogel, J., Schuurmans, J., Gladstone, T., Bradford, N., . . . Van Voorhees, B. W. (2011). Randomized controlled trial of primary care physician motivational interviewing versus brief advice to engage adolescents with an Internet-based depression prevention intervention: 6-month outcomes and predictors of improvement. *Translational Research, 158*(6), 315–25.

Hollis, J. F., Polen, M. R., Whitlock, E. P., Lichtenstein, E., Mullooly, J. P., Vellicer, W. F., & Redding, C. A. (2005). Teen Reach: Outcomes from a randomized, controlled trial of a tobacco reduction programs for teens seen in primary medical care. *Pediatrics, 115*, 981–89. doi:10.1542/peds.2004–0981

Horn, K., Dino, G., Kalsekar, I., & Mody, R. (2005). The impact of not on tobacco on teen smoking cessation: End-of-program evaluation results, 1998 to 2003. *Journal of Adolescent Research, 20*(6), 640–61. doi:10.1177/0743558405274891

Hutton, H. E., Wilson, L. M., Apelberg, B. J., Avila Tang, E., Odelola, O., Bass, E. B., & Chander, G. (2011). A systematic review of randomized controlled trials: Web-based interventions for smoking cessation among adolescents, college students, and adults. *Nicotine & Tobacco Research, 13*(4), 227–38. doi:10.1093/ntr/ntq252

James, A. C., James, G., Cowdrey, F. A., Soler, A., & Choke, A. (2013). Cognitive behavioural therapy for anxiety disorders in children and adolescents. *Cochrane Database of Systematic Reviews, 6*, Cd004690. doi:10.1002/14651858.CD004690.pub3

Jones, M., Luce, K. H., Osborne, M. I., Taylor, K., Cunning, D., Doyle, A. C., . . . Taylor, C. B. (2008). Randomized, controlled trial of an internet-facilitated intervention for reducing binge eating and overweight in adolescents. *Pediatrics, 121*(3), 453–62. doi:10.1542/peds.2007–1173

Koning, I. M., Vollebergh, W. A. M., Smit, F., Verdurmen, J. E. E., Van Den Eijnden, R. J. J. M., Ter Bogt, T. F. M., . . . Engels, R. C. M. E. (2009). Preventing heavy alcohol use in adolescents (PAS): Cluster randomized trial of a parent and student intervention offered separately and simultaneously. *Addiction, 104*(10), 1669–78. doi:10.1111/j.1360–0443.2009.02677.x

Koutakis, N., Stattin, H., & Kerr, M. (2008). Reducing youth alcohol drinking through a parent-targeted intervention: The Orebro Prevention Program. *Addiction, 103*(10), 1629–37. doi:10.1111/j.1360–0443.2008.02326.x

Madden, M., Lenhart, A., Duggan, M., Cortesi, S., & Gasser, U. (2013). *Teens and technology.* Washington DC: Pew Research Center Internet & American Life Project.

Merikangas, K. R., He, J. P., Burstein, M., Swanson, S. A., Avenevoli, S., Cui, L., . . . Swendsen, J. (2010). Lifetime prevalence of mental disorders in US adolescents: Results from the National Comorbidity Survey Replication—Adolescent Supplement (NCS-A). *Journal of the American Academy of Childhood and Adolescent Psychiatry, 49*(10), 980–9. doi:10.1016/j.jaac.2010.05.017

Merikangas, K. R., He, J. P., Burstein, M., Swendsen, J., Avenevoli, S., Case, B., . . . Olfson, M. (2011). Service utilization for lifetime mental disorders in US adolescents: Results of the National Comorbidity Survey-Adolescent Supplement (NCS-A). *Journal of the American Academy of Childhood and Adolescent Psychiatry, 50*(1), 32–45. doi:10.1016/j.jaac.2010.10.006

Mermelstein, R., & Turner, L. (2006). Web-based support as an adjunct to group-based smoking cessation for adolescents. *Nicotine & Tobacco Research, 8*(Suppl 1), S69–76. doi:10.1080/14622200601039949

Merry, S. N., Stasiak, K., Shepherd, M., Frampton, C., Fleming, T., & Lucassen, M. F. G. (2012). The effectiveness of SPARX, a computerised self help intervention for adolescents seeking help for depression: Randomised controlled non-inferiority trial. *BMJ (Online), 344*(7857).

Montaño, D. M., Kasprzyk, D., & Taplin, S. H. (1997). The theory of reasoned action and the theory of planned behavior. In K. Glanz, F. M. Lewis, & B. K. Rimer (Eds.), *Health behavior and health education: Theory, research and practice* (pp. 85–112). San Francisco: Jossey-Bass.

Muris, P., Merckelbach, H., Holdrinet, I., & Sijsenaar, M. (1998). Treating phobic children: Effects of EMDR versus exposure. *Journal of Consulting and Clinical Psychology, 66*(1), 193–8.

National Collaborating Centre for Mental Health. (2014). E-therapies: Systematic review for children and young people with mental health problems. https://www.minded.org.uk/pluginfile.php/1287/course/section/579/e-Therapies%20link2%20-%20Full%20Review%20-%20v0.2%2021.3.14.pdf

Norman, C. D., Maley, O., Li, X., & Skinner, H. A. (2008). Using the internet to assist smoking prevention and cessation in schools: A randomized, controlled trial. *Health Psychology, 27*(6), 799–810. doi:10.1037/a0013105

O'Kearney, R., Kang, K., Christensen, H., & Griffiths, K. (2009). A controlled trial of a school-based internet program for reducing depressive symptoms in adolescent girls. *Depression and Anxiety, 26*(1), 65–72.

Park, E., & Drake, E. (2014). Systematic review: Internet-based program for youth smoking prevention and cessation.

Journal of Nursing Scholarship, 47: 43–50. doi:10.1111/jnu.12104

Patten, C. A., Croghan, I. T., Meis, T. M., Decker, P. A., Pingree, S., Colligan, R. C., . . . Gustafson, D. H. (2006). Randomized clinical trial of an internet-based versus brief office intervention for adolescent smoking cessation. *Patient Education and Counseling, 64*(1–3), 249–58. doi:10.1016/j.pec.2006.03.001

Pretorius, N., Arcelus, J., Beecham, J., Dawson, H., Doherty, F., Eisler, I., . . . Schmidt, U. (2009). Cognitive-behavioural therapy for adolescents with bulimic symptomatology: The acceptability and effectiveness of internet-based delivery. *Behaviour Research and Therapy, 47*(9), 729–36.

Price, M., Yuen, E. K., Goetter, E. M., Herbert, J. D., Forman, E. M., Acierno, R., & Ruggiero, K. J. (2013). mHealth: A mechanism to deliver more accessible, more effective mental health care. *Clinical Psychology & Psychotherapy, 21*(5), 427–36. doi:10.1002/cpp.1855

Prochaska, J. O., Redding, C. A., & Evers, K. E. (1997). The transtheoretical model and stages of change. In K. Glanz, F. M. Lewis, & B. K. Rimer (Eds.), *Health behavior and health education: Theory, research, and practice* (2nd ed., pp. 60–84). San Francisco: Jossey-Bass Publishers.

Prokhorov, A. V., Kelder, S. H., Shegog, R., Murray, N., Peters, R., Agurcia-Parker, C., . . . Marani, S. (2008). Impact of A Smoking Prevention Interactive Experience (ASPIRE), an interactive, multimedia smoking prevention and cessation curriculum for culturally diverse highschool students. *Nicotine & Tobacco Research, 10*(9), 1477–85. doi:10.1080/14622200802323183

Redding, C. A., Prochaska, J. O., Pallonen, U. E., Rossi, J. S., Velicer, W. F., Rossi, S. R., . . . Plummer, B. A. (1999). Transtheoretical individualized multimedia expert systems targeting adolescents' health behaviors. *Cognitive and Behavioral Practice, 6*(2), 144–53. doi:10.1016/S1077-7229(99)80025-X

Reid, S. C., Kauer, S. D., Hearps, S. J., Crooke, A. H., Khor, A. S., Sanci, L. A., & Patton, G. C. (2013). A mobile phone application for the assessment and management of youth mental health problems in primary care: Health service outcomes from a randomised controlled trial of mobile type. *BMC Family Practice, 14*, 84. doi:10.1186/1471-2296-14-84

Reid, S. C., Kauer, S. D., Hearps, S. J. C., Crooke, A. H. D., Khor, A. S., Sanci, L. A., & Patton, G. C. (2011). A mobile phone application for the assessment and management of youth mental health problems in primary care: A randomised controlled trial. *BMC Family Practice, 12*: 131. doi:10.1186/1471-2296-12-131

Renton, T., Tang, H., Ennis, N., Cusimano, M. D., Bhalerao, S., Schweizer, T. A., & Topolovec-Vranic, J. (2014). Web-based intervention programs for depression: A scoping review and evaluation. *Journal of Medical Internet Research, 16*(9), e209.

Reynolds, S., Wilson, C., Austin, J., & Hooper, L. (2012). Effects of psychotherapy for anxiety in children and adolescents: A meta-analytic review. *Clinical Psychology Review, 32*(4), 251–262. doi:10.1016/j.cpr.2012.01.005

Rooke, S., Thorsteinsson, E., Karpin, A., Copeland, J. & Allsop, D. (2010). Computer-delivered interventions for alcohol and tobacco use : A meta-analysis. *Addiction, 105*(8), 1381–1390. doi:10.1111/j.1360-0443.2010.02975.x

Saulsberry, A., Marko-Holguin, M., Blomeke, K., Hinkle, C., Fogel, J., Gladstone, T., . . . Van Voorhees, B. W. (2013). Randomized clinical trial of a primary care internet-based intervention to prevent adolescent depression: One-year outcomes. *Journal of the Canadian Academy of Child and Adolescent Psychiatry, 22*(2), 106–17.

Schinke, S. P., Schwinn, T. M., Di Noia, J., & Cole, K. C. (2004). Reducing the risks of alcohol use among urban youth: Three-year effects of a computer-based intervention with and without parent involvement. *Journal on Studies of Alcohol, 65*(4), 443–9.

Schwinn, T. M., Schinke, S. P., & Di Noia, J. (2010). Preventing drug abuse among adolescent girls: Outcome data from an internet-based intervention. *Prevention Science, 11*(1), 24–32. doi:10.1007/s11121-009-0146-9

Sethi, S., Campbell, A. J., & Ellis, L. A. (2010). The use of computerised self-help packages to treat adolescent depression and anxiety. *Journal of Technology and Human Services, 28*(3), 144– 160. doi:10.1080/15228835.2010.508317

Spence, S. H., Donovan, C. L., March, S., Gamble, A., Anderson, R. E., Prosser, S., & Kenardy, J. (2011). A randomized controlled trial of online versus clinic-based CBT for adolescent anxiety. *Journal of Consulting and Clinical Psychology, 79*(5), 629–42. doi:10.1037/a0024512

Spirito, A., Esposito-Smythers, C., Wolff, J., & Uhl, K. (2011). Cognitive-behavioral therapy for adolescent depression and suicidality. *Child and Adolescent Psychiatric Clinics of North America, 20*(2), 191–204. doi:10.1016/j.chc.2011.01.012

Stallard, P., Richardson, T., Velleman, S., & Attwood, M. (2011). Computerized CBT (Think, Feel, Do) for depression and anxiety in children and adolescents: Outcomes and feedback from a pilot randomized controlled trial. *Behavioural and Cognitive Psychotherapy, 39*(3), 273–84. doi:10.1017/s135246581000086x

van der Zanden, R., Kramer, J., Gerrits, R., & Cuijpers, P. (2012). Effectiveness of an online group course for depression in adolescents and young adults: A randomized trial. *Journal of Medical Internet Research, 14*(3), e86. doi:10.2196/jmir.2033

Van Voorhees, B. W., Ellis, J. M., Gollan, J. K., Bell, C. C., Stuart, S. S., Fogel, J., . . . Ford, D. E. (2007). Development and process evaluation of a primary care internet-based intervention to prevent depression in emerging adults. *Primary Care Companion to the Journal of Clinical Psychiatry, 9*(5), 346–55.

Velicer, W. F., & Prochaska, J. O. (1999). An expert system intervention for smoking cessation. *Patient Education and Counseling, 36*(2), 119–29. doi:10.1016/S0738-3991(98)00129–3

Velicer, W. F., Prochaska, J. O., Bellis, J. M., DiClemente, C. C., Rossi, J. S., Fava, J. L., & Steiger, J. H. (1993). An expert system intervention for smoking cessation. *Addictive Behaviors, 18*(3), 269–90. doi:10.1016/0306–4603(93)90029–9

Walton, M. A., Chermack, S. T., Shope, J. T., Bingham, C. R., Zimmerman, M. A., Blow, F. C., & Cunningham, R. M. (2010). Effects of a brief intervention for reducing violence and alcohol misuse among adolescents: A randomized controlled trial. *Journal of the American Medical Association, 304*(5), 527–35. doi:10.1001/jama.2010.1066

Whittaker, R., Merry, S., Stasiak, K., McDowell, H., Doherty, I., Shepherd, M., . . . Rodgers, A. (2012). MEMO—a mobile phone depression prevention intervention for adolescents: Development process and postprogram findings on acceptability from a randomized controlled trial. *Journal of Medical Internet Research, 14*(1), e13. doi:10.2196/jmir.1857

Woodruff, S. I., Conway, T. L., Edwards, C. C., Elliott, S. P., & Crittenden, J. (2007). Evaluation of an internet virtual world chat room for adolescent smoking cessation. *Addictive Behaviors, 32*(9), 1769–86. doi:10.1016/j.addbeh.2006.12.008

Woodruff, S. I., Edwards, C. C., Conway, T. L., & Elliott, S. P. (2001). Pilot test of an internet virtual world chat room for rural teen smokers. *Journal of Adolescent Health, 29*(4), 239–43. doi:10.1016/S1054-139X(01)00262–2

Wuthrich, V. M., Rapee, R. M., Cunningham, M. J., Lyneham, H. J., Hudson, J. L., & Schniering, C. A. (2012). A randomized controlled trial of the Cool Teens CD-ROM computerized program for adolescent anxiety. *Journal of the American Academy of Child and Adolescent Psychiatry, 51*(3), 261–70. doi:10.1016/j.jaac.2011.12.002

CHAPTER

30 Digitally Assisted Interventions for the Treatment and Prevention of Risky Behavior in Adults

Incorporating the Transtheoretical Model

Janice M. Prochaska *and* James O. Prochaska

Abstract

To have a significant and sustainable impact on attaining and maintaining healthy behaviors, the Transtheoretical Model of Behavior Change addresses the needs of entire populations, not just the minority who are motivated to take immediate action for better health. The six stages of change are outlined as well as the 10 processes of change or strategies to progress from one stage to the next. Digitally assisted interventions tailored to specific stages of change allow programs supported by computer-based tools and methodologies to be interactive and individualized for treatment and prevention of entire populations with risk behaviors like smoking, inactivity, unhealthy diets, alcohol misuse, and ineffectively managed stress. Digitally assisted interventions include mobile phones, personal digital assistants, smartphones, portable media players, tablets, and smart books. The devices have a range of functions from mobile cellular communication using text messages, photos and videos, telephone, and worldwide web access to multimedia playback and software application support. They allow temporal synchronization of the intervention delivery and allow the intervention to engage people's attention when it is most relevant. The chapter presents examples of transtheoretical, digitally assisted interventions for use by both clients and coaches. Evidence is presented that compares the effectiveness of the digital programs.

Keywords: Transtheoretical Model, digital interventions, change, stages of change, healthy lifestyle

Importance of a Healthy Lifestyle

Health risk behaviors like smoking, inactivity, unhealthy diets, alcohol abuse, and ineffectively managed stress significantly contribute to a population's morbidity, disability, mortality, reduced functioning and productivity, and escalating healthcare costs. In contrast, accumulating evidence suggests that a healthy lifestyle including abstinence from smoking, eating five servings of fruits and vegetables each day, adequate physical activity (e.g., walking 10,000 steps a day or doing 150 minutes of moderate exercise a week), and striving to maintain a body mass index (BMI) of less than 25 increases life expectancy by up to 14 years (Khaw et al., 2008; van den Brandt, 2011; Pronk et al., 2010). However, having a healthy lifestyle of 0 (smoking), 5 (fruits and vegetables), 10 (10,000 steps), and 25 (<25 BMI) has been an elusive goal for 97% of the population (Reeves & Rafferty, 2005).

To have a significant and sustainable impact on attaining these healthy behaviors, a model of behavior change is needed to address the needs of entire populations, not just the minority who are motivated to take immediate action for better health. The Transtheoretical Model of Behavior Change (TTM) reframes change from equaling action to equaling progress through a series of stages. The TTM is integrated around the stages of change which can identify segments of populations in different stages of change (Prochaska & Prochaska, 2016). Then, principles and processes are applied to initiate movement through stages of change: Precontemplation (not ready to take action); Contemplation (getting ready); Preparation (ready); Action, and Maintenance.

Digitally assisted interventions tailored to specific needs allow programs supported by computer-based tools and methodologies to be interactive and individualized for treatment of entire populations. Digital interventions can provide new forms of access to self-care, including video and audio delivery for those with reading difficulties, and anonymous social support for those unable or unwilling to consult health professionals in person (Kraft, Dzrozd, & Olsen, 2009). Computer-tailored interventions (CTIs) delivered through various modalities, such as clinical guidance, telephonic counseling, and the Internet produce high impact on both single and multiple behaviors for disease management and prevention. These interventions involve new paradigms that complement existing ones, such as proactive stage-matched interventions for multiple behaviors delivered via computers, tablets, and handheld devices that are based on evidence from randomized population trials. These more inclusive and integrative paradigms have the potential to provide the foundation for a "well care system," one that will complement the existing "sick care system." They have the capability to engage patients in their self-care, increase patients' access to providers, and improve the quality of care while reducing costs (Pearl, 2014).

The Transtheoretical Model

The TTM uses stages of change to integrate principles and processes of change across major theories of intervention, hence the name "Transtheoretical." The TTM emerged from a comparative analysis of 25 leading theories of psychotherapy in an effort to integrate a field that had fragmented into more than 300 theories of psychotherapy (Prochaska & Norcross, 2018). Surprisingly, those theories had much more to say about *why* people do not change than about *how* they can change. They were really theories of behavior, such as theories of personality and psychopathology, rather than theories of behavior change.

Ten processes of change were identified that described key ways in which people changed their behaviors. These included consciousness raising from the Freudian tradition, contingency management from the Skinnerian tradition, and forming helping relationships from the Rogerian tradition. Next, among smokers and former smokers, a comparative analysis was performed on self-changers versus those in professional treatments since an integrative model of change should reflect how people change on their own as well as with professional guidance. The analysis examined how often each group used each of 10 processes (DiClemente & Prochaska, 1982). Participants used different processes of change at different times in their struggles to quit smoking. These naïve subjects taught researchers about a phenomenon that was not then a part of any therapy theories. They revealed that behavior change unfolds through a series of stages (Prochaska & DiClemente, 1983), with different change processes used at different stages. This profound insight changed the course of the research and led to development of the TTM.

Components of the Transtheoretical Model

The TTM includes six stages of change, decisional balance (the pros and cons of changing), self-efficacy, temptation, and the processes of change. *Stage of change* serves as the key integrating construct. Studies of change have shown that people move through a series of stages when modifying behavior. Although the time a person can stay in each stage is variable, the tasks required to move to the next stage are not. Certain principles and processes work best at each stage to reduce resistance, facilitate progress, and prevent relapse. Only a minority (usually <20%) of a population at risk is prepared to take action at any given time. Thus, action-oriented strategies are not helpful for those in the early stages of change. Strategies based on each of the TTM stages result in increased engagement in the change process because they are tailored to each individual in the whole population rather than the minority ready to take action.

Stages of Change

The stage construct implies progress occurring over time. Surprisingly, none of the leading theories of therapy contained a core construct representing time. Traditionally, behavior change was often construed as an event, such as quitting smoking, drinking, or overeating, but the TTM recognizes change as a process that unfolds over time and involving progress through a series of stages (see Figure 30.1).

PRECONTEMPLATION

People in the Precontemplation stage are not intending to take action in the foreseeable future, usually measured as the next 6 months. Being uninformed or underinformed about the consequences of one's behavior may cause a person to be in Precontemplation. Multiple, unsuccessful attempts at change can lead to demoralization about one's ability to change. Both the uninformed and underinformed tend to avoid reading, talking, or thinking about their high-risk behaviors. They are often characterized in other theories as resistant, unmotivated,

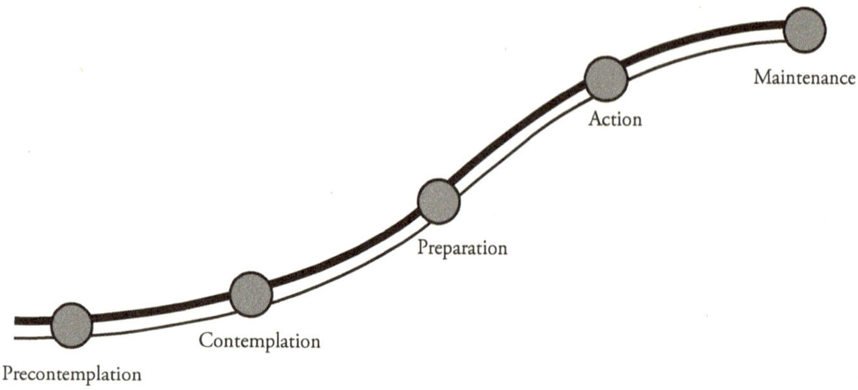

Figure 30.1 The stages of change.
From Pro-Change Behavior Systems, Inc. reprinted with permission.

or not ready for interventions, digitally assisted or otherwise. The fact is, action-oriented programs are not ready for such individuals and are not developed to meet their needs. Messages like "Wherever you are at, we can work with that"™ need to be delivered, and programs meeting that need ought to be developed.

CONTEMPLATION

Contemplation is the stage in which people are intending to change in the next 6 months. They are more aware of the pros of changing but are also acutely aware of the cons. In a meta-analysis across 48 health risk behaviors (Hall & Rossi, 2008), the pros and cons of changing were equal for people in Contemplation. This weighting between the costs and benefits of changing can produce profound ambivalence that can cause people to remain in this stage for long periods of time. This phenomenon is often characterized as chronic contemplation or behavioral procrastination. Individuals in Contemplation also are not ready for traditional action-oriented programs that expect participants to act immediately.

PREPARATION

Preparation is the stage in which people are intending to take action in the immediate future, usually measured as the next month. Typically, they have already taken some significant steps toward the healthier behavior in the past year. These individuals have a plan of action, such as joining an exercise class, consulting a counselor, talking to their physician, buying a self-help book, or relying on a self-change approach. These are the people who can be recruited for action-oriented programs such as Quitnet or Weight Watchers online.

ACTION

Action is the stage in which people have made specific overt modifications in their lifestyles within the past 6 months. Since action is observable, the overall process of behavior change often has been equated with action. But in the TTM, Action is only one of six stages. Not all modifications of behavior count as action in this model. In most applications, people have to attain a criterion that scientists and professionals agree is sufficient to reduce risk of disease. For example, reduction in the number of cigarettes or switching to low tar and nicotine cigarettes were formerly considered acceptable actions for smoking. Now the consensus is clear: only total abstinence counts because those other changes do not necessarily lead to quitting and do not lower the risks associated with smoking to zero.

MAINTENANCE

Maintenance is the stage in which people have made specific, overt modifications in their lifestyles and are working to prevent relapse, but they do not apply change processes as frequently as do people in Action. They are less tempted to relapse and grow increasingly more confident (have greater self-efficacy) that they can continue their changes. Based on self-efficacy and temptation data, researchers have estimated that Maintenance lasts from 6 months to about 5 years. Fitbit is a good example of a digital tool to help someone stay in Maintenance.

TERMINATION

Termination is the stage in which people are not tempted; they have 100% self-efficacy. Whether depressed, anxious, bored, lonely, angry, or stressed, individuals in this stage are sure they will not return to unhealthy habits as a way of coping. It is as if the habit was never acquired in the first place or their new behavior has become an automatic habit. Examples include people who have developed automatic seatbelt use or who automatically take their medications at the same time and place each day. In a study of former smokers and alcoholics, researchers found that fewer than 20% of each group had reached the criteria of zero temptation and total self-efficacy (Snow, Prochaska, & Rossi, 1992). The criterion of 100% self-efficacy may be too strict, or it may be that this stage is an ideal goal for population health efforts. In other areas, like exercise, consistent condom use, and weight control, the realistic goal for many people may be a lifetime of maintenance. Termination has not been given as much emphasis in TTM research since it may not be a practical reality for populations and it occurs long after interventions have ended.

Decisional Balance

The process of reflection and weighing of the pros and cons of changing is *decisional balance.* Sound decision making requires the consideration of the potential gains (pros) and losses (cons) associated with a behavior's consequences. For example, there are more than 65 scientifically established benefits of regular physical activity. One could be encouraged to make a list to see how many can be identified. One can also list the cons. The more the list of pros outweighs the cons, the better prepared one will be to take effective action.

Self-Efficacy

With TTM-based interventions, self-efficacy is operationalized as confidence to make and sustain changes. Confidence is low in the Precontemplation stage and increases across the stages (DiClemente et al., 1991). Given the importance of self-efficacy, it needs to be raised early by assisting individuals in setting and achieving small goals that will build their confidence for taking on increasingly difficult challenges. If, for example, someone is not exercising at all but is intending to do so in the next 6 months, it would be helpful to have them set a reasonable and achievable goal to begin exercising slowly (e.g., 10 minutes, three times a week) and increase the frequency and intensity once that goal has been mastered.

Temptation

Temptation reflects the intensity of urges to engage in a specific unhealthy habit while in the midst of difficult situations. Typically, three factors reflect the most common types of tempting situations: negative affect or emotional distress, positive social situations, and craving. People could ask themselves how they will cope with emotional distress (without relying on a cigarette or comfort foods) to help them cope more effectively and thereby build their confidence or self-efficacy.

Processes of Change

Table 30.1 illustrates the principles and processes of change by stage. Processes of change are the experiential and behavioral activities that people use to progress through the stages. They provide important guides for digital intervention programs, serving as activities that are applied to move from stage to stage. Ten processes have received the most scientific support to date. The processes will first be described with examples from clinical work, and later we will describe how digital technology can provide individualized and interactive guidance on the use of the processes.

CONSCIOUSNESS RAISING (GET THE FACTS)

Consciousness raising involves increased awareness about the causes, consequences, and cures for a particular problem behavior. Interventions that can increase awareness include feedback, interpretations, bibliotherapy (i.e., using self-help books or manuals), and media campaigns. Sedentary people, for example, may not be aware that their inactivity can have the same risk as smoking a pack of cigarettes a day.

DRAMATIC RELIEF (PAY ATTENTION TO FEELINGS)

Dramatic relief initially produces increased emotional experiences followed by reduced affect or anticipated relief if appropriate action is taken. Personal testimonies, social networks, and health risk feedback delivered by text messages are examples of techniques that can move people emotionally.

SELF-REEVALUATION (CREATE A NEW SELF-IMAGE)

Self-reevaluation combines both cognitive and affective assessments of one's self-image with and without a particular unhealthy habit, such as one's image as a couch potato versus an active person. Values clarification, identifying healthy role models, and imagery are techniques that can help people apply self-reevaluation. One might ask, "Imagine if

Table 30.1 Integration of the stages, principles and processes of change

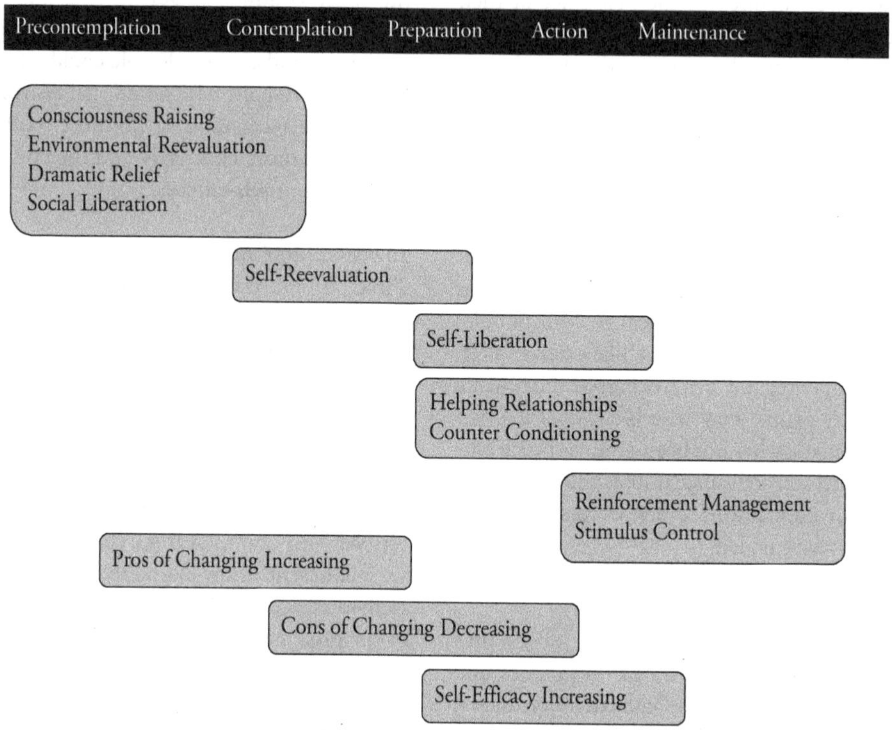

you were free from smoking. How would you feel about yourself?" Examples of what others have imagined can be shared via smartphones.

ENVIRONMENTAL REEVALUATION (NOTICE YOUR EFFECT ON OTHERS)

Environmental reevaluation combines both affective and cognitive assessments of how the presence or absence of a personal habit affects one's social environment, such as the effect of smoking on others. It can also include the awareness that one can serve as a positive or negative role model for others. Empathy training and documentaries can lead to such assessments.

SOCIAL LIBERATION (NOTICE SOCIAL TRENDS)

Social liberation involves realizing that social norms are changing to support the healthy behavior. Examples include recognizing smoke-free zones, salad bars at restaurants, and walking paths.

SELF-LIBERATION (MAKE A COMMITMENT)

Self-liberation is both the belief that one can change and the commitment as well as re-commitment to act on that belief. New Year's resolutions, public testimonies, or a contract are ways of enhancing what the public calls *willpower*. The intervention could state, "Telling others about my commitment to take action can strengthen my willpower. Who am I going to tell?" Today, with social networks, individuals can make commitments to many of their digital friends.

COUNTER CONDITIONING (USE SUBSTITUTES)

Counterconditioning requires learning healthy behaviors as substitutes for problem behaviors. Examples of counter conditioning include nicotine replacement as a safe substitution for smoking or walking as a healthier alternative than "comfort foods" as a way to cope with stress.

STIMULUS CONTROL (MANAGE YOUR ENVIRONMENT)

Stimulus control removes cues for unhealthy habits and adds prompts for healthier alternatives. Examples are removing all the ashtrays from the house and car or removing high-fat foods that are tempting cues for unhealthy eating.

REINFORCEMENT MANAGEMENT (USE REWARDS)

Reinforcement management provides positive consequences for taking steps in a positive direction. While reinforcement management can include the use of punishment, we found that self-changers rely on reward much more than punishment. Reinforcements are emphasized since a philosophy of the stage model is to work in harmony with how people change naturally. People expect to be reinforced by others more frequently than is actually the case, so they should be encouraged to reinforce themselves through self-statements like, "Nice going! You handled that temptation." They also can treat themselves at milestones as a reinforcement to increase the probability that healthy responses will be repeated.

HELPING RELATIONSHIPS (GET SUPPORT)

Helping relationships combine caring, trust, openness, and acceptance, as well as support for healthy behavior change. Guiding people on how to get social support through support groups, social media, and buddy systems can be sources of social support.

Critical Assumptions of the Transtheoretical Model

The TTM is based on critical assumptions about the nature of behavior change and interventions that can best facilitate such change. The following set of assumptions drive theory, research, and practice related to the TTM:

1. No single theory can account for all complexities of behavior change. A more comprehensive model is most likely to emerge from integration across major theories.
2. Behavior change is a process than unfolds over time through a sequence of stages.
3. Stages are both stable and open to change, just as chronic behavior risk factors are stable and open to change.
4. The majority of at-risk populations are not prepared for action and will not be served effectively by action-oriented behavior change programs.
5. Specific principles and processes of change should be emphasized at specific stages to maximize efficacy.

Digitally Assisted Interventions

Although it is an important function of healthcare services to encourage and support healthcare consumers to adopt healthy behaviors and to prevent and manage chronic diseases, the amount of information, encouragement, and support that can be conveyed during consultations, within existing service infrastructures, or through other traditional media, such as pamphlets, is limited.

Digitally assisted interventions (DAI) are a means for providing individual-level support to increase smoking cessation, activity levels, or adherence to prescribed medications. Digitally assisted interventions include mobile phones, personal digital assistants, smartphones, portable media players, tablets, and smart books. These devices have a range of functions from mobile cellular communication using text messages (SMS), photos and video, telephone, and World Wide Web access to multimedia playback and software application support. The features of DAI that may make them particularly appropriate for providing individual-level support relate to their popularity, mobility, ubiquity, and technological capabilities. This allows temporal synchronization of the intervention delivery and allows the intervention to claim people's attention when it is most relevant. For example, healthcare consumers can be sent messages designed to sustain their motivation to quit smoking near their quit date, interventions can be delivered at any time, and extra support can be requested. Current technological capabilities allow low-cost interventions. There are potential economics of scale as it is technically easy to deliver interventions to large populations. Motivational messages, monitoring, and tailored behavior change guidance used in face-to-face support can be modified for delivery via mobile phones. Interventions can be individualized, with the content tailored to stage of change, pros and cons, self-efficacy, and processes of change.

To evaluate the efficacy of computer-delivered interventions, Portnoy, Scott-Sheldon, Johnson, and Carey (2008) conducted a meta-analysis of the published literature. Studies examining health domains related to leading indicators outlined in *Healthy People 2010* were selected. Data from 75 randomized controlled trials, published between 1988 and 2007, with 35,685 participants and 82 separate interventions, were included. Compared with controls, participants who received a computer-delivered intervention improved several hypothesized antecedents of health behavior change (knowledge, attitudes, intentions); intervention recipients also improved health behavior (nutrition, tobacco use, substance use, safer sexual behavior, binge/purge behavior) and general health maintenance. This meta-analysis demonstrates the effects of digital interventions on antecedents of risk behaviors and improvements in those behaviors. Later in the section on comparing effectiveness, we will see the magnitude of effects from digital interventions and comparison of outcomes to other types of health behavior change programs.

Krishna, Boren, and Balas (2009) performed a systematic review to evaluate the research evidence related to the role of cell phones and text messaging interventions in improving health outcomes and processes of care. They identified 25 studies. Selected studies included 38,060 participants that covered 12 clinical areas and took place in 13 countries. Significant improvements were noted in compliance with medicine taking, asthma symptoms, HbA1C levels, stress levels, smoking quit rates, and self-efficacy. Process improvements were reported in lower failed appointments, quicker diagnoses, and treatment.

Digitally Assisted Interventions and the Transtheoretical Model

The following is an example of how TTM interventions can be supported by digitally assisted interventions. An expert system software program administers the assessments, scores them, and follows empirically derived decision rules to deliver individualized feedback and guidance efficiently, cost-effectively, and with fidelity. At Pro-Change Behavior Systems, Inc., a research and development company founded by James O. Prochaska, each mobile-optimized program is built on a flexible platform that can be incorporated into a variety of server environments, can be branded for various organizations, and can track utilization and participant outcomes based on organization codes. Standard aggregate reporting capabilities capture and display key outcomes. Given their capacity to reach individuals at all levels of readiness to change, digitally assisted TTM programs are population-based but provide a completely customized experience for each end user with feedback that is dynamically updated when users return to that program. The customized behavior change guidance is based on the comparison of the user's responses to reliable and valid assessment questions to preprogrammed, statistically derived decision rules.

Initially, individuals are given normative feedback that compares their current use of particular principles and process of change to their peers who have made the most progress to the next stage. Future interactions provide both normative feedback on how they are doing compared to their peers and ipsative feedback on how they are doing compared to their previous assessment. Feedback that they have significantly improved their pros and are ready to progress to the next stage can provide expert guidance and facilitate change as measured by progress. Without such digitally assisted guidance, people are left with guessing and with trial-and-error learning that is much less efficient and effective compared to evidence-based guided learning.

After participants complete the baseline assessment, they are transitioned immediately into the first CTI session. In the intervention session, individuals receive feedback on stage of change and on five to seven additional TTM constructs matched to stage of change.

1. *Decisional balance.* The pros of doing the new healthy behavior and how the participant's scores compare to those of others who have changed successfully; strategies for increasing the pros and decreasing the cons.
2. *Self-efficacy.* Situations in which the participant is most tempted to do the unhealthy behavior and ideas for coping with those situations.
3. *Processes of change.* How frequently the participant is using specific stage-matched processes of change and how he or she compares with others who were most successful in progressing to the next stage of change.
4. *Strategies.* Small steps for progressing to the next stage of change.

After the first CTI, participants can receive access to a printed report and an online Personal Activity Center. The printed report contains all the feedback received during the session and refers participants to specific activities in the Personal Activity Centers (PAC). The PAC, organized around stage of change, presents information and activities designed to elaborate on and reinforce ideas presented during the CTI. Stage-matched activities include listing the benefits of the new healthy behavior; examining self-image as it relates to the healthy behavior; developing a plan for action; getting support; substituting health changes and behaviors; avoiding people, places, and things that tempt the unhealthy behavior; and identifying intrinsic and extrinsic rewards for doing the healthy behavior. The PAC can be accessed at any time for as many times as desired.

At 30 days after the first CTI session, and 60 days after the second session, participants are prompted by up to eight text and/or email messages to return to the CTI program to complete a follow-up session. Our best practice of completing three sessions spaced out at least 1 month apart has been found to produce significant effects compared to controls across a broad range of problems and populations. (To view a demo of a program, visit www.prochange.com/products.) At follow-ups, the CTI readministers the TTM assessment measures, tracks and gives feedback on stage transitions and changes in stage-matched principles and processes of change, and provides access to an updated printed report.

In addition to the CTI feedback reports and the PAC, participants can receive tailored text messages every 1–3 days, depending on their current stage of change. Individuals in Precontemplation and Maintenance receive fewer messages, with a maximum of 30 messages between CTI sessions. Individuals in Contemplation receive a message every 2 days. And, individuals in Preparation and Action receive a message every day. All text message feedback is individually tailored to the participant's most recent stage of change and scores on the decisional balance, self-efficacy, and processes of change measures.

For example, a participant in the Precontemplation stage for smoking cessation might receive the following messages to facilitate Consciousness Raising: "Smoking facts: Smoking is the #1 preventable cause of death in America. 1 in 5 deaths in the US is caused by smoking. Can you think more about quitting?" A participant in Preparation might receive the following message to increase Self-Efficacy: "Read about relaxation techniques you can use to relax without smoking. It will make you more confident that you can quit. Login at [link to activity in the PAC]." And a participant in the Action stage might receive the following message to facilitate Counter Conditioning: "When you feel the urge to smoke, resist it by substituting healthier thoughts. Urges usually last only 3–5 minutes. You can do most anything for 3–5 minutes!"

Coaching

A digitally assisted coach-facing version of the assessment measures in the CTI can permit coaching to be evidence-based and completely tailored to the needs of each patient/consumer. Unlike many coaching protocols that are based only on clinical judgment, online programs provide telephone-based coaches with easy-to-read bulleted statements and directions that can link to online self-directed programs. A client could use the self-directed online program between coaching sessions for an even more tailored and consistent experience.

The *Clinical Dashboard*, another digitally assisted coaching intervention, offers a graphic representation of a patient's self-reported health status, behavior change challenges, and priorities on a single screen. The dashboard can be populated on demand with a patient's data from a Health Risk Appraisal. The dashboard's most important feature enables clinicians to provide evidence-based behavior change without extensive training. The dashboard can provide brief behavior change messages that the provider can deliver to guide the patient to a healthier lifestyle. The messages are matched to the patient's readiness to change.

Wireless Technologies

Mobile and wireless health technologies have grown exponentially in the past few years. Nearly 90% of US adults have a cell phone, and smartphone usage exceeds 60%. The ubiquity of mobile phone use has provided a platform for the delivery of health interventions previously unavailable to health research and practice. Although the number of mobile and wireless health tools grows each year, the majority of these tools need a more rigorous scientific foundation and have been inadequately validated in clinical research and practice. Developers have not incorporated many behavior change theories or techniques to date. Most incorporate fewer than four behavior change techniques. The most common involve providing instruction on how to perform exercises, feedback on performance, goal-setting assistance, and planning social support (Penn State, 2014). Adoption of these techniques requires more evaluation in clinical and behavioral research settings to examine their potential and the challenges of their use.

Comparing Effectiveness

The single most important question that individuals should ask when they are considering providing wellness programs to employees, patients, or other populations is "How does an approach that is being considered compare to other available approaches?" The second most important question is "What is the best way to compare approaches?" Here there is clear consensus among experts: Compare them on outcomes and the quality of experimental designs used to examine outcomes. A national task force on wellness programs for employee populations provided benchmarks for outcomes on four behaviors that account for a major percentage of chronic diseases: exercise, high-fat diets, diets low in fruits and vegetables, and smoking (Soler et al., 2010). Once the same criterion was applied (i.e., the percentage that progressed from being at-risk to not at-risk on public health criteria), results at long-term follow-up from 58 arms of randomized clinical trials and high-quality case studies became clear.

Johnson et al. (2013) recently compared the average outcomes of TTM-tailored digital programs from 26 arms of randomized population trials and one large case study to average outcomes on the same four behaviors with the same outcome criteria reported by the national task force (Soler et al., 2010). For exercise, the Soler results were 15.3% successful at 2- to 3-year follow-up compared to 47.5% in the TTM RCTs and 55.3% in the large case study (Johnson et al., 2013). For high-fat diets, the Solar results were 5.4% successful compared to 32.3% in the TTM RCTs and 44% in the case study. For fruits and vegetables, the average outcomes were 0% compared to 34.8% in the TTM RCTs and 54.4% in the case study. With smoking, the mean abstinence rates in the Soler review was 17.8% compared to 23.7% in the TTM RCTs and 33.7% in the case study.

The majority of individuals developing and delivering digital disease prevention and disease management programs do not have the resources to evaluate their programs using the gold standard of randomized population studies. They should, however, be able to evaluate their outcomes in case studies with their customers. If they used standard public health consensus outcomes, they can benchmark their results against the average outcomes in Soler et al.'s (2010) review and in TTM studies (Johnson et al., 2013). The developers and their potential adopters can then assess whether a particular program produces outcomes that are less than the average, average, greater than average, or in the highest performing range. These comparisons will have to take into account the percentage of the eligible population who participated in the program, since efficacy rates can be increased or inflated just through selectivity, such as including only motivated individuals in the Preparation stage.

With such benchmarking research, the field can identify innovative digital programs that appear to be producing breakthroughs. In a recent study (Jordan & Evers, 2012), adding TTM-tailored texting to online TTM tailoring for smoking cessation, a breakthrough was achieved, going from 26% abstinence for the best online practice to 38% for the enhanced program that included texting. Given the importance of change in populations, it is imperative that the bar continues to be raised so the field can fulfill the growing potential of digital technologies that are available to so many populations and providers.

References

DiClemente, C. C., & Prochaska, J. O. (1982). Self-change and therapy change of smoking behavior: A comparison of processes of change in cessation and maintenance. *Addictive Behaviors, 7,* 133–42.

DiClemente, C. C., Prochaska, J. O., Fairhurst, S., Velicer, W. F., Velasquez, M., & Rossi, J. S. (1991). The process of smoking cessation: An analysis of precontemplation, contemplation and preparation stages of change. *Journal of Consulting and Clinical Psychology, 59,* 295–304.

Hall, K. L., & Rossi, J. S. (2008). Meta-analytic examination of the strong and weak principles across 48 health behaviors. *Preventive Medicine, 46*(3), 266–74.

Johnson, J. L., Prochaska, J. O., Paiva, A. L., Fernandez, A. C., DeWees, S. J., & Prochaska, J. M. (2013). Advancing bodies of evidence for population-based health promotion programs: Randomized controlled trials and case studies. *Population Health Management, 16,* 373–80.

Jordan, P. J., & Evers, K. E. (2012). Cell phone enhanced expert systems to promote smoking cessation in veterans. *Telemedicine and e-Health, 18,* A-28.

Khaw, K. T., Wareham, N., Bingham, S., Welch, A., Luben, R., & Day, N. (2008). Combined impact of health behaviors and mortality in men and women: The EPIC-Norfolk Prospective Population Study. *PLOS Medicine, 5*(3), e70.

Kraft, P., Dzrozd, F., & Olsen, E. (2009). ePsychology: Designing theory-based health promotion interventions. *California Association of Independent Schools, 24,* 399–426.

Krishna, S., Boren, S. A., & Balas, E. A. (2009). Healthcare via cell phones: A systematic review. *TeleMedicine and e-Health, 15*(3), 231–40.

Pearl, R. (2014). Kiaser Permanente Northern California: Current experiences with internet, mobile and video technologies. *Health Affairs, 33*(2), 251–57.

Penn State. (2014). Mobile health apps lack behavior-change techniques. https://www.sciencedaily.com/releases/2014/05/140506120202.htm

Portnoy, D. B., Scott-Sheldon, L. A., Johnson, B. T., & Carey, M. P. (2008). Computer-delivered Interventions for health promotion and behavioral risk reduction: A meta-analysis of 75 randomized controlled trials, 1988–2007. *Preventive Medicine, 47*(1), 3–16.

Pronk, N. P., Lowry, M., Kottke, T. E., Austin, E., Gallagher, J., & Katz, A. (2010). The association between optimal lifestyle adherence and short-term incidence of chronic conditions among employees. *Population Health Management, 13,* 289–95.

Prochaska, J. O., & DiClemente, C. C. (1983). Stages and processes of self-change of smoking: Toward an integrative model of change. *Journal of Consulting and Clinical Psychology, 51,* 390–95.

Prochaska, J. O., & Norcross, J. (2018). Systems of psychotherapy: A transtheoretical analysis (9th ed.). Oxford, UK: Oxford University Press.

Prochaska, J. O., & Prochaska J. M. (2016). *Changing to thrive.* Center City, MN: Hazeldon.

Reeves, M. J., & Rafferty, A. P. (2005). Health lifestyle characteristics among adults in the United States, 2000. *Archives of Internal Medicine, 165*(8), 854–7.

Snow, M. G., Prochaska, J. O., & Rossi, J. S. (1992). Stages of change for smoking cessation among former problem drinkers: A cross-sectional analysis. *Journal of Substance Abuse, 4*, 107–16.

Soler, R. E., Leeks, K. D., Razi, S., Hopkins, D. P., Griffith, M., Aten, A., . . . Walker, A. M. (2010). A systematic review of selected interventions for worksite health promotion. The assessment of health risk feedback. *American Journal of Preventive Medicine, 38*, S237–62.

van den Brandt, P. A. (2011). The impact of a Mediterranean diet and healthy lifestyle on premature mortality in men and women. *American Journal of Clinical Nutrition, 94*, 913–20.

CHAPTER

31 Using Digital Technology for Cognitive Assessment and Enhancement in Older Adults

Sheida Rabipour *and* Patrick S. R. Davidson

Abstract

Digital technology is becoming increasingly prevalent in cognitive research and clinical applications for older adults. Innovations in web-based cognitive testing, digital tracking tools, and brain–computer interfaces show promise. Digital technology offers potentially safer, more effective, and less costly alternatives to pharmacological and behavioral methods. Computerized cognitive assessment and training show particular promise. However, a number of possible limitations must be kept in mind. This chapter outlines how digital technology shows promise for improving cognitive assessment and support of older adults while stressing caveats that researchers and clinicians should bear in mind. The chapter concludes with highlights of current challenges and practical guidelines for future research

Keywords: aging, brain–computer interface, cognitive assessment, computerized cognitive training, cognitive intervention, digital technology, research methods, web-based intervention

Introduction: Utopian Versus Dystopian Visions of the Future

We live in the Age of Information. You may feel awe-struck by how digital technology has improved our lives. Easier access to information and goods and services, instant communication, and simplification of many life tasks can make one feel that digital technology is nothing short of euthenic. You may feel this same sense of optimism when thinking about science and medicine. Digital innovation has led to the marriage of traditionally distinct domains, including clinical treatment and entertainment. The potential payoffs for cognitive aging are numerous. Older adults no longer need to rely as much on their deteriorating memories, for example, and can instead use digital reminders or life management programs to organize their daily tasks. Researchers and clinicians can employ sophisticated testing software and conduct larger scale studies, adapting entertainment software to render individual programs more user-friendly and engaging. Technology-mediated cognitive interventions can leverage computer- and web-based applications to become more convenient, efficient, cost-effective, and powerful. Increasingly complex algorithms can tailor cognitive exercises to the strengths and weaknesses of each individual, optimizing treatment. In short, you may feel that you are witnessing the coming of a Digital Utopia.

You may instead feel ambivalent or even harbor dystopian fears about digital technology: Unlimited access to information and digital multitasking can lead to overload and might limit opportunities for deep, uninterrupted intellectual contemplation (Carr, 2010). Relying on automated reminders and search engines instead of our own memories may dull the mind, depriving us of the cognitive exercise previous generations received naturally (Sparrow, Liu, & Wegner, 2011). Extensive experience with smartphones and the Internet may change brain activity in older adults (Gindrat, Chytiris, Balerna, Rouiller, & Ghosh, 2015; Small, Moody, Siddarth, & Bookheimer, 2009), but whether these changes are good or bad is unknown. In many cases, initial excitement surrounding a new computerized cognitive intervention—purported to increase intelligence or enhance memory, attention, or information processing speed—quickly turns into skepticism as critics point out weaknesses in the methods and the data.

Which of these two visions is more accurate? How do we ensure that the future of digital technology in cognitive aging is more utopian than dystopian? In this chapter, we outline the promise of digital technology for improving cognitive assessment and support of older adults while stressing caveats that researchers and clinicians should bear in mind. We conclude with highlights of current challenges and practical guidelines for researchers, clinicians, program developers, and other professionals aiming to integrate digital technology with cognitive assessment and intervention in older adults.

Digital Cognitive Assessment

For more than a century, we have measured different aspects of individuals' cognition to compare them to "average." This is particularly useful when aiming to know whether a person is having cognitive difficulty compared to someone of a similar age, education level, gender, and other demographic characteristics. Despite the continuous availability and occasional use of technology over the past century (Wesnes, 2014), cognitive assessment still relies heavily on paper-and-pencil tests administered by an evaluator in a one-on-one session, with results later scored by hand and compared to the performance of an archival standard comparison group. Obviously, this process is time-consuming and labor-intensive, and it relies on a potentially outdated or otherwise inappropriate comparison group.

Digital technology has the potential to improve cognitive assessment. Several computerized batteries have already given us reason for optimism. Leading candidates include the NIH Toolbox (National Institutes of Health and Northwestern University, 2006–2012; Weintraub et al., 2013) and the Penn Computerized Neurocognitive Battery (University of Pennsylvania, 2003–2013). In healthy young and older adults, these batteries have shown item consistency and construct validity (Gur et al., 2010; Heaton et al., 2014) and proved themselves reliable, inexpensive, and efficient—often taking less than half the time to administer and score relative to traditional paper-and-pencil methods. Many of the tasks comprising these batteries are face-valid adaptations of classical cognitive and neuropsychological measures; others are variants of online cognitive training and gaming (Hampshire, Highfield, Parkin, & Owen, 2012; Owen et al., 2010). Moreover, digital game-like tests such as the AttentionTrip (Hassan, Klein, & Wilson, 2015), a variation on the Attention Network Test (Fan, McCandliss, Sommer, Raz, & Posner, 2001), can offer more engaging and comprehensive alternatives to traditional measures and may permit more refined analyses of different cognitive abilities. Many computerized batteries run on desktop computers (either web-based or from the local hard drive), but tablet- and smartphone-based alternatives are being developed (Brouillette et al., 2013).

In addition, computerized cognitive batteries may provide more accurate information about someone's performance in relation to a comparison group. This group may represent typical performance (i.e., a normative comparison) or any other feature relevant to a particular study (i.e., a reference group comprised of a certain population or age group). Traditional cognitive measures often provide comparison data that were collected at one time, sometimes decades earlier, and in one place, usually where the test developers were located. The comparison group may only consist of a few dozen cases. The norms, therefore, may no longer be appropriate in the here-and-now. Further complicating matters, normative scores on many tests of cognition may change over time. If data collection for a comparison group can proceed with little cost and effort using these new computerized test batteries (perhaps through gamified crowd sourcing; e.g., Mitroff et al., 2014), developers can construct a large, up-to-date, local, and individualized comparison group for a more accurate assessment of an individual's performance.

Computerized cognitive assessment is no panacea, of course. It may prove most appropriate as a screening tool or for use with relatively high-functioning people. As work with computerized testing batteries moves forward, it is crucial to learn whether they are comparable to traditional cognitive testing in predicting cognitive decline and the onset of age-related neurological disorders, including dementia, and in differentiating among different cognitive disorders (Parsey & Schmitter-Edgecombe, 2013; Wild, Howieson, Webbe, Seelye, & Kaye, 2008). Computerized cognitive assessment offers enough potential benefits to merit optimism.

Digital Cognitive Support and Enhancement

Pharmacology Versus Technology

The Age of Information is also the Age of Pharmacology. Billions of dollars in marketing by pharmaceutical companies every year has led our society to embrace drugs wholeheartedly. Although good data are still scarce (Partridge, Bell, Lucke, Yeates, & Hall, 2011), preliminary evidence suggests that self-experimentation with nootropics ("smart drugs"), dietary supplements, and off-label use of prescription drugs is rising among students and young professionals (Bossaer et al., 2013; Emanuel et al., 2013; Franke, Bagusat, Rust, Engel, & Lieb, 2014). Depending on the substance, the goal is usually to heighten mood or enhance attentional focus, decision-making, or memory. Interestingly, a small survey by *Nature* magazine suggested that people over the age of 65 are not far behind 20-year-olds in using these substances for cognitive enhancement (Maher, 2008).

Even the use of conventional drugs for cognition presents problems. Medications thought to be cognitively beneficial, including antidepressants and acetylcholine agonists, often turn out to be less effective than expected (Schwarz, Froelich, & Burns, 2012). Furthermore, drugs aimed at providing cognitive benefits often have cognitively deleterious side effects: heart and blood pressure medications are meant to promote brain health via cardiovascular fitness, but these drugs are often anticholinergic and can therefore, ironically, lead to cognitive impairment themselves (Fox et al., 2011). Other dangers of cognitive enhancers, even when taken as prescribed, include depression, hallucinations, and delirium (Cancelli, Beltrame, Gigli, & Valente, 2009; Mintzer & Burns, 2000). Side effects are especially pronounced when people take multiple medications (polypharmacy), which becomes more common with age (Marcum, Peron, & Hanlon, 2012). Moreover, problems with the accessibility, delivery, and monitoring of medications have remained significant since the dawn of the medication era. Calls for better use of the current pharmacopeia (Murray & Callahan, 2003), including improved medication management and monitoring among older adults have, by-and-large, gone unheeded. Given that virtually all drugs have side effects and can be difficult to manage (leading to under- or overdose), wouldn't it be preferable to use technology as a safer—and potentially less expensive—substitute wherever possible?

Digital Cognitive Prosthetics: Technology as a Substitute for Declining Cognitive Functions

One alternative to medication is to use technology as a substitute or support for cognition. These supportive tools are useful for everyone (i.e., not only for people with cognitive impairment) and need not be high-tech: calendars, diaries, and pill organizers are classic methods of keeping track of past behavior and ensuring that one remembers to carry out specific tasks when one should in future. They are inexpensive, never crash, and rarely need to be replaced (for a review, see Kapur, Glisky, & Wilson, 2002).

Today, we can choose from among innumerable digital versions of these classic tools. Web-based digital calendars are commonplace, free, and can be accessed from anywhere and shared with anyone. One might be tempted to think of these digital tools as nothing more than old wine in new bottles, but they can incorporate small changes that provide major benefits to cognition and behavior. For example, although diaries and calendars are potentially useful to memory-impaired people, they are often not as effective as they could be because people with such disorders often forget to make regular reference to them. Something as simple as a chime or other reminder, which is built into most calendar and organizer software, is very useful to draw attention to an item. Today, most smartphones have free or low-cost applications that provide notifications and reminders not only at a certain time but—thanks to built-in global positioning systems—also in a specific place.

Memory support can also come in the form of cues to aid autobiographical memory retrieval. Low-tech versions—for example, the photo album—have always been available. However, advantages of digital photo collections include novelty, flexibility, interactivity, and the potential for sharing (van den Hoven, 2014). Instead of merely using digital technology for autobiographical memory cuing, new technologies show the potential to *replace* memory. Wearable cameras that capture still images at a high rate or record continuous video have been available for more than a decade (e.g., SenseCam; Microsoft Corporation, 2013), and more sophisticated systems (e.g., Google Glass; Google, 2014; Spectacles; Snap Inc., 2016) are emerging. This technology may be especially helpful to people with dementia or other forms of memory impairment (Seamon et al., 2014; Woodberry et al., 2014).

Digital technology also has the potential to revolutionize drug delivery. Numerous patents describe electronic delivery and real-time monitoring of medication (e.g., Katz & Nesbitt, 2014; van der Schaar et al., 2013; Walker, Evans, Hanson, & Burrow, 1997). The aim is greater accuracy and efficiency in regulating dosage. However, these innovations often rely on the patient, at least to some extent, for administration. In older adults with cognitive impairment, faulty memory can make this dangerous. As a solution, digital pill bottles can track when the bottle is opened and remind patients by lighting up or sending digital alerts. Initial results of a company-run randomized controlled trial evaluating one example (GlowCap; Vitality Inc., 2010-2013) reported 98% medication adherence in patients who used the technology, compared to 71% in patients who relied on their own memory. By monitoring medication-taking behavior and allowing offloading of cognitive functions such as memory, these technologies have the potential to increase adherence, minimizing the danger of over- or underdose without the need for on-site healthcare practitioners (Kvedar, Coye, & Everett, 2014).

The monitoring of health and behavior can be even more elaborate. Smartphone sensors can automatically track and transmit data on sleep duration, physical activity, and social interaction (Campbell & Choudhury, 2012). Such monitoring applications can extend to the entire home environment and may help identify declining cognitive capacities over time by tracking performance in activities of daily life (e.g., Dawadi, Cook, & Schmitter-Edgecombe, 2013). Futuristic devices may soon restore memory through implants that stimulate brain areas affected by injury or disease (Reardon, 2015).

Despite the convenience of digitally outsourcing many cognitive tasks, some argue that reducing the need for cognitive work is disadvantageous (Carr, 2010; Cellan-Jones, 2014). The more readily we integrate technology into daily life, the less often we have to draw on our own memory and other cognitive functions. Remembering directions, searching for knowledge in books, proofreading for errors in written works, and performing mental math may have helped maintain mental acuity in older adults in the past (Shimamura, Berry, Mangels, Rusting, & Jurica, 1995). If so, then outsourcing our cognitive work to digital proxies may, ironically, *contribute to* cognitive decline. This fear is powerful and goes back millennia: in the *Phaedrus*, Socrates described the concern that the introduction of the new technology of writing would harm memory and thinking. Yet this fear is difficult to justify with scientific evidence. In fact, some studies suggest the opposite, demonstrating that off-loading memories frees the mind to learn and remember new, more relevant information (Storm & Stone, 2014). Nevertheless, keeping the dystopian possibilities in mind, perhaps it would be best to err on the side of caution: rather than relying on the aforementioned "bottom-up" technological tools as proxies for cognition, it may be preferable to use technology for enhancing cognitive functions with digital exercises and games. If these technologies prove effective and gain acceptance among patients (Cruz et al., 2013), we may one day see doctors writing prescriptions for them (Dafnis, 2014; Wernick, 2014).

Digital Cognitive Enhancement

The general use of digital technology may support independence and perceived quality of life in older adults (Mynatt & Rogers, 2001). The cognitive abilities (Kaufman, Sauve, Renaud, & Duplaa, 2014; Tun & Lachman, 2010) and affective states (Cotten, Ford, Ford, & Hale, 2014) of older adults are positively associated with computer activity. Moreover, for improving speed of processing and episodic memory, small intervention studies suggest that learning to use digital social networks or electronic tablets may be as effective as—and perhaps even more effective than—taking part in stimulating activities of daily life and socializing (Chan, Haber, Drew, & Park, 2014; Myhre, Mehl, & Glisky, 2016).

High engagement and appropriate level of challenge are two important components of any cognitive intervention. The balance of these two parameters has been hypothesized to generate an optimal state of consciousness, also referred to as the state of *flow* (Csikszentmihalyi, 1990). This state of focused concentration involves complete absorption in a particular goal viewed as challenging yet attainable, distortion of one's perception of time, and the experience of engaging in an intrinsically rewarding activity. Digital media may be particularly well suited to promoting flow states by transforming mundane, repetitive cognitive tasks into enjoyable games and titrating difficulty to best suit a user's performance.

COMPUTERIZED COGNITIVE TRAINING: A BOOMING INDUSTRY

Cognitive training is big business. Targeted non-pharmacological cognitive enhancement methods largely focus on the deliberate practice of cognitive operations, such as those involved in memory or attention, through repetition of a particular type of task or activity (Martin, Clare, Altgassen, Cameron, & Zehnder, 2011; Rabipour & Raz, 2012). These interventions are often branded as "brain training" and have found their way beyond the clinic, embraced by individual consumers (and their employers) who wish to maintain or enhance mental acuity. Preserving mental functioning is of particular concern to middle-aged and older adults as they begin to fear the negative cognitive effects of growing older. This demographic is the strategic target of "anti-cognitive aging" advertising by a commercial industry that has a projected value of more than US$6 billion within the next few years (SharpBrains, 2013, 2016).

Among the most prevalent forms of digital cognitive intervention is computerized cognitive training (CCT), which generally involves computerized versions of behavioral tasks used in psychological or neuropsychiatric studies. Programs such as Lumosity (Lumos Labs Inc., n.d.), Cognifit (CogniFit Inc., n.d.), and Brain Age (Nintendo DS, n.d.) typify commercialized CCT and are becoming very popular: Lumosity, for example, was only launched in 2007, but boasted an annual growth rate of 150% in 2013 (Lumos Labs Inc., 2013) and is now used by more than 60 million people worldwide (Venkatesh, 2014).

Potential Benefits

CCT may lead to improvements in general cognitive functioning or in particular cognitive domains, such as working memory, long-term memory, attention, or speed of processing in healthy older adults (Kelly et al., 2014; Kueider, Parisi, Gross, & Rebok, 2012; Reijnders, van Heugten, & van Boxtel, 2013). Some studies have reported sustained enhancement of these functions compared to baseline or control groups following a no-contact period ranging from a few months (Anguera et al., 2013; Cheng et al., 2012; Zelinski et al., 2011) to several years (Wolinsky et al., 2006). Advanced Cognitive Training in Vital Elderly (ACTIVE; Rebok et al., 2014)—the most extensively studied program in healthy older adults to date—appears to yield measurable, small to medium-sized improvements as long as 10 years after initial testing. Reported real-world outcomes of the ACTIVE trial include the ability to continue driving in old age for people who scored lower on certain measures of cognitive function (Ross, Freed, Edwards, Phillips, & Ball, 2016). Moreover, older adults can still benefit from CCT without having prior experience with computers or specific consoles (Kueider et al., 2012).

The benefits of CCT may vary depending on the population that undergoes training and the conditions under which the training is administered. For high-functioning older adults, the most effective approach for improving executive function and information processing may involve training with game-based software that combines multiple types of tasks (Li et al., 2016). Sometimes drawing on a technique referred to as "core working memory training" (Morrison & Chein, 2011), the combination of training tasks can include complex digital media that require adaptive problem solving with rapid working memory encoding and retrieval demands, draw on multiple modalities, and demand concentration and perseverance. Such multimodal CCT is also more engaging and fun, potentially motivating players to adhere to the program and thereby enhancing training effectiveness (Boot, Champion, et al., 2013; Drobics & Smith, 2014). In the research laboratory, older adults have demonstrated improvements in a range of cognitive abilities—including memory, processing speed, and visuospatial skills—following training with various multimodal CCT programs, particularly those designed under the direction of independent research groups rather than commercial vendors (Lampit, Hallock, & Valenzuela, 2014). For example, a high-profile study reported improved distractibility, sustained attention, and working memory, along with enhanced patterns of neural activity related to cognitive control, following multitask training with Neuroracer, a virtual driving game (Anguera et al., 2013; see also Chadick, Zanto, & Gazzaley, 2014; Mayas, Parmentier, Andres, & Ballesteros, 2014; but for a list of insightful questions about the methods, data, and interpretations of the Neuroracer study, see Simons, 2013).

In addition to CCT programs developed in the laboratory, commercial video games may facilitate similar, albeit specific, enhancements in cognitive performance: Correlational studies have claimed that older adults who report solving certain types of brainteasers such as Sudoku or Tetris exhibit higher speeds of visual processing compared to non-gamers (Wilms & Nielsen, 2014). Nevertheless, older adults who regularly engage in these types of activities may be more open to new experiences (Jackson, Hill, Payne, Roberts, & Stine-Morrow, 2012), a personality trait which may account for differences in cognitive function rather than the puzzles themselves. Action video games—including complex action games such as Medal of Honour and Space Fortress—may facilitate improvements in cognitive abilities such as processing speed and executive control in older adults (for an early example using older games, see Clark, Lanphear, & Riddick, 1987). The magnitude of cognitive improvement experienced through video game training, moreover, has been argued to increase with age (Toril, Reales, & Ballesteros, 2014), but booster sessions may be necessary for sustained benefits (Ballesteros et al., 2015).

Another important influence on the degree to which people benefit from CCT might be the context in which the training occurs. Home-based programs appear less effective than trainer-facilitated training (Wadley et al., 2006), although the degree to which improvements arise from coaching versus the act of traveling to a facility is unclear. Some form of formal coaching nevertheless seems important to web-based applications; reports of significant improvement often describe interventions with at least one supervised weekly session (Lampit et al., 2014). Trainer-mediated programs that offer general support rather than dictate specific rules may help maintain participants' confidence and motivation and ensure their proper interaction with the program. Regularly administering CCT as part of a group or through multiplayer games that foster social interactions and a sense of competition may enhance the effectiveness of such programs in both healthy and cognitively impaired older adults (Drobics & Smith, 2014). An example of such an integrative CCT is the ElderGames Project (Gamberini et al., 2009), a European government initiative supported by independent companies, recreation centers, and universities. Designed to prevent age-related cognitive impairment, ElderGames encourages cross-cultural and intergenerational social relationships within a CCT program administered through an interactive, multiplayer tabletop. For adults with limited opportunities for regular face-to-face social interaction, virtual multiplayer games and social networks may offer at least some of the same benefits. In addition to providing social enjoyment, the added demands of communication and team-based problem-solving may increase the effectiveness of single-player programs.

Alternatively, CCT may focus on simpler, domain-specific strategy training (Morrison & Chein, 2011). Rather than exercising or restoring a general cognitive skill, strategy training often aims to circumvent deficits (e.g., in working memory) resulting from injury or disease. A number of applied memory strategies appear beneficial and are applicable to various contexts either within or independent of digital training platforms (McCabe, Redick, & Engle, 2016). For older adults, including those who are healthy (Mowszowski, Lampit, Walton, & Naismith, 2016) but especially those with cognitive impairment, strategy-based CCT may be more effective (Gross et al., 2012; Reijnders et al., 2013). In the domain of memory, for example, pure memory strategy training, compared to multimodal cognitive training, appears to have greater benefits for memory itself (Li et al., 2016). Teaching people domain-specific strategies yields circumscribed benefits that are unlikely to transfer to untrained abilities (Green & Bavelier, 2008); however, in rehabilitation, such specific improvement is often the primary goal. Strategy training mixed with use of engaging media, such as video games, may further benefit cognitively impaired people by increasing motivation and engagement with the task and encouraging the deep, enjoyable concentration of "flow states" (Astell et al., 2014).

Caveats

The current evidence on CCT for older adults is conflicting and has engendered a contentious debate among experts in the field ("Cognitive Training Data: An Open Letter," 2014; "A Consensus on the Brain Training Industry from the Scientific Community," 2014). Much of the controversy centers on the rigor with which researchers and program developers have gathered and interpreted evidence of CCT's effectiveness. Notably, a number of commercial CCT programs in today's market have *no* scientific evidence to support them. Even when studies of a particular CCT protocol exist, they are often too few or too low-quality for meaningful interpretation. The danger of a reporting bias exists among CCT companies and, perhaps more importantly, among academic journals, where positive effects are more likely to be published than null results.

Heterogeneity in design, training and outcome measures, and inclusion criteria hinder comparisons across individual studies. Moreover, the risk of "training-to-task" exists if training closely resembles the tests used to measure changes in performance before and after an intervention. Even when the training and outcome tasks differ, it is often unclear whether improvements occur for a circumscribed type of activity (i.e., near transfer) or generalize to a broad cognitive ability, with enhancement observed in real-world measures (i.e., far transfer). The largest effects of CCT are on trained tasks and, to a lesser extent, on tasks that closely resemble them (Karbach & Verhaeghen, 2014); evidence for sustained far transfer is weak (Melby-Lervag, Redick, & Hulme, 2016) and can be difficult to evaluate in the existing literature because of methodological problems in many studies (Simons et al., 2016). Many studies lack high-quality control conditions: Traditionally, studies have tended to include only a no-contact or wait-list control, which can account for practice effects and factors related to the passing of time or the natural progression of disease. However, studies using an "active" control requiring the control group to perform comparably engaging tasks under the same experimental conditions as the treatment group are methodologically superior. Use of active control groups can help isolate key components that contribute to a program's success. Unfortunately, the studies that do use an active control condition tend to compare dynamic CCT to repetitive and, arguably, less engaging control tasks (Walton et al., 2015).

In addition, active control groups are essential to account for psychological factors, including participant motivation, engagement in the task, and expectation of effectiveness (i.e., the placebo effect; Boot, Simons, Stothart, & Stutts, 2013). To date, studies largely attempt to minimize the influence of these psychological factors by blinding participants and experimenters to the conditions to which participants have been assigned in hopes that similar proportions of participants will assume they are in the "intervention" condition. This can be difficult to guarantee in the case of a no-contact or wait-list control, however. Furthermore, studies rarely assess participants' levels of expectations and motivation directly and, at most, use proxy measures of motivation such as percentage of program completed. Aside from these methodological limitations, variability exists in treatment adherence across studies on cognitive interventions, particularly those merging virtual reality or gaming systems with physical activity (Miller et al., 2014). These caveats limit the interpretability of reported results and likely account for the vexing pattern of unsuccessful replications of initial positive findings across the literature.

A final consideration is that, even when all of the aforementioned conditions are met, the majority of studies supporting CCT assess effects under ideal, artificial conditions. For example, a trial of a program that is purported to enhance visual attention will typically measure visual attention on a computer in a quiet research laboratory, perhaps in front of a precisely calibrated simulator. However, visual attention is not only used, but also extremely important, behind the wheel of a car driving through the real—unpredictable—world. In this regard, CCT companies and program developers should instead claim that their products show the potential for, rather than proof of, real-world effectiveness.

BEYOND COMPUTER GAMES: TECHNOLOGY-MEDIATED EXTENSIONS TO COGNITIVE TRAINING

The union of cognitive interventions with digital technology has numerous potential advantages. On a large scale, data mining techniques on social and other digital media can provide numerous types of information from thousands of people and help researchers better design individual programs while gleaning insights into human behavior and cognition (Ruths & Pfeffer, 2014). Within the scope of individual therapeutics, CCT software can calibrate the intervention to each person's capacities and change dynamically in response to performance. Digital game platforms offer the possibility of virtual coaching and immediate feedback and can create "desirable difficulty" in the program; in other words, digital media offer the possibility of tailoring cognitive exercise to individual strengths and weaknesses and attaining a level of challenge appropriate for each participant. Similar to the tracking of medications, CCT can discretely track treatment adherence. Furthermore, in comparison to traditional, face-to-face therapy sessions, CCT demands fewer resources, including time, money, and equipment (Wadley et al., 2006). Digital software permits multiple concurrent sessions to be directed by a single professional. Thus, web-based applications have the collective advantage of offering standardized care from the comfort and privacy of home or through group sessions while also increasing the accessibility of treatment. Moreover, web-based CCT enables researchers to examine larger samples using fewer resources. It is common for studies to now include hundreds (e.g., Smith et al., 2009) or even thousand of participants (e.g., Owen et al., 2010).

CCT can also incorporate technologies that enable self-directed changes in brain activity and physiological responses. Through the process of *neurofeedback*, participants actively learn to associate and control their own emotional reactions or behaviors with specific patterns of brain activity that are displayed on a screen in real time (Angelakis et al., 2007; deCharms, 2008). Different approaches rely on electrical brain activity (i.e., electroencephalogram [EEG]), blood oxygenation level (i.e., functional magnetic resonance imaging [fMRI] or functional near-infrared spectroscopy [fNIRS]), or a combination of these. Although the reported effects of neurofeedback are controversial and may result from placebo (Thibault, Lifshitz, & Raz, 2016; Thibault & Raz, 2016), older adults have improved on measures related to attention and executive function following various neurofeedback techniques (Gruzelier, 2014a). Similarly, *biofeedback techniques* pertaining to one's own cardiac, electrodermal, or breathing output during CCT may help control a plethora of physiological and emotional responses related to conditions such as stress, anxiety, and even cardiovascular or muscular conditions typically treated with medication (Peira, Pourtois, & Fredrikson, 2013; Prinsloo, Rauch, & Derman, 2014). Aside from monitoring brain activity, brain–computer interfaces (BCI) can couple patterns of brain activity associated with a particular command to an output on digital software and can incorporate common cognitive tasks as part of a gamified approach (Portugal, Ferreira, Reis, Pinho, & Dias, 2013). Streamlined versions of this technology include NeuralPhone, which uses EEG signals conveyed through a wireless, commercially available headset to drive smartphone applications (Campbell & Choudhury, 2012). Integrating neuro- or biofeedback into BCI may improve BCI functionality (Fazli et al., 2012). Influencing activity using these devices may improve learning conditions and increase the likelihood of training-related cognitive improvements. Modulation of one's own brain activity may be particularly beneficial for those who require assistance during learning.

Regardless of health status, older adults generally require more time and effort to improve on a practiced task (Rabbitt, 1993). Software-based cognitive interventions afford older adults the time to practice on their own. Creating user-friendly game platforms can also ease the process of adapting to new technologies and render game playing more enjoyable. In addition, noninvasive brain stimulation, including transcranial magnetic stimulation and transcranial direct-current stimulation (tDCS), have the potential to enhance plasticity while performing cognitively challenging tasks, thus decreasing the time necessary to acquire a particular cognitive skill and increasing the magnitude of improvement within a specific timeframe (Martin, Liu, Alonzo, Green, & Loo, 2014). For instance, preliminary studies have claimed improvements in cognitive control following such stimulation (Dityе, Jacobson, Walsh, & Lavidor, 2012). Relatively affordable, portable, and—if used properly—safe and painless (Bikson et al., 2016), tDCS and related approaches are a particularly appealing tool for home-based CCT or interventions involving large numbers of participants. Portable devices and mobile applications from commercial vendors such as Foc. Us (Transcranial Ltd., 2016), Thync (2016), and Halo (Halo Neuroscience, 2016) aim to leverage this technology to target consumers of all ages, promising improved mood, mental function (e.g., for gaming), and physical performance (e.g., for sports) using their headsets.

The unsupervised use of CCT and, especially, of brain stimulating devices can be problematic. What happens when experimental products appear prematurely on the commercial market? CCT applications are largely unregulated by governmental or third-party agencies (Schulke, 2013), often advertising themselves as entertainment products to avoid legal ramifications. Brain stimulation poses health risks if not used properly; however, universal guidelines do not currently exist. Short-term risks include scalp tenderness, headaches, dizziness and—however rare—mild burns or induced seizures (Davis, 2014). Potential long-term side effects related to prolonged exposure to the current (i.e., >30 minutes), repeated use, incorrect settings (e.g., high intensity of current), or use in inappropriate contexts are not currently documented but require more explicit evaluation (Bikson et al., 2016). Similarly, the safety of brain stimulation over unstudied brain areas and when used with children and certain clinical populations is unclear (Kadosh, Levy, O'Shea, Shea, & Savulescu, 2012). Furthermore, studies report inconsistent findings regarding polarity effects on cognitive function (Jacobson, Koslowsky, & Lavidor, 2012). Recurrent issues in CCT research, including lack of consensus regarding optimal frequency and duration of training, as well as trial design and controls, are also pertinent to brain stimulation (e.g., tDCS; see Berryhill, Peterson, Jones, & Stephens, 2014; Schambra, Bikson, Wager, DosSantos, & DaSilva, 2014) and to other approaches, including neurofeedback (Gruzelier, 2014b). A 2014 consensus statement—signed by more than 70 cognitive scientists—warns consumers against the overzealous claims of cognitive and lifestyle improvements made by companies ("A Consensus on the Brain Training Industry from the Scientific Community," 2014); the resulting counterstatement echoes many of the same concerns despite concluding on a more optimistic note ("Cognitive Training Data: An Open Letter," 2014). Thus, despite the potential of CCT and adjunct technologies in improving cognitive function, outstanding methodological questions and health concerns demand caution in using individual programs.

Researchers are increasingly noting flaws in CCT studies and making recommendations to promote higher quality research in future (e.g., Mowszowski et al., 2016; Simons et al., 2016). Navigating the sea of available products, however, is difficult for consumers. As marketers push the idea that CCT works for people of all ages, researchers rush to counter overzealous claims, feeling compelled to remind the public that these products often show potential for effectiveness, rather than definitive evidence ("A Consensus on the Brain Training Industry from the Scientific Community," 2014). In January 2016, Lumos Labs received a $50 million fine for "deceiv[ing] consumers with unfounded claims that Lumosity games can help users perform better at work and in school, and reduce or delay cognitive impairment associated with age and other serious health conditions" (Federal Trade Commission, 2016). Cases against CCT companies are nevertheless rare. Many companies skirt the legal ramifications of false advertising by leading consumers to infer certain claims, rather than stating them explicitly. Advertising, testimonials, and inaccurate causal implications are so common that they are difficult to combat. Since the 1990s, for example, scientific evidence has largely suggested that crosswords and other puzzles hardly improve intelligence or general cognitive function (Hambrick, Salthouse, & Meinz, 1999), yet the myth that they are helpful persists. In an effort to increase scientific rigor and combat criticism, CCT companies might opt to collaborate formally with independent researchers to evaluate their programs'effectiveness.

Technology and Aging: Methodological Considerations

Convenience and Its Costs

One of the greatest benefits of digital technology is the possibility for remote (often home-based) use. Digitally mediated programs offer not only convenience, but also peace of mind: older adults can log in regardless of physical or geographical limitations and need not face unpleasant or dangerous conditions to travel to a lab or clinic. Scheduling is rarely an issue since most programs allow participants to complete their cognitive assessment or exercises whenever they wish. Costs associated with traveling and meeting with a clinician or coach are minimized. Convenience, therefore, is the most evident advantage of computerized assessment and training.

What are the potential costs? Financially, while many CCT programs are initially free or low-cost, companies can limit access to services unless users upgrade their subscriptions. Furthermore, absent a researcher or clinician providing guidance and debriefing, there is no guarantee that participants truly understand the potential risks, benefits, and personal as well as communal implications of the program (Nosek, Banaji, & Greenwald, 2002). Finally, although password-protected accounts offer relative privacy, the security of digitally collected and stored information can never be guaranteed. Even if program administrators do their best to ensure discretion and confidentiality or anonymity, the possibility for hackers to extract information remains for all databases and software applications—even those on secured networks. Although standards of security and privacy for electronically transmitted health information exist, governing bodies and legislation such as the Health Insurance Portability and Accountability Act in the United States may be inadequate in ensuring that third-party developers adhere to proper data protection standards (Schulke, 2013). Moreover, guidelines on how to best protect and handle digital data differ based on jurisdiction. As a result, concerns about the protection of sensitive data remain far from trivial.

The Importance of Technology: Seniors Are Catching Up

Not surprisingly, today older adults do not use computers and virtual media as much as younger generations. According to a national survey in the United Kingdom, 13% of older adults had never used the Internet as of the first quarter of 2014, compared to a negligible percentage in younger age brackets (Office for National Statistics, 2014). The numbers are comparable in the United States, where the Pew Internet Project reported that 47% of adults over 65 years of age, and 66% of adults over 75 do not use the Internet or email (Zickuhr & Madden, 2012). Within the latter age group, perceived relevancy and lack of confidence in the ability to master new technologies are the leading reasons reported for Internet abstinence (Charness & Boot, 2009). Other factors that may contribute to technological aversion include ineffective communication and lack of accommodation for the changing cognitive and physical needs of older adults (Pew & Hemel, 2004).

Despite these statistics, the number of older adults using the Internet—including email and social networking—and electronic gadgets is increasing steadily. For example, a third of British seniors now use the Internet daily, three times more than a decade ago (Office for National Statistics, 2014; Statistics, 2013). The increases are similar across the Industrialized world (Statistics Canada, 2014; Zickuhr & Madden, 2012). Moreover, once online, many older adults will begin using the Internet on a daily basis. Organizations such as the Center for Research on Aging and Technology Enhancement (CREATE, 2012) aim to facilitate this process by studying the degree to which technological interfaces and instructional support offered by developers can be tailored to the capabilities of target users.

Do You See What I See? Cognitive and Perceptual Aspects of Aging

In healthy aging, cognitive decline is subtle and relatively specific (for a review, see Davidson & Winocur, 2017). Older adults mainly show declines in speed of perceptual and mental processing, and in aspects of attention, short- and long-term memory, and complex problem solving (i.e., aspects of executive function). These are the domains that receive the greatest focus in cognitive assessment and rehabilitation.

Several factors can exacerbate or mimic cognitive decline, even when cognitive capacities are normal. For example, low mood or depression can resemble memory impairment. Perceptual problems, such as visual or auditory limitations due to peripheral sensory loss, can masquerade as cognitive decline. In other words, older adults who have trouble seeing or hearing may be mislabeled as having cognitive difficulties. As with cognitive changes in aging, perceptual changes are relatively specific: in vision, common issues include loss of acuity and contrast sensitivity (Owsley, 2011). In hearing, loss of high-frequency acuity is especially prevalent, meaning that older adults will have greater difficulty hearing higher pitched sounds (e.g., having more difficulty understanding speech produced by a woman than speech produced by a man).

Two additional points regarding digital technology are worth mentioning. First, an overarching problem in cognitive aging is that the costs of multitasking appear to be greater for older adults than for the young. Thus, any assessment, rehabilitation, or other application that has "too much going on" risks underestimating the level of performance that older adults could achieve under less taxing circumstances. Second, in most aspects of cognitive and perceptual aging we see a wide range of individual differences: some older adults do as well as the best young people, but others perform far below that level. Factors related to personality (e.g., openness to experience) and beliefs about intelligence may also contribute to differences in adherence to and performance on CCT programs (Double & Birney, 2016). Cognitive assessment and rehabilitation tasks must therefore be constructed to allow for wide variability in performance, and extensive pilot testing might be required to ensure that scores are not at the ceiling or on the floor.

Practical Considerations for Researchers and Practitioners

What practices will help prevent, rectify, or overcome current methodological and practical challenges in providing cognitive assessment and intervention to older adults? The most fundamental considerations involve the physical and cognitive capabilities of older adults. In addition, researchers and practitioners must address the psychological barriers preventing older adults from using technology. Many older adults are intimidated by the rapid pace of digital media and may believe themselves incapable of mastering the novel techniques and terminology required to enjoy new technologies. Such perceptions may be amplified by societal stereotypes about older generations being incapable of mastering technology. Program developers often fail to take these fears into account and thus might not convey the potential benefits of specific programs in a language that appeals to the target population.

Together, these perceptual barriers often discourage older adults from investing the time needed to learn new technologies—even if they might have otherwise wanted to learn. On the other hand, if someone has lived an entire lifetime without computers, the Internet, and sophisticated mobile applications, explaining why such technology could improve his or her standard of living may mean little unless potential losses—becoming disconnected from the community, losing touch with loved ones, receiving suboptimal care, etc.—are effectively communicated. Minimizing age-related stereotypes as well as other cultural or demographic differences may help counteract the fears and lack of knowledge of older adults and ensure that as many participants as possible have an optimal experience.

For researchers, adopting scientifically rigorous methods is essential to ensuring that an intervention genuinely has the intended effects. The design of a program must, first and foremost, cater to a particular population. Older adults with cognitive or physical impairments have vastly different requirements from those who are high functioning and independent. To increase the applicability of programs to different needs and capacities, digital technologies can help monitor data on large scales (e.g., through web-based data mining) and facilitate comprehensive, retroactive analyses (e.g., meta-analytic reviews). Such analytic approaches may serve as a filter to identify which cognitive programs have shown the most potential and in what contexts, thereby optimizing investment in labor- and resource-intensive—but nevertheless essential—controlled trials for effectiveness (Howren, Vander Weg, & Wolinsky, 2014). When evaluating a particular program, researchers must select an appropriate number of participants; ensure they are matched for potential confounders such as age, education level, and health status; and randomize them into appropriate comparison groups (Boot & Kramer, 2014).

Understanding different participant profiles is also crucial. For instance, the vast majority of research on computerized cognitive assessment and interventions has used white, educated, industrialized, rich, democratic (WEIRD) participants (Henrich, Heine, & Norenzayan, 2010). However, many non-WEIRD individuals are using these technologies. Factors that contribute to cognitive aging and patterns of digital technology use—including age-related stereotypes or daily access to and dependence on digital media—may have varying influences in different cultures (e.g., Eastern cultures that, arguably, revere the aged) and geographic locations (e.g., urban vs. rural communities). Further research on cognitive aging and on digital technology for assessment and intervention with non-WEIRD older adults is needed.

Moreover, studies increasingly administer interventions using web-based media that do not require any participant or patient contact. Although convenient for both participants and researchers, remote administration of cognitive interventions introduces considerable variability in the environment in which the intervention is conducted. Given the value of offering participants such freedom, however, we argue that this is not a flaw as long as researchers can demonstrate program effectiveness under the same conditions during the study period. In order to ensure that participants are administering the intervention properly—an especially important consideration for potentially dangerous techniques such as tDCS—researchers and clinicians may consider holding a training phase during which participants learn the proper method by which to administer the intervention. Furthermore, researchers can impose a regular meeting date during which they observe participants during the intervention to ensure proper administration. These meetings can also serve as social gatherings and promote team-based training in groups.

Digital technologies offer efficient, noninvasive methods for assessing and enhancing cognitive function in older adults. Leveraging digital tools can broaden the range of data and help maximize the effectiveness of interventions. Considering these guidelines should help academics and practitioners overcome the challenges we have outlined and ensure that the future of older adults using digital technology is more likely to be utopian than dystopian.

Acknowledgments

We wish to thank Dr. David Faust and Annick Tanguay for helpful comments on an earlier draft of this chapter.

References

Angelakis, E., Stathopoulou, S., Frymiare, J. L., Green, D. L., Lubar, J. F., & Kounios, J. (2007). EEG neurofeedback: A brief overview and an example of peak alpha frequency training for cognitive enhancement in the elderly. *Clinical Neuropsychologist, 21*(1), 110–29.

Anguera, J. A., Boccanfuso, J., Rintoul, J. L., Al-Hashimi, O., Faraji, F., Janowich, J., . . . Gazzaley, A. (2013). Video game training enhances cognitive control in older adults. *Nature, 501*(7465), 97. doi:10.1038/Nature12486

Astell, A., Alm, N., Dye, R., Gowans, G., Vaughan, P., & Ellis, M. (2014). Digital video games for older adults with cognitive impairment. In K. Miesenberger, D. Fels, D. Archambault, P. Peňáz, & W. Zagler (Eds.), *Computers helping people with special needs* (pp. 264–71). New York: Springer International Publishing.

Ballesteros, S., Mayas, J., Prieto, A., Toril, P., Pita, C., de Leon, L. P., . . . Waterworth, J. A. (2015). A randomized controlled trial of brain training with non-action video games in older adults: Results of the 3-month follow-up. *Frontiers in Aging Neuroscience, 7*: Article 45, 1–12. doi:10.3389/fnagi.2015.00045

Berryhill, M. E., Peterson, D. J., Jones, K. T., & Stephens, J. A. (2014). Hits and misses: Leveraging tDCS to advance cognitive research. *Frontiers in Psychology, 5*: Article 800, 1–12. doi:10.3389/Fpsyg.2014.00800

Bikson, M., Grossman, P., Thomas, C., Zannou, A. L., Jiang, J., Adnan, T., . . . Woods, A. J. (2016). Safety of transcranial direct current stimulation: Evidence based update 2016. *Brain Stimulation, 9*(5), 641–61. doi:10.1016/j.brs.2016.06.004

Boot, W. R., Champion, M., Blakely, D. P., Wright, T., Souders, D. J., & Charness, N. (2013). Video games as a means to reduce age-related cognitive decline: Attitudes, compliance, and effectiveness. *Frontiers in Psychology*, 4: Article 31, 1–9. doi:10.3389/Fpsyg.2013.00031

Boot, W. R., & Kramer, A. F. (2014). The brain-games conundrum: Does cognitive training really sharpen the mind? http://www.dana.org/Cerebrum/2014/The_Brain-Games_Conundrum__Does_Cognitive_Training_Really_Sharpen_the_Mind_/-sthash.iPYa8y4b.dpuf

Boot, W. R., Simons, D. J., Stothart, C., & Stutts, C. (2013). The pervasive problem with placebos in psychology: Why active control groups are not sufficient to rule out placebo effects. *Perspectives on Psychological Science, 8*(4), 445–54. doi:10.1177/1745691613491271

Bossaer, J. B., Gray, J. A., Miller, S. E., Enck, G., Gaddipati, V. C., & Enck, R. E. (2013). The use and misuse of prescription stimulants as "cognitive enhancers" by students at one academic health sciences center. *Academic Medicine, 88*(7), 967–71. doi:10.1097/Acm.0b013e318294fc7b

Brouillette, R. M., Foil, H., Fontenot, S., Correro, A., Allen, R., Martin, C. K.,... Keller, J. N. (2013). Feasibility, reliability, and validity of a smartphone based application for the assessment of cognitive function in the elderly. *Plos One, 8*(6). doi:ARTN e65925 DOI 10.1371/journal.pone.0065925

Campbell, A., & Choudhury, T. (2012). From smart to cognitive phones. *IEEE Pervasive Computing, 11*(3), 7–11.

Cancelli, I., Beltrame, M., Gigli, G. L., & Valente, M. (2009). Drugs with anticholinergic properties: Cognitive and neuropsychiatric side-effects in elderly patients. *Neurological Sciences, 30*(2), 87–92. doi:10.1007/s10072-009-0033-y

Carr, N. G. (2010). *The shallows: What the Internet is doing to our brains* (1st ed.). New York: W. W. Norton.

Cellan-Jones, R. (2014). Stephen Hawking warns artificial intelligence could end mankind. *BBC News: Technology.* http://www.bbc.com/news/technology-30290540

Chadick, J. Z., Zanto, T. P., & Gazzaley, A. (2014). Structural and functional differences in medial prefrontal cortex underlie distractibility and suppression deficits in ageing. *Nature Communications, 5*(4223): 1–27. doi:10.1038/Ncomms5223

Chan, M. Y., Haber, S., Drew, L. M., & Park, D. C. (2014). Training older adults to use tablet computers: Does it enhance cognitive function? *Gerontologist, 56*(3): 475–84. doi:10.1093/geront/gnu057

Charness, N., & Boot, W. R. (2009). Aging and information technology use: Potential and barriers. *Current Directions in Psychological Science, 18*(5), 253–58.

Cheng, Y., Wu, W., Feng, W., Wang, J., Chen, Y., Shen, Y.,... Li, C. (2012). The effects of multi-domain versus single-domain cognitive training in non-demented older people: A randomized controlled trial. *BMC Medicine, 10,* 30. doi:10.1186/1741-7015-10-30

Clark, J. E., Lanphear, A. K., & Riddick, C. C. (1987). The effects of videogame playing on the response selection processing of elderly adults. *Journals of Gerontology, 42*(1), 82–5.

CogniFit Inc. CogniFit https://www.cognifit.com

Cognitive training data: An open letter. (2014). http://www.cognitivetrainingdata.org/.

Cotten, S. R., Ford, G., Ford, S., & Hale, T. M. (2014). Internet use and depression among retired older adults in the United States: A longitudinal analysis. *Journals of Gerontology Series B-Psychological Sciences and Social Sciences, 69*(5), 763–71. doi:10.1093/Geronb/Gbu018

CREATE. (2012). Center for Research and Education on Aging and Technology Enhancement http://www.create-center.org/

Cruz, V. T., Pais, J., Bento, V., Mateus, C., Colunas, M., Alves, I.,... Rocha, N. P. (2013). A rehabilitation tool designed for intensive web-based cognitive training: Description and usability study. *JMIR Research Protocols, 2*(2), e59. doi:10.2196/resprot.2899

Csikszentmihalyi, M. (1990). *Flow: The psychology of optimal experience* (1st ed.). New York: Harper & Row.

Dafnis, J. (2014). This neuroscientist wants to use video games like medicine. Game Informer, New York, NY: HarperCollins Publishers.

Davidson, P. S. R., & Winocur, G. (2017). Aging and cognition. *Reference Module in Neuroscience and Biobehavioral Psychology,* 1–7. doi:10.1016/B978-0-12-809324-5.00252–2

Davis, N. J. (2014). Transcranial stimulation of the developing brain: A plea for extreme caution. *Frontiers in Human Neuroscience,* 8, Article 600, 1–4. doi:10.3389/Fnhum.2014.00600

Dawadi, P. N., Cook, D. J., & Schmitter-Edgecombe, M. (2013). Automated cognitive health assessment using smart home monitoring of complex tasks. *IEEE Transactions on Systems, Man, and Cybernetics Systems, 43*(6), 1302–13. doi:10.1109/Tsmc.2013.2252338

deCharms, R. C. (2008). Applications of real-time fMRI. *Nature Reviews Neuroscience, 9*(9), 720–9. doi:10.1038/nrn2414

Ditye, T., Jacobson, L., Walsh, V., & Lavidor, M. (2012). Modulating behavioral inhibition by tDCS combined with cognitive training. *Experimental Brain Research, 219*(3), 363–8. doi:10.1007/S00221-012-3098-4

Double, K. S., & Birney, D. P. (2016). The effects of personality and metacognitive beliefs on cognitive training adherence and performance. *Personality and Individual Differences, 102,* 7–12. doi:10.1016/j.paid.2016.04.101

Drobics, M., & Smith, S. (2014). Game-based IT solutions for active and healthy aging. *Games for Training, Education, Health and Sports, 8395,* 8–11.

Emanuel, R. M., Frellsen, S. L., Kashima, K. J., Sanguino, S. M., Sierles, F. S., & Lazarus, C. J. (2013). Cognitive enhancement drug use among future physicians: Findings from a multi-institutional census of medical students. *Journal of General Internal Medicine, 28*(8), 1028–34. doi:10.1007/s11606-012-2249-4

Fan, J., McCandliss, B., Sommer, T., Raz, A., & Posner, M. (2001). Testing the efficiency and independence of attentional networks. *Journal of Cognitive Neuroscience,* 1(14): 340–47.

Fazli, S., Mehnert, J., Steinbrink, J., Curio, G., Villringer, A., Muller, K. R., & Blankertz, B. (2012). Enhanced performance by a hybrid NIRS-EEG brain computer interface. *Neuroimage, 59*(1), 519–29. doi:10.1016/j.neuroimage.2011.07.084

Federal Trade Commission. (2016). Lumosity to pay $2 million to settle FTC deceptive advertising charges for its "brain training" program. https://www.ftc.gov/news-events/press-releases/2016/01/lumosity-pay-2-million-settle-ftc-deceptive-advertising-charges

Fox, C., Richardson, K., Maidment, I. D., Savva, G. M., Matthews, F. E., Smithard, D.,... Brayne, C. (2011). Anticholinergic medication use and cognitive impairment in the older population: The Medical Research Council Cognitive Function and Ageing Study. *Journal of the American Geriatrics Society, 59*(8), 1477–83. doi:10.1111/J.1532–5415.2011.03491.X

Franke, A. G., Bagusat, C., Rust, S., Engel, A., & Lieb, K. (2014). Substances used and prevalence rates of pharmacological cognitive enhancement among healthy subjects. *European Archives of Psychiatry and Clinical Neuroscience, 264*(Suppl 1), S83–90. doi:10.1007/s00406-014-0537-1

Gamberini, L., Martino, F., Seraglia, B., Spagnolli, A., Fabregat, M., Ibanez, F.,... Andres, J. M. (2009). Eldergames project: An innovative mixed reality table-top solution to preserve cognitive functions in elderly people. In *2009 2nd Conference on Human System Interactions* (pp. 161–6).

Gindrat, A.-D., Chytiris, M., Balerna, M., Rouiller, E. M., & Ghosh, A. (2015). Use-dependent cortical processing from fingertips in touchscreen phone users. *Current Biology.* doi:http://dx.doi.org/10.1016/j.cub.2014.11.026

Google. (2014). The Glass Explorer Program. http://www.google.com/glass/start/

Green, C. S., & Bavelier, D. (2008). Exercising your brain: A review of human brain plasticity and training-induced learning. *Psychology and Aging, 23*(4), 692–701.

Gross, A. L., Parisi, J. M., Spira, A. P., Kueider, A. M., Ko, J. Y., Saczynski, J. S.,... Rebok, G. W. (2012). Memory training interventions for older adults: A meta-analysis. *Aging Mental Health, 16*(6), 722–34. doi:10.1080/13607863.2012.667783

Gruzelier, J. H. (2014a). EEG-neurofeedback for optimising performance. I: A review of cognitive and affective outcome in healthy participants. *Neuroscience and Biobehavioral Reviews, 44*, 124–41. doi:10.1016/J.Neubiorev.2013.09.015

Gruzelier, J. H. (2014b). EEG-neurofeedback for optimising performance. III: A review of methodological and theoretical considerations. *Neuroscience and Biobehavioral Reviews, 44*, 159–82. doi:10.1016/J.Neubiorev.2014.03.015

Gur, R. C., Richard, J., Hughett, P., Calkins, M. E., Macy, L., Bilker, W. B., . . . Gur, R. E. (2010). A cognitive neuroscience-based computerized battery for efficient measurement of individual differences: Standardization and initial construct validation. *Journal of Neuroscience Methods, 187*(2), 254–62. doi:10.1016/j.jneumeth.2009.11.017

Halo Neuroscience. (2016). Halo. https://www.haloneuro.com/

Hambrick, D. Z., Salthouse, T. A., & Meinz, E. J. (1999). Predictors of crossword puzzle proficiency and moderators of age-cognition relations. *Journal of Experimental Psychology General, 128*(2), 131–64.

Hampshire, A., Highfield, R. R., Parkin, B. L., & Owen, A. M. (2012). Fractionating human intelligence. *Neuron, 76*(6), 1225–37. doi:10.1016/J.Neuron.2012.06.022

Hassan, T. A., Klein, R. M., & Wilson, G. C. (2015). The AttentionTrip: A game-like task for assessment of attention networks. *Canadian Journal of Experimental Psychology, 69*(4), 374.

Heaton, R. K., Akshoomoff, N., Tulsky, D., Mungas, D., Weintraub, S., Dikmen, S., . . . Gershon, R. (2014). Reliability and validity of composite scores from the NIH Toolbox Cognition Battery in adults. *Journal of the International Neuropsychological Society, 20*(6), 588–98. doi:10.1017/S1355617714000241

Henrich, J., Heine, S. J., & Norenzayan, A. (2010). The weirdest people in the world? *Behavioral and Brain Sciences, 33*(2–3), 61. doi:10.1017/S0140525x0999152x

Howren, M. B., Vander Weg, M. W., & Wolinsky, F. D. (2014). Computerized cognitive training interventions to improve neuropsychological outcomes: Evidence and future directions. *Journal of Comparative Effectiveness Research, 3*(2), 145–54. doi:10.2217/Cer.14.6

Jackson, J. J., Hill, P. L., Payne, B. R., Roberts, B. W., & Stine-Morrow, E. A. L. (2012). Can an old dog learn (and want to experience) new tricks? Cognitive training increases openness to experience in older adults. *Psychology and Aging, 27*(2), 286–92. doi:10.1037/a0025918

Jacobson, L., Koslowsky, M., & Lavidor, M. (2012). tDCS polarity effects in motor and cognitive domains: A meta-analytical review. *Experimental Brain Research, 216*(1), 1–10. doi:10.1007/S00221-011-2891-9

Kadosh, R. C., Levy, N., O'Shea, J., Shea, N., & Savulescu, J. (2012). The neuroethics of non-invasive brain stimulation. *Current Biology, 22*(4), R108–11.

Kapur, N., Glisky, E. L., & Wilson, B. A. (2002). External memory aids and computers in memory rehabilitation. In A. D. Baddeley, M. D. Kopelman, & B. A. Wilson (Eds.), *Handbook of memory disorders* (2nd ed., pp. 757–83). Chichester, UK: Wiley.

Karbach, J., & Verhaeghen, P. (2014). Making working memory work: A meta-analysis of executive-control and working memory training in older adults. *Psychological Science, 25*(11), 2027–37. doi:10.1177/0956797614548725

Katz, H. H., & Nesbitt, M. T. (2014). US8777923 B2.

Kaufman, D., Sauve, L., Renaud, L., & Duplaa, E. (2014). *Cognitive benefits of digital games for older adults*. Paper presented at the EdMedia, Tampere, Finland.

Kelly, M. E., Loughrey, D., Lawlor, B. A., Robertson, I. H., Walsh, C., & Brennan, S. (2014). The impact of cognitive training and mental stimulation on cognitive and everyday functioning of healthy older adults: A systematic review and meta-analysis. *Ageing Research Reviews, 15*, 28–43. doi:10.1016/j.arr.2014.02.004

Kueider, A. M., Parisi, J. M., Gross, A. L., & Rebok, G. W. (2012). Computerized cognitive training with older adults: A systematic review. *PLoS One, 7*(7), e40588. doi:10.1371/journal.pone.0040588

Kvedar, J., Coye, M. J., & Everett, W. (2014). Connected health: A review of technologies and strategies to improve patient care with telemedicine and telehealth. *Health Affairs, 33*(2), 194–9. doi:10.1377/Hlthaff.2013.0992

Lampit, A., Hallock, H., & Valenzuela, M. (2014). Computerized cognitive training in cognitively healthy older adults: A systematic review and meta-analysis of effect modifiers. *PLoS Medicine, 11*(11), e1001756. doi:10.1371/journal.pmed.1001756

Levine, B., Bacopulos, A., Anderson, N. D., Black, S. E., Davidson, P. S., Fitneva, S. A., . . . Hampshire, A. (2013). Validation of a novel computerized test battery for automated testing. *Stroke, 44*(12), E196–206.

Li, B., Zhu, X. Y., Hou, J. H., Chen, T. J., Wang, P. Y., & Li, J. (2016). combined cognitive training vs. memory strategy training in healthy older adults. *Frontiers in Psychology, 7*. doi:10.3389/fpsyg.2016.00834

Lumos Labs Inc. (n.d.) Lumosity. http://www.lumosity.com/contact

Lumos Labs Inc. (2013). Lumosity grows 150 percent in the past year reaching over 35 million members worldwide: Mobile and international expansion planned in 2013. Lumosity Press.

Maher, B. (2008). Poll results: Look who's doping. *Nature, 452*(7188), 674–5. doi:10.1038/452674a

Marcum, Z. A., Peron, E. P., & Hanlon, J. T. (2012). Medication use in older adults. In A. B. Newman & H. A. Cauley (Eds.), *The epidemiology of aging* (pp. 317–26). Springer.

Martin, D. M., Liu, R., Alonzo, A., Green, M., & Loo, C. K. (2014). Use of transcranial direct current stimulation (tDCS) to enhance cognitive training: Effect of timing of stimulation. *Experimental Brain Research, 232*(10), 3345–51. doi:10.1007/S00221-014-4022-X

Martin, M., Clare, L., Altgassen, A. M., Cameron, M. H., & Zehnder, F. (2011). Cognition-based interventions for healthy older people and people with mild cognitive impairment. *Cochrane Database of Systematic Reviews* (1). doi:10.1002/14651858.Cd006220.Pub2

Mayas, J., Parmentier, F. B. R., Andres, P., & Ballesteros, S. (2014). Plasticity of attentional functions in older adults after non-action video game training: A randomized controlled trial. *Plos One, 9*(3), e92269. doi:10.1371/journal.pone.0092269

McCabe, J. A., Redick, T. S., & Engle, R. W. (2016). Brain-training pessimism, but applied-memory optimism. *Psychological Science in the Public Interest, 17*(3), 187–91. doi:10.1177/1529100616664716

Melby-Lervag, M., Redick, T. S., & Hulme, C. (2016). Working memory training does not improve performance on measures of intelligence or other measures of "far transfer": Evidence from a meta-analytic review. *Perspectives on Psychological Science, 11*(4), 512–34. doi:10.1177/1745691616635612

Microsoft Corporation. (2013). SenseCam. Microsoft Research. http://research.microsoft.com/en-us/um/cambridge/projects/sensecam/

Miller, K. J., Adair, B. S., Pearce, A. J., Said, C. M., Ozanne, E., & Morris, M. M. (2014). Effectiveness and feasibility of virtual reality and gaming system use at home by older adults for enabling physical activity to improve health-related domains: A systematic review. *Age and Ageing, 43*(2), 188–95. doi:10.1093/Ageing/Aft194

Mintzer, J., & Burns, A. (2000). Anticholinergic side-effects of drugs in elderly people. *Journal of the Royal Society of Medicine, 93*(9), 457–62.

Mitroff, S. R., Biggs, A. T., Adamo, S. H., Dowd, E. W., Winkle, J., & Clark, K. (2014). What can 1 billion trials tell us about visual search? *Journal of Experimental Psychology: Human Perception and Performance.*

Morrison, A. B., & Chein, J. M. (2011). Does working memory training work? The promise and challenges of enhancing cognition by training working memory. *Psychonomic Bulletin & Review, 18*(1), 46–60. doi:10.3758/S13423-010-0034-0

Mowszowski, L., Lampit, A., Walton, C. C., & Naismith, S. L. (2016). Strategy-based cognitive training for improving executive functions in older adults: A systematic review. *Neuropsychological Review, 26*(3), 252–70. doi:10.1007/s11065-016-9329-x

Murray, M. D., & Callahan, C. M. (2003). Improving medication use for older adults: An integrated research agenda. *Annals of Internal Medicine, 139*(5), 425–9.

Myhre, J. W., Mehl, M. R., & Glisky, E. L. (2016). Cognitive benefits of online social networking for healthy older adults. *Journal of Gerontol B Psychological Science and Social Science.* doi:10.1093/geronb/gbw025

Mynatt, E. D., & Rogers, W. A. (2001). Developing technology to support the functional independence of older adults. *Ageing International, 27*(1), 24–41.

National Institutes of Health and Northwestern University. (2006–2012). NIH Toolbox: For the assessment of neurological and behavioral function. http://www.nihtoolbox.org

Nintendo DS. Brain age. http://brainage.nintendo.com

Nosek, B. A., Banaji, M. R., & Greenwald, A. G. (2002). E-research: Ethics, security, design, and control in psychological research on the Internet. *Journal of Social Issues, 58*(1), 161–76. doi:10.1111/1540–4560.00254

Office for National Statistics. (2013). Internet access: Households and individuals, 2013. http://www.ons.gov.uk/ons/dcp171778_322713.pdf

Office for National Statistics. (2014). Internet access: Households and individuals 2014. Newport, Wales.

Owen, A. M., Hampshire, A., Grahn, J. A., Stenton, R., Dajani, S., Burns, A. S., . . . Ballard, C. G. (2010). Putting brain training to the test. *Nature, 465*(7299), 775-U776. doi:10.1038/nature09042

Owsley, C. (2011). Aging and vision. *Vision Research, 51*(13), 1610–22. doi:10.1016/J.Visres.2010.10.020

Parsey, C. M., & Schmitter-Edgecombe, M. (2013). Applications of technology in neuropsychological assessment. *Clinical Neuropsychologist, 27*(8), 1328–61. doi:10.1080/13854046.2013.834971

Partridge, B. J., Bell, S. K., Lucke, J. C., Yeates, S., & Hall, W. D. (2011). Smart drugs "As common as coffee": Media hype about neuroenhancement. *Plos One, 6*(11). doi:10.1371/journal.pone.0028416

Peira, N., Pourtois, G., & Fredrikson, M. (2013). Learned cardiac control with heart rate biofeedback transfers to emotional reactions. *PLoS One, 8*(7), e70004. doi:10.1371/journal.pone.0070004

Pew, R. W., & Hemel, S. B. V. (Eds.). (2004). *Technology for adaptive aging.* Washington, DC: National Academies Press.

Portugal, A. M., Ferreira, D. S., Reis, J. S., Pinho, F., & Dias, N. S. (2013, May). *Cognitive intervention protocol for age-related memory impairments.* 2013 IEEE 2nd International Conference on Serious Games and Applications for Health (SEGAH), Vilamoura, Portugal.

Prinsloo, G. E., Rauch, H. G. L., & Derman, W. E. (2014). A brief review and clinical application of heart rate variability biofeedback in sports, exercise, and rehabilitation medicine. *Physician and Sportsmedicine, 42*(2), 88–99. doi:10.3810/Psm.2014.05.2061

Rabbitt, P. M. A. (1993). Crystal quest: A search for the maintenance of practised skills into old age. In A. D. Baddeley & L. Weiskrantz (Eds.), *Attention, selection awareness and control. A tribute to Donald Broadbent* (pp. 188–230). Oxford: Clarendon Press.

Rabipour, S., & Raz, A. (2012). Training the brain: Fact and fad in cognitive and behavioral remediation. *Brain and Cognition, 79*(2), 159–79. doi:10.1016/j.bandc.2012.02.006

Reardon, S. (2015). Memory-boosting devices tested in humans. *Nature, 527*, 15–6.

Rebok, G. W., Ball, K., Guey, L. T., Jones, R. N., Kim, H. Y., King, J. W., . . . ACTIVE Study Group. (2014). Ten-year effects of the advanced cognitive training for independent and vital elderly cognitive training trial on cognition and everyday functioning in older adults. *Journal of the American Geriatrics Society, 62*(1), 16–24. doi:10.1111/Jgs.12607

Reijnders, J., van Heugten, C., & van Boxtel, M. (2013). Cognitive interventions in healthy older adults and people with mild cognitive impairment: A systematic review. *Ageing Research Reviews, 12*(1), 263–75. doi:10.1016/J.Arr.2012.07.003

Ross, L. A., Freed, S. A., Edwards, J. D., Phillips, C. B., & Ball, K. (2016). The impact of three cognitive training programs on driving cessation across 10 years: A randomized controlled trial. *Gerontologist, 00*(00), 1–9. doi:10.1093/geront/gnw143

Ruths, D., & Pfeffer, J. (2014). Social sciences. Social media for large studies of behavior. *Science, 346*(6213), 1063–4. doi:10.1126/science.346.6213.1063

Schambra, H. M., Bikson, M., Wager, T. D., DosSantos, M. F., & DaSilva, A. F. (2014). It's all in your head: Reinforcing the placebo response with tDCS. *Brain Stimulation, 7*(4), 623–4. doi:10.1016/J.Brs.2014.04.002

Schulke, D. F. (2013). The regulatory arms race: Mobile-health applications and agency posturing. *Boston University Law Review, 93*(5), 1699–752.

Schwarz, S., Froelich, L., & Burns, A. (2012). Pharmacological treatment of dementia. *Current Opinion in Psychiatry, 25*(6), 542–50. doi:10.1097/Yco.0b013e328358e4f2

Seamon, J. G., Moskowitz, T. N., Swan, A. E., Zhong, B., Golembeski, A., Liong, C., . . . Sosan, O. A. (2014). SenseCam reminiscence and action recall in memory-unimpaired people. *Memory, 22*(7), 861–6. doi:10.1080/09658211.2013.839711

SharpBrains. (2013). Executive Summary: Infographic on the digital brain health market 2012–2020.

SharpBrains. (2016). The digital brain health market 2012–2020: Web-based, mobile and biometrics-based technology to assess, monitor and enhance cognition and brain functioning.

In *Market intelligence: Digital platforms for brain training and cognitive assessment.*

Shimamura, A. P., Berry, J. M., Mangels, J. A., Rusting, C. L., & Jurica, P. J. (1995). Memory and cognitive-abilities in university professors—Evidence for successful aging. *Psychological Science, 6*(5), 271–7. doi:10.1111/J.1467–9280.1995.Tb00510.X

Simons, D. (2013). 19 questions about video games, multitasking, and aging (a HI-BAR commentary on a new Nature paper). http://blog.dansimons.com/2013/09/19-questions-about-video-games.html

Simons, D. J., Boot, W. R., Charness, N., Gathercole, S. E., Chabris, C. F., Hambrick, D. Z., & Stine-Morrow, E. A. L. (2016). Do "brain-training" programs work? *Psychological Science in the Public Interest, 17*(3), 103–86. doi:10.1177/1529100616661983

Small, G. W., Moody, T. D., Siddarth, P., & Bookheimer, S. Y. (2009). Your brain on Google: Patterns of cerebral activation during internet searching. *American Journal of Geriatric Psychiatry, 17*(2), 116–26. doi:10.1097/Jgp.0b013e3181953a02

Smith, G. E., Housen, P., Yaffe, K., Ruff, R., Kennison, R. F., Mahncke, H. W., & Zelinski, E. M. (2009). A cognitive training program based on principles of brain plasticity: Results from the Improvement in Memory with Plasticity-based Adaptive Cognitive Training (IMPACT) study. *Journal of the American Geriatrics Society, 57*(4), 594–603. doi:10.1111/j.1532–5415.2008.02167.x

Snap Inc. (2016). Snap Inc. https://www.snap.com/en-US/

Sparrow, B., Liu, J., & Wegner, D. M. (2011). Google effects on memory: Cognitive consequences of having information at our fingertips. *Science, 333*(6043), 776–8. doi:10.1126/Science.1207745

Stanford Center on Longevity. (2014). A consensus on the brain training industry from the scientific community.

Statistics Canada. (2014). Online activities of Canadian boomers and seniors. http://www.statcan.gc.ca/pub/11-008-x/2009002/article/10910-eng.htm

Storm, B. C., & Stone, S. M. (2014). Saving-enhanced memory: The benefits of saving on the learning and remembering of new information. *Psychological Science.* doi:10.1177/0956797614559285

Thibault, R. T., Lifshitz, M., & Raz, A. (2016). The self-regulating brain and neurofeedback: Experimental science and clinical promise. *Cortex, 74*, 247–61. doi:10.1016/j.cortex.2015.10.024

Thibault, R. T., & Raz, A. (2016). When can neurofeedback join the clinical armamentarium? *Lancet Psychiatry, 3*(6), 497–8. doi:10.1016/S2215-0366(16)30040–2

Thync. (2016). Thync, 2016. http://www.thync.com/

Toril, P., Reales, J. M., & Ballesteros, S. (2014). Video game training enhances cognition of older adults: A meta-analytic study. *Psychology and Aging, 29*(3), 706–16. doi:10.1037/A0037507

Transcranial Ltd. (2016). Foc.Us. http://www.foc.us/

Tun, P. A., & Lachman, M. E. (2010). The association between computer use and cognition across adulthood: Use it so you won't lose it? *Psychology and Aging, 25*(3), 560–8. doi:Doi 10.1037/A0019543

University of Pennsylvania. (2003–2013). The University of Pennsylvania Computerized Neuropsychological Testing. https://penncnp.med.upenn.edu/

van den Hoven, E. (2014). A future-proof past: Designing for remembering experiences. *Memory Studies, 7*(3), 370–84. doi:10.1177/1750698014530625

van der Schaar, P. J., Dijksman, J. F., Broekhuizen-de Gast, H., Shimizu, J., van Lelyveld, N., Zou, H., . . . Siersema, P. D. (2013). A novel ingestible electronic drug delivery and monitoring device. *Gastrointestinal Endoscopy, 78*(3), 520–8. doi:10.1016/J.Gie.2013.03.170

Venkatesh, G. (2014). Brain wave. *MyDigitalFC (Financial Chronicle).* http://www.mydigitalfc.com/knowledge/brain-wave-519

Vitality Inc. (2010–2013). Vitality: Products, 2014. http://www.vitality.net/glowcaps.html

Wadley, V. G., Benz, R. L., Ball, K. K., Roenker, D. L., Edwards, J. A., & Vance, D. E. (2006). Development and evaluation of home-based speed-of-processing training for older adults. *Archives of Physical Medicine and Rehabilitation, 87*(6), 757–63. doi:10.1016/J.Apmr.2006.02.027

Walker, R. B., Evans, R. F., Hanson, R., & Burrow, M. F. (1997). United States Patent No.

Walton, C. C., Kavanagh, A., Downey, L. A., Lomas, J., Camfield, D. A., & Stough, C. (2015). Online cognitive training in healthy older adults: A preliminary study on the effects of single versus multi-domain training *Translational Neuroscience, 6*, 13–9. doi:10.1515/tnsci-2015–0003

Weintraub, S., Dikmen, S. S., Heaton, R. K., Tulsky, D. S., Zelazo, P. D., Bauer, P. J., . . . Gershon, R. C. (2013). Cognition assessment using the NIH Toolbox. *Neurology, 80*, S54–64. doi:10.1212/Wnl.0b013e3182872ded

Wernick, A. (2014). Your video games may revolutionize health and scientific research. *Science, Tech & Environment*: Public Radio International.

Wesnes, K. A. (2014). Moving beyond the pros and cons of automating cognitive testing in pathological aging and dementia: The case for equal opportunity. *Alzheimers Research & Therapy, 6*(5). doi:10.1186/S13195-014-0058-1

Wild, K., Howieson, D., Webbe, F., Seelye, A., & Kaye, J. (2008). Status of computerized cognitive testing in aging: A systematic review. *Alzheimers and Dementia, 4*(6), 428–37. doi:10.1016/j.jalz.2008.07.003

Wilms, I. L., & Nielsen, S. (2014). Normative perceptual estimates for 91 healthy subjects age 60–75: Impact of age, education, employment physical exercise, alcohol, and video gaming. *Frontiers in Psychology, 5*. doi:10.3389/Fpsyg.2014.01137

Wolinsky, F. D., Unverzagt, F. W., Smith, D. M., Jones, R., Wright, E., & Tennstedt, S. L. (2006). The effects of the ACTIVE cognitive training trial on clinically relevant declines in health-related quality of life. *Journals of Gerontology—Series B Psychological Sciences and Social Sciences, 61*(5), S281–7.

Woodberry, E., Browne, G., Hodges, S., Watson, P., Kapur, N., & Woodberry, K. (2014). The use of a wearable camera improves autobiographical memory in patients with Alzheimer's disease. *Memory.* doi:10.1080/09658211.2014.886703

Zelinski, E. M., Spina, L. M., Yaffe, K., Ruff, R., Kennison, R. F., Mahncke, H. W., & Smith, G. E. (2011). Improvement in memory with plasticity-based adaptive cognitive training: Results of the 3-month follow-up. *Journal of the American Geriatrics Society, 59*(2), 258–65. doi:10.1111/J.1532–5415.2010.03277.X

Zickuhr, K., & Madden, M. (2012). Older adults and internet use: For the first time, half of adults ages 65 and older are online. In *Pew Internet & American Life Project.*

CHAPTER

32 Multicultural Considerations in Telepsychology

Jasmine A. Mena, Kyle A. Faust, Nathan E. Cook, David Faust, *and* Ryan Holt

Abstract

Although an expanding body of research demonstrates the potential benefits of telepsychology, little is known about its application with ethnoracial minority populations. Research with ethnoracial minority populations points to various factors that predict positive treatment outcomes; thus, it should be considered in multiculturally sensitive telepsychology practice. In this chapter, the authors discuss the multicultural telepsychology literature and provide recommendations for practice and research. The respective literature in multicultural psychology and telepsychology and their intersection suggest that multicultural telepsychology offers substantial promise for improving the lives of vulnerable and underserved ethnoracial minority populations by increasing access to health information and mental health treatment and reducing mental illness stigma. The chapter ends by discussing potentially fruitful avenues for research.

Keywords: multicultural, underserved, telepsychology, digital technology, behavioral telehealth

Multicultural Considerations in Telepsychology

Ethnoracial minority populations in the United States have grown considerably (US Census Bureau, 2012). The US Census Bureau projects that by 2043 non-Hispanic whites will no longer represent a majority population, although they will remain the largest of all racial groups (US Census Bureau, 2012). These demographic shifts are the results of the younger median age of ethnoracial minority populations, higher fertility rates (specifically among Hispanics/Latinxs and non-Hispanic blacks), and higher rates of interracial relationships resulting in multiracial children (Passel, Livingston, & Cohn, 2012). Demographic shifts have also been observed in Canada and many countries across Europe and have prompted increased attention to multicultural issues in mental health service delivery (European Commission, 2011; Malenfant, Lebel, & Martel, 2010). In the United States, ethnoracial minority groups experience health disparities due to differences in disease incidence, prevalence, morbidity, and mortality or survival rates attributed to social, economic, and/or environmental disadvantages (Minority Health and Health Disparities Research and Education Act US Public Law, 2000). Inequalities in health outcomes have also been observed among minority populations internationally (Bhopal, 2012; Missinne & Bracke, 2012).

Alongside these demographic shifts, telepsychology has increased and is likely to grow substantially in coming years (American Psychological Association [APA] Center for Workforce Studies, 2008). (Other terms commonly used to describe the delivery of mental health services by way of digital technology include "behavioral telehealth," "e-health," "telepsychiatry," and "distance counseling/therapy." The American Psychological Association uses the term "telepsychology," which we use in this chapter.) There is ample evidence that telepsychology is an effective vehicle for the treatment of many mental health issues (Barak, Hen, Boniel-Nissim, & Shapira, 2008; Rohland, Saleh, Rohrer, &

Romitti, 2000). Unfortunately, little is known about the efficacy of telepsychology with ethnoracial minority populations and whether, or the extent to which, alterations in content and modes of delivery might be needed to achieve optimal outcomes. Given the growing scientific support for the efficacy of telepsychology, this intervention tool offers considerable promise for reducing health disparities.

In contrast to telepsychology, there is considerable scientific knowledge about factors promoting favorable outcomes when delivering traditional face-to-face psychotherapy services to ethnoracial minorities. Here, we briefly summarize this knowledge base and then examine its potential application to telepsychology with ethnoracial minorities. We then offer recommendations for practice and research in this important and growing interface.

Multicultural Psychology and Telepsychology Interface

Multicultural psychology is the systematic study of how culture influences affect, cognition, and behavior; in other words, how culture influences the way people feel, think, and act. Beyond individual factors, multicultural psychology also considers the interaction between systems (i.e., family, organizations, community, larger society) when seeking to understand how culture impacts psychological processes. It seems self-evident that the development of effective population-based psychological services, such as those that might be delivered through digital technology, requires an adequate understanding of influential cultural factors.

More than three decades later, Hall's (1997) statement that "Psychology is at a critical junction in its lifecycle; it can adapt to the changing demographics of the United States or risk obsolescence" is still applicable (p. 650). In fact, the Agency for Healthcare Research and Quality (AHRQ) reaffirmed previous findings that ethnoracial minority populations in the United States receive unequal mental health treatment (AHRQ, 2012; United States Department of Health and Human Services, 2001). Unequal mental health access and treatment have also contributed to substantial disparities along ethnoracial lines in many nations globally (World Health Organization [WHO], 2010). An increased emphasis on multiculturalism across mental health training, service delivery, and outcomes research promises to protect the relevance of mental health treatment.

The various calls for mental health practitioners to embrace the multicultural imperative have been met with a proliferation of scholarly activity. A growing theoretical and empirically based literature exploring multicultural issues has helped shape and inform treatment guidelines and conceptions of ethical practice across organizations, which direct the practice of mental health practitioners (American Psychological Association, 2017; American Psychological Association Practice Organization, 2010; American Association for Marriage and Family Therapy [AAMFT], 2012; American Psychiatric Association, 2013a; Qureshi, Collazos, Ramos, & Casas, 2008). Multicultural psychology best practices are anchored by the American Psychological Association's *Multicultural Guidelines: An Ecological Approach to Context, Identity, and Intersectionality* (APA Guidelines) and the APA code of ethics (American Psychological Association, 2010, 2017). The APA Guidelines acknowledges the harmful effects of societal discrimination, which limits access to resources and services. They also challenge mental health practitioners to take steps to ensure they are working in culturally appropriate ways.

The APA Guidelines works in concert with the APA Ethics Code. Listed under the principle of Justice, the Ethics Code indicates, "Fairness and justice entitle all persons access to and benefit from the contributions of psychology and to equal quality in the processes, procedures, and services being conducted by psychologists" (American Psychological Association, 2010, p. 3). The principle of Respect for People's Rights and Dignity urges psychologists to be "aware of and respect cultural, individual, and role differences, including those based on age, gender, gender identity, race, ethnicity, culture, national origin, religion, sexual orientation, disability, language, and socioeconomic status (SES) and consider these factors when working with members of such groups" (American Psychological Association, 2010, p. 3). In addition to psychology, the ethics codes of various other mental health groups and organizations echo the expectation of culturally sensitive practice (AAMFT, 2012; American Psychological Association, 2002; American Psychiatric Association, 2013a). Taken together, the multicultural psychology scientific knowledge base, practice guidelines, and the ethics codes make a compelling case that practitioners should address multicultural issues across all aspects of service delivery, the latter of which almost surely includes telepsychology.

Practice guidelines were developed to inform digital technologies applied to self-assessments and monitoring, real-time two-way communication, and dissemination of psychoeducation resources (American Psychological Association, 2013; America Telemedicine Association, 2014). Successful implementation of distance healthcare interventions for both rural and urban underserved residents have been disseminated (Griffiths & Christensen, 2007). Healthy People 2020, a federal plan designed to improve the health of the American population, included goals for computer-mediated health communication (Healthy People, 2014). Considering that ethnoracial minorities, vulnerable, and underserved populations have limited access to health information and treatment and higher levels of morbidity and mortality (Kreps et al., 2007), expanding access to health information and treatment via telepsychology is a promising development.

Key Multicultural Psychotherapy Factors

Historically, individuals from ethnoracial minority groups have had limited access to mental health services and have faced several significant barriers to accessing quality mental healthcare (AHRQ, 2012; Holden et al., 2014; US Department of Health and Human Services, 2001; WHO, 2010). Prior research indicates that ethnoracial minority groups may hold stigmatized beliefs and attitudes toward individuals with mental illness (including self-stigma) that create a barrier to service utilization (Rao, Feinglass, & Corrigan, 2007). Cultural mistrust of organizations providing mental health services also hinders service use (Gary, 2005; Whaley, 2001). The quality of the services available to ethnoracial minorities also warrants attention. Smedley, Stith, and Nelson (2003) found that, even after statistically controlling for SES, ethnoracial minority populations received poorer quality services compared to whites. These barriers may be overcome by considering the key factors shown to increase treatment effectiveness, discussed in the following brief review.

Multicultural Treatment Effectiveness: Determinant Factors

Researchers have identified various multicultural adaptations critical to effective therapy. Griner and Smith's (2006) meta-analysis found that tailoring to a specific cultural group was the most important factor in treatment efficacy. For instance, multicultural group therapy consisting solely of Latinx clients is far more effective than multicultural group therapy including both Latinx clients and Asian clients. The effect size for interventions tailored to a specific culture indicates that such interventions were, on average, four times more effective ($d = .49$) than interventions using mixed-race groups ($d = .12$). Measures of effectiveness included treatment retention, symptom reduction, substance use/abuse, pro-social, behavior and treatment satisfaction, or a combination of these variables.

Benish, Quintana, and Wampold's (2011) subsequent meta-analysis identified cultural concepts of distress (also known as illness myths) as the most important factor in cultural adaptations. Adaptations of cultural concepts of distress involve explaining a clients' mental disorders in ways that are congruent with their cultural beliefs. For example, McCabe and Yeh (2009) made culturally specific modifications throughout the provision of a parent–child interaction therapy program for Mexican American families by referencing cultural concepts congruent with the participants' belief system (e.g., *familismo* and *personalismo*). Adaptations involving cultural concepts of distress was the only moderator of superior outcomes via culturally adapted psychotherapy (Benish et al., 2011). This seeming inconsistency between meta-analyses is likely due to the study inclusion method. Specifically, Griner and Smith only included studies comparing culturally adapted psychotherapy to nonadapted psychotherapy. Nevertheless, cultural adaptations involving cultural concepts of distress and tailoring therapy/interventions to a specific cultural group appear to be the two best predictors of successful therapeutic outcome.

Griner and Smith (2006) identified several individual-level characteristics that also led to improved multicultural treatment outcomes. For example, studies involving older clients yielded moderately higher effect sizes than studies with younger clients. The authors theorized that these findings were due to acculturation, given that this variable was also a strong predictor of treatment efficacy. Clients, especially Hispanic/Latinx clients, benefited more substantially if they had low levels of acculturation. The authors reasoned that this was because the interventions were specifically tailored to clients with low levels of acculturation compared to clients who grew up in the United States and were more Americanized. Notably, Huey and Polo's (2008) meta-analysis also resulted in weaker evidence for the efficacy of multicultural interventions for ethnic minority youth, possibly due to the comparatively rapid acculturation experienced by youth versus adults (Schwartz, Pantin, Sullivan, Prado, & Szapocznik, 2006).

Acculturation refers to psychological-level changes resulting from contact between two or more distinct cultures and is usually applied to migrants (Gibson, 2001, Schwartz, Unger, Zamboanga, & Szapocznik, 2010). The bidimensional model of acculturation associated with simultaneously receiving the host culture and retaining the heritage culture at varying levels is most widely accepted (Berry, 1980). As previously noted, researchers have documented differences in acculturation experiences largely associated with depth of exposure to the host and heritage cultures (Portes & Rumbaut, 2006). Additionally, individuals residing in ethnic enclaves where new migrants can easily engage in daily activities with others from a similar or closely related heritage-cultural background may remain largely unacculturated to the host culture for much of their lives (Schwartz et al., 2006). Youth are typically immersed in a mainstream environment (e.g., school) soon after migration, which partly explains their rapid acculturation. Various assessments have been developed to measure acculturation (Stephenson, 2000; Unger et al., 2002). It may be prudent to measure level of acculturation pretreatment to help determine the appropriateness of culturally modified treatment.

Griner and Smith (2006) also reported an association between language and outcome. If the intervention was conducted in a client's native versus secondary language, treatment effects were about twice as large, although it is unknown whether the use of interpreters would have attenuated this differential impact. Adequate levels of language proficiency are critical for accessible and effective treatment. Individuals with limited English language proficiency in the United States encounter barriers such as limited access to mental health services and mental health disparities partly due to lack of perceived need for treatment and substantial delays in accessing services (Bauer, Chen, & Alegría, 2010). According to the results of Keller, Gangnon, and Witt's (2014) study, upon accessing services for depression, non–English-speaking women were 50% less likely to receive adequate services compared to English-speaking women. Furthermore, conducting mental health evaluations in a patient's nonprimary language can easily result in incomplete and distorted information that impedes treatment (Bauer & Alegría, 2010).

When communicating in a second language the difference between conversational and proficient language capabilities should be considered. Although one can develop conversational capabilities in a second language in approximately 2 years, full proficiency is often not achieved for as many as 7 years (Demie, 2012). See Hulstijn (2010) and Halle, Hair, Wandner, McNamara, and Chien (2012) for more detailed coverage of acquired language proficiency.

One potential solution to the limited access to client–practitioner language congruence includes the use of interpreters. In addition to attending to issues of proficiency, proper interpretation requires attention to differences associated with client–interpreter–practitioner dialects and knowledge of culturally based idioms of distress and cultural assumptions (Lopez, 2002). Some believe that the interpreter should personally identify with the culture of the client in order to ensure that the interpreter possesses sufficient knowledge to also act as a "cultural broker" (Borchgrevink, 2003). For instance, Paone and Malott (2008) stated in their review of the literature on interpreters for mental health treatment that "interpreters can bridge existing cultural gaps by educating counselors regarding the client's culture and culturally informed behaviors" (p. 131).

Practitioners should be aware that interpretation gaps could occur as a result of differences in the meaning of words and phrases across cultures. In addition, other culturally based communication gaps can occur when using proverbs, humor, or language with emotional undertones (Paone & Malott, 2008). An interpreter with adequate knowledge of the relevant languages, cultures, and professional terminology is in the best position to interpret mental health treatments when client–practitioner language congruence is lacking. The client, however, should not have a personal relationship with the interpreter in order to prevent discomfort and bias (Murray & Wynne, 2001).

When evidence-based multicultural treatments are not available, practitioners should consider the best methods of adapting multicultural psychotherapy for various ethnic groups. In some instances, treatments that incorporate the factors that lead to the best outcomes have already been adapted for specific ethnic groups (based on the findings that Benish et al. [2011] and Griner & Smith [2006] reported).

One could speculate that, all else being equal, almost any culturally tailored intervention that incorporates cultural concepts of distress, level of acculturation, and age—and that is intended for a specific ethnicity and delivered in an individual's native language—would yield better treatment outcomes. Scholars have developed numerous treatment adaptation models and guidelines for use when there are no preexisting culturally tailored treatment adaptations for a specific cultural group (Bernal, Bonilla, & Bellido, 1995; Hwang, 2006; Morales & Norcross, 2010). Morales and Norcorss's (2010) guidelines emphasize applying the best available research; accounting for client characteristics, culture, and preferences; and incorporating clinical expertise. Instead of using years of experience as a measure of clinical expertise, we propose that practitioners assess the congruence between their training, knowledge, and skill and the best treatment option available, considering that the association between years of experience and accuracy (Faust & Faust, 2012) or treatment effectiveness is minimal or less than robust (Leon, Martinovich, Lutz, & Lyons, 2005; Öst, Karlstedt, & Widén, 2012; Smith & Glass, 1977; Smith, Glass, & Miller, 1980; Shapiro & Shapiro, 1982).

Therapeutic Relationship Factors and Cultural Competence

Decades of research with wide-ranging client populations and therapeutic approaches have reported a positive and often robust relationship between strength of therapeutic alliance and treatment outcomes (Arnow et al., 2013; Del Re, Flückiger, Horvath, Symonds, & Wampold, 2012; Norcross, 2011). Some research indicates that alliance can be strengthened by a client's perception of the practitioner's multicultural orientation (Owen, Leach, Tao, & Rodolfa, 2011). According to Owen and colleagues (2011), *multicultural orientation* refers to a practitioner's overall positive philosophy or values about one's own and the client's cultures. *Multicultural competency* typically refers to a practitioner's capabilities with cultural awareness and beliefs, cultural knowledge, and skills delivering interventions in a culturally sensitive and relevant manner (Sue, Zane, Hall, & Berger, 2009). According to Owen and colleagues (2011), client perception of practitioner multicultural orientation was positively related to working alliance as well as psychological improvement. Numerous other studies have reported similar findings pertaining to multicultural competence (Constantine, 2002; Fuertes, Stracuzzi, Bennett, Scheinholtz, & Mislowack, 2006; Kim, Li, & Liang, 2002). Owen and colleagues (2011) speculated that if a client believed the practitioner was more oriented toward cultural issues, the client would also believe the practitioner was more credible, thus leading to more comfort with the therapeutic process. Smith and Trimble (2016a) confirmed this speculation in their meta-analysis which indicated that when client—not therapist—ratings of multicultural competence were used, they predicted 44% of the variance in client participation in treatment and 16% of clinical outcomes for ethnoracial minority clients.

Other research seeking to understand factors that contribute to improved client outcomes have examined client–practitioner match. Griner and Smith's (2006) meta-analysis indicated that although language match made a significant difference in multicultural therapeutic outcome, shared ethnicity and race had little to no impact. Similarly, a meta-analysis of 53 studies that matched clients and practitioners based on race or ethnicity indicated that this practice yielded slightly improved engagement in treatment; however, the authors noted that this finding was moderated by language match (Smith & Trimble, 2016b). These results suggest that, for many clients, an effective therapeutic alliance is more important to treatment outcome than client–practitioner ethnic or racial match. In the meantime, based on the best available evidence, matching clients and practitioner on language seems to be a greater priority than matching along such factors as race and ethnicity.

Discussions about psychotherapy effectiveness have generated debates about the preeminence of general competency versus multicultural competency. Scholars and practitioners have emphasized the need to distinguish between general and multicultural competency; some argue that practitioners can be generally competent without having multicultural competency (Imel et al., 2011). Along these lines, some believe general competence aids in developing an effective therapeutic alliance and improves therapeutic outcomes. However, general competence may be insufficient if a practitioner is lacking specific knowledge, awareness, and skills about a client's culture. Critics of an exclusive general competence approach to psychotherapy argue this practice is steeped in ethnocentric monoculturalism (Sue, 2004) and verges on "cultural malpractice" (Hall, 1997). Moreover, in Constantine's (2002) study, although general and multicultural competencies overlapped considerably, multicultural competence was distinguishable from general competency and made a unique contribution to client satisfaction with psychotherapy services. These findings indicate that general and multicultural competencies are distinguishable and practitioners may need to use both simultaneously (Sue et al., 2009). In other words, while client–practitioner "match" does not seem critical to developing a strong therapeutic alliance, specific cultural knowledge, awareness, and skills can improve treatment outcomes.

Multicultural Treatment Access

A treatment, no matter how effective, is of no use if it is not accessible to clients. Organizational factors may impact service utilization due to cultural mistrust and limited access to services. According to Berger, Zane, and Hwang's (2014) study, if mental health practitioners become more involved in communities of diverse populations, those practitioners will become more culturally aware and will have better relationships with their diverse clients. Effective community outreach to diverse populations using culturally sensitive descriptions of mental illnesses will likely reduce mental illness stigma and help these groups obtain needed services. Berger and colleagues (2014) further note that ethnic- and racial-specific service organizations are more successfully treating ethnic minorities compared to mainstream clinics.

The individual, practitioner, and organizational factors just discussed improve psychotherapy experiences and outcomes for ethnoracial minority populations and should be considered and integrated into multicultural psychotherapy. However, little is known about how these factors translate to telepsychology contexts, which is the focus of the next section.

Multicultural Considerations Applied to Telepsychology

The overrepresentation of ethnoracial minorities with low SES has contributed to a "digital divide." The "digital divide" refers to the limited Internet health information accessed by vulnerable and underserved populations compared to those with higher SES (Kreps et al., 2007). For example, Wang, Bennett, and Probst (2011) reported less Internet access and use among rural compared to urban residents as well as lower Internet use among African American and Hispanic respondents compared to white respondents. The recent expansion of access to handheld digital technology (e.g., smartphones) has permeated SES categories, and, with it, new possibilities for telepsychology have emerged.

As described in the previous section, a large and growing body of research demonstrates the efficacy of multicultural psychotherapy and provides insights into conditions that seem to enhance treatment effectiveness, including the need to tailor interventions (see Benish et al., 2011). It seems rather improbable that none of this research has potential application to telepsychological services with ethnoracial minorities, and it seems most sensible at present to take these multicultural findings as working hypotheses or premises subject to modification as more research data are gathered.

Unfortunately, research studies and conceptual considerations of multicultural issues pertinent to telepsychology are scant. Most telepsychology research has focused predominantly on technological issues (e.g., security of health information and encryption considerations when using smartphones to deliver mental health treatment). A sizable body of telepsychology research has focused on the unique needs of individuals residing in geographically isolated communities. These underserved individuals, for whom mental health services are often inaccessible due to issues such as cost and location, piqued the interest of telepsychology researchers and have offered many important insights (e.g., Bischoff, Hollist, Smith, & Flack, 2004; Farrell & McKinnon, 2003; Reed, Messler, Coombs, & Quevillon, 2014; although our discussion focuses exclusively on telepsychology, research in the related area of telepsychiatry has directed considerable attention to the use of digital technology to address the mental health needs of rural populations). These studies suggest or demonstrate how several cultural factors identified in the general psychotherapy outcome literature (summarized earlier) relate to telepsychology in geographically isolated communities. Such findings are certainly germane and important, although few researchers have investigated multicultural telepsychology issues with ethnoracial minority populations.

Multicultural Telepsychology Treatment: Potential Determinant Factors

Multicultural psychology research summarized earlier clearly indicates that culturally relevant therapy offers advantages over approaches that accord little attention to cultural factors. There is a pressing need to extend the principles of culturally relevant and effective psychotherapy to telepsychology applications. This might include modifying telepsychology applications to specific cultural groups. It might also involve developing new, culturally specific telepsychology services for particular racial or ethnic groups.

For example, telepsychology delivery might be offered regularly or primarily via community technology centers. Kreps and colleagues (2007) reported that such computer centers successfully engaged low-income, predominately Latinx and

African American families in computer training courses with hopes of increasing access to health information. Furthermore, Kreps and colleagues noted that households with computers became "hubs" of computer activity in their apartment complexes and neighborhoods. This type of positive response and apparent increase in access to digital technology and Internet-based health information provides a promising model for implementation and delivery of telepsychology interventions.

As with traditional psychotherapy, telepsychology applications need to account for cultural concepts of distress and incorporate information about a client's mental health problems in a culturally congruent manner. For instance, at times, cultural conceptualizations of mental illnesses do not fit neatly with psychiatric nosology (Lewis-Fernández & Díaz, 2002). An example found in the "Glossary of Cultural Concepts of Distress" in the *Diagnostic and Statistical Manual of Mental Disorders* (DSM-5; American Psychiatric Association, 2013b) consists of *ataque de nervios* which is the second most prevalent psychological malady identified in Puerto Rico. *Ataque de nervios* is defined as, "intense emotional upset, including acute anxiety, anger, or grief; screaming and shouting uncontrollably; attacks of crying; trembling; heat in the chest rising into the head; and becoming verbally and physically aggressive" (American Psychiatric Association, 2013b, p. 833). Clients who are presented with conceptions of mental illnesses that are not culturally congruent are unlikely to identify with the treatment and, consequently, will remain untreated. It is highly likely that many current presentations and programs are not optimally suited, or are ill-suited, to various ethnoracial minority groups.

Age and acculturation are also important considerations. Older age is associated with lower digital technology use (Fox & Vitak, 2008). As such, psychological services delivered through digital technology would likely be a greater challenge on average for older ethnoracial minority adults (Wang et al., 2011). Furthermore, lower levels of acculturation are associated with decreased digital technology use for certain cultural groups (Li & Livingston, 2011). Telepsychology services for older and less acculturated populations should therefore provide additional support to encourage and facilitate use (Barak et al., 2008).

Additionally, Griner and Smith's (2006) findings that language match between practitioner and client is a critical factor in successful psychotherapy would seem to be similarly important for telepsychology. As previously noted, the complexities of language are many and require careful consideration. When printed content is concerned, such as in computer-generated messages, one consideration entails the issue of translation versus interpretation of content. Literal translation may not capture the essential message, which requires interpretation that incorporates cultural meaning (Searight & Searight, 2009). Future work in this area should examine the impact of language on telepsychology applications, and newly developed telepsychology applications should provide services in the consumer's preferred language.

Culture also influences the understanding and interpretation of visual materials (Ardila, 2007; Heaton, Ryan, & Grant, 2009), which are often used extensively in digital technology programs. Crilly, Moultrie, and Clarkson (2004) conducted a review of visual response to product design wherein they discussed culture as an influential factor in the appraisal of visual material. They noted that cognition, affect, and behavior are all involved in appraisal of visual stimuli and all represent culturally based processes. Taking beauty as an example, Crozier (1994) indicated that there is no universal standard of beauty; rather, beauty is a social construction based on cultural, economic, technological, and historical forces.

Therapeutic Relationship Factors, Cultural and Digital Competence

Meta-analyses of multicultural psychotherapy consistently show that language match is more critical than racial or ethnic match. Still, clients may sometimes prefer and benefit from a racial or ethnic match. Evidence from physical health literature suggests that ethnic match can support a strong working alliance. For example, a study of patient–physician communication reported that race-concordant dyads resulted in longer visits and higher ratings of patient positive affect, though match did not result in higher ratings of care (Cooper et al., 2003). These findings indicate that race concordance is a complex phenomenon with some desirable effects in some cases. Furthermore, Lisetti and colleagues (2012) evaluated an avatar-delivered intervention aimed at enhancing motivation to change unhealthy lifestyle, including problematic alcohol use, and reported a 91% rate of acceptance of diverse avatars. Specifically, the intervention allowed participants to choose avatars from a variety of races, genders, and physical appearances (Lisetti et al., 2012). These findings suggest that participants liked the ability to select the avatar with which to interact, thus building a client–practitioner concordance that led to a stronger working alliance (Lisetti et al., 2012).

It is unclear how much and under what circumstances racial or ethnic match might impact interactions via digital technology. For example, Quackenbush and Krasner (2012) described a case study of avatars delivering psychotherapy in a virtual environment. The case study highlighted that practitioners of "avatar therapy" will likely work with highly culturally diverse clients, which will make issues of cultural competence all the more salient (Quackenbush & Krasner, 2012).

Digital technology may also enhance trust between the client and practitioner and thereby facilitate a stronger therapeutic alliance. Aguilera and Muñoz (2011) conducted a pilot study testing the use of text messaging to augment a cognitive-behavioral intervention for depression. Participants, a diverse group of low-income outpatient clients who mostly spoke Spanish, received two to three text messages each day to assess and monitor their mood. According to the authors, 90% of clients indicated that the text messages made them feel cared for and closer to the group and the practitioner.

Digital technology may prove beneficial in promoting practitioner multicultural competence. Barnett (2011) introduced a special section in the journal *Psychotherapy* that included seven articles related to using technology in psychotherapy training and supervision. In one article, Abbass and colleagues (2011) discussed the provision of clinical supervision via web conferencing and video recordings of sessions. In much the same way, clinical supervisors with demonstrated expertise and competency in multicultural psychotherapy could provide supervision via digital technology applications with the hope of enhancing trainee's multicultural competence.

McKay and colleagues (2013) described the development of a psychology doctoral program in Alaska that infused technology throughout all aspects of the curriculum and training. The program was developed following a needs assessment that identified the lack of qualified professionals to meet the needs of Alaskan residents, particularly those in rural areas (McKay et al., 2013). Thus, the program was specifically designed to train doctoral-level psychologists to provide culturally competent services to rural Alaskan residents and Alaskan Natives, especially via telepsychology (McKay et al., 2013). As this example suggests, digital technology not only provides an opportunity to enhance and support students' and professionals' training, but also to foster technological proficiencies that can assist in effective delivery of telepsychology services.

Multicultural Treatment Access

A primary concern for minority populations is access to care. Farrell and McKinnon (2003) summarized several studies suggesting that computer-based psychoeducation efforts can be implemented successfully, thus supporting telepsychology as a useful tool for addressing the mental health needs of rural populations. Also, pilot work aimed at increasing Internet access in low-income populations reported positive effects (Kreps et al., 2007). Telepsychology may also be leveraged to address important cultural barriers to accessing care. For example, a pilot program in Nebraska found that providing care through the existing telecommunication infrastructure in rural high schools helped reduce or offset various cultural obstacles to treatment. Such benefits included lessened time demands when care was far away; potential negation of prohibitive costs, such as the need to take days off from work to travel great distances; and reduced stigma associated with receiving mental healthcare, which appears to be a particular concern among rural populations (Bischoff et al., 2004). Reduction in mental health self-stigma associated with help-seeking has been documented as a significant barrier for ethnoracial minority populations (Rao et al., 2007). Relatedly, telepsychology using smartphones appears promising given that the smartphone is inconspicuous (Eonta et al., 2011) and usually in the possession of the user (Boschen & Casey, 2008).

Despite multicultural telepsychology's potential, it should be emphasized that access to technology does not automatically dismantle extant social inequities (Kvasny, 2006). Thoughtful and deliberate action to make certain that multicultural telepsychology practice and research are culturally appropriate and in line with the best evidence will ensure its quality and effectiveness. For example, there are various issues which, if unknown to the practitioner or researcher, might well compromise the success of the technology/treatment. A case in point is the finding that ethnoracial minorities access computers outside the home more frequently than do whites due to the lack of home-based broadband Internet service (Ennis, Rose, Denis, Pandit, & Wykes, 2012). As a result, blacks and Latinxs are more likely than whites to use cell phones to access the Internet in lieu of home-based Internet (Li & Livingston, 2011).

Recommendations and Future Directions

Multicultural telepsychology has the potential to reach a broad clientele and, in doing so, can improve the practice of psychology. Although nascent, the extant multicultural telepsychology literature illuminates a number of promising strategies and provides a foundation for the recommendations given here.

Although treatments designed for specific cultural groups are more efficacious than treatments designed for mixed groups, some cultural adaptation results in more effective treatments than no adaptation at all (Griner & Smith, 2006). We recommend that researchers and practitioners consider the possible cultural values and norms of specific groups when designing and delivering treatments, rather than adopting a purely universal perspective. This recommendation extends to considering the client's cultural concepts of distress in the conceptualization of the client's mental disorder, as noted earlier. It is also important to note that while mental health practitioners need to learn general multicultural competence skills, including awareness of how culture influences one's attitudes, beliefs, and biases, general multicultural competence skills alone are insufficient since one cannot assume transferability of cultural knowledge from one group to another (Hall, 2001). As such, mental health practitioners must also gain sufficient culturally specific knowledge in the development of treatments and utilize *dynamic sizing* skills during the application of treatments (Sue, 1998). Sue (1998) used "dynamic sizing" to "mean that the therapist has appropriate skills in knowing when to generalize and be inclusive and when to individualize and be exclusive" (p. 446). This approach allows for a valuing of cultural characteristics while avoiding stereotyping.

The importance of language match between treatment and clients cannot be understated. Treatments must be delivered in a manner that clients can comprehend. In fact, in the United States legal requirements apply (Eighty-Eighth Congress, 1964), and, notably, interpreter error resulted in a US$71,000,000 medical negligence case (Harsham, 1984). In the event of a language mismatch, mental health practitioners are encouraged to evaluate the interpreter's competence to ensure appropriate skills since mental health practitioners may be held responsible for the competence of interpreters. Researchers and practitioners need to consider that, as noted previously, *translations* (the term used in reference to written text) and *interpretations* (the term used in reference to spoken language) of telepsychological treatments can be further complicated by differences in dialects and inaccuracies. Hence, practitioners should take steps to ensure that any individual recruited to serve in the capacity of translator/interpreter has the proper training and knowledge (Searight & Searight, 2009). For example, a mental health practitioner may contact references to inquire about the quality of translations/interpretations, employ a bilingual consultant to evaluate an interpreter's language proficiency, and assess the interpreter's familiarity with mental health interpreter guidelines and the culture of the patient population. Mental health interpreter training programs are few and trained interpreters are scarce, though attention to their need is rising. Searight and Searight (2009) and Paone and Malott (2008) provided additional recommendations for working with interpreters in psychological practice.

As previously noted, access to psychotherapy is a major barrier for ethnoracial minority, vulnerable, and underserved populations. The rise of telepsychology may grant individuals greater access to culturally appropriate services. Additionally, improved access could be achieved via collaborations with credible community organizations. Given the available evidence for telepsychology's effectiveness, we recommend its use to alleviate the access barrier experienced by vulnerable and underserved populations.

Collaborations with institutions with access to large numbers of underserved populations (e.g., Medicaid), including hospitals, public health agencies, and other programs targeting underserved populations have yielded fruitful results (Kreps et al., 2007). Grassroots organizations such as places of worship as well as community and cultural centers can serve as technology/training hubs from which mental health practitioners can launch multicultural telepsychology initiatives. Notably, different types of digital outreach may be more effective for some environments compared to others and can be considered. For example, the Computerized Health Education and Support System (CHESS) partnered with the Wisconsin Well Women Program (a community-based program that offers health-based services for women with limited insurance coverage) to provide an effective Internet-based delivery system for up-to-date information on cancer treatment (Kreps, 2005). This collaboration proved an effective recruitment vehicle for women in the Wisconsin area to access health services. However, other outlets, such as radio and television broadcasts, had more impact on densely populated areas (e.g., Detroit) compared to rural areas (Kreps, 2005). Practitioners and researchers using digital technology are encouraged to reach out to and maintain long-term relationships with community-based organizations with access to vulnerable and underserved populations in order to better serve them. Practitioners and researchers are also encouraged to tailor their messages to the specific needs and characteristics of the target population and geographic community.

Consideration of client comfort with technology is advised. Individuals with higher levels of technological familiarity and proficiency may find it easier to utilize telepsychology. For example, college students, on average, have high levels of technological familiarity and might be considerably more likely to use and benefit from multicultural telepsychology. Ethnoracial minority college students underutilize psychotherapy services available at their colleges and universities (Kearney, Draper, & Baron, 2005). We suspect that multicultural telepsychology could be implemented expediently in college/university counseling centers to reach ethnoracial minority students and might improve access to services among the general student body. University-based counseling centers are encouraged to consider telepsychology's potential for outreach and research with their student populations.

Although health and wellness centers stand to benefit from the integration of digital technology, members of these organizations may be unfamiliar with these emerging tools. Health practitioners who started practicing prior to the use of telepsychology are more likely to have difficulty recognizing the opportunities associated with incorporating digital technologies into their practice. In an educational context, practitioners may be reluctant to demonstrate telepsychology in the classroom because they may know less about technology than their students. As stated previously, competence is necessary for the use of telepsychology and especially for teaching telepsychology. We recommend that practitioners with less digital technology familiarity collaborate with more knowledgeable individuals who could provide instruction on basic and advanced telepsychology topics. Regardless of one's initial level of familiarity with a particular technology, adequate training can promote proficiency. As integration of technology becomes standard practice, reticence toward this area should diminish.

Integrating practice with a variety of digital technologies into graduate training programs should facilitate the expansion of telepsychology among future generations of mental health professionals. Although specific technologies and applications can have a short half-life and alternate programs could be developed by the completion of a student's degree, such training breaks away from the in-person-only tradition, thus creating a more flexible and accessible practitioner. Additionally, general familiarity and proficiency with telepsychology and associated technologies can make learning new applications and methods easier.

In addition to enhancing the education of current and future practitioners, training should also be provided for clients of practitioners who use telepsychology. We recommend that practitioners provide clients with a basic tutorial for the digital technology that the mental health practitioner uses. Moreover, including a training period will ensure that clients can competently engage with the practitioner through the technology with fidelity (Aguilera & Munoz, 2011). We recommend careful client training, especially with individuals who have lower levels of acculturation and comfort with technology.

The use of customizable avatars within virtual reality therapy or augmented reality therapy has already been developed and utilized successfully in treatments for individuals with schizophrenia (Leff, Williams, Huckvale, Arbuthnot, & Leff, 2013; Quackenbush & Krasner, 2012). As gaming platforms move toward greater degrees of virtual reality immersion, therapy may one day take place in a virtual setting. One device that has received a fair amount of attention, the Oculus Rift, is a virtual reality headset that tracks a user's head movements. This technology provides the player with a greater sense of immersion through visual feedback that accurately corresponds with the user's head movements. Advantages of using virtual reality therapy include the ability to control the stimuli with precision and deliver the treatment in a safe environment, thus providing more realistic treatments in instances where, for example, in vivo exposures might be dangerous or impractical.

Virtual technology research has been conducted in the areas of biometric research, attention deficit hyperactivity disorder intervention, and exposure therapy (Gavrilova, & Yampolskiy, 2011; Parsons, Bowerly, Buckwater, & Rizzo, 2007; Rothbaum, Hodges, Smith, Lee, & Price, 2000). For instance, virtual reality immersion has demonstrated effectiveness in treating combat veterans with posttraumatic stress disorder by exposing them to the feared stimuli, resulting in habituation and subsequent extinction of the fear response (Gerardi, Rothbaum,

Ressler, Heekin, & Rizzo, 2008). Given their promise, virtual environments or augmented environments may become more common, resulting in an expansion of effective treatment options.

Although there is great potential in multicultural telepsychology, a note of caution is in order. According to the ethics codes for psychologists, psychiatrists, and couple and family therapists, practitioners are expected to work within their scope of knowledge and training and attempt to maintain competence within emerging fields (AAMFT, 2012; American Psychiatric Association, 2002, 2013a). This mandate applies to telepsychology. In addition, maintaining client confidentiality and protecting client data are particularly salient given the use of technology and the history of cultural mistrust experienced by ethnoracial minorities toward mental health organizations. Mental health professionals are encouraged to limit unintended access to client data and collaborate with data-oriented security specialists. The American Psychological Association's *Guidelines for the Practice of Telepsychology* (2013) indicates that the dynamic turnover of technologies creates an environment where creating specific prescribed actions can quickly become outdated. It is recommended that practitioners and researchers frame ethical issues in multicultural telepsychology as an active and dynamic process if they are to keep up with the torrid pace of telepsychology.

Conclusion

In this chapter, we sought to identify the multicultural factors known to influence psychotherapy outcomes, apply these factors to the burgeoning field of telepsychology, and offer recommendations and future directions for practice and research. The growing research literature indicates that the use of digital technology in concert with or as a replacement for traditional face-to-face psychotherapy has great potential (Eonta et al., 2011).

Research points to various multicultural factors that should be considered in psychotherapy service delivery; these include culturally tailoring interventions to a specific ethnicity; delivering intervention in the client's preferred language whenever possible; and attending to cultural concepts of distress, level of acculturation, and age. Although the application of multicultural issues to telepsychology is a relatively new endeavor, a review of the multicultural telepsychology literature highlights a number of promising culturally sensitive strategies that should foster client as well as professional engagement. Such strategies include establishing technology centers in trusted organizations in the community; attending to relationships between age, acculturation, and digital literacy; ensuring clients' preferred language is used; considering cultural concepts of distress in the treatment; and incorporating digital technology training into mental health practitioners' training programs. Overall, we believe that, taken together, the literature in multicultural psychology and telepsychology supports multicultural telepsychology as a viable area of practice and as a high research priority, developments which have the potential to positively impact the lives of ethnoracial minority, vulnerable, and underserved populations by improving access to health information and mental health treatment and reducing mental illness stigma.

References

Abbass, A., Arthey, S., Elliott, J., Fedak, T., Nowoweiski, D., Markovski, J., & Nowoweiski, S. (2011). Web-conference supervision for advanced psychotherapy training: A practical guide. *Psychotherapy, 48*(2), 109–18.

Agency Healthcare Research and Quality (AHRQ). (2012). *National health disparities report.* https://archive.ahrq.gov/research/findings/nhqrdr/nhdr12/index.html

Aguilera, A., & Muñoz, R. F. (2011). Text messaging as an adjunct to CBT in low-income populations: A usability and feasibility pilot study. *Professional Psychology: Research and Practice, 42*(6), 472–8.

American Association for Marriage and Family Therapy (AAMFT). (2012). *Code of ethics.* http://www.aamft.org/iMIS15/AAMFT/Content/legal_ethics/code_of_ethics.aspx

American Psychological Association. (2002). Ethical principles of psychologists and code of conduct. *American Psychologist, 57,* 1060–73.

American Psychological Association. (2010). *Ethical principles of psychologists and code of conduct 2010 amendments.* Washington, DC: Author.

American Psychiatric Association. (2013a). *Ethics.* http://www.psychiatry.org/practice/ethics

American Psychiatric Association. (2013b). Diagnostic and *Statistical Manual of Mental Disorders* (5th ed.). Washington, DC: Author.

American Psychological Association. (2013). *Guidelines for the practice of telepsychology.* http://www.apapracticecentral.org/ce/guidelines/telepsychology-guidelines.pdf

American Psychological Association. (2017). *Multicultural guidelines: An ecological approach to context, identity, and intersectionality.* http://www.apa.org/about/policy/multicultural-guidelines.pdf

American Psychological Association Center for Workforce Studies. (2008). *2008 APA survey of psychology health service providers.* http://www.apa.org/workforce/publications/08-hsp/telepsychology/

American Psychological Association Practice Organization. (2010). Telehealth: Legal basics for psychologists. *Good Practice, 41,* 2–7.

American Telemedicine Association. (2014). *Practice guidelines for live, on demand primary and urgent care.* http://www.americantelemed.org/resources/telemedicine-practice-guidelines/telemedicine-practice-guidelines.VLBbZlq_v8E

Ardila, A. (2007). The impact of culture on neuropsychological test performance. In B. P. Uzzell, M. O. Pontón, & A. Ardila (Eds.), *International handbook of cross-cultural neuropsychology* (pp. 23–44). Mahwah, NJ: Erlbaum.

Arnow, B. A., Steidtmann, D., Blasey, C., Manber, R., Constantino, M. J., Klein, D. N., . . . Kocsis, J. H. (2013). The relationship between the therapeutic alliance and treatment outcome in two distinct psychotherapies for chronic depression. *Journal of Consulting and Clinical Psychology, 81*(4), 627–38.

Barak, A., Hen, L., Boniel-Nissim, M., & Shapira, N. (2008). A comprehensive review and a meta-analysis of the effectiveness of Internet-based psychotherapeutic interventions. *Journal of Technology in Human Services, 26,* 109–60.

Barnett, J. E. (2011). Utilizing technological innovations to enhance psychotherapy supervision, training, and outcomes. *Psychotherapy, 48*(2), 103–8.

Bauer, A. M., & Alegría, M. (2010). Impact of patient language proficiency and interpreter service use on the quality of psychiatric care: A systematic review. *Psychiatric Services, 61,* 765–73.

Bauer, A. M., Chen, C. N., & Alegría, M. (2010). English language proficiency and mental health service use among Latino and Asian Americans with mental disorders. *Medical Care, 48*(12), 1097–104.

Benish, S., Quintana, S., & Wampold, B. (2011). Culturally adapted psychotherapy and the legitimacy of myth: A direct comparison meta-analysis. *Journal of Counseling Psychology, 58*(3), 279–89.

Berger, L., Zane, N., & Hwang, W. (2014). Therapist ethnicity and treatment orientation differences in multicultural counseling competencies. *Asian American Journal of Psychology, 5*(1), 53–65.

Bernal, G., Bonilla, J., & Bellido, C. (1995). Ecological validity and cultural sensitivity for outcome research: Issues for cultural adaptation and development of psychosocial treatments with Hispanics. *Journal of Abnormal Child Psychology, 23,* 67–82.

Bhopal, R. S. (2012). Research agenda for tackling inequalities related to migration and ethnicity in Europe. *Journal of Public Health, 34*(2), 167–173.

Berry, J. W. (1980). Acculturation as varieties of adaptation. In A. M. Padilla (Ed.), *Acculturation: Theory, models, and some new findings* (pp. 9–26). Boulder, CO: Westview.

Bischoff, R. J., Hollist, C. S., Smith, C. W., & Flack, P. (2004). Addressing the mental health needs of the rural underserved: Findings from a multiple case study of a behavioral telehealth project. *Contemporary Family Therapy, 26*(2), 179–98.

Boschen, M. J., & Casey, L. M. (2008). The use of mobile telephones as adjuncts to cognitive behavioral psychotherapy. *Professional Psychology: Research and Practice, 39*(5), 546–552.

Borchgrevink, A. (2003). Silencing language: Of anthropologists and interpreters. *Ethnography, 4,* 95–121.

Constantine, M. (2002). Predictors of satisfaction with counseling: Racial and ethnic minority clients' attitudes toward counseling and ratings of their counselors' general and multicultural counseling competence. *Journal of Counseling Psychology, 49*(2), 255–63.

Cooper, L. A., Roter, D. L., Johnson, R. L., Ford, D. E., Steinwachs, D. M., & Powe, N. R. (2003). Patient-centered communication, ratings of care, and concordance of patient and physician race. *Annals of Internal Medicine, 139*(11), 907–15.

Crilly, N., Moultrie, J., & Clarkson, P. J. (2004). Seeing things: Consumer response to the visual domain in product design. *Design Studies, 25*(6), 547–77.

Crozier, W. R. (1994). *Manufactured pleasures: Psychological response to design.* Manchester, UK: Manchester University Press.

Del Re, A. C., Flückiger, C., Horvath, A. O., Symonds, D., & Wampold, B. E. (2012). Therapist effects in the therapeutic alliance–outcome relationship: A restricted-maximum likelihood meta-analysis. *Clinical Psychology Review, 32*(7), 642–9.

Demie, F. (2012). English as an additional language pupils: How long does it take to acquire English fluency? *Language and Education, 27*(1), 59–69.

Eighty-Eighth Congress. (1964). *PL 88–352, January 7.* Washington, DC.

Ennis, L., Rose, D., Denis, M., Pandit, N., & Wykes, T. (2012). Can't surf, won't surf: The digital divide in mental health. *Journal of Mental Health, 21*(4), 395–403.

Eonta, A. M., Christon, L. M., Hourigan, S. E., Ravindran, N., Vrana, S. R., & Southam-Gerow, M. A. (2011). Using everyday technology to enhance evidence-based treatments. *Professional Psychology: Research and Practice, 42*(6), 513–20.

European Commission. (2011). *Demography report 2010—Older, more numerous and diverse Europeans.* http://ec.europa.eu/social/main.jsp?catId=738&langId=en&pubId=5936&furtherPubs=yes

Farrell, S. P., & McKinnon, C. R. (2003). Technology and rural mental health. *Archives of Psychiatric Nursing, 17*(1), 20–6.

Faust, D., & Faust, K. A. (2012). Experts' experience and diagnostic and predictive accuracy. In D. Faust (Ed.), *Coping with psychiatric and psychological testimony* (6th ed., pp. 131–46). New York: Oxford University Press.

Fox, S., & Vitak, J. (2008). *Degrees of access.* Washington, DC: Pew Internet & American Life Project.

Fuertes, J., Stracuzzi, T., Bennett, J., Scheinholtz, J., & Mislowack, A. (2006). Therapist multicultural competency: A study of therapy dyads. *Psychotherapy, Theory Resistance, Practice, Training, 43*(4), 480–90.

Gary, F. A. (2005). Stigma: Barrier to mental health care among ethnic minorities. *Issues in Mental Health Nursing, 26,* 979–99.

Gavrilova, M. L., & Yampolskiy, R. (2011). Applying biometric principles to avatar recognition. In *Transactions on computational science XII* (pp. 140–58). Berlin: Springer.

Gerardi, M., Rothbaum, B. O., Ressler, K., Heekin, M., & Rizzo, A. (2008). Virtual reality exposure therapy using a virtual Iraq: Case report. *Journal of Traumatic Stress, 21*(2), 209–13.

Gibson, M. A. (2001). Immigrant adaptation and patterns of acculturation. *Human Development, 44,* 19–23.

Griffiths, K. M., & Christensen, H. (2007). Internet-based mental health programs: A powerful tool in the rural medical kit. *Australian Journal of Rural Health, 15*(2), 81–7.

Griner, D., & Smith, T. B. (2006). Culturally adapted mental health intervention: A meta-analytic review. *Psychotherapy: Theory, Research, Practice, Training,* 43(4), 531–48.

Hall, C. C. I. (1997). Cultural malpractice: The growing obsolescence of psychology with the changing US population. *The American Psychologist, 52*(6), 642–51.

Hall, G. C. N. (2001). Psychotherapy research with ethnic minorities: Empirical, ethical, and conceptual issues. *Journal of Consulting and Clinical Psychology, 69*(3), 502.

Halle, T., Hair, E., Wandner, L., McNamara, M., & Chien, N. (2012). Predictors and outcomes of early vs. later English language proficiency among English language learners. *Early Childhood Research Quarterly, 27*(1), 1–20.

Harsham, P. (1984). A misinterpreted word worth $71 million. *Medical Economics, 61*(12), 289–92.

Healthy People 2020. (2014). *Health communication and health information technology.* http://www.healthypeople.gov/2020/topicsobjectives2020/overview.aspx?topicid=18

Heaton, R. K., Ryan, L., & Grant, I. (2009). Demographic influences and use of demographically corrected norms in neuropsychological assessment. In I. Grant & K. M. Adams (Eds.), *Neuropsychological assessment of neuropsychiatric and neuromedical disorders* (pp. 127–55). New York: Oxford University Press.

Holden, K., McGregor, B., Thandi, P., Fresh, E., Sheats, K., Belton, A., . . . Satcher, D. (2014). Toward culturally centered integrative care for addressing mental health disparities among ethnic minorities. *Psychological Services, 11*(4), 357–68.

Huey, S., & Polo A. (2008). Evidence-based psychosocial treatments for ethnic minority youth: A review and meta-analysis. *Journal of Clinical Child Adolescence Psychology, 37*(1), 262–301.

Hulstijn, J. H. (2010). Measuring second language proficiency. In E. Blom & S. Unsworth (Eds.), *Experimental methods in language acquisition research* (pp. 185–99). Amsterdam: John Benjamins.

Hwang, W. (2006). The psychotherapy adaptation and modification framework. *American Psychologist, 61*(7), 702–15.

Imel, Z., Atkins, D., Baldwin, S., Owen, J., Baardseth, T., & Wampold, B. (2011). Racial/ethnic disparities in therapist effectiveness: A conceptualization and initial study of cultural competence. *Journal of Counseling Psychology, 58*(3), 290–8.

Kearney, L. K., Draper, M., & Barón, A. (2005). Counseling utilization by ethnic minority college students. *Cultural Diversity and Ethnic Minority Psychology, 11*(3), 272–85.

Keller, A., Gangnon, R., & Witt, W. P. (2014). The impact of patient-provider communication and language spoken on adequacy of depression treatment for US women. *Health Communication, 29*(7), 646–55.

Kim, B., Li, L., & Liang, C. (2002). Effects Asian American client adherence to Asian cultural values, session goal, and counselor emphasis of client expression on career counseling process. *Journal of Counseling Psychology, 49*, 342–54.

Kreps, G. L. (2005). Disseminating relevant health information to underserved audiences: Implications of the Digital Divide Pilot Projects. *Journal of the Medical Library Association, 93*(4 Suppl), S68–73.

Kreps, G. L., Gustafson, D., Salovey, P., Perocchia, R. S., Wilbright, W., Bright, M. A., & Muha, C. (2007). The NCI digital divide pilot projects: Implications for cancer education. *Journal of Cancer Education, 22*(S1), S56–60.

Kvasny, L. (2006). Cultural (re) production of digital inequality in a US community technology initiative. *Information, Communication & Society, 9*(02), 160–81.

Leff, J., Williams, G., Huckvale, M., Arbuthnot, M., & Leff, A. P. (2013). Avatar therapy for persecutory auditory hallucinations: What is it and how does it work? *Psychosis, 6*(2), 166–76.

Leon, S. C., Martinovich, Z., Lutz, W., & Lyons, J. S. (2005). The effect of therapist experience on psychotherapy outcomes. *Clinical Psychology and Psychotherapy, 12*, 417–26.

Lewis-Fernández, R., & Díaz, N. (2002). The cultural formulation: A method for assessing cultural factors affecting the clinical encounter. *Psychiatric Quarterly, 73*(4), 271–95.

Li, L., & Livingston, G. (2011). *Latinos and digital technology, 2010.* Washington, DC: Pew Hispanic Center.

Lisetti, C. L., Yasavur, U., De Leon, C., Amini, R., Visser, U., & Rishe, N. (2012, May). Building an on-demand avatar-based health intervention for behavior change. *Proceedings of the 25th International Florida Artificial Intelligence Research Society conference (FLAIRS-25>).* https://www.aaai.org/ocs/index.php/FLAIRS/FLAIRS12/paper/viewPaper/4481

Lopez, E. C. (2002). Best practices in working with school interpreters lo deliver psychological services to children and families. In A. Thomas & J. Grimes (Eds.), *Best practices in school psychology* (pp. 1419–32). Washington, DC: National Association of School Psychologists.

Malenfant, E. C., Lebel, A., & Martel, L. (2010). *Projections of the diversity of the Canadian population: 2006 to 2031.* http://www.statcan.gc.ca/pub/91-551-x/91-551-x2010001-eng.pdf

McCabe, K., & Yeh, M. (2009). Parent-child interaction therapy for Mexican Americans: A randomized clinical trial. *Journal of Clinical Child and Adolescent Psychology, 38*, 753–9.

McKay, J. C., Vásquez, Á. R., Chipp, C. L., Ford, T. J., Robinson, R. V., Sharma, D. K. B., . . . Dulin, P. L. (2013). Divided by miles, connected by purpose: Telepsychology technology in a graduate training program. *Training and Education in Professional Psychology, 7*(3), 166–73.

Minority Health and Health Disparities Research and Education Act, Pub. L. No. 106-525 (2000). Retrieved from https://www.govinfo.gov/app/details/PLAW-106publ525

Missinne, S., & Bracke, P. (2012). Depressive symptoms among immigrants and ethnic minorities: A population based study in 23 European countries. *Social Psychiatry and Psychiatric Epidemiology, 47*(1), 97–109.

Morales, E., & Norcross, J. (2010). Evidence-based practices with ethnic minorities: Strange bedfellows no more. *Journal of Clinical Psychology, 66*(8), 821–9.

Murray, C. D., & Wynne, J. (2001). Researching community, work and family with an interpreter. *Community, Work & Family 4*, 157–70.

Norcross, J. (2011). *Psychotherapy relationships that work: Evidence-based responsiveness.* New York: Oxford University Press.

Öst, L. G., Karlstedt, A., & Widén, S. (2012). The effects of cognitive behavior therapy delivered by students in a psychologist training program: An effectiveness study. *Behavior Therapy, 43*(1), 160–73.

Owen, J., Leach, M., Tao, K., & Rodolfa, E. (2011). Clients perceptions on their psychotherapists' multicultural orientation. *Psychotherapy, 48*(3), 274–82.

Paone, T. R., & Malott, K. M. (2008). Using interpreters in mental health counseling: A literature review and recommendations. *Journal of Multicultural Counseling and Development (36)*3, 130–42.

Parsons, T. D., Bowerly, T., Buckwalter, J. G., & Rizzo, A. A. (2007). A controlled clinical comparison of attention performance in children with ADHD in a virtual reality classroom compared to standard neuropsychological methods. *Child Neuropsychology, 13*(4), 363–81.

Passel, J. S., Livingston, G., & Cohn, D. (2012). Explaining why minority births now outnumber White births. Washington, DC: Pew Research Center. http://www.pewsocialtrends.org/2012/05/17/explaining-why-minority-births-now-outnumber-white-births/

Portes, A., & Rumbaut, R. G. (2006). *Immigrant America: A portrait.* (3rd ed.). Berkeley: University of California Press.

Quackenbush, D. M., & Krasner, A. (2012). Avatar therapy: Where technology, symbols, culture, and connection collide. *Journal of Psychiatric Practice, 18*(6), 451–9.

Qureshi, A., Collazos, F., Ramos, M., & Casas, M. (2008). Cultural competency training in psychiatry. *European Psychiatry, 23,* 49–58.

Rao, D., Feinglass, J., & Corrigan, P. (2007). Ethnoracial disparities in mental illness stigma. *The Journal of Nervous and Mental Disease, 195,* 1020–3.

Reed, R. N., Messler, E. C., Coombs, T. E., & Quevillon, R. P. (2014). Social media use and the acceptability of telepsychological services in rural populations. *Journal of Rural Mental Health, 38*(1), 2–8.

Rohland, B. M., Saleh, S. S., Rohrer, J. E., & Romitti, P. A. (2000). Acceptability of telepsychiatry to a rural population. *Psychiatric Services, 51*(5), 672–674.

Rothbaum, B. O., Hodges, L., Smith, S., Lee, J. H., & Price, L. (2000). A controlled study of virtual reality exposure therapy for the fear of flying. *Journal of Consulting and Clinical Psychology, 68*(6), 1020–6.

Schwartz, S. J., Pantin, H., Sullivan, S., Prado, G., & Szapocznik, J. (2006). Nativity and years in the receiving culture as markers of acculturation in ethnic enclaves. *Journal of Cross-Cultural Psychology, 37,* 345–53.

Schwartz, S. J., Unger, J. B., Zamboanga, B. L., & Szapocznik, J. (2010). Rethinking the concept of acculturation: Implications for theory and research. *American Psychologist, 65*(4), 237–51.

Searight, H. R., & Searight, B. K. (2009). Working with foreign language interpreters: Recommendations for psychological practice. *Professional Psychology: Research and Practice, 40*(5), 444.

Shapiro, D. A., & Shapiro, D. (1982). Meta-analysis of comparative therapy outcome studies: A replication and refinement. *Psychological Bulletin, 92,* 581–604.

Smedley, B. D., Stith, A. Y., & Nelson, A. R. (Eds.). (2003). *Unequal treatment: Confronting racial and ethnic disparities in health care.* Washington, DC: National Academies Press.

Smith, M. L., & Glass, G. V. (1977). Meta-analysis of psychotherapy outcome studies. *American Psychologist, 32,* 752–60.

Smith, M. L., Glass, G. V., & Miller, T. I. (1980). *The benefits of psychotherapy.* Baltimore, MD: Johns Hopkins University Press.

Smith, T. B., & Trimble, J. E. (2016a). Therapist multicultural competence: A meta-analysis of client experiences in treatment. In T. B. Smith and J. E. Trimble (Eds.), *Foundations of multicultural psychology: Research to inform effective practice* (pp. 49–64). Washington, DC: American Psychological Association.

Smith, T. B., & Trimble, J. E. (2016b). Matching clients with therapists on the basis of race or ethnicity: A meta-analysis of clients' level of participation in treatment. In T. B. Smith and J. E. Trimble (Eds.), *Foundations of multicultural psychology: Research to inform effective practice* (pp. 115–28). Washington, DC: American Psychological Association.

Stephenson, M. (2000). Development and validation of the Stephenson Multigroup Acculturation Scale (SMAS). *Psychological Assessment, 12,* 77–88.

Sue, D. W. (2004). Whiteness and ethnocentric monoculturalism: Making the "invisible" visible. *American Psychologist. Special Issue: Awards Issue 2004, 59*(8), 761–9.

Sue, S. (1998). In search of cultural competence in psychotherapy and counseling. *American Psychologist, 53*(4), 440–8.

Sue, S., Zane, N., Nagayama, H. Berger, L. K. (2009). The case for cultural competency in psychotherapeutic interventions. *Annual Review of Psychology, 60,* 525–48.

Unger, J. B., Gallagher, P., Shakib, S., Ritt-Olson, A., Palmer, P. H., & Johnson, C. A. (2002). The AHIMSA acculturation scale: A new measure of acculturation for adolescents in a multicultural society. *Journal of Early Adolescence, 22,* 225–51.

US Census Bureau. (2012). US Census Bureau projections show a slower growing, older, more diverse nation a half century from now. https://www.census.gov/newsroom/releases/archives/population/cb12-243.html

US Department of Health and Human Services. (2001). *Mental health: Culture, race, and ethnicity—a supplement to mental health: A report of the surgeon general.* Rockville, MD: US Department of Health and Human Services, Substance Abuse and Mental Health Services Administration, Center for Mental Health Services.

Wang, J. Y., Bennett, K., & Probst, J. (2011). Subdividing the digital divide: Differences in Internet access and use among rural residents with medical limitations. *Journal of Medical Internet Research, 13*(1), e25.

Whaley, A. L. (2001). Cultural mistrust: An important psychological construct for diagnosis and treatment of African Americans. *Professional Psychology: Research and Practice, 32,* 555–62.

World Health Organization (WHO). (2010). *A conceptual framework for action on the social determinants of health.* http://www.who.int/sdhconference/resources/ConceptualframeworkforactiononSDH_eng.pdf

PART 7

Use of Digital Technologies to Treat Specific Disorders

CHAPTER

33 Use of Digital Technology and Mobile Applications to Treat Anxiety Disorders

Dawn Delfin McDaniel, Marat V. Zanov, Michael Van Ameringen, Jasmine Turna, *and* Barbara Olasov Rothbaum

Abstract

The societal burden of anxiety disorders is enormous in the United States and in many other countries. A quarter of the US population will experience an anxiety disorder at some point in their lives. Although cognitive-behavioral therapy is effective at treating anxiety disorders, most individuals with anxiety disorders will go untreated as a consequence of several barriers to accessing treatment. Technology may serve as a means of addressing such barriers. This chapter reviews the application of technology for psychoeducation, training, screening, tracking, treatment, homework, and aftercare in anxiety disorders. More research is needed to evaluate the efficacy of these applications in controlled trials, but preliminary evidence is promising.

Keywords: anxiety, mobile, technology, Internet, computer, cognitive-behavioral therapy

The societal burden of anxiety disorders is enormous in the United States and in many other countries. The prevalence of anxiety and related disorders varies by condition, with specific phobias (6–12%), social anxiety disorder (10%), and posttraumatic stress disorder (PTSD) (6–9%) being the most common, followed by generalized anxiety disorder (GAD) (3–5%) and obsessive-compulsive disorder (OCD) (2–5%) and then agoraphobia (2%) and separation anxiety disorder (2–3%) (Kessler, Ruscio, Shear, & Wittchen, 2010). (Note that, as of the fifth edition of the *Diagnostic and Statistical Manual of Mental Disorders* [DSM-5, 2013], OCD and PTSD no longer classify as anxiety disorders.) Overall, approximately 1 in 4 individuals will experience an anxiety disorder at some point in their lives (Gunter & Whittal, 2010). Cognitive-behavioral therapy (CBT) is an effective treatment for anxiety disorders (Butler, Chapman, Forman, & Beck, 2006; Hofmann & Smits, 2008), yet more than 70% of individuals with anxiety disorders are not receiving treatment (Andrews, Henderson, & Hall, 2001; Lepine, 2002).

There are a number of reasons therapists are not able to reach individuals with anxiety. Major barriers to treatment include cost, time, and convenience. The cost of treatment for anxiety is often more than $100 an hour in the United States (Anxiety and Depression Association of America, 2014). Also, medical utilization rates for individuals with an anxiety disorder are inflated as their anxiety is often misdiagnosed, especially in those individuals who have panic attacks (Deacon, Lickel, & Abramowitz, 2008). Consequently, the economic cost for those individuals who seek medical services and do not receive mental health services is high. In the United States, healthcare expenditures for anxiety disorders were approximately $42.3 billion a year in the 1990s (Greenberg et al., 1999).

CBT is considered one of the faster modalities of anxiety treatment; however, the time commitment associated with CBT is significant. Individuals treated with CBT often attend more than 10 sessions and each session may extend beyond the typical 50-minute treatment time. For example, when CBT includes exposures, a 90-minute session is often required in order to allow sufficient time for the client to habituate during the session. Additionally, CBT commonly includes homework that is assigned between sessions, thus requiring a greater time commitment specifically for the patient. Finally, scheduling of CBT sessions requires an agreed-upon time for both the therapist and the client for each contact.

Despite the issues of lengthy time commitment and high cost of treatment, the greatest barrier to treatment may be the lack of therapists trained in CBT. In rural and remote areas, there may not be enough therapists, and, because of this, wait-lists for treatment can be long. Additionally, clients may need to travel long distances to find available therapists trained in CBT or specialized in the treatment of anxiety disorders. An anxious individual may have additional worries that make it difficult to seek treatment, such as concerns regarding social stigma, fears that others will negatively evaluate them, and difficulty leaving their house if they suffer from agoraphobia.

The use of digital technology and mobile applications ("apps") is a potential means of addressing many of these barriers to treatment. These technologies can automate many aspects of treatment, such as providing psychoeducation or training in CBT, which may make the treatments more efficient to deliver. Not only does this have the potential to reduce the cost of treatment, but because these technologies are often available on standard personal computers, mobile devices, and tablets, individuals may no longer need to leave their homes to access mental health care. Furthermore, these technologies deliver the content in interactive ways, ranging from text-based content to very immersive three-dimensional, audio-visual graphics, which may be more engaging and appealing to clients. Technology may also improve the quality of treatment or augment treatments in a way that increases effectiveness.

This chapter provides a review of the literature examining the use of technology in treating anxiety disorders. The review is organized by application of the technology, including its use for psychoeducation, training, screening, treatment, homework, and aftercare. We discuss ethnical issues of, challenges with, and limitations to the use of technology for the treatment of anxiety disorder. Finally, we offer suggestions for future directions by which researchers and therapists can use technology to advance their understanding of anxiety, their work, and the dissemination of effective interventions.

Psychoeducation on Anxiety

In 2012, three out of four US households reported having Internet access and about 80% reported having a computer (US Census Bureau, 2014). Given the convenience and ease of access, websites are likely the first way that individuals with anxiety learn about services and resources. These websites may improve an individual's knowledge of anxiety, including symptoms of anxiety, treatments for anxiety, and rationales for treatments. A number of websites are available that provide psychoeducation on anxiety (Table 33.1). A meta-analysis on psychoeducational interventions providing information similar to these websites (i.e., education, feedback, and advice in a passive manner) concluded that these resources can be effective at reducing symptoms of psychological distress and depression (Donker, Griffiths, Cuijpers, & Christensen, 2009).

Although the effect sizes of these studies were small, the findings from the meta-analysis suggest that passive psychoeducation is likely an important first step toward treatment for anxiety. Psychoeducational interventions are often cost-effective, may reduce the stigma of seeking treatment, and can easily be tailored to target a wide array of individual's needs. However, many psychoeducational tools, especially websites, do not offer high-quality, evidence-based information; therefore, their effectiveness is likely limited by their content.

To assure the quality of psychoeducational websites, organizations are developing critical reviews of this information (Christensen, Batterham, & Calear, 2014). For example, in Australia, the Beacon website at the Australian National University provides a portal for individuals seeking information on mental health. This portal includes information on phobias, generalized anxiety disorder, OCD, PTSD, and social anxiety disorder. Although Beacon can still be accessed by the public, it is no longer being updated.

In the United States, PsyberGuide.org provides a similar service for individuals seeking information on mobile apps. Apps are evaluated by three criteria: credibility, user experience, and transparency.

Examples of evaluated apps include Breathe2Relax, T2 MoodKit, and PE Coach (Table 33.2). Breathe2Relax is an example of an app that provides psychoeducation on stress, teaches diaphragmatic breathing, and provides opportunities for skill rehearsal (Media Kit: Breathe2Relax Mobile Application, 2014). Breathe2Relax was developed by the National Center for PTSD and the National Center for Telehealth and Technology (known as "T2"). This app is available for free on the App Store and Google Play. This chapter reviews several evaluated mobile apps, along with other apps and digital technologies (see Table 33.2). While all of the apps

Table 33.1 Digital resources for anxiety

Psychoeducation resources	
Anxiety and Depression Association of America	http://www.adaa.org
The National Institute of Mental Health	http://www.nimh.nih.gov/health/topics/anxiety-disorders/index.shtml
National Center for PTSD	http://www.ptsd.va.gov/index.asp
The Beacon	https://beacon.anu.edu.au/
International OCD Foundation	http://iocdf.org
Training Resources	
Trauma Focused Cognitive Behavioral Therapy	www.musc.edu/tfcbt2
American Psychological Association (APA)'s Advanced Training Institutes (ATI)	http://www.apa.org/science/resources/ati
Assessment Resources	
Liebowitz Social Anxiety Scale	http://asp.cumc.columbia.edu/SAD/
Yale-Brown Obsessive Compulsive Scale	http://psychology-tools.com/yale-brown-obsessive-compulsive-scale/
Treatment Resources	
FearFighter™	http://fearfighter.cbtprogram.com/

Table 33.2 Mobile apps for anxiety

Mobile app	Targeted anxiety disorder	Recommended clinical application						
		Psychoeducation	Training	Screening	Self-administered treatment	Therapist-assisted treatment	Homework	Aftercare
Breathe2Relax	PTSD	◆						
PE Coach	PTSD		◆	◆		◆	◆	◆
PTSD Coach	PTSD	◆		◆				◆
Anxiety Coach	SAD, OCD, GAD, SP, PD, PTSD	◆		◆	◆			
LiveOCDFree	OCD	◆				◆	◆	
T2 Mood Tracker	All Anxiety Disorders			◆			◆	

OCD, obsessive-compulsive disorder; SAD, social anxiety disorder; GAD, generalized anxiety disorder; SP, specific phobia; PD, panic disorder; PTSD, posttraumatic stress disorder.

discussed in this chapter are informed by evidence-based treatments, it is important to note that the apps themselves have not been scientifically validated.

Training Therapists in the Treatment of Anxiety Disorders

Because the need for therapists trained in evidence-based approaches such as CBT exceeds their availability, there are a growing number of digital resources for training therapists. For instance, Trauma-Focused Cognitive-Behavioral Therapy (TF-CBT) offers a free web-based training course called TF-CBTWeb2.0 that provides a program of study for the treatment of PTSD in children (Cohen, Mannarino, & Deblinger, 2006; Deblinger & Heflin, 1996). TF-CBTWeb covers the key components to TF-CBT including psychoeducation, stress management, affect expression and modulation, cognitive coping, creating the trauma narrative, cognitive processing, and behavior management training. TF-CBTWeb2.0 was specifically developed for practitioners who have limited availability to attend formal trainings. Therefore, the training is presented in interactive modules that allow therapists to learn at their own pace. Since its initial roll-out, this course has generated much interest among therapists and contributed to an increase in therapists adequately trained in evidence-based trauma treatment for children.

PE Coach is a mobile app that was developed to serve as a training tool for therapists and an aid to prolonged exposure (PE) treatment to be used by both patients and therapists. It was developed in collaboration with the National Center for PTSD, the Center for Deployment Psychology, and T2. For training purposes, it has various built-in tutorials and a clinician's guide to improve therapist fidelity to the treatment protocol. In addition, this app contains a number of useful tools including an audio recorder for imaginal exposures, symptom assessments, and calendar integration for therapy appointment reminders. Usability and app satisfaction were evaluated in a small within-subjects crossover trial (Reger, Skopp, Edwards-Stewert, & Lemus, 2015). This app is available free of charge at the Android marketplace or the Apple App Store.

Assessment and Screening for Anxiety Disorders

Many rating scales, screening tools, real-time self-monitoring, symptom checklists, and other assessment tools for anxiety disorders are now available in digital formats to be used on personal computers, mobile devices, and tablets. Having these tools available digitally means that they can often be assessed more conveniently at any time, no matter where the therapist or client is located. Many of the available digital assessment and screening tools allow clients to share their assessment information securely with their therapists or export their information so that it can be printed. In addition, these assessments can be programmed to notify therapists if critical values have been identified. The clients could then be connected to resources or the therapist can follow up (Luxton, McCann, Bush, Mishkind, & Reger, 2011). Examples of widely available digital versions of assessment and screening tools include the Hamilton Anxiety Rating Scale (HAM-A), Liebowitz Social Anxiety Scale (LSAS), PTSD Checklist (PCL), and Yale-Brown Obsessive Compulsive Scale (Y-BOCS).

Compared to the pen-and-paper versions, many of the digital versions of assessments can reduce problems with missing data by making the client select a response on each item. While increasing the efficiency of data collection, these digital assessment methods also simplify scoring, storage, and data analyses. For example, therapists no longer have to hand-score many of these tests or enter test results manually into a database. Finally, digital assessments often provide instant feedback, making reporting outcomes much less cumbersome and time-consuming for the therapist.

When using digital assessments it is important that the psychometric properties of the tool are not compromised. Results from a study comparing Internet versus paper-and-pencil delivered measures commonly used in research on social anxiety disorder found that the following measures maintained their psychometric properties when administered via the Internet: Liebowitz Social Anxiety Scale-Self-Report, Social Interaction and Anxiety Scale, and the Social Phobia Scale (Hedman et al., 2010). Other scales have not been evaluated.

PTSD Coach is an example of an app that incorporates assessment and rating scales. PTSD Coach includes the PTSD Checklist (PCL), which is a reliable and valid self-report measure of PTSD symptomatology. The PCL has also been tested on the iPhone and was considered comparable to paper and computer formats (Bush, Skopp, Smolenski, Crumpton, & Fairall, 2013). According to its website, this app is widely used, with more than 100,000 downloads in more than 74 countries (US Department of Veterans Affairs, 2014). PTSD Coach was developed by the VA's National Center for PTSD in partnership with T2. Beyond its assessment tools, PTSD Coach includes psychoeducation on PTSD, tools to manage symptoms, and ways to find support. It is currently available for free on the Apple App Store and Google Play.

Self-Administered Interventions for Anxiety

Technological innovations that maintain clinical outcomes but reduce or eliminate the need for a therapist's time have the potential benefit of increasing access to treatment. Because little is known about whether therapist contact is essential for the treatment of anxiety disorder, Newman, Szkodny, Llera, and Przeworski (2011) conducted a systematic review and meta-analysis of technology-based anxiety interventions that used minimal therapist contact to explore this question. They used four categories to describe these technologies: (a) "self-administered therapy," in which therapist contact was limited to assessment; (b) "predominately self-help," in which therapist contact was limited to less than 1.5 hours of the therapist's time; (c) "minimal contact therapy," in which the therapist is involved less than standard approaches, but more than 1.5 hours; and (d) "predominately therapist administered treatments," in which the technology augments standard therapy.

The results of this meta-analysis showed that self-administered and predominately self-help therapy were most effective for motivated clients. When technologies are used at home and/or with little therapist contact, there are issues with compliance and attrition. Also, these results vary by type of anxiety disorder. Self-administered therapy and predominately self-help therapy seemed most promising for social phobia and panic disorder.

FearFighter is one example of a computer-based program that uses a minimal contact treatment of phobias/panic disorder (Marks, Kenwright, McDonough, Whittaker, & Mataix-Cols, 2004). FearFighter is available for €99.00–179.00 in the United Kingdom (see Table 33.1 for the website). The program involves video modules, practice exercises, and downloadable content. It is available for any personal computer with an Internet connection.

When compared to a clinician-guided group, FearFighter required 73% less clinician time, yet showed similar improvement in clinical outcomes and satisfaction (Marks et al., 2004). Treatments like FearFighter, which require limited therapist contact, may be key to a "stepped care" approach to mental health (Lewis, Pearce, & Bisson, 2012). This stepped care approach may be particularly suitable to clients who otherwise would have difficulty accessing care because of their concerns with stigma, negative evaluation, or agoraphobia.

Anxiety Coach is an example of predominately self-administered treatment app. Anxiety Coach was developed by researchers at the Mayo Clinic and is currently available for download on the iPhone and iPad for $6.99. This app provides users with a self-test to rate which anxiety disorder (i.e., social anxiety disorder, GAD, panic disorder, OCD, PTSD, and specific phobia) is most in line with their overall level of anxiety. This app also includes psychoeducational resources, exposure exercises, and the ability to graphically view progress in their anxiety over select periods of time. However, it may also have use in situations where therapist contact is interrupted, as suggested by a case report of two pediatric OCD patients (Whiteside, Ale, Vickers Douglas, Tiede, & Dammann, 2014).

Therapist-Assisted Apps and Internet-Delivered Interventions

Internet-delivered interventions can increase the accessibility and availability of CBT by eliminating the need for face-to-face contact with a therapist. Unlike self-administered interventions, Internet-delivered interventions that are therapist-assisted include therapist contact through email, text messaging, or telephone. In these interventions the treatment content is consistent with that of typical in-person CBT. However, the clients work through the content on their own at anytime, in any place, with minimal therapist contact.

On average, the therapists provide 20 minutes of their time weekly per client instead of the typical 45- to 60-minute weekly CBT session (Lenhard et al., 2014). More research is needed to understand the impact of therapist assistance on these interventions (Newman et al., 2011). It is expected that therapist involvement may increase treatment adherence and improve treatment outcomes (Lenhard et al., 2014).

A meta-analysis of Internet-delivered CBT reported large effect sizes in the treatment of social phobia and panic disorder (Hedman, Ljotsson, & Lindefors, 2012). Internet-delivered CBT was found to be equivalent to standard CBT in two well-designed, randomized controlled trials for panic disorder and in three well-designed, randomized controlled trials for social phobias. Four randomized controlled trials looked at the effects of Internet-based CBT for PTSD; the results were classified as "probably efficacious" because an active control group was used in only one of the studies.

Lenhard and colleagues' (2014) work provides an example of an Internet-delivered CBT intervention for pediatric OCD. As these researchers noted, although many Internet-based CBT interventions were created for adult populations, few were developed for child and adolescent populations. Therefore, they designed an intervention for adolescents and their parents that included age-appropriate interactive materials, films, and animations. The therapists spent a total of 20 minutes per participant per week, assisting with treatment, selecting homework assignments, and problem-solving. Their efficacy trial showed that the participants experienced a significant decrease in symptom severity at post-treatment.

LiveOCDFree is an example of an app designed to increase the efficiency of treatment for OCD. This app was developed by Pocket Therapist LLC and Dr. Kristen Mulcahy. This app uses techniques from exposure and response prevention, which is an evidence-based treatment. It is currently available on the Apple App Store for $29.99. With versions for both children and adults, the app helps users set up an exposure hierarchy, practice goals, and use rewards to offer immediate relief for OCD symptoms. The adult version is equipped with a toolbox including motivational scripts and relaxation and meditation recordings in addition to specific strategies for contamination and checking rituals. The app allows users to track their progress. The children's version provides the same basic functions as the adult version; however, the content includes songs, stories, visuals, mechanics, and voice-overs that are age-appropriate.

Exposure Therapy Using Virtual Reality

Exposure therapy using virtual reality has been employed with various conditions, including fear of flying, fear of heights, fear of public speaking, and PTSD (Parsons & Rizzo, 2008). Unlike traditional exposure therapy, *virtual reality exposure* (VRE) offers a flexible and cost-effective alternative for some patients. For example, completing in vivo exposure with a patient who is fearful of flying would require a significant investment of time and resources (going to the airport and flying on a real airplane). Such treatment would have to include therapist time for the drive to the airport, standing in lines to check in for the flight, going through security checkpoints, and so forth. Moreover, the cost of round-trip airfare for the clinician and the patient, particularly considering the multiple exposure sessions that may be needed, could be prohibitive. In VRE therapy, exposure sessions are conducted in the clinician's office and can include several round-trip "flights" all within the therapy hour.

Perhaps one of the stronger arguments in favor of VRE therapy is its potential utility in treating PTSD. Emergence of programs such as Bravemind (Rizzo, Hartholt, Grimani, Leeds, & Liewer, 2014) has offered clinicians an opportunity to "place" their combat veteran patients into virtual Afghanistan or Iraq environments. Depending on their individual trauma, patients may be exposed to a variety of scenarios, including convoys, foot patrols, roadside explosions, and ambush situations. The patient is engaged in imaginal exposure, repeatedly recounting the worst moments of the index trauma. Unlike traditional prolonged imaginal exposure, however, their eyes are open and they are viewing stimuli in the head-mounted display that matches what they are describing.

Although VRE therapy may be a robust, versatile, and convenient approach, it is neither intended to be used as a stand-alone treatment, nor should it be self-administered. Ideally, VRE would be integrated in a comprehensive treatment package that is designed to address individual-specific cognitive and behavioral aspects of the patient's anxiety disorder.

Homework Tools

Digital technology and mobile apps have functionality that may increase homework compliance, patient accountability, and treatment adherence. This functionality includes the capability of integrating with calendar and phone contacts, recording a time and date stamp, texting homework reminders, and emailing homework feedback. These technologies have the capability of notifying therapists if their clients have not opened an email, visited a webpage, or proceeded in the software program. The audio, photo, and video capability of digital devices are also tools that can be useful for homework. For instance, therapists can ask their client to take photos of feared stimuli, videos of exposures, or to make audio recordings of social interactions. Rather than clients completing a homework worksheet at the end of the day, homework done on a digital device may be easier to complete in real time (Aguilera & Muench, 2012). Finally, some homework tools provide clients with instantaneous feedback on their progress that may enhance motivation to complete homework assignments (Aguilera & Muench, 2012).

The T2 Mood Tracker is an example of an app that could be used in conjunction with CBT for homework. Developed by the National Center for PTSD and T2, T2 Mood Tracker allows an individual to track ratings on anxiety, depression, general well-being, head injury, posttraumatic stress, and stress, or to build custom rating scales. Items for the anxiety scale include worried/untroubled, pressured/calm, tense/relaxed, sleepless/rested, distracted/focused, irritable/cheerful, unsafe/safe, fearful/fearless, panicked/content, and anxious/peaceful. Clients can rate their level of anxiety and then view a graphical representation of their results over time. T2 Mood Tracker allows the client to save results as CSV or PDF files, which could be sent to a therapist. T2 Mood tracker is available for free on Google Play, the Apple App Store, and Amazon.

Aftercare

Whereas a traditional approach for aftercare may include a remotely scheduled session or a telephone consultation, there are many resources, including those already discussed, that can be used to maintain or extend the clinical gains made in treatment. Some of the earlier steps in utilizing technology to this end involved text messaging between the clinician/clinic and the patient. For example, Bauer and colleagues (2003) obtained promising results when using text messaging to follow-up on patients recently discharged from inpatient hospitalization treatment for bulimia nervosa. Specifically, patients are asked to send weekly reports on their symptomatic status and receive personalized feedback in response. For instance, a patient who is not feeling well may receive the following feedback: "If you feel desperate, it may be helpful to talk to friends, not just about problems, but also about nice things. Don't give up."

Therapists could use the PE Coach and PTSD Coach app described earlier to assign continued, self-guided homework assignments upon completion of in-person treatment. In PE Coach, clients could continue to proceed through their steps in the Exposure Hierarchy, do ongoing breathing retraining exercises, and revisit the psychoeducational materials. In PTSD Coach, clients could use coping tools, symptom management information, and available support resources, based on their specific location, allowing them to feel supported and connected.

Discussion

This chapter has reviewed various forms of digital technologies and mobile apps used to treat anxiety disorders. These types of technologies are becoming a common component of mental health services. Although the technologies reviewed show promise, it is important that we fully consider the ethical issues of, challenges with, and limitations to the use of this technology.

A major concern in applying technology to treat anxiety disorders is the lack of rigorous research on many new technologies. A recent review summarizing the existing app literature suggests that apps for anxiety and related disorders have limited empirical support, although the mood disorder app literature is more developed (Van Ameringen et al., 2017). Specifically, meta-analyses have indicated that these studies have used small sample sizes, have high dropout rates, and use designs that are not well-controlled (Newman et al., 2011). Another concern is that some anxiety interventions are growing out of a technology-driven focus and do not adequately consider clinical needs or gaps in the field. Thus, these technologies may not take advantage of the evidence base surrounding the topic. To foster or maintain the quality of anxiety interventions, more rigorous designs are needed that evaluate these technologies against standard treatments.

Data security and patient privacy are key concerns when incorporating technology into clinical practice. These types of threats come in many forms. If an individual loses his or her mobile device or that device in accessed by another user, there could be a serious violation of that individual's privacy. To prevent unauthorized access to personal information, apps often include password protection that adds an additional level of security above and beyond the password to access the device. However, as described in the end-user agreement of PTSD Coach, "Any data created by the user of th[e] app are only as secure as the phone/device itself" (US Department of Veterans Affairs, 2014). Therefore, therapists and clients need to understand the security limitations of not just the apps, but also of the devices they use.

When a therapist transmits protected health information to a client or a client to the therapist, then the Health Insurance Portability and Accountability Act (HIPAA) is evoked. HIPAA requires a certain level of encryption and protection of digital transmission of information, which includes sources such as cloud storage, computer faxes, mobile devices, Wi-Fi networks, flash drives, and websites (American Psychological Association Practice Organization, 2013). When using technology in clinical practice, therapists might want to review HIPAA rules to ensure compliance (American Psychological Association Practice Organization, 2013).

Other privacy legislation, including the Electronic Communications Privacy Act, which contains an exception for user consent where third parties may access their information, and the Computer Fraud and Abuse Act, which protects against unauthorized accessing of data from a person's computer (but not mobile phone), may have loopholes in their privacy protection for health apps. Other issues such as potential installation of malware and the apps' use of GPS to track the user's location are also important to consider when advising clients to use a mobile app (Yang & Silverman, 2014).

In 2013, the US Food and Drug Administration (FDA) published a guidance document for mobile medical apps for industry and FDA staff. The FDA now regulates any app that is an accessory to a medical device, is a free-standing medical device app, or includes clinical decision software. Health and wellness apps that provide users with the ability to log life events, retrieve medical content, or communicate with clinicians or health centers will not be regulated. Therefore, most mental health apps will not be subject to regulation (Hamel, Cortez, Cohen, & Kesselheim, 2014).

Unfortunately, the accessibility of technology has the potential to blur boundaries between individuals and their therapists. With high-risk patients or with patients in remote areas, boundary setting needs to be considered, especially in regards to use of technology that is not time dependent. Technology can create the illusion that therapists are available 24 hours a day, 7 days a week. This extension of the typical therapy hour beyond the confines of a particular time and place can be useful as clients can feel they have increased access to a therapy, but it can also be problematic if not appropriately considered. Therapists might want to explain their policy for email responses or for when they check business email (Tate & Zabinski, 2004). Typical technology failures, such as difficulty with dropped calls, unreliable Internet, and battery failure, which may ordinarily just be a nuisance, can create major challenges in treatments that rely on these resources. It may be important to have multiple ways to communicate with a client in order to overcome these potential problems.

In the treatment of anxiety disorders, it is important for therapists to consider whether or not digital technologies are enabling any of their client's presenting problems or serving as a safety signal. In the treatment of some disorders, such as agoraphobia or social anxiety disorder, technology may increase social isolation and avoidance of social situations. If clients use VR for exposure, it is important, when possible, to have them also expose themselves to the fear outside the virtual world to ensure generalizability of the treatment.

Clinicians may be intimidated by or uncomfortable with the constantly changing landscape of digital technologies and mobile apps. To stay current with technologies, clinicians may need to become familiar with a number of different devices (i.e., mobile, tablet, and person computer), configurations, and software solutions. Most psychology programs provide little to no training in technology, although the American Psychological Association (APA) has created the Advanced Training Institutes (ATI), which focus on emerging technologies.

Beyond the barrier of comfort with technology, the technologies offered may not match the specifics of the client's anxiety issues. For example, a client might find VR cues to produce mild levels of anxiety but not produce the levels of anxiety they experience in real life. Given these issues, therapists should carefully vet any technologies they suggest to their clients. Similarly, therapists should assess client's technological aptitude. Clients who have limited technological experience may not be well-suited for technological interventions.

Conclusion

As digital technologies continue to advance, they will likely become more interactive, convenient, and tailored to the individual user. A clinician's own competence with technology is important for his or her uptake of new technologies. Therefore, the inclusion of technology in the training of therapists who are learning to treat anxiety disorders will be important for the dissemination of these new tools. In addition, it is important for therapists to be able to evaluate new technologies and understand their utility for their client populations. Technology has the potential to help therapists transcend typical time and location constraints in order to have a greater impact. While promising, therapists must combine systematic review of the scientific literature and state of knowledge with reasoned judgment to ensure that these technologies are applied in a way that will be most helpful for their clients.

References

Aguilera, A., & Muench, F. (2012). There's an app for that: Information technology applications for cognitive behavioral practitioners. *Behavioral Therapist*, *35*(4), 65–73.

American Psychological Association Practice Organization. (2013). *HIPAA privacy rule: A primer for psychologists*. Washington, DC: Author.

Andrews, G., Henderson, S., & Hall, W. (2001). Prevalence, comorbidity, disability and service utilisation: Overview of the Australian National Mental Health Survey. *British Journal of Psychiatry*, *178*(2), 145–153. doi:10.1192/bjp.178.2.145

Anxiety and Depression Association of America. (2014). *Low-cost treatment*. http://www.adaa.org/finding-help/treatment/lowcost-treatment%3E

Bauer, S., Okon, E., Meermann, R., & Kordy, H. (2012). Technology-enhanced maintenance of treatment gains in eating disorders: Efficacy of an intervention delivered via text messaging. *Journal of Consulting and Clinical Psychology*, *80*(4), 700–706. doi:10.1037/a0028030

Breathe2Relax Mobile Application. (2014). https://apps.apple.com/us/developer/national-center-for-telehealthtechnology/id499648345

Bush, N. E., Skopp, N., Smolenski, D., Crumpton, R., & Fairall, J. (2013). Behavioral screening measures delivered with a smartphone app. *Journal of Nervous and Mental Disease*, *201*(11), 991–5. doi:10.1097/NMD.0000000000000039

Butler, A. C., Chapman, J. E., Forman, E. M., & Beck, A. T. (2006). The empirical status of cognitive-behavioral therapy: A review of meta-analyses. *Clinical Psychology Review*, *26*(1), 17–31. doi:10.1016/j.cpr.2005.07.003

Christensen, H., Batterham, P., & Calear, A. (2014). Online interventions for anxiety disorders. *Current Opinions in Psychiatry, 27*(1), 7–13. doi:10.1097/YCO.0000000000000019

Cohen, J. A., Mannarino, A. P., & Deblinger, E. (2006). Treating trauma and traumatic grief in children and adolescents. *Treating Trauma and Traumatic Grief in Children and Adolescents., 16*: 256.

Deacon, B., Lickel, J., & Abramowitz, J. S. (2008). Medical utilization across the anxiety disorders. *Journal of Anxiety Disorders, 22*(2), 344–50. doi:10.1016/j.janxdis.2007.03.004

Deblinger, E., & Heflin, A. H. (1996). *Treating sexually abused children and their nonoffending parents: A cognitive behavioral approach (1996-98952-000).* Thousand Oaks, CA: Sage Publications, Inc.

Donker, T., Griffiths, K. M., Cuijpers, P., & Christensen, H. (2009). Psychoeducation for depression, anxiety and psychological distress: A meta-analysis. *BMC Medicine, 7,* 79. doi:10.1186/1741-7015-7-79

Greenberg, P. E., Sisitsky, T., Kessler, R. C., Finkelstein, S. N., Berndt, E. R., Davidson, J. R., . . . Fyer, A. J. (1999). The economic burden of anxiety disorders in the 1990s. *Journal of Clinical Psychiatry, 60*(7), 427–35.

Gunter, R. W., & Whittal, M. L. (2010). Dissemination of cognitive-behavioral treatments for anxiety disorders: Overcoming barriers and improving patient access. *Clinical Psychology Review, 30*(2), 194–02. doi:10.1016/j.cpr.2009.11.001

Hamel, M. B., Cortez, N. G., Cohen, I. G., & Kesselheim, A. S. (2014). FDA regulation of mobile health technologies. *New England Journal of Medicine, 371*(4), 372–9.

Hedman, E., Ljotsson, B., & Lindefors, N. (2012). Cognitive behavior therapy via the Internet: A systematic review of applications, clinical efficacy and cost-effectiveness. *Expert Reviews of Pharmacoecon Outcomes Research, 12*(6), 745–64. doi:10.1586/erp.12.67

Hedman, E., Ljótsson, B., Rück, C., Furmark, T., Carlbring, P., Lindefors, N., & Andersson, G. (2010). Internet administration of self-report measures commonly used in research on social anxiety disorder: A psychometric evaluation. *Computers in Human Behavior, 26*(4), 736–40. doi:10.1016/j.chb.2010.01.010

Hofmann, S. G., & Smits, J. A. (2008). Cognitive-behavioral therapy for adult anxiety disorders: A meta-analysis of randomized placebo-controlled trials. *Journal of Clinical Psychiatry, 69*(4), 621–32.

Kessler, R. C., Ruscio, A. M., Shear, K., & Wittchen, H. U. (2010). Epidemiology of anxiety disorders. *Current Topics in Behavioral Neuroscience, 2,* 21–35.

Lépine, J.-P. (n.d.). The Epidemiology of Anxiety Disorders: Prevalence and Societal Costs. *J Clin Psychiatry,* 5.

Lenhard, F., Vigerland, S., Andersson, E., Ruck, C., Mataix-Cols, D., Thulin, U.,... Serlachius, E. (2014). Internet-delivered cognitive behavior therapy for adolescents with obsessive-compulsive disorder: An open trial. *PLoS One, 9*(6), e100773. doi:10.1371/journal.pone.0100773

Lewis, C., Pearce, J., & Bisson, J. I. (2012). Efficacy, cost-effectiveness and acceptability of self-help interventions for anxiety disorders: Systematic review. *British Journal of Psychiatry, 200*(1), 15–21. doi:10.1192/bjp.bp.110.084756

Luxton, D. D., McCann, R. A., Bush, N. E., Mishkind, M. C., & Reger, G. M. (2011). mHealth for mental health: Integrating smartphone technology in behavioral healthcare. *Professional Psychology: Research and Practice, 42*(6), 505.

Marks, I. M., Kenwright, M., McDonough, M., Whittaker, M., & Mataix-Cols, D. (2004). Saving clinicians' time by delegating routine aspects of therapy to a computer: A randomized controlled trial in phobia/panic disorder. *Psychological Medicine, 34*(1), 9–17.

Newman, M. G., Szkodny, L. E., Llera, S. J., & Przeworski, A. (2011). A review of technology-assisted self-help and minimal contact therapies for anxiety and depression: Is human contact necessary for therapeutic efficacy? *Clinical Psychology Review, 31*(1), 89–103. doi:10.1016/j.cpr.2010.09.008

Parsons, T. D., & Rizzo, A. A. (2008). Affective outcomes of virtual reality exposure therapy for anxiety and specific phobias: A meta-analysis. *Journal of Behavioral Therapy and Experimental Psychiatry, 39*(3), 250–61. doi:10.1016/j.jbtep.2007.07.007

Reger, G. M., Skopp, N. A., Edwards-Stewert, A., & Lemus, E. L. (2015). Comparison of prolonged exposure (PE) coach to treatment as usual: A case series with two active duty soldiers. *Military Psychology,* 27(5), 287–96.

Rizzo, A., Hartholt, A., Grimani, M., Leeds, A., & Liewer, M. (2014). Virtual reality exposure therapy for combat-related posttraumatic stress disorder. *Computer, 47*(7), 31–7.

Tate, D. F., & Zabinski, M. F. (2004). Computer and Internet applications for psychological treatment: Update for clinicians. *Journal of Clinical Psychology, 60*(2), 209–20. doi:10.1002/jclp.10247

US Census Bureau (Producer). (2014). *Computer and Internet access in the United States: 2012.* https://www.census.gov/data/tables/2012/demo/computer-internet/computer-use-2012.html

US Department of Veterans Affairs. (2014). *Mobile app: PTSD coach.* http://www.ptsd.va.gov/public/materials/apps/PTSDCoach.asp

Van Ameringen, M., Turna, J., Khalesi, Z., Pullia, K., & Patterson, B. (2017). There is an app for that! The current state of mobile applications (apps) for DSM-5 obsessive-compulsive disorder, posttraumatic stress disorder, anxiety and mood disorders: VAN AMERINGEN et al. *Depression and Anxiety, 34*(6), 526–539. doi:10.1002/da.22657

Whiteside, S. P. H., Ale, C. M., Vickers Douglas, K., Tiede, M. S., & Dammann, J. E. (2014). Case examples of enhancing pediatric OCD treatment with a smartphone application. *Clinical Case Studies, 13*(1), 80–94. doi:10.1177/1534650113504822

Yang, Y. T., & Silverman, R. D. (2014). Mobile health applications: The patchwork of legal and liability issues suggests strategies to improve oversight. *Health Affairs, 33*(2), 222–7.

CHAPTER

34 Digital Technologies in the Assessment and Treatment of Impulsivity and Problematic Alcohol and Drug Use

Frederick Muench, Rachel P. Vitale, *and* Marc N. Potenza

Abstract

Digital health technologies (DHTs) are coming of age in improving the assessment, treatment, and continuing care of individuals struggling with problem substance use and impulsive behavior. While many of these methods are still being tested and continue to evolve, DHTs constitute a powerful new way of enhancing traditional treatment models and offer the opportunity to meet individuals in their natural environments to combat reductions in self-regulation with just-in-time tailored interventions. This chapter provides readers with a general overview of DHTs in the context of the treatment of substance use disorders, detailing a brief history of computer-based interventions for substance use, the core mechanisms of mobile and wireless technologies, a review of how specific technology components (e.g., video chat, text messaging) can be used to assess and treat substance use disorders and self-regulation failures, and potential concerns surrounding the integration of DHTs into addiction care.

Keywords: digital health technologies DHTs, impulsivity, substance use, adaptive interventions, mobile technologies, telemedicine

Digital health technologies (DHTs) have tremendous potential to improve nearly every facet of substance abuse assessment and treatment. DHTs include assessments and interventions delivered via computers, mobile phones, tablets, and wireless or wearable device technologies. DHTs have the potential to enhance both the quality of care within treatment and the reach of care beyond the treatment setting to any individual with access to a computer or mobile phone. Digital screening tools can assess thousands of people a day, offer targeted interventions including medication recommendations and referrals, and follow individuals, including the most disenfranchised populations, for extended periods. Beyond their tangible reach and promise as platforms for disseminating more personalized care, they have the capacity to provide a therapeutic resource that most healthcare practitioners cannot: using automated and self-report indicators, they can identify and respond to self-regulation failures as they occur, thereby reinforcing therapeutic salience and providing just-in-time support and skills.

Many DHTs for substance use-related behaviors have been developed and made immediately available to the consumer outside of treatment settings. Such resources include web-based screening and feedback programs, blood-alcohol concentration (BAC) calculators, mobile applications, coping skills programs, and computer-based group self-help programs such as online self-help groups and peer recovery apps. While few of these programs have been tested using even quasi-experimental methods, they represent the powerful and potentially disruptive impact that new technologies can have on traditional treatment models. However, recent evidence from empirical studies is highlighting the opportunity for consumer-based and treatment-guided mobile interventions in reducing substance use while focusing on ease of use and convenience to reach more individuals than previously imagined (Kazemi et al., 2017). This chapter provides a general overview of DHTs in the assessment and treatment of substance use disorders, starting with a brief historical overview of computer-based interventions for substance use and abuse, followed by a discussion of the core mechanisms of mobile and wireless technologies, a review of how specific technology components (e.g., video, text messaging, transdermal sensors, etc.) can be used to assess and treat substance use disorders and self-regulation failures, and a brief review of potential concerns surrounding the integration of DHTs into addiction care.

Traditional Computer-Based Self-Report Assessment and Interventions

Computer-Based Assessment and Interventions

The benefits of computer-based digital assessments compared to both paper-and-pencil and face-to-face assessment have been supported by a literature spanning the past 40 years. These benefits are especially salient in the context of assessing addictive behaviors. Some of the earliest feasibility studies comparing computer-based to alternative assessment modalities showed that nearly half of psychiatric problems were missed during in-person clinical interviews (Davenport, Goldberg, & Millar, 1987) and that computerized interviews may reveal more data than paper-based questionnaires (Maitland & Mandel, 1994; Paperny, Aono, Lehman, Hammar, & Risser, 1990; Robinson & West, 1992). These early studies also offered evidence that computer-assisted interviews may be better platforms for collecting sensitive information than face-to-face interviews (Weisband & Kiesler, 1996), perhaps in that a less personal format may overcome issues related to embarrassment, guilt, or feelings of being judged. Specific examples include collection of information related to suicide (Petrie & Abell, 1995), alcohol use (Lucas, 1977), psychiatric conditions (Bachman, 2003), HIV screening (Locke et al., 1992), sexual behavior and drug use (Skinner, 1982; Tourangeau & Smith 1996; Turner et al., 1998), sexual risk behavior and same-sex sexual activity (Des Jarlais et al., 1999), and domestic violence (Lapham, Kring, & Skipper, 1991). More recently, Kang and Gratch (2010) found that individuals seeking treatment for social phobia revealed more information to a virtual avatar than to a personal counselor. While the mechanisms of this are not entirely clear, it appears that the fear of judgment and negative feedback that comes from revealing sensitive information to a human does not apply to the same degree when disclosing to a digital system. This mechanism has been highlighted as especially important in substance abuse-related disclosing. Interestingly, analysis of computer and mobile health searches reveal that searches on the mobile phone pertained to more sensitive topics (i.e., mental health and sexually transmitted diseases) than computer-based health searches. These findings suggest that even the simplest computerized assessments may allow some individuals to feel more comfortable disclosing crucial sensitive health information, thereby enhancing the personalized intervention process.

Computer-Based Prevention and Early Intervention

The field of treatment for substance abuse was one of the earliest adopters of simple computerized brief assessment and feedback systems that used automated decision support algorithms to personalize interventions based on data. Approaches have primarily been computer- and Internet-based interventions (CIBIs) for individuals not seeking specialty care, either via the Internet or in opportunistic settings such as colleges and primary care medical centers. The goal of CIBIs for prevention and early intervention is to raise awareness, provide normative feedback, and foster harm reduction–based behavioral change (Doumas & Andersen, 2009; Saitz et al., 2004). Several meta-analyses and comprehensive reviews have revealed that CIBIs may be superior to wait-list or no-treatment controls and roughly equivalent to alternative interventions for problem drinking, but less robust for more severe users. While CIBIs typically have small to medium effect sizes compared to control conditions, longer interventions appear to have larger effect sizes than one-time brief feedback interventions (Bewick et al., 2008; Carey, Scott-Sheldon, Elliott, Bolles, & Carey, 2009; Cunningham, Humphreys, Kypri, & van Mierlo, 2006; Elliott, Carey, & Bolles, 2008; Riper et al., 2011; Rooke, Thorsteinsson, Karpin, Copeland, & Allsop, 2010). When compared to in-person interventions, self-referred Internet-based CIBIs tend to attract more participants who are female, score lower on measures of severity and readiness for change, and report higher socioeconomic status (SES) and more education, thus highlighting the reach and engagement potential of these interventions to those who traditionally are less likely to seek in-person treatment. There are numerous CIBIs primarily for alcohol use problems available to individuals (Riper et al., 2011). They represent a "low-hanging fruit" approach to engaging individuals interested in learning more about their substance use and offering comprehensive skills training for those motivated to take action to change.

Within-Treatment Computer-Based Interventions

Relatively few studies have been conducted investigating the use of CIBIs within treatment settings, but these studies are significantly more likely to target both drug and alcohol use. The majority of studies on CIBIs primarily assess computerized systems that deliver all or a portion of care that would traditionally be delivered by a counselor (Marsch, Lord, & Dallery, 2014). A recent study of the computerized therapeutic education system (TES) skills program for substance abuse (Bickel, Marsch, Buchhalter, & Badger, 2008), in which 2 hours of in-person therapy time were substituted with a digital intervention, yielded better outcomes than treatment as usual (Campbell, Muench, & Nunes, 2014). Carroll and Rounsaville (2010) integrated a digital cognitive-behavioral therapy (CBT) intervention into outpatient treatment and saw a significant reduction in positive urine samples and an increase in coping skills usage when compared to treatment as usual. The CBT program in this study included multiple modules that could be delivered flexibly and tailored to the individual. As Carroll and Rounsaville (2010) suggest, the CBT component of therapy is essentially "subcontracted" to the digital treatment program. While the mechanism of why these systems may improve outcomes is not entirely clear, it has been suggested that because computers can deliver standardized empirically supported information with "perfect" fidelity, they may be better suited to deliver certain interventions—especially those that involve skills training. Overall, there is evidence that treatment-based CIBIs are highly acceptable to patients and enhance efficacy during treatment, even yielding some post-treatment continuation effects (Campbell et al., 2014). Moreover, this research has revealed that CIBIs with therapist support are as effective as completely therapist-delivered versions of the same intervention.

Overall, CIBIs may be best suited for providing brief one-time assessment and feedback or as supplementary interventions within treatment settings or other existing services. While CIBIs have many distinct advantages from perspectives of public health and personal finance, including their ability to be tailored to specific subgroups using decision-support algorithms, their capacity for data progress monitoring, and their cost-effectiveness once systems are developed, CIBIs have several limitations that reduce their promise as stand-alone interventions. First, stand-alone CIBIs often have high attrition rates. For example, Klein, Slaymaker, Dugosh, and McKay (2012) examined the impact of a computerized continuing-care intervention following inpatient treatment and found that engagement dropped to 50% after 1 month. By the end of the program, compliance was only 5%. It has been suggested that this may result from a combination of lack of human support, lack of proactive digital outreach (e.g., alerts), and the need for the user to proactively engage in the intervention after sign-up. A second limitation is that they are often poorly equipped to deal with in vivo self-regulatory failures that might lead to excess intake and relapse. Fortunately, both limitations can be addressed by using mobile and wireless technologies and new digital coaching paradigms that integrate text chat support with automated services.

Mobile Technologies and Substance Abuse Treatment

The promise of mobile DHTs for the treatment of substance use disorders can best be described through the lens of prevailing theories of initiation of substance use and development of substance use disorders. These theories include biological, social learning, and self-regulation considerations. Traditional treatments and early CIBIs primarily targeted the former two components through the prescription of medication, education, skills training, feedback, and psychotherapy. CIBIs essentially expanded these components by standardizing, personalizing, and extending the reach of these existing services. The emergence of mobile phone and wireless sensors has resulted in the opportunity to reach and provide services to individuals "in the moment." This availability has led to newer treatment initiatives that focus on the process of self-regulation. Self-regulation failures may occur when inhibitory-behavioral-control systems in the body become overwhelmed by the demand of substance use cues, resulting in the suppression of change goals, minimization of consequence salience, and increased craving (Wiers & Stacy, 2013).

Self-regulation theories (Carver & Scheier, 2001; Vohs & Baumeister, 2004) and implicit-regulation research (Field & Wiers, 2012; Wiers & Stacy, 2013) stress the relationship between "top-down" and "bottom-up" processes and the efforts made by individuals to override or manage impulsive systems using a range of tools from environmental reengineering to reflective processing. Mobile and wireless device-based interventions appear well suited to facilitate regulation by triggering top-down reflective processes in the face of impulsive bottom-up demands. Such outcomes may be achieved by (1) increasing salience of change goals using reinforcement in one's natural environment, (2) providing proactive engagement, and (3) continually assessing one's world and intervening at those critical moments when environmental and internal cues are driving an individual toward unhealthy behavior. While these treatment targets are not new, the combination of mobile data collection and intervention capabilities allow for the creation of personalized, adaptive, data-driven interventions that promote goals with greater precision (Riley et al., 2011). The following section will provide an overview of these themes and of research that harnesses available technologies to assess and intervene with individuals with substance use problems in their natural environments.

Mobile Assessment

The DHT feature that spans nearly all tools is the ability to collect and analyze large amounts of data for diagnostic and interventional purposes. Whether it be utilizing data to provide more accurate diagnoses through multiple data streams, using real-time data to anticipate changes in symptoms over time, understanding how context or location triggers certain behaviors, providing an intervention based on self-report feedback data, or gathering information in other domains, the opportunity to collect and analyze these data is perhaps the greatest opportunity DHTs provide to improve health and well-being. While static diagnostic assessments (e.g., intakes) offer the ability to tailor care, mobile assessment (MA) is the primary means to assess individuals in their natural environment and trigger just-in-time adaptive interventions. We will use the term "MA" to encapsulate all assessment methods that are designed to collect individual data in one's natural environment, including ecological momentary assessment, experience sampling (Larson & Csikszentmihalyi, 1983), and the daily diary method (Bolger, Davis, & Rafaeli, 2003). MA will also be used to refer to all forms of sampling that use mobile tools, including measures of subjective states such as craving and confidence (Shiffman, 2009) and objective parameters that utilize mobile and wireless sensors. There now exists a range of noninvasive user-friendly passive MA tools embedded in the mobile phone. These tools allow for ongoing continuous passive monitoring without active participation by the user in the data collection processes (aside from ensuring that the phone and its sensors are active). They also combat the limitation of excessive user burden or the loss of important assessment opportunities. Passive data collection tools typically fall into several general categories including but not limited to location (e.g., global positioning system [GPS], geographic information system [GIS]); motion/activity (e.g., accelerometers, gyroscope); sound, visual, and light capture; and psychophysiology (e.g., heart rate, heart rate variability, galvanic skin response, temperature, electromyography). Some tools have been used with respect to substance use and abuse and addiction treatment, and these include context and location sensing (Vahabzadeh, Mezghanni, Lin, Epstein, & Preston, 2010), physiological assessment (Schulze et al., 2013), and transdermal sensing (Hawthorne & Wojcik, 2006). We discuss these passive assessment technologies in further detail later in the chapter.

Subjective MA has revolutionized how the use of alcohol and other substances may be measured in the user's natural environment (Ferguson & Shiffman, 2011). MA captures in vivo data spanning a range of factors to avoid potential problems associated with retrospective recall and forgetting and to enhance our understanding of temporal dynamics through repeated assessments at predetermined, random, or event-specific times (Shiffman & Stone, 1998). Shiffman (2009) concisely underscores the benefits of MA for assessing the natural course of substance use as an episodic behavior based on both external/situational experiences and internal experiences that cannot be captured wholly via retrospective reports or laboratory-based study. Over the past 10 years, multiple studies have used MA to assess patterns of substance use in participants' natural environments, including studies of smokers (Berkman, Dickenson, Falk, & Lieberman., 2011), heroin and cocaine users (Johnson, Barrault, Nadeau, & Swendsen, 2009), alcohol-dependent individuals (Chih et al., 2014), and problem drinkers (Kuerbis, Armeli, Muench, & Morgenstern, 2013). Subjective MA studies have revealed discrepancies between retrospective reports and MA, such that people using retrospective recall may under- or overreport (Homma et al., 2002; Shiffman et al., 2007) behaviors or cognitions. For example, while there is fairly good correspondence between lab-based measures of substance use and MA for frequency or quantity of substance use in the short term, there is poor correspondence for more complex judgments and appraisals and long-term recall (Shiffman, Stone, & Hufford, 2008). For example, Kuerbis et al. (2013) revealed that, compared to self-efficacy judgments collected via static baseline assessments, self-efficacy judgments collected via mobile assessment during the first week of treatment were significantly associated with prospective reductions in problem drinking (Kuerbis, Armeli, Muench, & Morgenstern, 2014).

In addition to yielding more reliable and valid data about substance use, MA may permit better understanding of the temporal relationships between affect, craving, context, and social circle and the onset, use, abuse, and recovery from substances (Chih et al., 2014; Holt, Litt, & Cooney, 2012). A particularly interesting finding is that simple continued MA monitoring in one's natural environment can be an intervention in itself for many substance users (Collins & Muraven, 2007; Freedman, Lester, McNamara, Milby, & Schumacher, 2006), perhaps by increasing self-awareness around patterns of use and making the change process more salient. Interestingly, Shiffman (2009) emphasizes the utility of MA to collect data from drinking and substance-abusing populations and highlights that while some have yielded mild intervention effects (Collins et al., 1998), most show little reactivity. However, "self-monitoring" or self-tracking, which is simply MA that has been framed to the participant as an intervention, yields significant outcomes across health behaviors (Abraham & Michie, 2008). For example, in a recent study on a mobile application to reduce problem drinking, Dulin, Gonzalez, and Campbell (2014) found that the alcohol-tracking feature was perceived to be the most helpful feature and that use of the app was associated with improved outcomes. Therefore, it appears that MA in the hands of individuals with intrinsic motivation to change their drinking may function as an intervention in and of itself, while MA usage in the absence of any desire to change may result in little reactivity.

Therapeutic Salience

Creating therapeutic salience is one of the core mechanisms of mobile DHTs. The ability to self-regulate is determined by multiple factors, but a core component of impulsivity and regulation of substance use behaviors involves the incentive salience of internal and environmental substance-related stimuli. Leigh and Stacy (1998) reported that positive thoughts about substance use may be more readily accessible in a user's memory than thoughts about recovery when they are cued by situational factors and events. Because therapy occurs in a specific, removed setting, a possible explanation for high rates of relapse is that the learning that occurs in a care setting does not readily generalize to the naturalistic environment. Brooks and Bouton (1994) reported that spontaneous recovery and renewal of addiction are greatly reduced when a cue presented during therapy (extinction) is presented again just before the recovery test. This reduces the likelihood that patients will relapse in the context in which the substance use historically occurred (Bouton, 2002). Prior to the existence of mHealth, Bouton (2002) suggested that, in principle, stimulus generalization might be achieved through strategies that help a person remember "some things about therapy when you feel a lapse or relapse about to occur," such as retrieval cues like reminder cards or phone calls. He added that extinction done in multiple temporal contexts may also safeguard more effectively against relapse. Mobile therapies can extend the therapeutic environment beyond the clinic, thereby enhancing therapeutic salience. From telephone therapy (McKay, 2009), to telehealth (Young, 2012), to skills training apps (Dulin et al., 2014) and videos, to interactive virtual reality (Hone-Blanchet, Eensing, & Fecteau, 2014), among others, individuals can use multiple mobile mediums and mechanisms to access therapeutic content in the moment and reinforce their commitment to behavior change.

Proactive Engagement

Careful examination of the self-help DHT literature highlights the limitation of user engagement in all such systems, from CIBIs to mobile apps. This has been termed the "law of attrition" because it is so common to all media and therapeutic targets where an individual must engage on his or her own without prompting (Brendryen et al., 2014; Cunningham, Wild, Cordingley, van Mierlo, & Humphreys, 2009). This is true even when the interventions are an extension of formal treatment with highly motivated clients (Klein et al., 2012). A potential problem with offering therapeutic tools to an individual with impulse control problems is that such programs may require the individual to proactively self-regulate in precisely those situations in which he or she may be most vulnerable. Numerous studies on delay discounting suggest that this is likely to be very difficult for substance users. Combating this has been a primary goal of real-world peer-driven interventions, proactive care coordination, and recovery-management therapies. Fortunately, mobile technologies offer the opportunity for prompting and therapeutic reminders through a variety of mechanisms such as push alerts, text messages, emails, and context-sensitive applications. Such triggers engage individuals in treatment beyond the traditional healthcare setting (Muench & Baumel, 2017). Reviews suggest that the addition of mobile messaging and other prompts improves the impact of web-based interventions (Fry & Neff, 2009; Riley et al., 2011; Webb, Joseph, Yardley, & Michie, 2010). In a recent study, text messaging was found to be more effective in helping young smokers achieve abstinence over a 12-week period than was a smartphone app. Investigators posited that text messaging may have been more effective because it was familiar and proactively delivered to the mobile phone without the user needing to open an application or engage in the intervention on his or her own (Buller, Borland, Bettinghaus, Shane, & Zimmerman, 2014).

Just-in-Time

In their formative concept paper, Riley et al. (2011) highlight that mobile technology's greatest strength may be its ability to apply "dynamical system models needed to transform our current health behavior theories into the dynamic theories required for the time-intensive, interactive, and adaptive health behavior interventions" (p. 11). Thus, the treatment of substance use disorders may be vastly enhanced by the use of DHTs to create therapeutic salience through proactive engagement of the end user and adaptability to the changing needs of the user from moment to moment. The mechanisms of *just-in-time adaptive interventions* (JITAIs) can range from tailoring the timing of an intervention to be delivered based on a baseline assessment of usual patterns (e.g., usual drinking times; Muench et al., 2017) to continual passive sensing and data analysis using machine learning approaches to develop true real-time interventions that can respond to the individual's current state (Chakraborty & Murphy, 2014). While these interventions are still in their infancy and require significant resources, predictive modeling, and machine learning to reach their full potential, even the most basic tailored adaptive interventions offer significant promise. In a study comparing an adaptive to a static intervention, Muench and colleagues found that while many types of text messages outperform assessment messaging only over a 12-week period, the messaging intervention that adapted to individuals' drinking goals each week had the largest effect sizes over the 90-day period. Moreover, across all reasons that participants believed the messaging program helped them, receiving messages at the time an individual was most likely to drink was a predictor of outcome (Muench et al., 2017). When taken together, mobile capabilities have allowed the therapeutic mechanisms of salience, proactive engagement, and timely adaptive interventions to be more fully realized.

DHT Interventions

Telephone Therapy

The first true mobile intervention for substance abuse was telephonic outreach. Numerous studies have been conducted that reveal that telephone-based stepped-care therapies can improve the efficacy of brief-screening, stepped-care, and continuing-care interventions (Brown, Saunders, Bobula, Mundt, & Koch, 2007) and assist in fostering a return to care where necessary (Bischof et al., 2008; McKay, 2009). For example, several studies have revealed that motivational interviewing and CBT can be effectively delivered over the phone to improve substance use outcomes. McKay and colleagues revealed that an 18-month telephone intervention consisting of semi-monthly phone calls delivering personalized CBT resulted in significantly reduced alcohol use at 18 months compared to treatment as usual (McKay et al., 2010). Gates and Albertella (2016) compiled a literature review of current opinion pieces, editorials, case studies, and more supporting the treatment of problem alcohol use via short-term telephone counseling. Similar results have been found for telephone-based treatments for use of illicit drugs (McKay, 2009). Other studies have revealed that telephone-based therapies are as effective as in-person interventions for other issues like depression (Mohr, 2012), are well accepted by participants, and require significantly fewer resources (McKay, 2009). Despite the promise of telephone interventions, there is also evidence that they may work best as adjuncts to initial in-person services and that they yield poorer outcomes over the long term when compared to face-to-face interventions in other domains (Mohr et al., 2012).

Telehealth Treatments

Video-based telehealth interventions are a natural extension of telephone-based therapies but offer the potential for face-to-face contact and the sharing of information (e.g., decisional balance) using video chat and web-based tools in real time (Santa Ana & Jardin, 2013). Video-based person-to-person therapies have empirical support across multiple conditions (Godleski, Darkins, & Peters, 2012). In arguably the most comprehensive study to date, Godleski et al. (2012) found that patients in Veteran's Affairs

(VA) hospitals who used telemental health services were significantly less likely to be hospitalized for mental health concerns than those in traditional treatment only. In 2011, the VA conducted more than 140,000 video mental health sessions, and telehealth has now replaced in-person sessions as the standard of care due to its therapeutic reach, cost savings, and improved outcomes in veterans. Studies within substance abuse treatment reveal positive outcomes for individual and group therapies for methadone-maintained patients conducted via video conferencing (King et al., 2009; King, Brooner, Peirce, Kolodner, & Kidorf, 2014). Consumer-based self-help programs such as *In the Rooms*, which hosts video-based 12-step groups, are also becoming much more commonplace. These programs allow for face-to-face communication and can be especially helpful to populations—such as those in rural areas—that lack in-person resources, those who fear stigmatization from participation in in-person care, and those who face time-related complications (e.g., inflexible work schedules) to attending traditional care. The promise of telehealth practice is driving organizations and providers to adopt the necessary resources to harness its benefits, but preparation to practice extends far beyond simply installing Skype on one's computer. Practitioners must be trained in unique procedures for handling emergencies in telehealth settings, the legal and ethical rules and regulations for providing therapy remotely, and how to troubleshoot or circumvent hardware and software limitations (Doarn & Merrell, 2014).

Text Messaging

Although the number of empirical studies is significantly smaller than the number of studies on computer-based and telephone-based assessment, the use of text messaging or short message service (SMS) has also been examined for a range of mental and behavioral health conditions, including addictions (Free et al., 2011, 2013; Heron & Smyth, 2010). In general, SMS interventions have been found to have small to moderate effects against no-treatment controls, with the largest effect being for smoking cessation and HIV medication adherence (Free et al., 2013). Interestingly, recent studies have revealed that text messaging is more effective than app-based interventions for smoking cessation (Buller et al., 2014) and is preferred by patients in medical settings over apps (Wendling, 2014). Text messaging has been used to facilitate physician–patient communication during from-home treatment between clinical appointments, thus minimizing the burden to clinical personnel and patients and extending care outside the clinical setting (Tofighi, Grossman, Sherman, Nunes, & Lee, 2016). While research is still in its nascent stages, the greatest efficacy findings for mobile messaging in the addictions have been for reducing heavy drinking days in young people in university settings (Weitzel, Bernhardt, Usdan, Mays, & Glanz, 2007; Muench et al., 2017), patients in emergency care (Suffoletto, Hu, Guyette, & Callaway, 2014), and adult heavy drinkers seeking to reduce their drinking recruited from the Internet. However, these studies have primarily assessed short-term outcomes. There are also several studies with substance-dependent individuals in which text messages are designed to enhance in-person treatment, appointment attendance, and/or medication adherence rather than explicitly to reduce substance use (Ingersoll et al., 2014; Tofighi, Nicholson, McNeely, Muench, Lee, 2016). In our own work, problem drinkers reduced their drinking significantly when they received automated daily text messages to help them reduce their drinking compared to messages sent only once per week, thus underscoring the benefits of continuous contact with individuals via text (Muench et al., 2017). Overall, these studies reveal that while there is short-term engagement in these interventions and positive results, those few studies with longer follow-up periods (i.e., 3 months) show less efficacy, suggesting the need for more comprehensive interventions (Tofighi, Nicholson, McNeely, Muench, Lee, 2016).

Regardless of the content of the intervention they are receiving, people with substance abuse problems both in and out of treatment report text messaging as being highly acceptable and feasible. The emerging literature on the use of text messaging to capture ecological momentary assessment (EMA) data reveals similar outcomes to personal digital assistants (PDAs) and interactive voice response (IVR; Berkman et al., 2011), highlighting its benefits for both data collection and adaptive intervention development. It also appears that text messaging is regularly perceived as interactive personal communication even when it is automated. For example, we found that individuals in a study to improve adherence to methadone treatment responded to automated messages even though participants were explicitly informed that all messages were sent by an automated system and that they would have no text-based human contact. Interestingly, the response messages from users stopped within 2 weeks as the participants became more acclimatized to the fact that the system was automated, thus highlighting the need for reciprocal communication between the user and the system to maintain engagement and engender a sense of accountability. Survey findings reveal that individuals like the idea of staying connected to care and having reminders of the therapeutic encounter outside of the treatment setting (Muench, Weiss, Kuerbis, & Morgenstern, 2013).

Audio and Video

IVR has primarily been used as a mobile assessment tool, but it has also been used as an intervention platform for substance use disorders (Moore et al., 2013). The early benefit of IVR was that it allowed individuals to use their own phones regardless of the type of phone. While there is less need for IVR in the assessment of substance use with the rise of mobile/web data collection and text messaging, it has certain advantages such as accessibility by less technologically advanced populations and, unlike text messaging, it harnesses the unique characteristics of speech (e.g., emotional tone) in intervention delivery. Recently, Moore et al. (2013) created an IVR Recovery Line to treat secondary drug use in methadone-maintained individuals (N = 36). The Recovery Line provided IVR coping modules to promote abstinence as well as daily assessments. Overall results were promising, with those who accessed the recovery line yielding significantly better drug use outcomes than those who did not. Other studies, such as the Alcohol Therapeutic IVR program (Rose, Skelly, Badger, Naylor, & Helzer, 2012), used a comprehensive decision-support intervention to treat alcohol and other substance use disorders to great effect, particularly in the realm of coping skills practice and review. In both of these studies, the benefit of IVR appeared to be the adaptive tailoring of content to the person's current state, while the weakness was the lack of proactive engagement in the systems by end users. Rose et al. (2012) also underscore the benefits of using audio features to enhance emotional responding beyond text-based therapies.

One of the earliest DHTs designed to teach coping skills for substance abuse prevention and treatment used prerecorded videos for skills training and modeling (Marsch, Carroll, & Kiluk, 2014). Video-based modules have been integrated into drink refusal skills programs and used as treatment modules in formal care to teach users a range of skills (see earlier discussion on computer-based DHTs). In addition, orientation videos can be used to introduce large groups to therapy and are as effective as in-person orientations for many health and behavior problems (Walitzer, Dermen, & Connors, 1999; Zwick & Attkisson, 1985). Standardized videos reduce human error and bias and can also enhance learning (Aronson, Marsch, & Acosta, 2012) as videos can be standardized but also tailored to specific groups to match learning styles and goals.

Virtual Reality

Some extensions of video-based skills training include virtual reality cue exposure, drink refusal, and avatar-based therapies. Reviews indicate that virtual reality is an excellent means by which to assess cue reactivity across substances (Bordnick, Carter, & Traylor, 2011; Hone-Blanchet et al., 2014) and represents an opportunity to include social interactions in traditional cue-exposure assessments. Unlike the robust literature on VR to understand craving by enhancing cue reactivity, there is less evidence for its effectiveness when combined with cue exposure treatment, perhaps because of the dearth of studies on this topic or because of the poor graphics of VR delivered via older technologies. In one study with alcohol use disorders, Lee et al. (2009) found a reduction in alcohol cravings after 10 sessions of VR therapy. Other studies have used VR environments to recreate individuals' natural environments and simulate situations that they might encounter in everyday life in order to enhance coping responses (Gustafson, Shaw, Isham, Dillon, & Spartz, 2009). Similarly, there are 12-step groups that individuals can join in VR environments that allow for anonymity and distancing to help people engage in care at their own pace. Results of these early studies are promising and more research is needed. With the rise of technologies like *augmented reality* to create actual real-world simulations of one's environment, interactive avatars and machine-learning agents (e.g., Siri meets Watson), and truly immersive environments (e.g., Oculus Rift), there appears to be tremendous promise in developing interactive avatars, augmented reality-cue paradigms, adaptive virtual worlds, and virtual diagnostic tools to assess and treat substance use disorders (Hone-Blanchet et al., 2014). As with many burgeoning technologies, it will be some time before virtual reality can truly mimic real-world settings. Although they require significant time and resources to program and warrant frequent updating, these technologies may eventually constitute one of the greatest departures from our current treatment models.

Mobile and Web-Based Support Groups

There are numerous online and web-based support groups for individuals or loved ones of an individual with a substance use problem. The Partnership for Drug-Free Kids, SMART Recovery, and Moderation Management, among many others, have online discussion groups moderated by professionals. Programs like In the Rooms offer online 12-step groups, thus eliminating the justification that meetings are too far or inconvenient. Overall, these programs offer individuals the opportunity to connect at their own pace with a group of individuals experiencing similar issues. While research on these online groups is mixed across disorders (Griffiths, Calear, & Banfield, 2009), it appears that there are subgroups who use these services more than others. For example, Hester, Lenberg, Campbell, and Delaney (2013) found that a subgroup of participants who enrolled in a DHT with an online group component did not choose to participate in the group but had equivalent drinking outcomes to those who opted to participate in the group component along with the other features. Moreover, they found that there was no difference between online-only groups and in-person groups on outcomes.

In addition to moderated online groups, there are several open mobile applications on which a group leader can create a closed mini-group that group members can use to stay connected to each other. Social media sites such as Facebook allow for closed discussion groups that can be created and used with relative ease by individual therapeutic programs or groups. A primary problem with these groups is they that are often unmoderated and are typically an adjunctive feature of a larger therapy, making them difficult for most populations to access. The absence of a moderator enhances the risk that impulsive individuals might send messages in the moment that could be harmful to others, reduce participation, or even reduce the therapeutic effect of the group. Groups should be carefully moderated for safety, but requiring a moderator can reduce the real-time back-and-forth interaction potential of the resource. While there are limitations to these support groups, they continue to expand and be offered as part of a range of DHTs for substance abuse treatment.

Smartphone Applications for Substance Use

While there are hundreds of applications available to consumers that are specific to substance use and abuse, most are untested and have minimal uptake. With the rise of mobile web applications that "mobilize" websites, it is difficult to differentiate between native traditional apps on the mobile phone (e.g., for Android) and those hosted on the Internet alone that do not have to be downloaded from an app store. For example, the Overcoming Addictions SMART Recovery program could easily be considered a multicomponent smartphone app if it was designed using mobile development tools on a specific platform. There are also numerous untested direct-to-consumer substance abuse treatment apps for the smartphone that are simple regurgitations of web-based programs, such as BAC calculators (Cohn, Hunter-Reel, Hagman, & Mitchell, 2011). For individuals in recovery, there are 12-step meeting-finder apps, virtual sponsors and recovery coaches, and a range of tools with which to watch online meetings.

Little research has been done on smartphone apps to treat substance use problems, with a few notable exceptions. Gajecki, Berman, Sinadinovic, Rosendahl, and Andersson (2014) tested two features of some of the most widely available smartphone apps in an effort to reduce risky drinking in college students, comparing a real-time estimated BAC calculator, a BAC calculator with drink planning and follow-up risk avoidance instructions, and a no-treatment control. There were no significant reductions in drinking between the two experimental groups and the control group, and men in the BAC-only group actually increased their drinking. Engagement in the interventions was low among all groups and attrition was particularly high among higher severity drinkers. Overall, results suggest that app features that require proactive engagement are rarely used by participants, and certain components of widely available apps (such as BAC calculators) may not provide any benefits to end users. In another study, Dulin et al. (2014) examined the use of a comprehensive application called Location-Based Monitoring and Intervention System for Alcohol Use Disorders (LBMI-A) to help adults seeking to reduce their drinking without abstaining. Results revealed that participants rated the alcohol-tracking feature (not to be confused with the BAC calculator) as the most helpful feature. Moreover, these authors found that more intensive use of the smartphone app was associated with improved outcomes—results that correspond to the web-based alcohol research literature (Cunningham, Kypri, & McCambridge, 2011) and the self-monitoring literature across behavior change interventions (Heron & Smyth, 2010). Other comprehensive interventions that combine multiple media to reduce problem drinking include an app for college students (Witkiewitz et al., 2014) and the Scandinavian combined web- and mobile-based alcohol intervention (Brendryen et al., 2014), which has text messaging, mobile web, and Internet-based components.

While there are several mobile apps for recovery management (e.g., Hazeldon's Mobile More), arguably the most comprehensive mobile smartphone app for addictive disorders is the A-CHESS system developed by Gustafson et al. (2011a, 2014), which is designed to continually assess and support individuals following treatment. The program provides extensive skills training, offers a panic button for high-risk situations, and assesses individuals for relapse risk based on their assessment results and/or when they are entering a high-risk environment via geolocation. Based on risk, it first sends the client reminders of his or her therapeutic goals, self-modeling audio and image reminders, and tailored educational and therapeutic materials and then triggers in-person peer and provider support if the individual is unresponsive or requests additional assistance. When compared to a treatment-as-usual aftercare condition following inpatient alcohol treatment, the A-CHESS mobile app significantly reduced the number of risky drinking days and increased the number of abstinent days in an alcohol use disorder sample 8 months after treatment. These results were maintained for 4 months after the app was removed from users' phones, indicating that users were not overly dependent on the DHT. It is likely that many programs will eventually work like A-CHESS, using subjective and objective parameters and a range of assessment tools to trigger interventions that help individuals either become more aware of risky patterns that could lead to relapse or connect them to support networks in the event of an emergency. Chih et al. (2014) revealed that weekly check-ins of recovery progress collected by the system were the best predictors of relapse, and the team is now using machine learning to build in alerts to help individuals manage risk of relapse.

Self-report and geolocation are the most commonly cited mobile assessment tools in addictions, but the smartphone and wearable sensor movement allow for development of mobile assessment tools that were once available exclusively in laboratory settings. These include implicit assessments, attentional bias tasks (Field & Cox, 2008), psychophysiology (Baskett, Shang, Patterson, & Trull, 2013), transdermal and sweat-based wireless sensors (Marques & McKnight, 2007), voice-based assessments (Sigmund & Zelinka, 2011), and text-based natural language processing and analytics (Westgate, Neighbors, Heppner, Jahn, & Lindgren, 2014), among others. These assessments harness the passive sensing features embedded in wearable devices and smartphones. For example, there is substantial research to suggest that cue reactivity leads to poor inhibitory control among those high in impulsivity. Therefore, traditional lab-based impulsivity tasks like go/no-go and implicit associations tasks can be (and are being) developed on mobile phones to assess individuals when they are most vulnerable, rather than exclusively in controlled lab settings. For example, our group (Wen et al., submitted) have recently created a mobile assessment of impulsivity comprised of mobile self-report, cognitive attentional and risk-taking tasks, and passive assessment (e.g., battery life, screen on/off display, incoming/outgoing call frequency) on the mobile phone via ResearchSuite, which is supported on both Android and iOS platforms. Users were tested both in-lab (one-time) and in the real world for 3 weeks, completing surveys and game-like tasks (e.g., researcher-developed mobile version of the Balloon Analogue Risk Task [mBART]; Lejuez et al., 2002) in the morning and evening, thus allowing researchers the opportunity to collect and compare data both in-lab and in the real world. Preliminary results reveal that excessive phone checking and irregular battery charging were associated with the Barratt Impulsiveness Scale (BIS-15; Spinella, 2007) nonplanning structure.

As noted earlier, perhaps the most promising but unexplored area of research to be born from the rise of smartphone technology is the utilization of noninvasive passive assessment tools that do not require significant user input (e.g., GPS) (Pentland, Lazer, Brewer, & Heibeck, 2009; Wen et al., submitted). While these tools are designed to be passive, they require significant "training" to become validated tools and often suffer from large amounts of missing data. Validating passive data collection has also proved challenging in that individuals are skeptical about giving consent to what they perceive to be invasive (Wen et al., submitted). Nevertheless, these tools represent the future of mobile assessment. Simply watching the rigor with which massive companies such as Apple and Google are pursuing these passive tools for health highlights how much potential these technologies have for revolutionizing medicine. Next, we will briefly review some of the most widely used passive assessment methodologies that have been used to assess substance use, as well as methodologies with significant potential.

Geolocation

Geolocation has been integrated into several smartphone apps for addiction (Dulin et al., 2014; Gustafson et al., 2014; Vahabzadeh et al., 2010). In most cases, individuals have geotagged high-risk areas where drinking or drug use is most likely to occur, and alerts have been created to either warn or check-in with clients when they enter those areas. Gustafson et al. (2011b, 2014) outline a stepped system that eventually leads to a counselor being called based on geotagging. In addition to geolocation warning systems, there are many apps that assist individuals in finding 12-step or other groups in their area. For example, rather than calling AA, an individual can click "find a meeting" on his or her phone and will be directed to the nearest meetings or individuals in recovery who have signed up to be a part of the group. This is one of the fastest growing areas of technology development in substance abuse and will continue to grow as we gain more specificity in care.

Environmental Noise and Speech

The mobile phone can now collect data on vocal and ambient noise. Within the alcohol use field, multiple laboratory-based studies have examined changes in vocal parameters from baseline to intoxication, or compared alcohol-induced intake speech to no-alcohol-intake controls (Chin & Pisoni, 1997; Hollien, Harnsberger, Martin, Hill, & Alderman, 2009; Sigmund & Zelinka, 2011). Studies reveal that intoxication generally produces changes such as slower speech, elongated syllable length, increased loudness, and increased pitch variability. When analyzing a range of prosodic features in the laboratory, Sigmund and Zelinka (2011) revealed a 69.3–77.0% recognition rate of intoxication. Several studies within stress and depression assessment also have expanded vocal analysis to mobile audio sensors within the phone. Lu et al. (2012) were able to identify stress with 81% and 76% accuracy in indoor and outdoor environments, respectively, with the phone microphone. Similar results have been found using vocal parameters to identify depression using the mobile phone and specifically to characterize the affect of the speaker (Chang, Fisher, & Canny, 2011). The results of this research underscore the promise of using passive auditory sensing as another means to assist in identifying intoxication and environmental sounds associated with substance use through intermittent mobile sampling (Trull & Ebner-Priemer, 2013).

Psychophysiology

With the increased availability of wearable devices that measure a range of physiological parameters, there is enthusiasm for monitoring indices such as heart rate, heart rate variability (HRV), and skin conductance in real time. Similar to voice analysis, there is significant laboratory-based research on how these metrics may predict craving states or later substance use. For example, studies have found a positive cross-sectional relationship between low HRV, substance use, and craving (Ingjaldsson, Laberg, & Thayer, 2003), and these physiological parameters often prospectively relate to later lapses. For example, Garland, Franken, and Howard (2012) revealed that post-treatment HRV cue reactivity related prospectively to relapse 6 months later. However, the relationship between psychophysiology and addiction is complex as multiple physiological parameters and patterns are associated with various states. For example, although HRV decreases with cue exposure in dependent patients, one study found that moderate alcohol intake increased HRV in nondependent social drinkers (Quintana, McGregor, Guastella, Malhi, & Kemp, 2013). Therefore, systems will need to incorporate multiple sensors and self-report measures so that researchers or care providers can accurately understand the data. For example, Baskett et al. (2013) created a full-body sensing system and self-report mobile assessment designed to detect alcohol craving. These nuances, the potential confounds associated with ambulatory assessment (e.g., controlling for respiration and movement), and data cleaning and data analysis needs make physiological assessment a complex approach to the ambulatory evaluation of self-regulation. To that end, significantly more research is needed to validate physiological assessment in real-world settings (Houtveen & de Geus, 2009; Kumar, Al'Absi, Beck, Ertin, & Scott, 2014).

Substance Use Sensing Devices

Wearable substance abuse sensors have been used in criminal justice settings for many years, and they are gaining traction with researchers and clinicians. They work by objectively measuring the actual outcome of interest rather than a derivative such as HRV. Arguably, the most robust literature is on assessing alcohol consumption using transdermal sensors (Barnett, Meade, & Glynn, 2014; Swift, 1993). *Transdermal sensing* involves assessing alcohol through vaporous perspiration from the skin. Studies reveal that transdermal sensing may accurately and objectively predict alcohol use and warn individuals of impending intoxication in the hope of reducing the harmful consequences of heavy drinking. These sensors have significant potential to provide objective data to better understand how people change and the proximal and distal triggers for relapse and heavy drinking. While beyond the scope of this chapter, DHTs may also include a range of biomarkers that may eventually be assessed and analyzed continuously through wearable devices and mobile sensors.

Social Media and Text-Based Assessments

There is emerging research on the potential of social networking site (SNS) text and image analysis to predict mental health states and risk for future problems and relapse. For example, studies reveal that natural-language processing can differentiate the Twitter posts of depressed versus nondepressed individuals. Additionally, posting alcohol-related images and text has been linked to risky drinking behaviors in young people (Ridout, Campbell, & Ellis, 2012). In another study, Westgate et al. (2014) found that alcohol-related posts were associated with drinks per week, alcohol-related problems, alcohol use disorders, and alcohol cravings, and friends' alcohol-related posts were associated with alcohol use disorders. In a study examining digital alcohol marketing efforts, college students' use of alcohol-related social media predicted their own problem drinking behaviors (Hoffman et al., 2017). Other studies have suggested that the influence of SNS on alcohol use may be due to a combination of factors, including social norms (Miller, Pritchard, Hutchinson, & Wilson, 2014). Overall, there are an increasing number of studies that assess how SNS and other tools can be used to target substance use and self-regulation problems (Hoffman, Pinkleton, Weintraub, & Reys-Velázquez et al., 2014). Other methods include analysis of actual text-based communication, social analytics, and proximity measures on the mobile phone to help predict heavy drinking episodes.

Limitations and Cautions

Like any potentially disruptive and promising technology, healthcare DHTs come with cautions, limitations, and weaknesses that vary in salience between stakeholders (e.g., organizations, providers, researchers, and patients). Rather than discuss implementation and workflow barriers to integration, we will highlight some of the global concerns related to the use and management of DHT entities.

Data Security

Integrating technology into treatment poses significant challenges related to data privacy and confidentiality. Understanding where and how the data are being entered, transmitted, and stored and what types of data are being collected (e.g., personal health information vs. appointment reminders) requires careful consideration. For example, social media-based support groups for addiction are emerging as a wonderful medium for interactive support, but participants need to be informed that social media sites such as Facebook will then have the information about their support group activity and participation at its disposal. Similarly, sending a text message is perhaps the least secure form of communication as texts are stored in multiple databases. Using these technology-based services requires creativity and caution, such as using code words or general goal-directed assessments and messaging or other forms of communication that do not expose the client to a broad digital footprint unnecessarily. Similarly, the consent process must be transparent in presenting the types of data storage and transmission breach risks to which a participant might be vulnerable, as well as which organizations might have access to the participant's data. DHT consent forms will likely need to include information such as the scope of digital communication, what information will be communicated and how, inherent privacy risks of communication, security and storage of communication, the use of outside vendors who have access to communication, security of external vendor applications, procedures for lost provider devices, training on how to secure communication devices, lack of control over timing of digital communication, missed communication interaction likelihood, the inappropriateness of digital communication as an emergency platform, recorded digital communication as part of the client's health record, risk of misinterpretation in text-based communication (e.g., cryptic tone or context), possible charges incurred by the client, protection of agency and agency staff devices, and opt-out and help options (Muench, 2014). Understanding each of these components takes careful consideration.

Technology and Data Management

DHTs require technologists to develop and manage the technology. Technology outages, glitches, and bugs often derail programs and require ongoing management. A similar but more tangible barrier is the need to manage and analyze the massive streams of data being collected. For example, a month-long

24/7 heart rate monitoring program with event-based self-report mobile assessment likely yields more data than 100 separate self-report paper-and-pencil assessments. This type of information needs to be cleaned, managed, and analyzed in very different ways. In addition to data cleaning, the process of "training" these systems to understand how heart rate is related to stress requires knowledge of statistical and mathematical modeling of longitudinal data. Truly interdisciplinary teams are needed to build and manage DHTs—a requirement that is not currently supported by many existing treatment and research models.

Efficacy and Feasibility

The hype surrounding DHTs can at times mask their usefulness and efficacy limitations. Recent reviews of computer-based interventions found significant methodological flaws in research designs, evaluations of treatment exposure and adherence, rates of follow-up assessment, and conformity to intention-to-treat principles (Kiluk et al., 2011). As in direct-to-consumer computer-based interventions, mobile apps have extremely low retention rates. Perhaps due to the combination of proactive outreach and supportive accountability, only text messaging, within-treatment computer-based interventions, and DHTs with a human support component (e.g., A-CHESS) have shown positive effects to date. Clients may also have issues with using technology, which can limit interpretation of results. For example, is the lack of use of a smartphone app due to burden, a participant's failure to charge or turn on their device or pay their phone bill, or because the participant did not understand the instructions? Likewise, many types of DHTs require specific technologies (e.g., smartphones) that are available to only a portion of clients. Many of these concerns can be overcome with proper training and management of client perceptions and preferences. Despite these concerns, much of the current research highlights the high user acceptability of DHTs. Thus, the concerns of researchers may not reflect those of clients who are more accepting of technology failures. As a colleague once noted, providers want to help and clients want to get better, but lawyers sometimes get in the way.

Future Directions

It is likely that the promise of DHTs will be realized and our systems of care will be continuously transformed through ongoing iteration. New data yield new opportunities to build better models. New models using multiple sensor systems may be developed to passively predict substance abuse relapse and heavy drinking and drug use periods. Impulsive individuals may be identified earlier and may be taught self-regulation strategies personalized to their environment. Big data may promote personalization. Before these feedback loops may be optimized, however, significant research will be needed to disentangle the multiple streams of data and isolate the mechanisms of action within interventions. While it is very difficult to predict what will happen to our current models of research and care and how new technologies will help versus hurt these models, the coming years will likely be an exciting time of both uncertainty and rapid discovery.

References

Abraham, C., & Michie, S. (2008). A taxonomy of behavior change techniques used in interventions. *Health Psychology, 27*(3), 379–87.

Aronson, I. D., Marsch, L. A., & Acosta, M. C. (2012). Using findings in multimedia learning to inform technology-based behavioral health interventions. *Translational Behavioral Medicine, 3*(3), 234–43.

Bachman, J. W. (2003). The patient-computer interview: A neglected tool that can aid the clinician. *Mayo Clinic Proceedings, 78*(1), 67–78.

Barnett, N. P., Meade, E. B., & Glynn, T. R. (2014). Predictors of detection of alcohol use episodes using a transdermal alcohol sensor. *Experimental and Clinical Psychopharmacology, 22*(1), 86–96.

Baskett, P., Shang, Y., Patterson, M. V., & Trull, T. (2013). Towards a system for body-area sensing and detection of alcohol craving and mood dysregulation. In *2013 IEEE 10th Consumer Communications and Networking Conference, CCNC 2013*. pp. 875–6.

Berkman, E. T., Dickenson, J. Falk, E. B., & Lieberman, M. D. (2011). Using SMS text messaging to assess moderators of smoking reduction: Validating a new tool for ecological measurement of health behaviors. *Health Psychology, 30*(2), 186–94.

Bewick, B. M., Trusler, K., Barkham, M., Hill, A. J., Cahill, J., & Mulhem, B. (2008). The effectiveness of web-based interventions designed to decrease alcohol consumption: A systematic review. *Preventive Medicine, 47*(1), 17–26.

Bickel, W. K., Marsch, L. A., Buchhalter, A. R., & Badger, G. J. (2008). Computerized behavior therapy for opioid-dependent outpatients: A randomized controlled trial. *Experimental and Clinical Psychopharmacology, 16*(2), 132–43.

Bischof, G., Grothues, J. M., Reinhardt, S., Meyer, C., John, U., & Rumpf, H. J. (2008). Evaluation of a telephone-based stepped care intervention for alcohol-related disorders: A randomized controlled trial. *Drug and Alcohol Dependence, 93*(3), 244–51.

Bolger, N., Davis, A., & Rafaeli, E. (2003). Diary methods: Capturing life as it is lived. *Annual Review of Psychology, 54*(1), 579–16.

Bordnick, P. S., Carter, B. L., & Traylor, A. C. (2011). What virtual reality research in addictions can tell us about the future of obesity assessment and treatment. *Journal of Diabetes Science and Technology*, *5*(2), 265–71.

Bouton, M. E. (2002). Context, ambiguity, and unlearning: Sources of relapse after behavioral extinction. *Biological Psychiatry*, *52*(10), 976–86.

Brendryen, H., Lund, I. O., Johansen, A. B., Riksheim, M., Nesvåg, S., & Duckert, F. (2014). Balance: A pragmatic randomized controlled trial of an online intensive self-help alcohol intervention. *Addiction*, *109*(2), 218–26.

Brooks, D. C., & Bouton, M. E. (1994). A retrieval cue for extinction attenuates response recovery (renewal) caused by a return to the conditioning context. *Journal of Experimental Psychology: Animal Behavior Processes*, *20*(4), 366–79.

Brown, R. L., Saunders, L. A., Bobula, J. A., Mundt, M. P., & Koch, P. E. (2007). Randomized-controlled trial of a telephone and mail intervention for alcohol use disorders: Three-month drinking outcomes. *Alcoholism: Clinical and Experimental Research*, *31*(8), 1372–9.

Buller, D. B., Borland, R., Bettinghaus, E. P., Shane, J. H., & Zimmerman, D. E. (2014). Randomized trial of a smartphone mobile application compared to text messaging to support smoking cessation. *Telemedicine and e-Health*, *20*(3), 206–14.

Campbell, A. N. C., Muench, F., & Nunes, E. V. (2014). Technology-based behavioral interventions for alcohol and drug use problems. In L. A. Marsch, S. E. Lord, & J. Dallery (Eds.), *Behavioral healthcare and technology: Using science-based innovations to transform practice* (pp. 40–57). New York: Oxford University Press.

Carey, K. B., Scott-Sheldon, L. A., Elliott, J. C., Bolles, J. R., & Carey, M. P. (2009). Computer-delivered interventions to reduce college student drinking: A meta-analysis. *Addiction*, *104*(11), 1807–19.

Carroll, K. M., & Rounsaville, B. J. (2010). Computer-assisted therapy in psychiatry: Be brave–it's a new world. *Current Psychiatry Reports*, *12*(5), 426–32.

Carver, C. S, & Scheier, M. F. (2001). *On the self-regulation of behavior*. Cambridge, UK: Cambridge University Press.

Chakraborty, B., & Murphy, S. A. (2014). Dynamic treatment regimes. *Annual Review of Statistics and Its Application*, *1*(1), 447–64.

Chang, K., Fisher, D., & Canny, J. (2011). AMMON: A speech analysis library for analyzing affect, stress, and mental health on mobile phones. *Proceedings of PhoneSense*.

Chih, M, Patton, T., McTavish, F. M., Isham, A., Judkins-Fisher, C. L., Atwood, A. K., & Gustafson, D. H. (2014). Predictive modeling of addiction lapses in a mobile health application. *Journal of Substance Abuse Treatment*, *46*(1), 29–35.

Chin, S. B., & Pisoni, D. B. (1997). *Alcohol and speech*. Cambridge, MA: Academic Press.

Cohn, A. M., Hunter-Reel, D., Hagman, B. T., & Mitchell, J. (2011). Promoting behavior change from alcohol use through mobile technology: The future of ecological momentary assessment. *Alcoholism: Clinical and Experimental Research*, *35*(12), 2209–15.

Collins, R. L., Morsheimer, E. T., Shiffman, S., Paty, J. A., Gnys, M., & Papandonatos, G. D. (1998). Ecological momentary assessment in a behavioral drinking moderation training program. *Experimental and Clinical Psychopharmacology*, *6*(3), 306–15.

Collins, R. L., & Muraven, M. (2007). Ecological momentary assessment of alcohol consumption. In A. A. Stone, S. Shiffman, A. Atienza, L. Nebeling (Eds.) *The science of real-time data capture: Self-reports in health research* (pp. 189–203). New York: Oxford University Press.

Cunningham, J. A., Humphreys, K., Kypri, K., & van Mierlo, T. (2006). Formative evaluation and three-month follow-up of an online personalized assessment feedback intervention for problem drinkers. *Journal of Medical Internet Research*, *8*(2), e5.

Cunningham, J. A., Kypri, K., & McCambridge, J. (2011). The use of emerging technologies in Alcohol Treatment. *Alcohol Research & Health*, *33*(4), 320–6.

Cunningham, J. A., Wild, T. C., Cordingley, J., van Mierlo, T., & Humphreys, K. (2009). A randomized controlled trial of an Internet-based intervention for alcohol abusers. *Addiction*, *104*(12), 2023–32.

Davenport, S., Goldberg, D., & Millar, T (1987). How psychiatric disorders are missed during medical consultations. *The Lancet*, *330*(8556), 439–41.

Des Jarlais, D. C., Paone, D., Milliken, J., Turner, C. F., Miller, H., Gribble, J., . . . Friedman, S. R. (1999). Audio-computer interviewing to measure risk behaviour for HIV among injecting drug users: A quasi-randomised trial. *The Lancet*, *353*(9165), 1657–61.

Doarn, C. R., & Merrell, R. C. (2014). Standards and guidelines for telemedicine: An evolution. *Telemedicine and e-Health*, *20*(3), 187–9.

Doumas, D. M., & Andersen, L. L. (2009). Reducing alcohol use in first-year university students: Evaluation of a Web-based personalized feedback program. *Journal of College Counseling*, *12*(1), 18–32.

Dulin, P. L., Gonzalez, V. M., & Campbell, K. (2014). Results of a pilot test of a self-administered smartphone-based treatment system for alcohol use disorders: Usability and early outcomes. *Substance Abuse*, *35*(2), 168–75.

Elliott, J. C., Carey, K. B., & Bolles, J. R. (2008). Computer-based interventions for college drinking: A qualitative review. *Addictive Behaviors*, *33*(8), 994–1005.

Ferguson, S. G., & Shiffman, S. (2011). Using the methods of ecological momentary assessment in substance dependence research–smoking cessation as a case study. *Substance Use & Misuse*, *46*(1), 87–95.

Field, M., & Cox, W. M. (2008). Attentional bias in addictive behaviors: A review of its development, causes, and consequences. *Drug and Alcohol Dependence*, *97*(1), 1–20.

Field, M., & Wiers, R. (2012). Automatic and controlled processes in the pathway from drug abuse to addiction. In J. Verster, K. Brady, M. Galanter, & P. Conrod (Eds.) *Drug abuse and addiction in medical illness* (pp. 35–45). New York: Springer.

Free, C., Knight, R., Robertson, S., Whittaker, R., Edwards, P., Zhou, W., . . . Roberts, I. (2011). Smoking cessation support delivered via mobile phone text messaging (txt2stop): A single-blind, randomised trial. *The Lancet*, *378*(9785), 49–55.

Free, C., Phillips, G., Watson, L., Galli, L., Felix, L., Edwards, P., . . . Haines, A. (2013). The effectiveness of mobile-health technologies to improve health care service delivery processes: A systematic review and meta-analysis. *PLOS Medicine*, *10*(1), e1001363.

Freedman, M. J., Lester, K. M., McNamara, C., Milby, J. B., & Schumacher, J. E. (2006). Cell phones for ecological momentary assessment with cocaine-addicted homeless patients in treatment. *Journal of Substance Abuse Treatment*, *30*(2), 105–11.

Fry, J. P., & Neff, R. A. (2009). Periodic prompts and reminders in health promotion and health behavior interventions: Systematic review. *Journal of Medical Internet Research*, *11*(2), e16.

Gajecki, M., Berman, A. H., Sinadinovic, K., Rosendahl, I., & Andersson, C. (2014). Mobile phone brief intervention applications for risky alcohol use among university students: A randomized controlled study. *Addiction Science & Clinical Practice, 9*(1), 11.

Gates, P., & Albertella, L. (2016). The effectiveness of telephone counselling in the treatment of illicit drug and alcohol use concerns. *Journal of Telemedicine and Telecare*, 22(2), 67–85. doi:10.1177/1357633X15587406.

Garland, E. L., Franken, I. H., & Howard, M. O. (2012). Cue-elicited heart rate variability and attentional bias predict alcohol relapse following treatment. *Psychopharmacology, 222*(1), 17–26.

Godleski, L., Darkins, A., & Peters, J. (2012). Outcomes of 98,609 US Department of Veterans Affairs patients enrolled in telemental health services, 2006–2010. *Psychiatric Services, 63*(4), 383–5.

Griffiths, K. M., Calear, A. L., & Banfield, M. (2009). Systematic review on Internet support groups (ISGs) and depression (1): Do ISGs reduce depressive symptoms? *Journal of Medical Internet Research, 11*(3), e40.

Gustafson, D. H., Boyle, M. G., Shaw, B. R., Isham, A., McTavish, F. M., Richards, S., . . . Johnson, K. (2011b). An e-health solution for people with alcohol problems. *Alcohol Research & Health, 33*(4), 327–37.

Gustafson, D. H., McTavish, F. M., Chih, M. Y., Atwood, A. K., Johnson, R. A., Boyle, M. G., . . . Shah, D. (2014). A smartphone application to support recovery from alcoholism: A randomized clinical trial. *JAMA Psychiatry, 71*(5), 566–72.

Gustafson, D. H., Shaw, B. R., Isham, A., Baker, T., Boyle, M. G., & Levy, M. S. (2011a). Explicating an evidence-based, theoretically informed, mobile technology-based system to improve outcomes for people in recovery for alcohol dependence. *Substance Use & Misuse, 46*(1), 96–111.

Gustafson, D. H., Shaw, B. R., Isham, A., Dillon, D., & Spartz, J. (2009). *Exploring the potential of the Web-based virtual world of second life to improve substance abuse treatment outcomes.* Madison: Network for the Improvement of Addiction Treatment, University of Wisconsin.

Hawthorne, J. S., & Wojcik, M. H. (2006). Transdermal alcohol measurement: A review of the literature. *Canadian Society of Forensic Science Journal, 39*(2), 65–71.

Heron, K. E., & Smyth, J. M. (2010). Ecological momentary interventions: Incorporating mobile technology into psychosocial and health behaviour treatments. *British Journal of Health Psychology, 15*(1), 1–39.

Hester, R. K., Lenberg, K. L., Campbell, W., & Delaney, H. D. (2013). Overcoming addictions, a Web-based application, and SMART recovery, an online and in-person mutual help group for problem drinkers, Part 1: Three-month outcomes of a randomized controlled trial. *Journal of Medical Internet Research, 15*(7), e134.

Hoffman, E. W., Austin, E. W., Pinkleton, B. E., & Austin, B. W. (2016). An exploration of the associations of alcohol-related social media use and message interpretation outcomes to problem drinking among college students. *Health Communication, 32*(7), 864–71.

Hoffman, E. W., Pinkleton, B. E., Weintraub Austin, E., & Reyes-Velázquez, W. (2014). Exploring college students' use of general and alcohol-related social media and their associations with alcohol-related behaviors. *Journal of American College Health, 62*(5), 328–35.

Hollien, H., Harnsberger, J. D., Martin, C. A., Hill, R., & Alderman, G. A. (2009). Perceiving the effects of ethanol intoxication on voice. *Journal of Voice, 23*(5), 552–9.

Holt, L. J., Litt, M. D., & Cooney, N. L. (2012). Prospective analysis of early lapse to drinking and smoking among individuals in concurrent alcohol and tobacco treatment. *Psychology of Addictive Behaviors, 26*(3), 561–72.

Homma, Y., Ando, T., Yoshida, M., Kageyama, S., Takei, M., Kimoto, K., . . . Hashimoto, T. (2002). Voiding and incontinence frequencies: Variability of diary data and required diary length. *Neurourology and Urodynamics, 21*(3), 204–309.

Hone-Blanchet, A., Wensing, T., & Fecteau, S. (2014). The use of virtual reality in craving assessment and cue-exposure therapy in substance use disorders. *Frontiers in Human Neuroscience, 8*, 844.

Houtveen, J. H., & de Geus, E. J. C. (2009). Noninvasive psychophysiological ambulatory recordings: Study design and data analysis strategies. *European Psychologist, 14*(2), 132–41.

Ingersoll, K., Dillingham, R., Reynolds, G., Hettema, J., Freeman, J., Hosseinbor, S., & Winstead-Derlega, C. (2014). Development of a personalized bidirectional text messaging tool for HIV adherence assessment and intervention among substance abusers. *Journal of Substance Abuse Treatment, 46*(1), 66–73.

Ingjaldsson, J. T., Laberg, J. C., & Thayer, J. F. (2003). Reduced heart rate variability in chronic alcohol abuse: Relationship with negative mood, chronic thought suppression, and compulsive drinking. *Biological Psychiatry, 54*(12), 1427–36.

Johnson, E. I., Barrault, M., Nadeau, L., & Swendsen, J. (2009). Feasibility and validity of computerized ambulatory monitoring in drug-dependent women. *Drug and Alcohol Dependence, 99*(1), 322–6.

Kazemi, D. M., Borsari, B., Levine, M.J., J., LI, S., Lamberson, K. A., & Matta, L. A. (2017). A systematic review of the mHealth interventions to prevent alcohol and substance abuse. *Journal of Health Communication*, 22(5), 413–32.

Kang, S., & Gratch, J. (2010). Virtual humans elicit socially anxious interactants' verbal self-disclosure. *Computer Animation and Virtual Worlds, 21*(3-4), 473–82.

Kiluk, B. D., Sugarman, D. E., Nich, C., Gibbons, C. J., Martino, S., Rounsaville, B. J., & Carroll, K. M. (2011). A methodological analysis of randomized clinical trials of computer-assisted therapies for psychiatric disorders: Toward improved standards for an emerging field. *Perspectives, 168*(8), 790–9.

King, V. L., Brooner, R. K., Peirce, J. M., Kolodner, K., & Kidorf, M. S. (2014). A randomized trial of web-based videoconferencing for substance abuse counseling. *Journal of Substance Abuse Treatment, 46*(1), 36–42.

King, V. L., Stoller, K. B., Kidorf, M., Kindbom, K., Hursh, S., Brady, T., & Brooner, R. K. (2009). Assessing the effectiveness of an Internet-based videoconferencing platform for delivering intensified substance abuse counseling. *Journal of Substance Abuse Treatment, 36*(3), 331–8.

Klein, A. A., Slaymaker, V. J., Dugosh, K. L., & McKay, J. R. (2012). Computerized continuing care support for alcohol and drug dependence: A preliminary analysis of usage and outcomes. *Journal of Substance Abuse Treatment, 42*(1), 25–34.

Kuerbis, A., Armeli, S., Muench, F., & Morgenstern, J. (2013). Motivation and self-efficacy in the context of moderated drinking: Global self-report and ecological momentary assessment. *Psychology of Addictive Behaviors, 27*(4), 934–43.

Kuerbis, A., Armeli, S., Muench, F., & Morgenstern, J. (2014). Profiles of confidence and commitment to change as predictors of moderated drinking: A person-centered approach. *Psychology of Addictive Behaviors, 28*(4), 1065–76.

Kumar, S., Al'Absi, M., Beck, G., Ertin, E., & Scott, M. S. (2014). Behavioral monitoring and assessment via mobile sensing technologies. *Behavioral healthcare and technology: Using science-based innovations to transform practice* (pp. 27 –39). New York: Oxford University Press.

Lapham, S. C., Kring, M. K., & Skipper, B. (1991). Prenatal behavioral risk screening by computer in a health maintenance organization-based prenatal care clinic. *American Journal of Obstetrics and Gynecology, 165*(3), 506–14.

Larson, R., & Csikszentmihalyi, M. (1983). The experience sampling method. *New Directions for Methodology of Social & Behavioral Science, 15*, 41–56.

Lee, S. H., Han, D. H., Oh, S., Lyoo, I. K., Lee, Y. S., Renshaw, P. F., & Lukas, S. E. (2009). Quantitative electroencephalographic (qEEG) correlates of craving during virtual reality therapy in alcohol-dependent patients. *Pharmacology Biochemistry and Behavior, 91*(3), 393–7.

Leigh, B. C., & Stacy, A. W. (1998). Individual differences in memory associations involving the positive and negative outcomes of alcohol use. *Psychology of Addictive Behaviors, 12*(1), 39–46.

Lejuez, C. W., Read, J. P., Kahler, C. W., Richards, J. B., Ramsey, S. E., Stuart, G. L., . . . Brown, R. A. (2002). Evaluation of a behavioral measure of risk taking: The Balloon Analogue Risk Task (BART). *Journal of Experimental Psychology: Applied, 8*(2), 75–84.

Locke, S., Kowaloff, H. B., Hoff, R. G., Safran, C., Popovsky, M. A., Cotton, D. J., . . . Slack, W. V. (1992). Computer-based interview for screening blood donors for risk of HIV transmission. *JAMA, 268*(10), 1301–5.

Lu, H., Frauendorfer, D., Rabbi, M., Mast, M. S., Chittaranjan, G. T., Campbell, A. T., . . . Choudhury, T. (2012). Stresssense: Detecting stress in unconstrained acoustic environments using smartphones. In *Proceedings of the 2012 ACM Conference on Ubiquitous Computing*, pp. 351–60.

Lucas, R. W. (1977). A study of patients' attitudes to computer interrogation. *International Journal of Man-Machine Studies, 9*(1), 69–86.

Maitland, M. E., & Mandel, A. R. (1994). A client-computer interface for questionnaire data. *Archives of Physical Medicine and Rehabilitation, 75*(6), 639–42.

Marques, P. R., & McKnight, A. S. (2007). *Evaluating transdermal alcohol measuring devices*. www.nhtsa.gov.

Marsch, L., Lord, S., & Dallery, J. (2014). *Behavioral healthcare and technology: Using science-based innovations to transform practice*. New York: Oxford University Press.

Marsch, L. A., Carroll, K. M., & Kiluk, B. D. (2014). Technology-based interventions for the treatment and recovery management of substance use disorders: A JSAT special issue. *Journal of Substance Abuse Treatment, 46*(1), 1–4.

McKay, J. R. (2009). Continuing care research: What we've learned and where we're going. *Journal of Substance Abuse Treatment, 36*(2), 131–45.

McKay, J. R., Van Horn, D., Oslin, D., Lynch, K. G., Ivey, M., Ward, K., . . . Coviello, D. (2010). A randomized trial of extended telephone-based continuing care for alcohol dependence: Within treatment substance use outcomes. *Journal of Consulting and Clinical Psychology, 78*(6), 912–23.

Miller, J., Prichard, I., Hutchinson, A., & Wilson, C. (2014). The relationship between exposure to alcohol-related content on Facebook and predictors of alcohol consumption among female emerging adults. *Cyberpsychology, Behavior, and Social Networking, 17*(12), 735–41.

Mohr, D. C. (2012). Mobilyze! Context sensing mobile intervention for depression. *Medicine 2.0 Conference*.

Mohr, D. C., Ho, J., Duffecy, J., Reifler, D., Sokol, L., Burns, M. N., . . . Siddique, J. (2012). Effect of telephone-administered vs face-to-face cognitive behavioral therapy on adherence to therapy and depression outcomes among primary care patients: A randomized trial. *JAMA, 307*(21), 2278–85.

Moore, B. A., Fazzino, T., Barry, D. T., Fiellin, D. A., Cutter, C. J., Schottenfeld, R. S., & Ball, S. A. (2013). The recovery line: A pilot trial of automated, telephone-based treatment for continued drug use in methadone maintenance. *Journal of Substance Abuse Treatment, 45*(1), 63–9.

Muench, F. (2014). The promises and pitfalls of integrating technology into alcohol treatment. *Alcohol Research: Current Reviews, 36*(1), 131–42.

Muench, F., & Baumel, A. (2017). More than a text message: Dismantling digital triggers to curate behavior change in patient-centered health interventions. *Journal of Medical Internet Research, 19*(5), 147.

Muench, F., van Stolk-Cooke, K., Kuerbis, A., Stadler, G., Baumel, A., Shao, S., . . . Morgenstern, J. (2017). A randomized controlled pilot trial of different mobile messaging interventions for problem drinking compared to weekly drink tracking. *PLoS One*. http://journals.plos.org/plosone/article?id=10.1371/journal.pone.0167900

Muench, F., Weiss, R. A., Kuerbis, A., & Morgenstern, J. (2013). Developing a theory driven text messaging intervention for addiction care with user driven content. *Psychology of Addictive Behaviors, 27*(1), 315–21.

Paperny, D. M., Aono, J. Y., Lehman, R. M., Hammar, S. L., & Risser, J. (1990). Computer-assisted detection and intervention in adolescent high-risk health behaviors. *Journal of Pediatrics, 116*(3), 456–62.

Pentland, A., Lazer, D., Brewer, D., & Heibeck, T. (2009). Improving public health and medicine by use of reality mining. *Studies in Health Technology Informatics, 149*, 93–102.

Petrie, K., & Abell, W. (1995). Responses of parasuicides to a computerized interview. *Computers in Human Behavior, 10*(4), 415–8.

Quintana, D. S., McGregor, I. S., Guastella, A. J., Malhi, G. S., & Kemp, A. H. (2013). A meta-analysis on the impact of alcohol dependence on short-term resting-state heart rate variability: Implications for cardiovascular risk. *Alcoholism: Clinical and Experimental Research, 37*, e23–9.

Ridout, B., Campbell, A., & Ellis, L. (2012). 'Off your Face(book)': Alcohol in online social identity construction and its relation to problem drinking in university students. *Drug and Alcohol Review, 31*(1), 20–6.

Riley, W. T., Rivera, D. E., Atienza, A. A., Nilsen, W., Allison, S. M., & Mermelstein, R. (2011). Health behavior models in the age of mobile interventions: Are our theories up to the task? *Translational Behavioral Medicine, 1*(1), 53–71.

Riper, H., Spek, V., Boon, B., Conijn, B., Kramer, J., Martin-Abello, K., & Smit, F. (2011). Effectiveness of e-self-help interventions for curbing adult problem drinking: A meta-analysis. *Journal of Medical Internet Research, 13*(2), e42.

Robinson, R., & West, R. (1992). A comparison of computer and questionnaire methods of history-taking in a genito-urinary clinic. *Psychology and Health, 6*(1–2), 77–84.

Rooke, S., Thorsteinsson, E., Karpin, A., Copeland, J., & Allsop, D. (2010). Computer-delivered interventions for alcohol and tobacco use: A meta-analysis. *Addiction, 105*(8), 1381–90.

Rose, G. L., Skelly, J. M., Badger, G. J., Naylor, M. R., & Helzer, J. E. (2012). Interactive voice response for relapse prevention following cognitive-behavioral therapy for alcohol use disorders: A pilot study. *Psychological Services, 9*(2), 174–84.

Saitz, R., Helmuth, E. D., Aromaa, S. E., Guard, A., Belanger, M., & Rosenbloom, D. L. (2004). Web-based screening and brief intervention for the spectrum of alcohol problems. *Preventive Medicine, 39*(5), 969–75.

Santa Ana, E. J., & Jardin, B. (2013). Treatment-as-usual for substance abuse in community Settings. *Interventions for Addiction: Comprehensive Addictive Behaviors and Disorders, 3*, 245–53.

Schulze, M., Scharnweber, C., Janke, E., Leitmeier, V., Ulrich, T., Frieling, H.,... Marschollek, M. (2013). An interdisciplinary workshop to identify alcohol craving based on psychophysiological sensor data. *Biomedical Engineering/Biomedizinische Technik, 58*.

Shiffman, S. (2009). Ecological Momentary Assessment (EMA) in studies of substance use. *Psychological Assessment, 21*(4), 486–97.

Shiffman, S., Balabanis, M. H., Gwaltney, C. J., Paty, J. A., Gnys, M., Kassel, J. D.,... Paton, S. M. (2007). Prediction of lapse from associations between smoking and situational antecedents assessed by ecological momentary assessment. *Drug and Alcohol Dependence, 91*(2), 159–68.

Shiffman, S., & Stone, A. A. (1998). Introduction to the special section: Ecological momentary assessment in health psychology. *Health Psychology, 17*(1), 3–5.

Shiffman, S., Stone, A. A., & Hufford, M. R. (2008). Ecological momentary assessment. *Annual Review of Clinical Psychology, 4*, 1–32.

Sigmund, M., & Zelinka, P. (2011). Analysis of voiced speech excitation due to alcohol intoxication. *Information Technology and Control, 40*(2), 143–50.

Skinner, H. A. (1982). The drug abuse screening test. *Addictive Behaviors, 7*(4), 363–71.

Spinella, M. (2007). Normative data and a short form of the Barratt Impulsiveness Scale. *International Journal of Neuroscience, 117*(3), 359–68.

Suffoletto, B., Hu, J., Guyette, M., & Callaway, C. (2014). Factors contributing to emergency department care within 30 days of hospital discharge and potential ways to prevent it: Differences in perspectives of patients, caregivers, and emergency physicians. *Journal of Hospital Medicine, 9*(5), 315–9.

Swift, R. M. (1993). Transdermal measurement of alcohol consumption. *Addiction, 88*(8), 1037–9.

Tofighi, B., Grossman, E., Buirkle, E., McNeely, J., Gourevitch, M., & Lee, J. D. (2015). Mobile phone use patterns and preferences in safety net office-based buprenorphine patients. *Journal of Addiction Medicine, 9*(3), 217–21.

Tofighi, B., Grossman, E., Sherman, S., Nunes, E. V., & Lee, J. D. (2016). Mobile phone messaging during unobserved home induction to buprenorphine. *Journal of Addiction Medicine, 10*(5), 309–13.

Tofighi, B., Nicholson, J. M., McNeely, J., Muench, F., & Lee, J. D. (2016). Mobile phone messaging for illicit drug and alcohol dependence: A review of the literature. *Drug and Alcohol Review, 36*(4), 477–91.

Tourangeau, R., & Smith, T. W. (1996). Asking sensitive questions: The impact of data collection mode, question format, and question context. *Public Opinion Quarterly, 60*(2), 275–304.

Trull, T. J., & Ebner-Priemer, U. (2013). Ambulatory assessment. *Annual Review of Clinical Psychology*, 9, 151–76.

Turner, C. F., Ku, L., Rogers, S. M., Lindberg, L. D., Pleck, J. H., & Sonenstein, F. L. (1998). Adolescent sexual behavior, drug use, and violence: Increased reporting with computer survey technology. *Science, 280*(5365), 867–73.

Vahabzadeh, M., Mezghanni, M., Lin, J., Epstein, D. H., & Preston, K. L. (2010). PGIS: Electronic diary data integration with GPS data initial application in substance-abuse patients. In *Computer-Based Medical Systems, 2010 IEEE 23rd International Symposium*, pp. 474–9.

Vohs, K. D., & Baumeister, R. F. (2004). Understanding self-regulation: An introduction. *Handbook of self-regulation: Research, theory, and applications* (pp. 1–9). New York: Guilford.

Walitzer, K. S., Dermen, K. H., & Connors, G. J. (1999). Strategies for preparing clients for treatment: A review. *Behavior Modification, 23*(1), 129–51.

Webb, T., Joseph, J., Yardley, L., & Michie, S. (2010). Using the Internet to promote health behavior change: A systematic review and meta-analysis of the impact of theoretical basis, use of behavior change techniques, and mode of delivery on efficacy. *Journal of Medical Internet Research, 12*(1), e4.

Weisband, S., & Kiesler, S. (1996). Self disclosure on computer forms: Meta-analysis and implications. In *Proceedings of the SIGCHI Conference on Human Factors in Computing Systems*, pp. 3–10.

Weitzel, J. A., Bernhardt, J. M., Usdan, S., Mays, D., & Glanz, K. (2007). Using wireless handheld computers and tailored text messaging to reduce negative consequences of drinking alcohol. *Journal of Studies on Alcohol and Drugs, 68*(4), 534–7.

Wen, H., Sobolev, M., Pollak, J. P., Estrin, D., Vitale, R. P., & Muench, F. (submitted). Continuous monitoring and assessment for impulsivity: An exploratory study.

Westgate, E. C., Neighbors, C., Heppner, H., Jahn, S., & Lindgren, K. P. (2014). I will take a shot for every 'like' I get on this status: Posting alcohol-related Facebook content is linked to drinking outcomes. *Journal of Studies on Alcohol and Drugs, 75*(3), 390–8.

Wiers, R. W., & Stacy, A. W. (2013). Implicit and associative processes in addiction. In P. Miller (Eds.) *Principles of addiction: Comprehensive addictive behaviors and disorders* (pp. 405 –11). Amsterdam: Elsevier.

Witkiewitz, K., Falk, D. E., Kranzler, H. R., Litten, R. Z., Hallgren, K. A., O'Malley, S. S., & Anton, R. F. (2014). Methods to analyze treatment effects in the presence of missing data for a continuous heavy drinking outcome measure when participants drop out from treatment in alcohol clinical trials. *Alcoholism: Clinical and Experimental Research, 38*(11), 2826–34.

Young, L. B. (2012). Telemedicine interventions for substance-use disorder: A literature review. *Journal of Telemedicine and Telecare, 18*(1), 47–53.

Zwick, R., & Attkisson, C. C. (1985). Effectiveness of a client pretherapy orientation videotape. *Journal of Counseling Psychology, 32*(4), 514–24.

CHAPTER

35 Use of Digital Technology to Provide or Enhance the Delivery of Psychotherapeutic Interventions for Addictions

Computer-Based Cognitive Behavioral Therapies

Kathleen M. Carroll *and* Brian D. Kiluk

Abstract

Cognitive-behavioral therapy (CBT) is effective across a range of substance use disorders yet implementation in many substance use treatment settings is comparatively rare due to multiple challenges, including the costly resources needed for appropriate training and supervision of clinicians. Digital technology is one strategy to address these challenges, potentially making such evidence-based therapies more broadly available to those in need of treatment. This chapter provides an overview of the development of a computerized version of CBT (CBT4CBT) as a means of exposing patients to basic CBT skills and strategies in an engaging and user-friendly manner while also allowing clinicians and treatment programs to be more efficient and effective. Empirical evidence supporting CBT4CBT from four randomized trials at the time of writing is reviewed, as well as a description of the potential benefits and applications of computerized therapies. Given their flexibility, relative ease of dissemination, and lower cost compared to clinician-delivered treatment, computerized versions of CBT (and other behavioral therapies) might be used to enhance and extend psychiatric treatment for addictions. Moreover, the level of standardization and control that characterizes computerized therapies may be useful in understanding mechanisms of effective treatments and in development of personalized interventions. While there is tremendous optimism regarding the potential of computerized therapies, such as CBT4CBT, systematic evaluation of these interventions and the methodological standards for evaluating them is still in very early stages relative to the more established behavioral and pharmacologic interventions for addictions.

Keywords: cognitive behavioral therapy, computer-based therapies, computer-assisted therapy, CBT4CBT, substance use disorders

Introduction

Enormous scientific effort has been devoted in the past 30 years to the development of effective treatments for addiction, a public health problem affecting more than 25 million Americans and their families with an estimated annual cost of more than US$180 billion (Hoffman & McCarty, 2013), including medical care, lost productivity, and criminal justice system costs. Important advances have been made in the development of effective pharmacotherapies and behavioral therapies, but it is estimated that only a fraction of individuals with substance use disorders receive appropriate evidence-based therapies (Institute of Medicine, 2001). Digital technology is thus an important strategy for making evidence-based therapies more broadly available. This chapter provides an overview of web-based delivery of cognitive-behavioral therapies (CBT), a form of behavioral therapy that has been demonstrated to be effective across a range of both substance use and mental health disorders (Tolin, 2010). After a brief overview of CBT, the chapter covers the development and current state of empirical support of technology-based CBT for substance use disorders. Finally, we review the possible range of settings and applications where computerized CBT might be implemented to broaden, strengthen, and make this empirically based form of treatment more widely available.

Overview of Cognitive-Behavioral Therapy for Addictions

CBT has been shown to be effective across a wide range of substance use disorders, including alcohol, marijuana, cocaine, and nicotine dependence (Carroll & Onken, 2005; Dutra et al., 2008; Magill & Ray, 2009). It is compatible with a number of other treatment approaches, including pharmacotherapy (Anton et al., 1999; O'Malley et al., 1992) and traditional counseling approaches (Morgenstern, Mrogan, McCrady, Keller, & Carroll, 2001) and thus can be implemented in a wide range of settings. CBT is also a widely used platform for pharmacotherapy trials; that is, the "base" treatment provided to all participants to improve retention in treatment and assure that all participants are receiving an adequate and standard level of behavioral intervention (Carroll, Kosten, & Rounsaville, 2004b). Notably, CBT has been evaluated in virtually all of the landmark multisite of addiction treatment trials, including Project MATCH and Project COMBINE for alcohol (Anton et al., 2006; Project MATCH Research Group, 1997), the National Institute on Drug Abuse (NIDA) Cooperative Cocaine Treatment Study (Crits-Christoph et al., 1999), and the Marijuana Treatment Project (MTP Research Group, 2004), as well as numerous single-site trials.

As applied to the addictions, two key defining features of CBT are (1) an emphasis on functional analysis of drug use (i.e., understanding drug use with respect to its antecedents and consequences) and (2) emphasis on skills training (Carroll, 1998). These typically include strategies for (1) understanding the patterns that maintain drug use and developing strategies for changing these patterns; (2) understanding craving, craving cues, and the development of skills for coping with craving; (3) recognizing and challenging the cognitions that accompany and maintain patterns of substance use; (4) increasing awareness of the consequences of even small decisions (e.g., which route to take home from work) and the identification of "seemingly irrelevant" decisions which can culminate in high-risk situations; (5) development of problem-solving skills and practicing application of those skills to substance-related and more general problems; and (6) developing skills for assertively refusing offers of drugs, as well as reducing exposure to drugs and drug-related cues.

These skills are useful in their application to helping patients control and stop substance use, but these basic skills are also the building blocks of effective behavior in multiple contexts (Carroll, Ball, & Martino, 2004a). For example, skills used to cope with craving can easily be applied to other aspects of regulation of affect and ability to temporize behavior; the principles used in the sessions on seemingly irrelevant decisions can easily be adapted to improve decision making skills and reduce exposure to high-risk situations; and substance use refusal skills can easily be transferred to more effective and assertive responding in a number of situations.

A key distinguishing feature of CBT for addictions includes its relative durability of effects. Several groups have demonstrated that, unlike most pharmacotherapies and many behavioral therapies, the effects of CBT tend to be much longer lasting, in some cases with individuals continuing to improve even after treatment ends (Carroll et al., 2000; Carroll et al., 1994; Hollon, 2003). This "sleeper effect" is thought to be associated with CBT's emphasis on learning and implementing new skills and strategies and the generalization of these skills to new behaviors and problems. Since the durability of CBT is one of its most salient features, efforts have focused on acquisition of cognitive and behavioral control skills as a likely mediator of CBT's effects and durability. Practice and mastery of skills outside of sessions is another key feature of CBT; virtually all forms of CBT emphasize the importance of "homework" in effective implementation of CBT. A number of researchers have found that patients who do homework assignments tend to have better extended outcomes relative to those who do not practice skills outside of sessions (Burns & Nolen-Hoeksema, 1991; Burns & Spangler, 2000; Carroll, Nich, & Ball, 2005; Gonzalez, Schmitz, & DeLaune, 2006; Neimeyer, Kazantzis, Kassler, Baker, & Fletcher, 2008).

Challenges in Implementing CBT

Although clinical acceptability of CBT is relatively high, multiple lines of evidence suggest that effective implementation of CBT in many substance abuse treatment settings is comparatively rare. This is the case for multiple reasons. First, compared with typical counseling approaches, CBT when effectively implemented is comparatively more structured, active, and cognitively demanding for patients and clinicians alike. Effective CBT therapies establish agendas for sessions, work to maintain session focus, and teach complex skills. Patients who benefit from CBT must pay attention to complex new ideas and skills, retain them, and practice them in challenging circumstances. Simply said, CBT is a lot of work, particularly when it is implemented at the levels of fidelity and skill characterizing the trials establishing its efficacy.

Second, clinicians tend to overestimate the degree to which they focus on CBT interventions. In multiple studies, correspondence of clinicians' versus independent raters' assessments of treatment fidelity was low, with therapists consistently reporting much higher levels of adherence and integrity compared with their supervisors as well as with those independent raters' reviewing identical sessions (Carroll, Nich, & Rounsaville, 1998; Martino, Ball, Nich, Frankforter, & Carroll, 2009a). Similarly, data from analyses of clinicians participating in several trials conducted as part of the NIDA Clinical Trials Network, a national partnership of treatment providers and clinical researchers (Tai et al., 2010), suggest that although clinicians reported CBT was a key component of the treatment they routinely provided (Ball et al., 2002), when independent fidelity raters reviewed audiotapes of their sessions, interventions associated with CBT and other empirically validated therapies were virtually undetectable (Santa Ana et al., 2008). Instead, clinician-initiated conversations regarding topics unrelated to the symptoms or problems for which the individual sought treatment (or "chat") was more common than most evidence-based interventions and practices (Bamatter et al., 2010; Martino, Ball, Nich, Frankforter, & Carroll, 2009b).

Third, there is a scarcity of well-trained CBT clinicians; there are no national training programs or accreditation standards for CBT. Doctoral and master's level counseling programs have begun integrating training evidence-based therapies like CBT only recently (Beidnas & Kendall, 2010; Weissman et al., 2006), and most community-based specialty programs neither require or offer training in CBT (Olmstead, Abraham, Martino, & Roman, 2012). Relatedly, it is fairly time-consuming to offer the type of training that brings clinicians to adequate levels of competence; moreover, the most commonly used approach to training (brief workshops) has been shown to be insufficient to bring clinicians to needed levels. For example, randomized trials evaluating strategies in training community-based clinicians to implement evidence-based therapies like CBT and motivational interviewing (MI) have demonstrated that (1) exposure to manuals or workshops alone has little effect on readiness to implement treatment effectively, (2) training needs to be comparatively intensive (e.g., 3–4 days of didactic training with ample opportunity for role-play and practice), and (3) intensive ongoing supervision is essential in bringing most clinicians to adequate levels of fidelity and skill (Beidnas & Kendall, 2010; Miller & Mount, 2001; Miller, Yahne, Moyers, Martinez, & Pirritano, 2004; Sholomskas et al., 2005). Thus, appropriate training and supervision in CBT remains comparatively costly, time-consuming, and may be difficult for many small programs to justify given the high rate of turnover that characterizes the current specialty treatment system (Knudsen, Ducharme, & Roman, 2008; Schoenwald, Sheidow, & Chapman, 2009).

There are other barriers to making evidence-based therapies more widely available, many of them inherent in the current US system for healthcare delivery (McLellan & Meyers, 2004). Trained clinicians are rare in many geographic locations in the United States, and most payors still do not require that clinicians implement evidence-based interventions, much less require evidence that they do so (Hoffman & McCarty, 2013). The substance abuse treatment system continues to rely on "soft" indicators of program performance such as retention, rather than more meaningful evidence of patient improvement in functioning and reduction in drug use (Humphreys & McLellan, 2011). Healthcare reform via the Affordable Care Act may foster greater emphasis on performance standards and accountability within the specialty treatment system (Stewart, Horgan, Garnick, Ritter, & McLellan, 2013) and hence drive greater focus on treatment outcomes and evidence-based treatments. At the same time, however, higher demand for substance abuse prevention and intervention services and implementation of substance use treatment in primary care settings is a likely result of these reforms (McLellan & Woodworth, 2014), further increasing the demand for evidence-based treatment and the consequent shortage of appropriate services and trained clinicians.

Development and Validation of CBT4CBT

The issues just outlined led, in part, to our development of a computer-assisted version of CBT (CBT4CBT; Carroll et al., 2008a; Carroll et al., 2009a; Carroll & Kiluk, 2017; Carroll & Rounsaville, 2010), a project which began in 2002. The fundamental goal of our efforts to develop an engaging, user-friendly, computerized version of CBT was to capitalize on the multimedia features and wide availability of the Internet to provide a form of CBT that could be delivered much more broadly than traditional clinician-delivered CBT.

CBT4CBT was conceived as a means of exposing patients to basic CBT skills and strategies that would also allow clinicians and treatment programs to be more efficient and effective. That is, the clinician would continue to provide key components of care to his or her patients (urine monitoring, pharmacotherapy, case management, support, and assessment/treatment of co-occurring medical and psychological problems) while the delivery of CBT skills training is "subcontracted" to the computer. This would allow providers to save considerable clinician time while still providing their patients with exposure to a form of an evidence-based approach. Moreover, the program, delivered through the Internet, could be available at anytime and anywhere the patient had access to the Internet.

In developing a computer-assisted version of CBT that could be used with minimal clinician or staff assistance, it was necessary to very clearly specify what the program was intended to convey; in our case we conceived of CBT4CBT as a "cognitive coping skills training machine." The program capitalizes on the use of multimedia features to demonstrate implementation of targeted coping skills in realistic settings, with emphasis on how these coping skills can be generalized to address a range of behaviors and problems in addition to addiction. The CBT4CBT program, delivered as an adjunct to treatment as a clinician "extender" (Carroll & Rounsaville, 2010), provides a standardized means of conveying specific components of CBT with a high, consistent level of fidelity.

CBT4CBT was designed to be as engaging as possible as well as user-friendly, requiring no previous experience with computers, no reading skills (any material presented in text was also read aloud by a narrator), and it collects no personal health information (PHI). The program is media-rich, using games, cartoons, and exercises to illustrate points. At its core is a series of videos which, for each module, present connected scenes of engaging characters (portrayed by professional actors) who, first, experience a common, difficult situation then demonstrate using the targeted skill how to successfully negotiate that situation without resorting to drug use.

CBT4CBT consists of seven modules, covering seven core components of CBT as described in the NIDA CBT manual (Carroll, 1998). These include (1) the basics of CBT and understanding patterns of substance use, (2) identifying and coping with craving, (3) recognizing and changing thoughts associated with substance use, (4) problem-solving skills, (5) temporizing behavior and decision-making skills, (6) dealing with offers to use drugs and assertiveness skills, and (7) HIV/HCV risk reduction, focusing on both drug and sexual risk behaviors. Each module takes about an hour to complete and follows a similar format. First, the program "checks in" regarding the patient's experience with last practice exercise; next, the narrator introduces the skill that will be the focus of that session. A short video then plays that demonstrates the problem to be addressed by that skill (e.g., a woman comes home from a difficult day to her husband offering her alcohol, a man who is under pressure at work makes a series of impulsive decisions that result in a very high-risk situation). The skill topic is then described using a mix of animation, graphics, and narration. The video then repeats, but this time showing the character using the skill to resolve the situation without use of drugs or alcohol. The program also emphasizes homework in multiple ways: homework is introduced by the characters in each of the videos, and they provide detailed examples of how to do the practice exercise based on the situation illustrated in the video and then walk the patient through the practice exercise based on their own experience. Other characters emphasize the value of practice of skills, and the check-in component of each module conducts a detailed review of the patient's experience with the assignment.

As of this writing, four randomized trials of CBT4CBT have been completed in community-based settings (Carroll et al., 2008b; Carroll, DeVito, Shi, Nich, & Sofuoglu, 2017; Carroll et al., 2014; Kiluk et al., 2016), with multiple trials ongoing or in press. The first, conducted in an outpatient addiction treatment setting, evaluated outcomes among treatment-seeking individuals with a range of substance use problems (Carroll et al., 2008a). Participants were predominantly alcohol, cocaine, marijuana, or opioid dependent, with use of multiple substances reported by 80% of participants (i.e., this protocol was designed to take "all comers"), and they were randomly assigned to receive standard outpatient treatment with or without access to the CBT4CBT program. At the end of the 8-week trial, participants assigned to the CBT4CBT condition submitted significantly fewer urine specimens that were positive for any type of drug (34% vs. 53%) and tended to have longer continuous periods of abstinence during treatment compared to those assigned to standard outpatient treatment only (22 vs. 15 days). A 6-month follow-up of 82% of the intention-to-treat sample indicated significantly better durability of effects of CBT4CBT over standard treatment for both self-report and urinalysis data (Carroll et al., 2009b), suggesting the "sleeper effect" of clinician-delivered CBT was retained in its transition to computer delivery.

An evaluation of the extent to which participants acquired the cognitive and behavioral control skills emphasized by the program indicated that (1) participants assigned to CBT4CBT had larger improvements in the quality of their skills as assessed by independent raters in a role-play task, (2) level of skill acquisition mediated treatment outcome and level of drug use during follow-up, and, (3) for the participants assigned to CBT4CBT, quality of skills continued to increase in the follow-up period (Kiluk, Nich, Babuscio, & Carroll, 2010). Thus, not only was the "sleeper effect" found for drug use during the follow-up period, but it was also seen in the demonstrated quality of the patients' coping skills. This suggests that the CBT4CBT program appears to have been successful in its goal of teaching generalizable skills and strategies. Self-reported coping skills showed a similar pattern (Sugarman, Nich, & Carroll, 2010).

The second randomized trial was conducted with a larger, more homogeneous but challenging population; that is, methadone maintained individuals with cocaine use disorders. As with the first study, acceptance of and satisfaction with the CBT4CBT program by the participants was high, and significantly more individuals assigned to the CBT4CBT condition maintained at least 3 weeks of continuous abstinence during treatment compared to standard treatment only (36% vs. 17%). As with the initial trial, the CBT4CBT program was associated with better outcomes through a 6-month follow-up than standard methadone maintenance treatment (Carroll et al., 2014), again suggesting that the durability of traditional, clinician-delivered CBT also occurs in this web-based version. Individuals in this trial also rated a positive level of working alliance (a.k.a., "therapeutic alliance") with the CBT4CBT program similar to that of their working alliance with a clinician, without evidence of a negative impact on the clinician–patient relationship for those individuals who received both forms of treatment (Kiluk, Serafini, Frankforter, Nich, & Carroll, 2014). Recent data also indicate that completion of homework is associated with improved outcomes in both the clinician- and computer-delivered forms of CBT (Decker et al., 2016).

A major potential advantage of technology-based interventions like CBT4CBT is their relatively low cost (compared to clinician-delivered therapies), as access to computers and the Internet continues to grow even in rural and remote locations (Hedman, Ljotsson, & Lindefors, 2012; Marks, Cavanagh, & Gega, 2007; McCrone et al., 2004). While there have been few economic evaluations of computerized therapies thus far, the data do suggest that while they carry some costs, as all effective therapies do, these costs appear to be justified by outcomes. For example, using the same methods to evaluate cost and efficacy as were used in evaluations of other evidence-based behavioral therapies (see Olmstead, Carroll, Canning-Ball, & Martino., 2011; Olmstead, Sindelar, & Petry, 2007; Yates, 1994), Olmstead reported that, as practiced in the trial, the incremental cost effectiveness ratio (ICER) for producing an additional drug-free urine specimen cost $21 for CBT4CBT compared with standard outpatient treatment (Olmstead, Ostrow, & Carroll, 2010). This compared favorably to identically calculated ICERs for Petry's contingency management (CM) in methadone programs in the studies ($70), CM in outpatient programs in the CTN ($146), and traditional clinician-delivered CBT ($159) for the same outcome. Furthermore, when taken to scale (a single computer used by many patients), CBT4CBT quickly "dominated" treatment as usual; that is, it could produce better outcomes at lower cost (Olmstead et al., 2010).

Summary of Current Level of Empirical Support

Systematic evaluation of Internet-based interventions like CBT4CBT is in very early stages relative to the more established areas of behavioral and pharmacologic interventions for the addictions. Thus, methodological standards for evaluating Internet-based therapies are also at a relatively early stage. In general terms, the early efficacy data from many of these approaches are seen as promising (e.g., Bickel, Christensen, & Marsch, 2011; Cuijpers et al., 2009; Kaltenthaler, Pary, & Beverley, 2004; Marks & Cavanagh, 2009; Portnoy, Scott-Sheldon, Johnson, & Carey, 2008; Titov, 2007) but should be interpreted with caution due to multiple methodological problems that characterize much of the existing literature (Copeland & Martin, 2004; Gibbons et al., 2009; Kaltenthaler, Parry, Beverley, & Ferriter, 2008; Postel, de Haan, & DeJong., 2008; Tumur, Kaltenthaler, Ferriter, Beverley, & Parry, 2007).

While optimism regarding the potential of these approaches is warranted, it should be tempered by awareness that few of the existing studies meet the current methodological quality standards required for determining that a behavioral therapy is empirically supported. In particular, the most common control conditions used in randomized controlled trials of computer-assisted therapies are wait-list or assessment-only controls (Portnoy et al., 2008), which constitute weak tests of the efficacy of an approach. This problem is further magnified for the multiple studies in which outcome measures are based solely on participants' unblinded, subjective self-reports. Similarly, many of the existing studies rely almost exclusively on participant self-report of symptoms without independent clinician interview or review of change. A review by Postel and colleagues of Internet treatment studies for mental health disorders characterized the methodological quality of the literature as low (Postel et al., 2008): only 5 of the 14 studies reviewed met minimal criteria for study quality as defined by the Cochrane criteria (Higgins & Green, 2006; Postel et al., 2008), with consistent weaknesses noted across studies in terms of monitoring treatment compliance, high levels of attrition, inadequate application of intention-to-treat principles, insufficient attention paid to issues such as treatment credibility, failure to protect the integrity of the independent variable, reliance on nonvalidated or subjective self-reports of outcome, and failure to comply with CONSORT principles, such as intention-to-treatment analyses (Altman et al., 2001). The nature of the computer-assisted intervention itself, as in the early psychotherapy research literature, is too often an underspecified or poorly defined "black box," the components or integrity of which are difficult to evaluate or replicate. Our 2011 review of the methodological quality of 75 randomized trials evaluating web-based interventions for a range of psychiatric disorders, including substance use disorders, found that no existing program met current standards for consideration as an evidence-based practice nor was demonstrated to be as effective as the clinician-delivered version of that treatment (Kiluk et al., 2011).

In this context, the empirical evidence supporting CBT4CBT as an add-on to standard care is comparatively strong: four randomized trials in different populations have indicated its relative efficacy to standard care alone, with outcomes validated by biological measures (Carroll et al., 2008b; Carroll et al., 2017; Carroll et al., 2014; Kiluk et al., 2016). In all studies, there was evidence of durability of CBT4CBT's effects relative to control over a 6-month follow-up (Carroll et al., 2009b; Carroll et al., 2014). There is evidence to support CBT4CBT's proposed mechanism of action in that we have demonstrated that quality of coping skills increased in CBT4CBT relative to standard treatment, showing an increase in quality-mediated self-reported outcomes as well as percentage of drug-negative urine specimens submitted (Kiluk et al., 2010). Evidence is also emerging regarding the types of individuals who appear to respond particularly well to CBT4CBT versus standard treatment. For example, we have found that individuals higher in alexithymia, which is characterized by difficulty expressing affect and appears to be prevalent among individuals with substance use disorders (Taylor, Parker, & Babgby, 1990) may have better outcomes when treated with CBT4CBT rather than standard counseling (Morie, Nich, Hunkele, Potenza, & Carroll, 2015). It is important to recognize that CBT4CBT's efficacy in the early studies was evaluated as an add-on to standard specialty substance abuse treatment and was not yet evaluated as a stand-alone treatment or compared directly with clinician-delivered CBT. However, the recent trial indicating that the alcohol-specific version of CBT demonstrated superiority to standard counseling is promising (Kiluk et al., 2016) and suggests that CBT4CBT may be used as a "virtual stand-alone" under some conditions (Carroll & Kiluk, 2017). These issues and possible new applications for CBT4CBT are addressed in the following sections.

Ongoing Work with CBT4CBT and Potential Applications of Computer-Assisted Therapies

With support from the NIDA and the National Institute on Alcoholism and Alcohol Abuse (NIAAA), new versions of CBT4CBT have been developed and are being evaluating in randomized clinical trials. A version designed specifically for individuals with alcohol use disorders is being tested as both an addition to standard care as well as a "virtual stand-alone" (i.e., delivered with only very brief clinical monitoring). Retention data collected thus far suggest that this approach appears to be safe and effective for many individuals and is worth evaluating in larger trials. Another ongoing trial evaluating web-based CBT4CBT for drug use disorders includes a CBT4CBT-only condition (provided with brief weekly clinical monitoring), as well as a standard clinician-delivered CBT condition. This trial offers the potential to evaluate CBT4CBT in comparison to a "gold standard" CBT treatment (i.e., master's and PhD-level clinicians who receive 2-day didactic workshop with practice and ongoing supervision), which may help elucidate the mechanisms of action of CBT in general as well as allow further investigation of the client characteristics that influence how the mechanisms operate in each form of treatment delivery. Particularly exciting is our culturally adapted version of the program for Spanish-speaking individuals, which, if demonstrated to be effective, could have significant impact in bringing this form of CBT to Latino/a populations and hence address health disparities in this important group (Wells, Klap, Koike, & Sherbourne, 2001). In addition to these ongoing randomized controlled trials, we are also conducting secondary analyses of our completed trials focusing on the types of individuals who respond particularly well or poorly to computerized versions of CBT (e.g., evaluating factors such as cognitive function, motivation, addiction severity, etc.).

Given their flexibility, relative ease of dissemination, and lower cost (compared with clinician-delivered treatment), computerized versions of CBT might be used in any number of ways to enhance and extend psychiatric treatment, some of which we outline later. It should be noted, however, that this is very much a list of possibilities rather than existing options, and computer-assisted therapies have not yet been validated for many of these applications (Carroll & Rounsaville, 2010).

As "Clinician Extenders"

The most common strategy for evaluating computer-assisted therapies, and the model with the strongest level of empirical support at present, is as an adjunct to clinician-supervised treatment. In this model, the patient receives assessment, support, monitoring, and intervention as usual from the clinician; however, the patient also accesses the computer-assisted treatment to either receive an additional intervention or to complement standard care. This is exemplified by our work on CBT4CBT as described earlier, as well as by others, such as the Therapeutic Education System (TES) developed by Bickel, Marsch, and colleagues (Bickel, Marsch, Buchhalter, & Badger, 2008; Marsch et al., 2014), a multicomponent system which uses the Community Reinforcement Approach including contingency management to address illicit substance use. TES was recently found in a large multisite study to enhance within-treatment outcomes in a range of community-based programs across the United States (Campbell et al., 2014).

A similar model might involve using computer-assisted therapies to help clinicians better meet the needs of patients with complex or multiple disorders. That is, most clinicians can only specialize in a few disorders, and most have expertise in a limited number of empirically supported approaches. Thus, it is unrealistic for any single clinician to master the almost overwhelming number of empirically supported therapies (Carroll & Rounsaville, 2007). Therefore, it is possible that computer-assisted therapies could play a role in extending clinicians' expertise and enable them to offer more integrated, comprehensive treatments that address multiple issues. For instance, depression specialists might complement treatment by offering computer-assisted addiction treatment to their depressed patients who also drink or use drugs, or a specialty addiction clinic could integrate computerized posttraumatic stress disorder (PTSD) treatments to broaden the scope of services offered to the many individuals with comorbid addiction and PTSD, and so on. Given the high rates of smoking and associated morbidities among individuals with mental health disorders (Anthony, Warner, & Kessler, 1994; Lawrence, Mitrou, & Zubrick, 2009), it should arguably become standard practice to refer all patients to a computerized smoking cessation program, which could be done at virtually no cost but with extraordinary benefit and healthcare cost savings.

This leads to the possibility that the role of the individual clinician could eventually evolve into one which involves, in addition to providing treatment for the presenting complaint or problem, assessing his or her patients for a range of psychiatric disorders and related problems, including behavioral health issues (insomnia, obesity) (Gibbons et al., 2009; Portnoy et al., 2008). The clinician could then provide the patient with links to the appropriate, validated computer-assisted resource for the identified comorbid problems, acting in a sense as the patient's "general contractor" for mental and behavioral health to integrate, individualize, and enhance care (Carroll & Rounsaville, 2010).

To Extend the Benefits of Treatment

Computer-assisted therapies might also be used to extend the benefit of acute treatment episodes. Individuals completing intensive outpatient or inpatient hospitalizations too often fail to follow through on referrals for aftercare or continuing care, which is exacerbated in cases where patients live far from the hospital. Given that the majority of psychiatric disorders are characterized by a chronic or relapsing course, computer-assisted therapies could thus be used to extend care and thus improve long-term outcomes. Furthermore, as approximately 87% of the US population can access the Internet via computer or mobile device within their home (www.internetlivestats.com), the potential reach of computer-assisted aftercare or continuing care interventions is much greater than for any other existing system. Thus, individuals completing an episode of care or hospitalization could be provided with links to computer-assisted approaches that could be used to help them manage and monitor their symptoms and to alert their clinicians to early signs of relapse. Thus, web-based CBT may be able to provide a form of "relapse prevention" for some individuals.

Linking Systems of Care

Recognizing that many more individuals with psychiatric disorders access primary care rather than the mental health system, extensive efforts have been made in recent years to bridge the mental health, substance abuse, and healthcare delivery systems. In the area of substance use and addiction, these approaches are referred to as *screening, brief intervention, and referral to treatment* (SBIRT), in which individuals at risk for substance use problems are systematically identified at a primary care setting such as an emergency room or general practice and provided a brief intervention with advice to stop their smoking, alcohol, or drug use; those who are identified to be at higher risk are referred to specialty addiction treatment (Babor et al., 2007; Saitz, Svikis, D'Onofrio, Kraemer, & Perl, 2006). These efforts have had success in a number of settings, and screening and brief intervention is now reimbursable under Medicare in some locations, although recent trials indicate limited success for users of illicit drugs in primary care and emergency department settings (Bogenschutz et al., 2014; Saitz et al., 2014). This implies that, unlike individuals with alcohol use disorders, individuals with drug use disorders may need more intensive intervention than brief motivational interventions alone. At the same time, however, one factor limiting the success of SBIRT programs is that individuals at risk often fail to follow through on referrals to specialty care (Babor et al., 2007). Integration of web-based therapies in primary care settings, and even initiating treatment at the primary care visit, may be one strategy for fostering stronger links between these systems of care.

As Behavioral Platforms

In most areas of psychiatry, combined treatments encompassing both medication and behavioral therapy are seen as the ideal. In many settings, this ideal is prohibitively costly and difficult to achieve or maintain over the course of treatment, given time constraints on clinicians and the logistical issues of patients. Thus, offering computer-assisted therapy to complement pharmacotherapy for depression, anxiety, or addictive disorders may be one means of broadening the benefits of pharmacotherapy for these disorders. Some pharmaceutical companies have already made access to computer-assisted therapy available to patients who are prescribed specific medications for those disorders.

Similarly, the benefits in terms of cost, statistical power, and addressing ethical concerns of offering some form of behavioral therapy to individuals participating in placebo-controlled trials of pharmacotherapies are now widely acknowledged (Carroll, 1997). However, it remains a challenge, particularly in multisite trials, to train and supervise clinicians to provide the behavioral therapy platform and to do so at a consistent, standardized level to reduce risk of therapist or site effects. Thus, offering all participants in a clinical pharmacotherapy trial access to an empirically validated computer-assisted treatment in conjunction with close monitoring and clinical management in the protocol is another key potential role for these approaches.

Prevention for Mild Cases/Introduction to Treatment

While many psychiatric disorders are more effectively treated before they become severe and intractable, individuals early in the course of a disorder rarely seek formal treatment or specialty care. Thus, one particularly exciting application of computer-assisted interventions is to offer early, and thus possibly preventative, intervention. A number of web-based therapies have been evaluated and have been demonstrated to show some promise in early intervention and prevention with general, nonclinical populations as well as with hard-to-reach populations (Postel, de Jong, & de Haan, 2005). Similarly, there are a wide variety of web-based screening and brief intervention approaches targeting heavy and at-risk drinkers (e.g., Collins, Kirouac, Lewis, Witkiewitz, & Carey, 2014; Hester, Delaney, & Campbell, 2011; Palfai, Winter, Lu, Rosenbloom, & Saitz, 2014; Witkiewitz et al., 2014). Computerized CBT has not yet been evaluated in this context for substance users, but it is possible that a web-based program may be sufficient for individuals with milder forms of addiction or who wish for some assistance in making changes in their behavior before seeking formal treatment.

As a Step Toward Powerful and Personalized Interventions

Although web-based therapies like CBT4CBT may be one strategy for making some therapies more widely available and less expensive, another potential benefit is that the level of standardization and control that characterizes computerized therapies may prove to be useful in understanding the mechanisms of effective treatments and enhancing their effectiveness. Compared with the high level of variability that characterizes clinician-delivered treatments, computerized therapies are relatively standard, delivering a form of treatment with less variability. More standardization in delivery may confer important advantages in identifying treatment mechanisms. For example, a major challenge in behavioral therapies research has been to identify specific effects of therapies and link them causally to treatment outcomes (Morgenstern & Longabaugh, 2000), particularly because the specific effects are inseparable from "relational" effects (e.g., therapeutic alliance) when treatments are delivered in the context of an interpersonal relationship (Miller & Moyers, 2015). Standardization via computerized delivery may reduce the level of variability in common elements of therapy (e.g., empathy, support) and thus make specific effects of treatment more easily detected. Our work on evaluating acquisition of coping skills in computerized CBT may be one example of this, where lower variability in treatment delivery may have made it easier to detect changes in skill acquisition across groups and link these to outcome (Kiluk et al., 2010; Longabaugh, 2010). Moreover, in our most recent trial, we've found that although the working alliance was related to treatment outcomes for those assigned to standard treatment (consistent with the general psychotherapy literature), the same was not true for those assigned to CBT4CBT, which suggests that the specific treatment ingredients may be more salient in computer-delivered versions of CBT (Kiluk et al., 2014).

Another promising line of research that capitalizes on standardization of delivery of treatment is the growing body of work on understanding effects of specific therapies in terms of potential neural mechanisms through integrating neuroimaging with treatment outcome research (Morgenstern, Naqvi, Debellis, & Breiter, 2013; Potenza, Sofuoglu, Carroll, & Rounsaville, 2011; Witkiewitz, Lustyk, & Bowen, 2013). This translational approach attempts to identify changes associated with treatment and abstinence and is beginning to yield some preliminary glimpses at what might prove to be the neurobiology of successful abstinence (Garavan, Brennan, Hester, & Whelan, 2013). As an example, we conducted pre- and post-treatment functional magnetic resonance imaging (fMRI) using the Stroop task for individuals participating in our initial trial of CBT4CBT. Although based on a small sample, there was some evidence of changes in Stroop-related blood oxygen level-dependent (BOLD) signal in regions including the anterior cingulate, inferior frontal gyrus, and midbrain at post-treatment relative to pre-treatment. While preliminary, these data suggest potential changes in indices of cognitive control and impulsivity that may be associated with changes related to treatment (DeVito et al., 2012).

Standardization via computerized delivery of treatment may also prove useful in evaluating the effectiveness of specific components of interventions. For example, rather than evaluating web-based therapies like CBT4CBT as a "package," where it is difficult to evaluate the efficacy, or lack thereof, of specific components, computerized delivery of treatment may facilitate evaluation of specific components. That is, does training in skills for coping with craving actually reduce craving? Does training in problem solving improve problem-solving skills? By understanding the contribution of each component to the whole of a complex array of interventions like CBT, we may be better able to identify individuals who respond differentially to specific components of treatment, eventually delivering only those components from which a given individual is most likely to achieve benefit and hence delivering more potent and efficient treatments.

Similarly, we may eventually be able to build effective interventions from the "neuroscience up," that is, developing specific tasks or modules to most efficiently target an individual's own patterns of strengths and weaknesses. Examples might include Bickel's approach to addressing delayed discounting in substance users by offering computerized cognitive training focusing on working memory (Bickel, Yi, Landes, Hill, & Baxter, 2011) or the approaches used by Wiers and others by offering training to reduce attentional bias to drug cues (Marissen et al., 2006; Schoenmakers, Wiers, Jones, Bruce, & Jansen, 2007; Waters & Feyerabend, 2000; Wiers, Eberl, Rinck, Becker, & Lindenmeyer, 2011). Another example from our Yale group is Kober's expansion of a task developed to evaluate the neural correlates of craving, the regulation of craving (ROC) task (Kober, Kross, Mischel, Hart, & Ochsner, 2010a; Kober, Mende-Siedlecki et al., 2010). While these translational approaches are yielding exciting findings regarding the potential of highly focused single modules to address important aspects of addiction, the complexity of addiction suggests that none of these approaches will be sufficient treatment for the majority of individuals with substance use disorders. Rather, carefully constructed combinations of such approaches, possibly in combination with new pharmacotherapies, may eventually become tailored, technology-based approaches in the near future.

Conclusion

Evaluation of CBT4CBT, as well as numerous other computerized therapies, is still in early stages, but this line of research is quite promising for making a form of empirically validated therapies more broadly available to individuals who might benefit from it. The vast evidence demonstrating the effectiveness of CBT for substance use disorders in clinical trials over the past several decades has not fully translated to broad implementation in clinical practice. The majority of community substance abuse treatment settings do not have sufficient resources to provide the level of clinician training and supervision required to ensure adequate delivery of CBT. Thus, computerized delivery of CBT offers the potential to overcome many of the challenges to successful implementation of this empirically validated treatment. Furthermore, this mode of treatment may free up clinician time to address other patient needs (without impacting the therapeutic alliance), may assist with the linkage of addiction treatment in primary care settings, and may extend the reach of aftercare treatment to better fit the needs of a chronic, relapsing condition such as substance abuse. These, as well as the other many benefits of computer-assisted therapies such as CBT4CBT highlighted in this chapter, suggest great promise for the future of addiction treatment. Even so, there is still far to go before these promises can be realized. More rigorous trials are needed to evaluate the efficacy of these therapies in broader populations with clinician-delivered versions as comparison conditions and with greater emphasis on understanding how the treatment works (i.e., mechanisms), as well as for whom it does or does not work. The hope is that this line of research (in accordance with the work of behavioral and pharmacotherapies) will ultimately lead to a more personalized approach to addiction treatment, one in which computer-assisted therapies, such as CBT4CBT, may play a vital role.

Acknowledgments

We gratefully acknowledge the support of NIDA (P50 DA09241, U10 DA015831, R37/01 DA15969, R01 DA030369) and NIAAA (R01 AA024122, R21 AA021405) for this work.

References

Altman, D. G., Schulz, K. F., Moher, D., Egger, M., Davidoff, F., Elbourne, D., . . . Lang, T. (2001). The revised CONSORT statement for reporting randomized trials: Explanation and elaboration. *Annals of Internal Medicine, 134*, 663–94.

Anthony, J. C., Warner, L. A., & Kessler, R. C. (1994). Comparative epidemiology of dependence on tobacco, alcohol, controlled substances and inhalants. Basic findings from the National Comorbidity Study. *Experimental and Clinical Psychopharmacology, 2*, 244–68.

Anton, R. F., Moak, D. H., Waid, L. R., Latham, P. K., Malcolm, R. J., & Dias, J. K. (1999). Naltrexone and cognitive-behavioral therapy for the treatment of outpatient alcoholics: Results of a placebo-controlled trial. *American Journal of Psychiatry, 156*, 1758–64.

Anton, R. F., O'Malley, S. S., Ciraulo, D. A., Cisler, R. A., Couper, D., Donovan, D. M., . . . Zweben, A. (2006). Combined pharmacotherapies and behavioral interventions for alcohol dependence: The COMBINE study: A randomized controlled trial. *Journal of the American Medical Association, 295*, 2003–17.

Babor, T. F., McKee, B. G., Kassenbaum, P. A., Grimaldi, P. L., Ahmed, K., & Bray, J. (2007). Screening, Brief Intervention, and Referral to Treatment (SBIRT): Toward a public health approach to the management of substance abuse. *Substance Abuse, 28*, 7–30.

Ball, S., Bachrach, K., DeCarlo, J., Farentinos, C., Keen, M., McSherry, T., . . . Carroll, K. (2002). Characteristics, beliefs, and practices of community clinicians trained to provide manual-guided therapy for substance abusers. *Journal of Substance Abuse Treatment, 23*, 309–18.

Bamatter, W., Carroll, K. M., Anez, L. M., Paris, M., Jr., Ball, S. A., Nich, C., . . . Martino, S. (2010). Informal discussions in substance abuse treatment sessions with Spanish-speaking clients. *Journal of Substance Abuse Treatment, 39*, 353–63.

Beidnas, R. S., & Kendall, P. C. (2010). Training therapists in evidence-based practice: A critical review of studies from a systems-contextual perspective. *Clinical Psychology: Science and Practice, 17*, 1–30.

Bickel, W. K., Christensen, D. R., & Marsch, L. A. (2011). A review of computer-based interventions used in the assessment, treatment, and research of drug addiction. *Substance Use & Misuse, 46*, 4–9.

Bickel, W. K., Marsch, L. A., Buchhalter, A. R., & Badger, G. J. (2008). Computerized behavior therapy for opioid-dependent outpatients: A randomized controlled trial. *Experimental and Clinical Psychopharmacology, 16*, 132–43.

Bickel, W. K., Yi, R., Landes, R., Hill, P. F., & Baxter, C. (2011b). Remembering the future: Working memory training decreases delay discounting among stimulant addicts. *Biological Psychiatry, 69*, 260–5.

Bogenschutz, M. P., Donovan, D. M., Mandler, R. N., Perl, H. I., Forcehimes, A. A., Crandall, C., . . . Douaihy, A. (2014). Brief intervention for patients with problematic drug use presenting in emergency departments: A randomized clinical trial. *JAMA Internal Medicine, 174*(11), 1736–45. doi:10.1001/jamainternmed.2014.4052.

Burns, D. D., & Nolen-Hoeksema, S. (1991). Coping styles, homework compliance, and the effectiveness of cognitive-behavioral therapy. *Journal of Consulting and Clinical Psychology, 59*, 305–11.

Burns, D. D., & Spangler, D. L. (2000). Does psychotherapy homework lead to improvements in depression in cognitive-behavioral therapy or does improvement lead to increased homework compliance? *Journal of Consulting and Clinical Psychology, 68*, 46–56.

Campbell, A. N., Nunes, E. V., Matthews, A. G., Stitzer, M., Miele, G. M., Polsky, D., . . . Ghitza, U. E. (2014). Internet-delivered treatment for substance abuse: A multisite randomized controlled trial. *The American Journal of Psychiatry, 171*, 683–90.

Carroll, K. M. (1997). Manual guided psychosocial treatment: A new virtual requirement for pharmacotherapy trials? *Archives of General Psychiatry, 54*, 923–8.

Carroll, K. M. (1998). *A cognitive-behavioral approach: Treating cocaine addiction*. Rockville, MD: NIDA.

Carroll, K. M., Ball, S. A., & Martino, S. (2004a). Cognitive, behavioral, and motivational therapies. In M. Galanter & H. D. Kleber (Eds.), *The American psychiatric publishing textbook of substance abuse treatment* (pp. 365–376). Washington, DC: American Psychiatric Publishing.

Carroll, K. M., Ball, S. A., Martino, S., Nich, C., Babuscio, T., Gordon, M. A., . . . Rounsaville, B. J. (2008a). Computer-assisted cognitive-behavioral therapy for addiction: A randomized clinical trial of 'CBT4CBT'. *American Journal of Psychiatry, 165*, 881–88.

Carroll, K. M., Ball, S. A., Martino, S., Nich, C., Babuscio, T. A., Nuro, K. F., . . . Rounsaville, B. J. (2008b). Computer-assisted delivery of cognitive-behavioral therapy for addiction: A randomized trial of CBT4CBT. *The American Journal of Psychiatry, 165*, 881–8.

Carroll, K. M., Ball, S. A., Martino, S., Nich, C., Babuscio, T. A., & Rounsaville, B. J. (2009a). Enduring effects of a computer-assisted training program for cognitive-behavioral therapy: A six-month follow-up of CBT4CBT. *Drug and Alcohol Dependence, 100*, 178–81 PMCID: PMC274(2309).

Carroll, K. M., Ball, S. A., Martino, S., Nich, C., Babuscio, T. A., & Rounsaville, B. J. (2009b). Enduring effects of a computer-assisted training program for cognitive behavioral therapy: A 6-month follow-up of CBT4CBT. *Drug and Alcohol Dependence, 100*, 178–81.

Carroll, K. M., Nich, C., DeVito, E. E., Shi, J. M., & Sofuoglu, M. (2017). Galantamine and computerized cognitive behavioral therapy for cocaine dependence: A randomized clinical trial. *Journal of Clinical Psychiatry, 79*(1). doi: 10.4088/JCP.17m11669.

Carroll, K. M., & Kiluk, B. D. (2017). Cognitive behavioral interventions for alcohol and drug use disorders: Through the stage model and back again. *Psychology of Addictive Behaviors, 31*, 847–61.

Carroll, K. M., Kiluk, B. D., Nich, C., Gordon, M. A., Portnoy, G. A., Marino, D. R., & Ball, S. A. (2014). Computer-assisted delivery of cognitive-behavioral therapy: Efficacy and durability of CBT4CBT among cocaine-dependent individuals maintained on methadone. *The American Journal of Psychiatry, 171*, 436–44.

Carroll, K. M., Kosten, T. R., & Rounsaville, B. J. (2004b). Choosing a behavioral therapy platform for pharmacotherapy of substance users. *Drug and Alcohol Dependence, 75*, 123–34.

Carroll, K. M., Nich, C., & Ball, S. A. (2005). Practice makes progress? Homework assignments and outcome in treatment of cocaine dependence. *Journal of Consulting and Clinical Psychology, 73*, 749–55.

Carroll, K. M., Nich, C., Ball, S. A., McCance-Katz, E. F., Frankforter, T. F., & Rounsaville, B. J. (2000). One year follow-up of disulfiram and psychotherapy for cocaine-alcohol abusers: Sustained effects of treatment. *Addiction, 95*, 1335–49.

Carroll, K. M., Nich, C., & Rounsaville, B. J. (1998). Use of observer and therapist ratings to monitor delivery of coping skills treatment for cocaine abusers: Utility of therapist session checklists. *Psychotherapy Research, 8*, 307–20.

Carroll, K. M., & Onken, L. S. (2005). Behavioral therapies for drug abuse. *The American Journal of Psychiatry, 162*, 1452–60.

Carroll, K. M., & Rounsaville, B. J. (2007). A vision of the next generation of behavioral therapies research in the addictions. *Addiction, 102*, 850–62; discussion 863–859.

Carroll, K. M., & Rounsaville, B. J. (2010). Computer-assisted therapy in psychiatry: Be brave-it's a new world. *Current Psychiatry Reports, 12*, 426–32.

Carroll, K. M., Rounsaville, B. J., Nich, C., Gordon, L. T., Wirtz, P. W., & Gawin, F. H. (1994). One-year follow-up of psychotherapy and pharmacotherapy for cocaine dependence: Delayed emergence of psychotherapy effects. *Archives of General Psychiatry, 51*, 989–97.

Collins, S. E., Kirouac, M., Lewis, M. A., Witkiewitz, K., & Carey, K. B. (2014). Randomized controlled trial of web-based decisional balance feedback and personalized normative feedback for college drinkers. *Journal of Studies on Alcohol and Drugs, 75*, 982–92.

Copeland, J., & Martin, G. (2004). Web-based interventions for substance use disorders: A qualitative review. *Journal of Substance Abuse Treatment, 26*, 109–16.

Crits-Christoph, P., Siqueland, L., Blaine, J., Frank, A., Luborsky, L., Onken, L. S., . . . Beck, A. T. (1999). Psychosocial treatments for cocaine dependence: National Institute on Drug Abuse Collaborative Cocaine Treatment Study. *Archives of General Psychiatry, 56*, 493–502.

Cuijpers, P., Marks, I. M., Van Straten, A., Cavanagh, K., Gega, L., & Andersson, G. (2009). Computer-aided psychotherapy for anxiety disorders: A meta-analytic review. *Cognitive Behavioural Therapy, 38*, 66–82.

Decker, S. E., Kiluk, B. D., Frankforter, T., Babuscio, T., Nich, C., & Carroll, K. M. (2016). Just showing up is not enough: Homework adherence and outcome in cognitive-behavioral therapy for cocaine dependence. *Journal of Consulting and Clinical Psychology, 84*, 907–12.

DeVito, E. E., Worhunsky, P. D., Carroll, K. M., Rounsaville, B. J., Kober, H., & Potenza, M. N. (2012). A preliminary study of the neural effects of behavioral therapy for substance use disorders. *Drug and Alcohol Dependence, 122*, 228–35.

Dutra, L., Stathopoulou, G., Basden, S. L., Leyro, T. M., Powers, M. B., & Otto, M. W. (2008). A meta-analytic review of psychosocial interventions for substance use disorders. *American Journal of Psychiatry, 165*, 179–87.

Garavan, H., Brennan, K., Hester, R., & Whelan, R. (2013). The neurobiology of successful abstinence. *Current Opinion in Neurobiology, 23*(4), 668–674. doi: 10.1016/j.conb.2013.01.029.

Gibbons, M. C., Wilson, R. F., Samal, L., Lehmann, C. U., Dickersin, K., Aboumatar, H., . . . Bass, E. B. (2009). Impact of consumer health informatics applications. *Evidence Report Technology Assessment, 188*, 1–546.

Gonzalez, V. M., Schmitz, J. M., & DeLaune, K. A. (2006). The role of homework in cognitive-behavioral therapy for cocaine dependence. *Journal of Consulting and Clinical Psychology, 74*, 633–7.

Hedman, E., Ljotsson, B., & Lindefors, N. (2012). Cognitive behavior therapy via the Internet: A systematic review of applications, clinical efficacy and cost-effectiveness. *Expert Review of Pharmacoeconomics & Outcomes Research, 12*, 745–64.

Hester, R. K., Delaney, H. D., & Campbell, W. (2011). ModerateDrinking.Com and moderation management: Outcomes of a randomized clinical trial with non-dependent problem drinkers. *Journal of Consulting and Clinical Psychology, 79*, 215–24.

Higgins, J. P. T., & Green, S. (2006). *Cochrane handbook for systematic reviews of interventions 4.2.6. The Cochrane Library, 4*. Chichester, UK: Wiley.

Hoffman, K. A., & McCarty, D. (2013). Improving the quality of addiction treatment. In P. M. Miller (Ed.), Interventions for addiction: Comprehensive addictive behaviors and disorders (pp. 579–88). San Diego: Academic Press.

Hollon, S. D. (2003). Does cognitive therapy have an enduring effect? *Cognitive Therapy and Research, 27*, 71–5.

Humphreys, K., & McLellan, A. T. (2011). A policy-oriented review of strategies for improving the outcomes of services for substance use disorder patients. *Addiction, 106*, 2058–66.

Institute of Medicine. (2001). *Crossing the quality chasm: A new mental health system for the 21st century*. Washington, DC: National Academy Press.

Kaltenthaler, E., Parry, G., & Beverley, C. (2004). Computerized cognitive behaviour therapy: A systematic review. *Behavioural and Cognitive Psychotherapy, 32*, 31–55.

Kaltenthaler, E., Parry, G., Beverley, C., & Ferriter, M. (2008). Computerized cognitive-behavioural therapy for depression: Systematic review. *The British Journal of Psychiatry, 193*, 181–4.

Kiluk, B. D., Devore, K. A., Buck, M. B., Nich, C., Frankforter, T. L., LaPaglia, D. M., . . . Carroll, K. M. (2016). Randomized trial of computerized cognitive behavioral therapy for alcohol use disorders: Efficacy as a virtual stand-alone and treatment add-on compared with standard outpatient treatment. *Alcoholism, Clinical and Experimental Research, 40*, 1991–2000.

Kiluk, B. D., Nich, C., Babuscio, T., & Carroll, K. M. (2010). Quality versus quantity: Acquisition of coping skills following computerized cognitive-behavioral therapy for substance use disorders. *Addiction, 105*, 2120–7.

Kiluk, B. D., Serafini, K., Frankforter, T., Nich, C., & Carroll, K. M. (2014). Only connect: The working alliance in computer-based cognitive behavioral therapy. *Behaviour Research & Therapy, 63*, 139–46.

Kiluk, B. D., Sugarman, D. E., Nich, C., Gibbons, C. J., Martino, S., Rounsaville, B. J., & Carroll, K. M. (2011). A methodological analysis of randomized clinical trials of computer-assisted therapies for psychiatric disorders: Toward improved standards for an emerging field. *The American Journal of Psychiatry, 168*, 790–9.

Knudsen, H. K., Ducharme, L. J., & Roman, P. M. (2008). Clinical supervision, emotional exhaustion, and turnover intention: A study of substance abuse treatment counselors in the Clinical Trials Network of the National Institute on Drug Abuse. *Journal of Substance Abuse Treatment, 35*, 387–95.

Kober, H., Kross, E. F., Mischel, W., Hart, C. L., & Ochsner, K. N. (2010). Regulation of craving by cognitive strategies in cigarette smokers. *Drug and Alcohol Dependence, 106*, 52–5.

Kober, H., Mende-Siedlecki, P., Kross, E. F., Weber, J., Mischel, W., Hart, C. L., & Ochsner, K. N. (2010). Prefrontal-striatal pathway underlies cognitive regulation of craving. *Proceedings of the National Academy of Sciences of the United States of America, 107*, 14811–6.

Lawrence, D., Mitrou, F., & Zubrick, S. R. (2009). Smoking and mental illness: Results from population surveys in Australia and the United States. *BMC Public Health*, 9, 285.

Longabaugh, R. (2010). Commentary on Kiluk et al. (2010): The emperor has some new clothes—coping is a mediator of cognitive-behavioral therapy's effectiveness. *Addiction, 105*, 2128–9.

Magill, M., & Ray, L. A. (2009). Cognitive-behavioral treatment with adult alcohol and illicit drug users: A meta-analysis of randomized controlled trials. *Journal of Studies on Alcohol and Drugs, 70*, 516–27.

Marissen, M. A., Franken, I. H., Waters, A. J., Blanken, P., van den Brink, W., & Hendriks, V. M. (2006). Attentional bias predicts heroin relapse following treatment. *Addiction, 101*, 1306–12.

Marks, I. M., & Cavanagh, K. (2009). Computer-aided psychological treatments: Evolving issues. *Annual Review of Clinical Psychology, 5*.

Marks, I. M., Cavanagh, K., & Gega, L. (2007). *Hands on help: Computer-aided psychotherapy*. Hove, UK: Psychology Press.

Marsch, L. A., Guarino, H., Acosta, M., Aponte-Melendez, Y., Cleland, C., Grabinski, M., . . . Edwards, J. (2014). Web-based behavioral treatment for substance use disorders as a partial replacement of standard methadone maintenance treatment. *Journal of Substance Abuse Treatment, 46*, 43–51.

Martino, S., Ball, S., Nich, C., Frankforter, T. L., & Carroll, K. M. (2009a). Correspondence of motivational enhancement treatment integrity ratings among therapists, supervisors, and observers. *Psychotherapy Research, 19*, 181–93.

Martino, S., Ball, S. A., Nich, C., Frankforter, T. L., & Carroll, K. M. (2009b). Informal discussions in substance abuse treatment sessions. *Journal of Substance Abuse Treatment, 36*, 366–75.

McCrone, P., Knapp, M., Proudfoot, J., Ryden, C., Cavanagh, K., Shapiro, D. A., . . . Tylee, A. (2004). Cost-effectiveness of computerized cognitive-behavioral therapy for anxiety and depression in primary care: Randomized controlled trial. *British Journal of Psychiatry, 185*, 55–62.

McLellan, A. T., & Meyers, K. (2004). Contemporary addiction treatment: A review of systems problems for adults and adolescents. *Biological Psychiatry, 56*, 764–70.

McLellan, A. T., & Woodworth, A. M. (2014). The affordable care act and treatment for "substance use disorders:" implications of ending segregated behavioral healthcare. *Journal of Substance Abuse Treatment, 46*, 541–5.

Miller, W. R., & Mount, K. A. (2001). A small study of training in motivational interviewing: Does one workshop change clinician and client behavior? *Behavioural and Cognitive Psychotherapy, 29*, 457–71.

Miller, W. R., & Moyers, T. B. (2015). The forest and the trees: Relational and specific factors in addiction treatment. *Addiction, 110*(3), 401–413. doi:10.1111/add.12693.

Miller, W. R., Yahne, C. E., Moyers, T. B., Martinez, J., & Pirritano, M. (2004). A randomized trial of methods to help clinicians learn motivation interviewing. *Journal of Consulting and Clinical Psychology, 72*, 1050–62.

Morgenstern, J., & Longabaugh, R. (2000). Cognitive-behavioral treatment for alcohol dependence: A review of the evidence for its hypothesized mechanisms of action. *Addiction, 95*, 1475–90.

Morgenstern, J., Morgan, T. J., McCrady, B. S., Keller, D. S., & Carroll, K. M. (2001). Manual-guided cognitive behavioral therapy training: A promising method for disseminating empirically supported substance abuse treatments to the practice community. *Psychology of Addictive Behaviors, 15*, 83–88.

Morgenstern, J., Naqvi, N. H., Debellis, R., & Breiter, H. C. (2013). The contributions of cognitive neuroscience and neuroimaging to understanding mechanisms of behavior change in addiction. *Psychology of Addictive Behaviors, 27*, 336–50.

Morie, K. P., Nich, C., Hunkele, K., Potenza, M. N., & Carroll, K. M. (2015). Alexithymia level and response to computer-based training in cognitive behavioral therapy among cocaine-dependent methadone-maintained individuals. *Drug and Alcohol Dependence, 152*, 157–63.

MTP Research Group. (2004). Brief treatments for cannabis dependence: Findings from a randomized multisite trial. *Journal of Consulting and Clinical Psychology, 72*, 455–66.

Neimeyer, R. A., Kazantzis, N., Kassler, D. M., Baker, K. D., & Fletcher, R. (2008). Group cognitive behavioural therapy for depression outcomes predicted by willingness to engage in homework, compliance with homework, and cognitive restructuring skill acquisition. *Cognitive and Behaviour Therapy, 37*, 199–215.

O'Malley, S. S., Jaffe, A. J., Chang, G., Schottenfeld, R., Meyer, R. E., & Rounsaville, B. J. (1992). Naltrexone and coping skills therapy for alcohol dependence: A controlled study. *Archives of General Psychiatry, 49*, 881–7.

Olmstead, T., Carroll, K. M., Canning-Ball, M., & Martino, S. (2011). Cost and cost-effectiveness of three strategies for training clinicians in motivational interviewing. *Drug and Alcohol Dependence, 116*, 195–202.

Olmstead, T. A., Abraham, A. J., Martino, S., & Roman, P. M. (2012). Counselor training in several evidence-based psychosocial addiction treatments in private US substance abuse treatment centers. *Drug and Alcohol Dependence, 120*, 149–54.

Olmstead, T. A., Ostrow, C. D., & Carroll, K. M. (2010). Cost-effectiveness of computer-assisted training in cognitive-behavioral therapy as an adjunct to standard care for addiction. *Drug and Alcohol Dependence, 110*, 200–7.

Olmstead, T. A., Sindelar, J. L., & Petry, N. M. (2007). Cost-effectiveness of prize-based incentives for stimulant abusers in outpatient psychosocial treatment programs. *Drug and Alcohol Dependence, 87*, 175–82.

Palfai, T. P., Winter, M., Lu, J., Rosenbloom, D., & Saitz, R. (2014). Personalized feedback as a universal prevention approach for college drinking: A randomized trial of an e-mail linked universal web-based alcohol intervention. *The Journal of Primary Prevention, 35*, 75–84.

Portnoy, D. B., Scott-Sheldon, L. A. J., Johnson, B. T., & Carey, M. P. (2008). Computer-delivered interventions for health promotion and behavioral risk reduction: A meta-analysis of75 randomized controlled trials, 1988–(2007). *Preventive Medicine, 47*, 3–16.

Postel, M. G., de Haan, H. A., & DeJong, C. A. J. (2008). E-therapy for mental health problems: A systematic review. *Telemedicine and E-Health, 14*, 707–14.

Postel, M. G., de Jong, C. A., & de Haan, H. A. (2005). Does e-therapy for problem drinking reach hidden populations? *American Journal of Psychiatry, 162*(12), 2393. doi:10.1176/appi.ajp.162.12.2393.

Potenza, M. N., Sofuoglu, M., Carroll, K. M., & Rounsaville, B. J. (2011). Neuroscience of behavioral and pharmacological treatments for addictions. *Neuron, 69*, 695–712.

Project MATCH Research Group. (1997). Matching Alcohol Treatments to Client Heterogeneity: Project MATCH posttreatment drinking outcomes. *Journal of Studies on Alcohol, 58*, 7–29.

Saitz, R., Palfai, T. P., Cheng, D. M., Alford, D. P., Bernstein, J. A., Lloyd-Travaglini, C. A., . . . Samet, J. H. (2014). Screening and brief intervention for drug use in primary care: The ASPIRE randomized clinical trial. *Journal of the American Medical Association, 312*, 502–13.

Saitz, R., Svikis, D., D'Onofrio, G., Kraemer, K. L., & Perl, H. (2006). Challenges applying alcohol brief intervention in diverse practice settings: Populations, outcomes, and costs. *Alcoholism, Clinical and Experimental Research, 30*, 332–8.

Santa Ana, E. J., Martino, S., Ball, S. A., Nich, C., Frankforter, T. L., & Carroll, K. M. (2008). What is usual about "treatment-as-usual"? Data from two multisite effectiveness trials. *Journal of Substance Abuse Treatment, 35*, 369–79.

Schoenmakers, T., Wiers, R. W., Jones, B. T., Bruce, G., & Jansen, A. T. (2007). Attentional re-training decreases attentional bias in heavy drinkers without generalization. *Addiction, 102*, 399–405.

Schoenwald, S. K., Sheidow, A. J., & Chapman, J. E. (2009). Clinical supervision in treatment transport: Effects on adherence and outcomes. *Journal of Consulting and Clinical Psychology, 77*, 410–21.

Sholomskas, D. E., Syracuse-Siewert, G., Rounsaville, B. J., Ball, S. A., Nuro, K. F., Carroll, & K. M. (2005). We don't train in vain: A dissemination trial of three strategies of training clinicians in cognitive-behavioral therapy. *Journal of Consulting and Clinical Psychology, 73*, 106–15.

Stewart, M. T., Horgan, C. M., Garnick, D. W., Ritter, G., & McLellan, A. T. (2013). Performance contracting and quality improvement in outpatient treatment: Effects on waiting time and length of stay. *Journal of Substance Abuse Treatment, 44*, 27–33.

Sugarman, D. E., Nich, C., & Carroll, K. M. (2010). Coping strategy use following computerized cognitive-behavioral therapy for substance use disorders. *Psychology of Addictive Behaviors, 24*, 689–95.

Tai, B., Straus, M. M., Liu, D., Sparenborg, S., Jackson, R., & McCarty, D. (2010). The first decade of the National Drug Abuse Treatment Clinical Trials Network: Bridging the gap between research and practice to improve drug abuse treatment. *Journal of Substance Abuse Treatment, 38*(Suppl 1), S4–13.

Taylor, G. J., Parker, J. D., & Babgby, R. M. (1990). A preliminary investigation of alexithymia in men with psychoactive substance dependence. *American Journal of Psychiatry, 147*, 1228–30.

Titov, N. (2007). Status of computerized cognitive behavioural therapy for adults. *The Australian and New Zealand Journal of Psychiatry, 41*, 95–114.

Tolin, D. F. (2010). Is cognitive-behavioral therapy more effective than other therapies? A meta-analytic review. *Clinical Psychology Review, 30*, 710–20.

Tumur, I., Kaltenthaler, E., Ferriter, M., Beverley, C., & Parry, G. (2007). Computerized cognitive behaviour therapy for obsessive-compulsive disorder: A systematic review. *Psychotherapy and Psychosomatics, 76*, 196–202.

Waters, A. J., & Feyerabend, C. (2000). Determinants and effects of attentional bias in smokers. *Psychology of Addictive Behaviors, 14*, 111–20.

Weissman, M. M., Verdeli, H., Gameroff, M. J., Bledsoe, S. E., Betts, K., Mufson, L., . . . Wickramaratne, P. (2006). National survey of psychotherapy training in psychiatry, psychology, and social work. *Archives of General Psychiatry, 63*, 925–34.

Wells, K., Klap, R., Koike, A., & Sherbourne, C. (2001). Ethnic disparities in unmet need for alcoholism, drug abuse, and mental health care. *American Journal of Psychiatry, 158*, 2027–32.

Wiers, R. W., Eberl, C., Rinck, M., Becker, E. S., & Lindenmeyer, J. (2011). Retraining automatic action tendencies changes alcoholic patients' approach bias for alcohol and improves treatment outcome. *Psychological Science, 22*, 490–7.

Witkiewitz, K., Desai, S. A., Bowen, S., Leigh, B. C., Kirouac, M., & Larimer, M. E. (2014). Development and evaluation of a mobile intervention for heavy drinking and smoking among college students. *Psychology of Addictive Behaviors, 28*, 639–50.

Witkiewitz, K., Lustyk, M. K., & Bowen, S. (2013). Retraining the addicted brain: A review of hypothesized neurobiological mechanisms of mindfulness-based relapse prevention. *Psychology of Addictive Behaviors, 27*, 351–65.

Yates, B. T. (1994). Toward the incorporation of costs, cost-effectiveness analysis, and cost-benefit analysis into clinical research. *Journal of Consulting and Clinical Psychology, 62*, 729–36.

CHAPTER

36 Smartphone Applications for Mindfulness Training in the Treatment of Substance Use Disorders

Kathleen A. Garrison, Stephanie O'Malley, Judson A. Brewer, *and* Marc N. Potenza

Abstract

There are presently more than 1,000 smartphone apps offering mindfulness or meditation in some form, marketed largely to improving one's health and well-being. At the same time, scientific credibility of most available mindfulness and meditation apps is considered low, and clinical testing of these apps is only in beginning stages. Nevertheless, initial work is under way and suggests that evidence-based mindfulness apps may have clinical benefits for mental health. This chapter reviews the state of the science of mindfulness apps, with a focus on the treatment of substance use disorders. Mindfulness training, in person, has been shown to be effective in the treatment of substance use disorders. Mobile technologies such as smartphone apps offer numerous advantages to delivering mindfulness training, conducting clinical studies, and potentially improving clinical outcomes in substance use treatment over in-person mindfulness training. This chapter outlines the advantages and some possible limitations of delivering mindfulness training via smartphone app, reviews available mindfulness apps for mental health, reviews scientific literature supporting these apps, and proposes areas of focus for further development of mindfulness apps. Findings indicate that mindfulness training is feasible to deliver by smartphone app and other mobile technologies, initial clinical testing of mindfulness apps for substance use treatment is promising, and larger randomized controlled trials are under way. Importantly, more mindfulness apps and trials are utilizing evidence-based clinical practice guidelines.

Keywords: mindfulness, meditation, smartphone app, application, mobile health, mobile technology, substance-use disorder, addiction, substance use treatment

Introduction

Mindfulness has been defined as "the awareness that emerges through paying attention on purpose, in the present moment, and nonjudgmentally to the unfolding of experience moment by moment" (Kabat-Zinn, 2003: p. 145). Mindfulness training has been adapted as a central component of some contemporary psychotherapies and has been shown to be effective in the treatment of psychiatric disorders including those relating to or involving pain, anxiety, and depression (Marchand, 2013), as well as in the treatment of substance use disorders and other (e.g., behavioral) addictions (Brewer, Elwafi, & Davis, 2013). However, in-person mindfulness training is challenged by limited access to treatment, potential financial burden, significant time demands, and variability in the experience and competence of therapists, among other limitations. Recent advances in mobile technologies offer potential solutions by enabling smartphone applications ("apps") for mindfulness training. After a brief overview of mindfulness training for the treatment of substance use disorders, this chapter outlines the major advantages, and some limitations, of mindfulness training (or substance abuse treatment more broadly) via smartphone app; reviews some of the available mindfulness training apps and studies of these and related apps; and proposes recommendations for further development of mindfulness apps for addictions treatment.

Mindfulness Training for the Treatment of Substance Use Disorders

Mindfulness has been operationalized as maintaining attention on immediate experience and maintaining an attitude of acceptance toward that experience (Bishop et al., 2004). As such, training in mindfulness is considered to alter one's relationship to aversive experiences such as suffering and craving (Black, 2014). Mindfulness training has been adapted in secular treatment programs such as *mindfulness-based stress reduction* (MBSR; Kabat-Zinn, 1982), *mindfulness-based cognitive therapy* (MBCT; Teasdale et al., 2000), and *mindfulness-based relapse prevention* (MBRP; Bowen et al., 2009). Studies suggest the efficacy of incorporating these mindfulness programs in the treatment of substance use disorders and behavioral addictions, including in relapse prevention (Chiesa & Serretti, 2014; Witkiewitz et al., 2014). In this context, mindfulness training may be used to modify addictive behaviors such as learned responses to substance-related cues and affective states. Individuals learn to pay attention to and work mindfully with cravings and affective states, rather than to react by pursuing addictive behaviors (Brewer et al., 2013).

Recent reviews have identified up to 42 distinct studies testing mindfulness interventions for substance use disorders and found that mindfulness interventions were associated with reduced consumption of substances of misuse including alcohol, cocaine, amphetamines, marijuana, cigarettes, and opiates, compared with several active and inactive controls (Chiesa & Serretti, 2014; Li et al., 2017). Several studies included in the reviews reported that mindfulness interventions were associated with reduced craving and stress and increased mindfulness, suggesting potential mechanisms contributing to outcomes. Several limitations of the studies were identified, notably small sample sizes, underreporting of methodological details, and lack of replication. A related review evaluated randomized clinical trials of meditation programs to improve stress-related outcomes, including only those trials with an active control, and found low to no effect of meditation, or insufficient evidence of an effect, on substance use, although only five trials measuring substance use (alcohol use or smoking) met the inclusion criteria (Goyal et al., 2014). Overall, these reviews highlight preliminary evidence supporting mindfulness as an intervention for the reduction of substance use and misuse and a critical need for larger randomized controlled trials (RCTs) of mindfulness-based addiction treatments.

Advantages of Smartphone Based Mindfulness Training

Dissemination

Mobile technologies are providing new and innovative ways to improve mindfulness training for the treatment of substance use disorders and behavioral addictions. A major advantage of "mobile mindfulness training" is improved dissemination or access to treatment, including for minority populations who are typically underserved and underrepresented in clinical trials (Burlew et al., 2011; Oh et al., 2015). In-person mindfulness training programs typically have limited resources and teachers, and individuals seeking treatment incur financial, scheduling, and time burdens of travel to treatment. However, most adults in the United States (77%; Pew Research Center, 2017) and the United Kingdom (72%; Pew Research Center, 2015) own a smartphone. Ownership rates are comparable among white, black, and Hispanic populations in the United States, and a growing number of individuals own smartphones who do not have Internet in their home (Pew Research Center, 2017). Furthermore, more than half of mobile phone users (58%) have downloaded a health-related mobile app (Krebs & Duncan, 2015). These demographics illustrate the accessibility of smartphone-based mindfulness training.

Standardization

As the demand for mindfulness training increases, there is concern about the appropriate training and competence of mindfulness teachers (Crane et al., 2012). It has been suggested that the quality of a mindfulness-based course is only as good as the instructor (Crane et al., 2012; Kabat-Zinn et al., 2014), and, in complementary medicine more generally, it is suggested that the practitioner should be recognized as a contributor to treatment (Mason, Tovey, & Long, 2002). Variability in the experience and competence of mindfulness program facilitators has been identified as a common quality issue in studies of mindfulness-based interventions (Shonin, Van Gordon, & Griffiths, 2013). Best practice guidelines are being developed for some mindfulness-based courses (e.g., Kabat-Zinn et al., 2014; UK Mindfulness-Based Teacher Trainer Network, 2011). In contrast, smartphone app-based mindfulness training is standardized. In the clinical research setting, standardization is critical in evaluating treatment outcomes. The lack of standardization of mindfulness training has been identified as a limitation of the current evidence on the impact of mindfulness, for example on cognitive functioning (Chiesa, Calati, & Serretti, 2011). One potential disadvantage of app-based mindfulness training is that it may lack the relational aspects of in-person training. Nevertheless, there is evidence that individuals learn well from computerized versions of behavioral training (Carroll et al., 2014).

Reduced Stigma

Offering treatment on mobile devices may help to reduce the stigma associated with mental healthcare, including treatment for substance use disorders and other addictions. Substance abuse recovery is affected by *perceived stigma*, such as beliefs about stigmatizing attitudes and actions in society; *enacted stigma*, such as social discrimination; and *self-stigma*, such as negative thoughts and feelings (Link et al., 2004). These forms of stigma can be barriers to treatment (Luoma et al., 2007). Stigmatization may be reduced by online or mobile health interventions, thus lowering barriers to seeking treatment (Morris & Aguilera, 2012). For example, individuals who might not otherwise seek treatment will consider an online intervention (Cunningham et al., 2009).

Adherence

Smartphone-based mindfulness training may improve adherence to treatment. Most meditation studies require home practice that is self-reported, and both participant adherence to home practice and an overreliance on self-report have been identified as common quality issues in studies of mindfulness-based interventions (Shonin et al., 2013). Adherence may be improved by tracking interactions with a mindfulness training app, including tracking timing and completion of meditation exercises, using guided meditations, meditation timers, and so on. A recent study (Wahbeh, Zwickey, & Oken, 2011) tested proof of concept for a tablet-based app, iMINDr, described as an objective adherence measurement system to help researchers more accurately track adherence to home practice of mindfulness meditation. In the study, 11 combat veterans with posttraumatic stress disorder (PTSD) were provided with a tablet and instructed to practice mindfulness using a 20-minute audio-guided meditation on the iMINDr app. Findings indicated that adherence information could be collected from the app and also demonstrated the utility of tracking adherence because subjects reported more meditation practice than was objectively tracked by iMINDr.

Adherence to home meditation practice components of mindfulness training may be critical to the treatment of substance use disorders. In a recent study of in-person mindfulness training for smoking cessation, greater home meditation practice significantly predicted lower smoking, and an informal home meditation exercise moderated a decrease in the association between craving and smoking at the end of treatment (Elwafi et al., 2013). Tracking adherence to mindfulness training might improve adherence to home practice and, thereby, outcomes and our understanding of the related psychological mechanisms contributing to outcomes.

Self-Management

Mobile health (as well as mindfulness training) can improve self-management of personal health and healthcare, including treatment. Self-management skills such as self-control, decision making, and self-reinforcement have been associated with lower substance use in a longitudinal study of adolescents (Lowe et al., 2013). Self-management is also emphasized in substance use relapse prevention (Carroll, Rounsaville, & Keller, 1991; Marlatt & Donovan, 2005). One way that mobile technologies support self-management is by enabling the tracking of real-time personal health information. Tracking health information has been identified as a key intervention strategy in mobile health (Klasnja & Pratt, 2012). A recent qualitative analysis of smartphone apps in supporting health behavior change found that young adults value the ability to monitor, track, and review health behavior and goals (Dennison et al., 2013). Another way that mobile technologies contribute to self-management is by providing on-hand access to health information. In the same qualitative study (Dennison et al., 2013), young adults reported that smartphones supported their adoption of healthy behaviors by increasing accessibility to health information and efficiency in obtaining it.

Health education can be achieved on mobile devices in the most basic way through Internet access and additionally through notifications and reminders related to health behaviors, with displays that regularly update personal health information, and by interaction with healthcare providers, support groups, or other resources, via text messaging, message boards, or direct calls, among other tools (Klasnja & Pratt, 2012).

Social Support

Mobile technology allows for peer-to-peer influence, facilitating social support from family, friends, and social networks, as well as peer modeling (Klasnja & Pratt, 2012). This is particularly relevant for mindfulness training as a major component of traditional mindfulness practice is *sangha*, or community. Peer support groups have been integrated into many in-person mindfulness-based programs, such as the group-based format of MBSR (Kabat-Zinn, 1982). Social networking is already an integral part of how we use our smartphones. For example, 75% of US smartphone owners reported using a social networking site on their phone at least once per week (Pew Research Center, 2014). The importance of social support in the treatment of substance use disorders and prevention of relapse is well-established (Havassy, Hall, & Wasserman, 1991), and active use of Internet-based social support has been associated with, for example, greater smoking cessation and continuous abstinence (Cobb et al., 2005). Increased access to social support via mobile devices and the inclusion of social support components in mobile interventions may benefit substance use outcomes, although this warrants direct testing.

Treatment in Context

Mobile mindfulness training gets treatment into the hands of the user, in context and potentially just in time. Smartphones are already an integral part of our daily routine; for example, 67% of mobile phone users check their device for messages, alerts, or calls without being prompted by an indicator, and 44% of mobile phone users sleep with their phone next to their bed to avoid missing calls, messages, or updates (Smith, 2012). This intensive daily use makes it possible to achieve enormous expansion in the points of care from the clinic to nearly any place and any time an individual needs support (Klasnja & Pratt, 2012). This may be especially useful in the treatment of substance use disorders and other addictions that are influenced by context-related cues and affective states. Smartphones can offer in-context access to the healthcare team, including remote coaching, remote symptom monitoring, automated feedback, and direct access by mobile phone, text message, and video calls (Klasnja & Pratt, 2012). Mobile devices can also provide "just-in-time" interventions. For example, the Alcohol Comprehensive Health Enhancement Support System (A-CHESS), a smartphone app to support recovery from alcohol use disorder (Gustafson et al., 2011), features a "panic button." That button can be used to initiate in-the-moment support, such as reminders of personal motivations for not drinking, specific tools in the app to help with urges, or to send an alert to self-identified key supporters such as counselors. The app also includes a global positioning system (GPS) patient locator to initiate "rescue" if the user approaches a high-risk location, such as triggering a call to a counselor if the user approaches a liquor store. A-CHESS has been found to be effective in reducing risky drinking days and increasing abstinence in a randomized clinical trial (Gustafson et al., 2014), and users appear to engage with these just-in-time features (Gustafson et al., 2014; McTavish et al., 2012). For mobile mindfulness training for substance use, an example of a just-in-time intervention is an in-the-moment mindfulness exercise to help cope with cravings or negative affective states (Brewer et al., 2013; Garrison et al., 2015).

Experience Sampling

Mobile devices enable *ecological momentary assessment* or *experience sampling*, the repeated sampling of an individual's behavior and experience in real time, in the real world. By sampling behavior and experience in real time, it is possible to minimize recall bias, maximize ecological validity, and document variation in behavior and experience over time (Shiffman, Stone, & Hufford, 2008). Experience sampling has become the gold standard method to assess real-world outcomes given its validity, and it has been applied successfully across disciplines. Furthermore, recent work suggests experience sampling by mobile device (e.g., text messaging) as compared with written assessments (e.g. diaries) leads to higher response rates and reduced latencies (Berkman, Giuliani, & Pruitt., 2014).

Related to mindfulness, a recent study used experience sampling by smartphone to provide evidence that individuals were less happy when their minds wandered regardless of the activity in which they were engaged in (Killingsworth & Gilbert, 2010). Experience sampling has also been used widely to study substance use, in particular smoking, and is considered to be well-suited for this research given the importance of momentary internal (e.g., cravings, affective states) and external (e.g., drug-related cues) experience to substance use disorders (Shiffman, 2009). One study of cigarette smokers sent text messages every 2 hours for 21 days of a quit attempt to assess smoking, mood, and craving and found that negative mood and craving predicted smoking, and craving mediated the mood–smoking relationship (Berkman et al., 2011). Multiple studies now support the feasibility and utility of experience sampling by mobile device to investigate substance use, craving, and affective states (Serre et al., 2015), including studies that pair experience sampling with other objective, mobile device–based measures of behavior and physiology such as biological sampling (e.g., breathalyzers), GPS tracking (e.g., to measure the influence of environmental characteristics), and wearable sensors (e.g., for physiological measures; see next section) (Bertz, Epstein, & Preston, 2017).

Wearables

Wearable technologies, devices that can be worn on the body and include sensors and an Internet connection, offer new ways to monitor and intervene in substance use and misuse and to track metrics related to mindfulness and potentially enhance mindfulness training. Wearable devices continue to be developed and currently include wristbands and smartwatches, headbands and head-mounted displays, glasses and contact lenses, smart fabrics and clothing, and other wearables that clip to the body or clothing or can be worn around the neck. Wearables can be used to monitor and detect instances of substance use. For example, SmokeBeat is an app that pairs with wristband sensors to detect the characteristic hand-to-mouth gestures associated with smoking a cigarette (Dar, 2017). Other wristband sensors have been developed to detect smoking (Parate et al., 2014), including StopWatch, a smoking detection app that runs entirely on a smartwatch (Skinner et al., 2017).

Automatic detection and alerting the user in real time may alone reduce substance use (Dar, 2017), and there is additionally great potential for wearables paired with just-in-time interventions (Naughton, 2017), including in predicting and attempting to prevent stress, craving, and drug use (Bertz et al., 2017). Wearables can be also used to monitor physiological data relevant to substance use (Leonard et al., 2017) and mindfulness (Steinhubl et al., 2015), such as skin conductance, respiratory rate, heart rate, blood pressure, and electroencephalography (EEG) measures of brain electrical activity as markers of stress, mood, affect, and, potentially, mindfulness. Few studies have tested wearables related to substance use or mindfulness, and multiple challenges to their utilization in these contexts exist, including the accuracy of measurements/detection, device functionality, data processing, and participant burden, including the conspicuousness of wearable devices (Bertz et al., 2017). It is also critical to develop and test specific biomarkers. For example, as of yet, there are no gold standard physiological measures from which to infer mindfulness or even stress (Hovsepian et al., 2015).

Retention

It is possible that mobile device–based treatments such as mobile mindfulness training may increase treatment retention as compared to in-person training largely due to treatment accessibility as well as ease of contacting patients, including contacting those who did not complete treatment, to obtain information about outcomes. For example, in a recent randomized controlled pilot trial of smartphone-based acceptance and commitment therapy for smoking cessation, retention to a 2-month follow-up survey was 84%, as compared with the 54% typically achieved in web-based trials (Bricker et al., 2014). However, more generally, many people download health apps and don't use them. For example, although about half of US adults in a recent survey had downloaded a health app, about half of those had also stopped using a health app, citing reasons such as high data entry burden, loss of interest, and hidden costs (Krebs & Duncan, 2015). A challenge moving forward with smartphone based-treatments for substance use and in mobile health more broadly will therefore be treatment retention.

Mobile Technology in Clinical Research

Multiple features of mobile devices are useful for clinical trials of substance abuse treatments, as mentioned earlier. Overall, it is now possible that all study procedures can be conducted using a mobile device, from recruitment, screening, informed consent, and randomization, to initial training and treatment itself, through to outcomes assessment, follow-up, and study compensation. Regarding recruitment, studies using mobile device–based interventions can recruit more broadly because treatment is not limited to participants local to a research center. Regarding outcomes assessment, biochemical verification of abstinence from substance use, such as alcohol or nicotine, can now be achieved by smartphone, either by using breath monitors that read directly into the mobile device or by using handheld breath monitors and either recording breath screening on video for upload or breath screening with a researcher on video chat in real time. These approaches have been used to monitor substance use in clinical trials to reduce smoking

(Dallery et al., 2017; Garrison et al., 2015) and alcohol use (Alessi & Petry, 2013).

Despite these advantages, several potential limitations of mobile device-based interventions in clinical research deserve consideration. On the user end, participants can turn off notifications or silence their phone. In addition, battery life, Internet access, and device functionality can be problematic. As discussed earlier, many people download health apps but never or rarely use them, thus posing a unique challenge for treatment retention and adherence. There are also important ethical considerations, including potential challenges in providing informed consent on a platform where users do not typically read software licensing agreements before agreeing, as well as participant privacy and anonymity issues (Miller, 2012).

On the research end, one limitation is that no clinical guidelines have yet been developed for smartphone-based treatments, and there is only a limited evidence basis to inform treatments and run clinical trials on this new platform. Even more generally, few currently available apps for mindfulness training or substance use treatment follow evidence-based guidelines. For example, a content analysis of smartphone apps for smoking cessation found low levels of adherence to the US Public Health Service's Clinical Practice Guidelines for Treating Tobacco Use and Dependence, such as providing a reference to quit lines and recommending quit-smoking medications (Abroms et al., 2013). Another potential limitation is that most smartphone apps are multi-featured, and thus it can be difficult to control for different features to determine the effective aspects of treatment. Additionally, expert programming skills are typically required to develop and maintain smartphone apps, and the resulting large and complex datasets can be challenging to manage and analyze (Miller, 2012).

Clinical Trials of Mindfulness Training Apps

New mindfulness training apps are being released daily, some directed at clinical populations, although most are not targeted to clinical populations and are therefore not evidence-based or tested in clinical trials. In an early review (Plaza et al., 2013), more than 1,000 meditation apps were available on the Android (Google, Inc.) platform alone, of which 203 were specific to mindfulness, whereas other apps were meditation timers, breathing exercises, meditation music, or more broadly related to health and well-being, and yet no clinical trials had been conducted to test the efficacy of any mindfulness app. More recently, only 23 mindfulness apps were identified on the Apple App Store (Apple, Inc.) when guided meditation apps, timers, and reminders were excluded, and very few of the mindfulness apps identified were rated highly on visual aesthetics, engagement, functionality, or information quality, and, again, no RCTs of mindfulness apps had been conducted (Mani et al., 2015).

Beginning work in testing mindfulness apps is now under way, mainly feasibility and other pilot studies, including testing mindfulness apps to reduce smoking (Bricker et al., 2017) and stress (Coulon, Monroe, & West, 2016; Gregoski et al., 2013) and to increase mindfulness (Garcia et al., 2017), among others. Only one pilot randomized clinical trial of a mindfulness-related intervention for substance use has been reported (Bricker et al., 2014). That trial tested SmartQuit, a smartphone app for smoking cessation using acceptance and commitment therapy (ACT), in which individuals learn to accept cravings, emotions, and thoughts and commit to value-guided behavior changes. SmartQuit includes motivational images and videos; a personalized quit plan; links to social networking and other social support; guidance for accessing available smoking cessation medications; audio, video, and text for teaching acceptance and self-compassion skills; and tools for self-monitoring of smoking habits. The trial tested the efficacy of 8 weeks use of SmartQuit compared with the National Cancer Institute's QuitGuide app to reduce smoking ($N = 196$). Findings suggest that ACT was feasible to deliver by smartphone, and quit rates were promising at 13% for the experimental app and 8% for the comparator.

Another relevant RCT tested the effectiveness of a smartphone app for mindfulness training to reduce symptoms of depression in individuals with major depressive disorder (Ly et al., 2014). Mindfulness training included web-based psychoeducation about the theoretical basis for mindfulness treatment of depression; a smartphone app-based mindfulness program with guided and unguided, short and long meditation exercises; email messages from therapists with encouraging or educational messages; and a weekly reflection email from patients to their therapists. The mindfulness app was compared to a web-based psychoeducation and smartphone app-based program for behavioral activation, an intervention that aims to teach patients about the relationship between mood and behavior and increase patient contact with potentially reinforcing experiences. Both apps were effective in reducing symptoms of depression, with only subgroup differences in outcomes; for example, the mindfulness app was more effective among individuals with lower initial depression severity. Findings lend additional support for the delivery of mindfulness training via smartphone.

These studies provide beginning evidence that smartphone-based mindfulness training may be feasible and effective for the treatment of psychiatric disorders including addictions. However, larger, well-controlled randomized clinical trials testing the efficacy of mindfulness training apps for the treatment of these disorders are needed. Several large-scale RCTs of smartphone app-based mindfulness interventions are currently under way. In the National Institutes of Health registry for clinical trials in the United States (https://clinicaltrials.gov; December 2017), a combined search for "smartphone" as the intervention/treatment and "mindfulness" or "meditation" as other terms revealed 35 studies, of which 8 include substance use as tested conditions, 7 testing smoking, and 1 testing food cravings. A similar search in the UK Clinical Trials Gateway (https://www.ukctg.nihr.ac.uk; December 2017) revealed 13 trials, primarily testing stress and mental health, but none testing substance use. Among the ongoing trials identified, several are testing Headspace (https://www.headspace.com), a smartphone app that teaches mindfulness through audio-guided meditations and supporting animations, including general meditation exercises; exercises targeted to specific activities such as sleeping, walking, eating, cooking, and running; and a short "SOS" meditation, as well as a meditation tracker and an option to link one's account with friends for social support. The ongoing trials test the effectiveness of 2–6 months of using the Headspace app to impact primary outcome measures of stress and well-being compared with a wait-list control, a matched relaxation app, or no control group. Although none tests substance use as a primary outcome, lapses in smoking cessation and overeating episodes are included as secondary outcomes in one trial utilizing Headspace in a 10-day supported quit attempt.

Also ongoing are several RCTs of Craving to Quit (www.cravingtoquit.com), a smartphone app for mindfulness training for smoking cessation developed by our research team. Craving to Quit was developed based on an in-person mindfulness training program found to be associated with increased smoking abstinence rates (Brewer et al., 2011). Craving to Quit teaches mindfulness for smoking cessation by helping users self-monitor their smoking habits, learn to recognize when and how often they smoke, identify triggers for smoking habits, and learn methods to become more mindful of cravings and ride them out. Mindfulness training is delivered using video, audio, and animations to reinforce key concepts, meditation exercises, and an online community for peer support. The app teaches three standard meditation practices: body scan, loving kindness, and breath awareness (Gunaratana, 2002), as well as an informal practice to work mindfully with cravings: Recognize, Accept, Investigate, and Note (RAIN) what cravings feel like as they arise and pass away. Experience sampling is used to query smokers' craving, smoking, mood, and mindfulness. One ongoing RCT tests the efficacy of Craving to Quit to increase smoking abstinence as compared with a control app that provides only experience sampling in order to disentangle the effects of mindfulness training from those of effective self-monitoring. A second, larger trial tests the efficacy of Craving to Quit to increase smoking abstinence as compared with another multifeatured quit-smoking app, the National Cancer Institute's QuitPal.

Other Informative Studies

Although there are only a very limited number of completed or ongoing clinical trials of mindfulness training smartphone apps, our understanding of the potential for mindfulness training apps to treat addictions can be informed by studies of other mobile device–based substance use interventions. Most current evidence in support of mobile device–based treatments for substance use is for text messaging, where the most promising findings are in RCTs of text messaging interventions for smoking cessation (Keoleian, Polcin, & Galloway, 2015; Watson, Simpson, & Hughes, 2016). For example, in an RCT of Text2Quit, a text-messaging program that provides automated, theoretically based, personalized, and interactive text messages to support smoking cessation, Text2Quit was found to increase smoking abstinence as compared with a control group receiving self-help material (Abroms et al., 2014).

In contrast, current findings suggest text messaging interventions may be insufficient to support recovery for alcohol use disorder (Quanbeck et al., 2014), and very few text messaging interventions for other substance use disorders have been tested (Keoleian et al., 2015). Moreover, typically in these trials, text messaging was combined with other treatment modalities such as counseling (Scott-Sheldon et al., 2016; Spohr et al., 2015). A recent review identified 12 RCTs of mobile health interventions (9 text messaging and 3 smartphone apps) to treat alcohol and substance use disorders (Kazemi et al., 2017), most providing evidence of reduced substance use. The smartphone app trials were focused on alcohol use (including A-CHESS, described earlier; Gustafson et al., 2014), an app for Location-Based Monitoring and Intervention for Alcohol Use Disorders (Gonzalez & Dulin, 2015), and an app delivering brief interventions targeting students' drinking choices on party occasions (Gajecki et al., 2014). In addition to methodological limitations such as small sample sizes and lack of adequate controls, some common limitations of clinical studies of smartphone apps identified by these studies include a lack of active participant engagement with the app and reduced app use over time, an inability to control for multiple app features, reliance on self-reported outcomes, and a lack of racial/ethnic diversity in the study sample.

Conclusion and Recommendations

Mobile technologies offer new and innovative ways to improve mindfulness training as a treatment for substance use disorders and other addictions, with potential treatment advantages in dissemination and accessibility, scalability, personalization or customization, adherence, retention, and relapse prevention, among others. Existing data suggest that mindfulness training may improve outcomes in the treatment of substance use disorders and that mindfulness training is feasible to deliver via smartphone app. Larger RCTs are under way testing mindfulness training apps in clinical settings including addiction treatment. Related studies using mobile technologies to deliver or support addiction treatment have shown considerable promise. However, there is a clear need for further development of mindfulness apps and for trials of these apps, particularly to follow evidence-based guidelines. As evidence-based guidelines specific to mobile health are being developed, mindfulness apps might well incorporate existing guidelines for substance abuse treatment and mindfulness training, as well as consider new findings reported from clinical trials in mobile health. Nevertheless, it is promising that these issues have been discussed in the literature and some new apps are being developed with these considerations.

References

Abroms, L. C., et al. (2013). A content analysis of popular smartphone apps for smoking cessation. *American Journal of Preventive Medicine*, *45*(6), 732–6. doi:10.1016/j.amepre.2013.07.008

Abroms, L. C., et al. (2014). A randomized trial of Text2Quit: A text messaging program for smoking cessation. *American Journal of Preventive Medicine*, *47*(3), 242–50. doi:10.1016/j.amepre.2014.04.010

Alessi, S. M., & Petry, N. M. (2013). A randomized study of cellphone technology to reinforce alcohol abstinence in the natural environment. *Addiction*, *108*(5), 900–9. doi:10.1111/add.12093

Berkman, E. T., Giuliani, N. R., & Pruitt, A. K. (2014). Comparison of text messaging and paper-and-pencil for ecological momentary assessment of food craving and intake. *Appetite*, *81*, 131–7. doi:10.1016/j.appet.2014.06.010

Berkman, E. T., et al. (2011). Using SMS text messaging to assess moderators of smoking reduction: Validating a new tool for ecological measurement of health behaviors. *Health Psychology*, *30*(2), 186–94. doi:10.1037/a0022201

Bertz, J. W., Epstein, D. H., & Preston, K. L. (2017). Combining ecological momentary assessment with objective, ambulatory measures of behavior and physiology in substance-use research. *Addictive Behaviors*. doi:10.1016/j.addbeh.2017.11.027

Bishop, S. R., Lau, M., Shapiro, S., Carlson, L., Anderson, N. D., Carmody, J.,... Devins, G. (2004). Mindfulness: A proposed operational definition. *Clinical Psychology-Science and Practice*, *11*(3), 230–41. doi:10.1093/Clipsy/Bph077

Black, D. S. (2014). Mindfulness-based interventions: An antidote to suffering in the context of substance use, misuse, and addiction. *Substance Use and Misuse*, *49*(5), 487–91. doi:10.3109/10826084.2014.860749

Bowen, S., et al. (2009). Mindfulness-based relapse prevention for substance use disorders: A pilot efficacy trial. *Substance Abuse*, *30*(4), 295–305. doi:10.1080/08897070903250084

Brewer, J. A., Elwafi, H. M., & Davis, J. H. (2013). Craving to quit: Psychological models and neurobiological mechanisms of mindfulness training as treatment for addictions. *Psychology of Addictive Behaviors*, *27*(2), 366–79. doi:10.1037/a0028490

Brewer, J. A., et al. (2011). Mindfulness training for smoking cessation: Results from a randomized controlled trial. *Drug and Alcohol Dependence*, *119*(1–2), 72–80. doi:10.1016/j.drugalcdep.2011.05.027

Bricker, J. B., et al. (2014). Randomized, controlled pilot trial of a smartphone app for smoking cessation using acceptance and commitment therapy. *Drug and Alcohol Dependence*, *143*, 87–94. doi:10.1016/j.drugalcdep.2014.07.006

Bricker, J. B., et al. (2017). Single-arm trial of the second version of an acceptance & commitment therapy smartphone application for smoking cessation. *Drug and Alcohol Dependence*, *170*, 37–42. doi:10.1016/j.drugalcdep.2016.10.029

Burlew, K., et al. (2011). Increasing ethnic minority participation in substance abuse clinical trials: Lessons learned in the National Institute on Drug Abuse's clinical trials network. *Cultural Diversity and Ethnic Minority Psychology*, *17*(4), 345–56. doi:10.1037/a0025668

Carroll, K. M., Rounsaville, B. J., & Keller, D. S. (1991). Relapse prevention strategies for the treatment of cocaine abuse. *American Journal of Drug and Alcohol Abuse*, *17*(3), 249–65.

Carroll, K. M., et al. (2014). Computer-assisted delivery of cognitive-behavioral therapy: Efficacy and durability of CBT4CBT among cocaine-dependent individuals maintained on methadone. *American Journal of Psychiatry, 171*(4), 436–44. doi:10.1176/appi.ajp.2013.13070987

Chiesa, A., Calati, R., & Serretti, A. (2011). Does mindfulness training improve cognitive abilities? A systematic review of neuropsychological findings. *Clinical Psychology Review, 31*(3), 449–64. doi:10.1016/j.cpr.2010.11.003

Chiesa, A., & Serretti, A. (2014). Are mindfulness-based interventions effective for substance use disorders? A systematic review of the evidence. *Substance Use and Misuse, 49*(5), 492–512. doi:10.3109/10826084.2013.770027

Cobb, N. K., et al. (2005). Initial evaluation of a real-world internet smoking cessation system. *Nicotine and Tobacco Research, 7*(2), 207–16. doi:10.1080/14622200500055319

Coulon, S. M., Monroe, C. M., & West, D. S. (2016). A systematic, multi-domain review of mobile smartphone apps for evidence-based stress management. *American Journal of Preventive Medicine, 51*(1), 95–105. doi:10.1016/j.amepre.2016.01.026

Crane, R. S., et al. (2012). Competence in teaching mindfulness-based courses: Concepts, development and assessment. *Mindfulness, 3*(1), 76–84. doi:10.1007/s12671-011-0073-2

Cunningham, J. A., et al. (2009). A randomized controlled trial of an internet-based intervention for alcohol abusers. *Addiction, 104*(12), 2023–32. doi:10.1111/j.1360–0443.2009.02726.x

Dallery, J., et al. (2017). Nationwide access to an internet-based contingency management intervention to promote smoking cessation: A randomized controlled trial. *Addiction, 112*(5), 875–83. doi:10.1111/add.13715

Dar, R. (2017). Effect of real-time monitoring and notification of smoking episodes on smoking reduction: A pilot study of a novel smoking cessation app. *Nicotine and Tobacco Research*. doi:10.1093/ntr/ntx223

Dennison, L., et al. (2013). Opportunities and challenges for smartphone applications in supporting health behavior change: Qualitative study. *Journal of Medical Internet Research, 15*(4), e86. doi:10.2196/jmir.2583

Elwafi, H. M., et al. (2013). Mindfulness training for smoking cessation: Moderation of the relationship between craving and cigarette use. *Drug and Alcohol Dependence, 130*(1–3), 222–9. doi:10.1016/j.drugalcdep.2012.11.015

Gajecki, M., et al. (2014). Mobile phone brief intervention applications for risky alcohol use among university students: A randomized controlled study. *Addiction Science and Clinical Practice, 9*, 11. doi:10.1186/1940-0640-9-11

Garcia, I. P., et al. (2017). Development and initial evaluation of a mobile application to help with mindfulness training and practice. *International Journal of Medical Informatics, 105*, 59–67. doi:10.1016/j.ijmedinf.2017.05.018

Garrison, K. A., et al. (2015). A randomized controlled trial of smartphone-based mindfulness training for smoking cessation: A study protocol. *BMC Psychiatry, 15*, 83. doi:10.1186/s12888-015-0468-z

Gonzalez, V. M., & Dulin, P. L. (2015). Comparison of a smartphone app for alcohol use disorders with an internet-based intervention plus bibliotherapy: A pilot study. *Journal of Consulting and Clinical Psychology, 83*(2), 335–45. doi:10.1037/a0038620

Goyal, M., et al. (2014). Meditation programs for psychological stress and well-being: A systematic review and meta-analysis. *JAMA Internal Medicine, 174*(3), 357–68. doi:10.1001/jamainternmed.2013.13018

Gregoski, M. J., et al. (2013). Tension tamer: Delivering meditation with objective heart rate acquisition for adherence monitoring using a smart phone platform. *Journal of Alternative and Complementary Medicine, 19*(1), 17–9. doi:10.1089/acm.2011.0772

Gunaratana, H. (2002). *Mindfulness in plain English*. Somerville, MA: Wisdom Publications.

Gustafson, D. H., et al. (2011). An e-health solution for people with alcohol problems. *Alcohol Research and Health, 33*(4), 327–37.

Gustafson, D. H., et al. (2014). A smartphone application to support recovery from alcoholism: A randomized clinical trial. *JAMA Psychiatry, 71*(5), 566–72. doi:10.1001/jamapsychiatry.2013.4642

Havassy, B. E., Hall, S. M., & Wasserman, D. A. (1991). Social support and relapse: Commonalities among alcoholics, opiate users, and cigarette smokers. *Addictive Behaviors, 16*(5), 235–46.

Hovsepian, K., et al. (2015). cStress: Towards a gold standard for continuous stress assessment in the mobile environment. *Proceedings of the ACM International Conference of Ubiquitous Computing, 2015*, 493–504. doi:10.1145/2750858.2807526

Kabat-Zinn, J. (1982). An outpatient program in behavioral medicine for chronic pain patients based on the practice of mindfulness meditation: Theoretical considerations and preliminary results. *General Hospital Psychiatry, 4*(1), 33–47.

Kabat-Zinn, J. (2003). Mindfulness-based interventions in context: Past, present, and future. *Clinical Psychology, 10*(2), 144–56. doi:10.1093/clipsy.bpg016

Kabat-Zinn, J., et al. (2014). *Training teachers to deliver mindfulness-based stress reduction principles and standards*. http://www.umassmed.edu/cfm/training/principles-standards

Kazemi, D. M., et al. (2017). A systematic review of the mhealth interventions to prevent alcohol and substance abuse. *Journal of Healthcare Communications, 22*(5), 413–32. doi:10.1080/10810730.2017.1303556

Keoleian, V., Polcin, D., & Galloway, G. P. (2015). Text messaging for addiction: A review. *J Psychoactive Drugs, 47*(2), 158–76. doi:10.1080/02791072.2015.1009200

Killingsworth, M. A., & Gilbert, D. T. (2010). A wandering mind is an unhappy mind. *Science, 330*(6006), 932. doi:10.1126/science.1192439

Klasnja, P., & Pratt, W. (2012). Healthcare in the pocket: Mapping the space of mobile-phone health interventions. *Journal of Biomedical Informatics, 45*(1), 184–98. doi:10.1016/j.jbi.2011.08.017

Krebs, P., & Duncan, D. T. (2015). Health app use among US mobile phone owners: A national survey. *JMIR Mhealth and Uhealth, 3*(4), e101. doi:10.2196/mhealth.4924

Leonard, N. R., et al. (2017). Mobile health technology using a wearable sensorband for female college students with problem drinking: An acceptability and feasibility study. *JMIR Mhealth and Uhealth, 5*(7), e90. doi:10.2196/mhealth.7399

Li, W., et al. (2017). Mindfulness treatment for substance misuse: A systematic review and meta-analysis. *Journal of Substance Abuse Treatment, 75*, 62–96. doi:10.1016/j.jsat.2017.01.008

Link, B. G., et al. (2004). Measuring mental illness stigma. *Schizophrenia Bulletin, 30*(3), 511–41.

Lowe, S. R., et al. (2013). Longitudinal relationships between self-management skills and substance use in an urban sample of predominantly minority adolescents. *Journal of Drug Issues, 43*(1), 103–18. doi:10.1177/0022042612462221

Luoma, J. B., et al. (2007). An investigation of stigma in individuals receiving treatment for substance abuse. *Addictive Behaviors, 32*(7), 1331–46. doi:10.1016/j.addbeh.2006.09.008

Ly, K. H., et al. (2014). Behavioural activation versus mindfulness-based guided self-help treatment administered through a smartphone application: A randomised controlled trial. *British Medical Journal Open, 4*(1), e003440. doi:10.1136/bmjopen-2013–003440

Mani, M., et al. (2015). Review and evaluation of mindfulness-based iphone apps. *JMIR Mhealth and Uhealth, 3*(3), e82. doi:10.2196/mhealth.4328

Marchand, W. R. (2013). Mindfulness meditation practices as adjunctive treatments for psychiatric disorders. *Psychiatric Clinics of North America, 36*(1), 141–52. doi:10.1016/j.psc.2013.01.002

Marlatt, G. A., & Donovan, D. M. (2005). *Relapse prevention: Maintenance strategies in the treatment of addictive behaviors.* New York: Guilford.

Mason, S., Tovey, P., & Long, A. F. (2002). Evaluating complementary medicine: Methodological challenges of randomised controlled trials. *British Medical Journal,* 325, 832–4. doi:10.1136/bmj.325.7368.832

McTavish, F. M., et al. (2012). How patients recovering from alcoholism use a smartphone intervention. *Journal of Dual Diagnosis, 8*(4), 294–304. doi:10.1080/15504263.2012.723312

Miller, G. (2012). The smartphone psychology manifesto. *Perspectives on Psychological Science, 7*(3), 221–37. doi:10.1177/1745691612441215

Morris, M. E., & Aguilera, A. (2012). Mobile, social, and wearable computing and the evolution of psychological practice. *Professional Psychology: Research and Practice, 43*(6), 622–6. doi:10.1037/a0029041

Naughton, F. (2017). Delivering 'just-in-time' smoking cessation support via mobile phones: Current knowledge and future directions. *Nicotine and Tobacco Research, 19*(3), 379–83. doi:10.1093/ntr/ntw143

Oh, S. S., et al. (2015). Diversity in clinical and biomedical research: A promise yet to be fulfilled. *PLoS Medicine, 12*(12), e1001918. doi:10.1371/journal.pmed.1001918

Parate, A., et al. (2014). RisQ: Recognizing smoking gestures with inertial sensors on a wristband. *MobiSys, 2014,* 149–61. doi:10.1145/2594368.2594379

Pew Research Center. (2014). *American trends panel experience sampling survey.* http://www.pewresearch.org/fact-tank/2015/04/01/6-facts-about-americans-and-their-smartphones/

Pew Research Center. (2015). *Spring 2015 global attitudes survey.* http://www.pewglobal.org/2016/02/22/smartphone-ownership-and-internet-usage-continues-to-climb-in-emerging-economies/

Pew Research Center. (2017). *Mobile fact sheet.* http://www.pewinternet.org/fact-sheet/mobile/

Plaza, I., et al. (2013). Mindfulness-based mobile applications: Literature review and analysis of current features. *Journal of Medical Internet Research mHealth and uHealth, 1*(2), e24. doi:doi:10.2196/mhealth.2733

Quanbeck, A., et al. (2014). Mobile delivery of treatment for alcohol use disorders: A review of the literature. *Alcohol Research, 36*(1), 111–22.

Scott-Sheldon, L. A., et al. (2016). Text messaging-based interventions for smoking cessation: A systematic review and meta-analysis. *JMIR mHealth and uHealth, 4*(2), e49. doi:10.2196/mhealth.5436

Serre, F., et al. (2015). Ecological momentary assessment in the investigation of craving and substance use in daily life: A systematic review. *Drug and Alcohol Dependence, 148,* 1–20. doi:10.1016/j.drugalcdep.2014.12.024

Shiffman, S. (2009). Ecological Momentary Assessment (EMA) in studies of substance use. *Psychological Assessment, 21*(4), 486–97. doi:10.1037/a0017074

Shiffman, S., Stone, A. A., & Hufford, M. R. (2008). Ecological momentary assessment. *Annual Review of Clinical Psychology, 4,* 1–32.

Shonin, E., Van Gordon, W., & Griffiths, M. D. (2013). Mindfulness-based interventions: Towards mindful clinical integration. *Frontiers in Psychology, 4,* 194. doi:10.3389/fpsyg.2013.00194

Skinner, A., et al. (2017). *Stopwatch: A smartwatch-based system for passive detection of cigarette smoking.* https://psyarxiv.com/75j57, doi:10.17605/OSF.IO/75J57

Smith, A. (2012). *The best (and worst) of mobile connectivity.* http://pewinternet.org/Reports/2012/Best-Worst-Mobile.aspx.

Spohr, S. A., et al. (2015). Efficacy of SMS text message interventions for smoking cessation: A meta-analysis. *Journal of Substance Abuse Treatment, 56,* 1–10. doi:10.1016/j.jsat.2015.01.011

Steinhubl, S. R., et al. (2015). Cardiovascular and nervous system changes during meditation. *Frontiers in Human Neuroscience, 9,* 145. doi:10.3389/fnhum.2015.00145

Teasdale, J. D., et al. (2000). Prevention of relapse/recurrence in major depression by mindfulness-based cognitive therapy. *Journal of Consulting and Clinical Psychology, 68*(4), 615–23.

UK Mindfulness-Based Teacher Trainer Network. (2011). *Good practice guidelines for teaching mindfulness-based courses.* http://mindfulnessteachersuk.org.uk/pdf/teacher-guidelines.pdf

Wahbeh, H., Zwickey, H., & Oken, B. (2011). One method for objective adherence measurement in mind-body medicine. *Journal of Alternative and Complementary Medicine, 17*(2), 175–7. doi:10.1089/acm.2010.0316

Watson, T., Simpson, S., & Hughes, C. (2016). Text messaging interventions for individuals with mental health disorders including substance use: A systematic review. *Psychiatry Research, 243,* 255–62. doi:10.1016/j.psychres.2016.06.050

Witkiewitz, K., et al. (2014). Mindfulness-based treatment to prevent addictive behavior relapse: Theoretical models and hypothesized mechanisms of change. *Substance Use and Misuse, 49*(5), 513–24. doi:10.3109/10826084.2014.891845

CHAPTER

37 mHealth Therapy for Problem and Pathological Gambling

Ardeshir S. Rahman *and* Timothy W. Fong

Abstract

Internet-enabled mobile devices (i.e., smartphones and tablets) are ubiquitous in the United States, with more than 250 million individuals owning one. These mobile devices offer researchers and clinicians new opportunities to diagnose disease, administer healthcare, and improve outcomes. Mental healthcare is particularly receptive to feature-rich mobile applications that can augment traditional therapies. This chapter provides an overview of one such application developed to treat problem/pathological gambling called Advanced Behavioral Management for Gambling (ABMG). The clinical basis for the application is described within the context of the technical considerations for mobile application development. Additionally, a feasibility study is described which outlines a methodology to assess the acceptability of, limited efficacy of, and demand for the ABMG platform. Finally, future developments for the ABMG platform and mHealth in general are discussed, as are unique challenges faced by current behavioral mHealth researchers.

Keywords: mHealth, smartphone app, pathological gambling, feasibility study, addiction, mental healthcare

Problem/Pathological Gambling, Ecological Momentary Interventions, and mHealth

Gambling is common, with more than two-thirds of the US adult population having gambled in the past year (Lynch, Maciejewski, & Potenza, 2004; Potenza, Kosten, & Rounsaville, 2001). Most adults gamble without problems, although an estimated 12 million individuals experience either problematic or pathological gambling (PPG; Lynch et al., 2004). PPG has been associated with substance use problems, legal troubles, and poor physical and mental health (Barry et al., 2011; Potenza, 2001; Shaffer & Korn, 2002; Toneatto & Wang, 2009). The costs to society of pathological gambling have been estimated to be close to US$5 billion per year in lost income, productivity, and time (Potenza & Charney, 2001). PPG is classified in the *Diagnostic and Statistical Manual of Mental Disorders* (DSM-IV) as an impulse-control disorder, clinically manifested as the failure to resist urges to gamble or to stop gambling (American Psychiatric Association, 2000). A core feature of PPG is difficulty resisting impulses to gamble along with a sense of relief from tension that is achieved only after the act has been committed. As these gambling urges are associated with self-destructive behaviors and negative health outcomes, they have been proposed and investigated as viable targets for therapeutic intervention (Petry & Roll, 2001; Potenza et al., 2003).

The characteristics of gambling urges suggest that interventions that are instantaneous and easily accessible may be particularly effective at reducing negative gambling behaviors among those with PPG. Researchers and clinicians refer to such ambulatory therapies as *ecological momentary interventions* (EMIs; Cohn et al., 2011; Heron & Smyth, 2010; Kaplan & Stone, 2013; Smith et al., 2012). Theoretically, EMIs are related to another clinical methodology called *ecological momentary assessments* (EMAs), though they are typically researched separately. The premise of both frameworks is to influence and/or study behaviors instantaneously within the subject's natural environment, making these approaches particularly suitable for addressing PPG behavior (Csikszentmihalyi & Hunter, 2003; Kaplan & Stone, 2013; Stone et al., 2007). A significant advantage of these approaches is generalizability and ecological validity of the intervention techniques and/or collected data (Csikszentmihalyi & Larson, 1987; Smyth & Stone, 2003). For example, EMIs offer opportunities for patients to utilize skills, behaviors, and techniques learned during therapy in their natural environment, and this may result in more ecologically valid outcomes that may be longer lasting (Heron & Smyth, 2010; Kalichman et al., 2002). Historically, EMIs have come in the form of clinical recommendations between therapy sessions; these may include practicing skills, reading educational materials, or completing paper assignments (Kazantzis, Deane, & Ronan, 2000). Similarly, EMAs were typically initiated by pagers and completed on paper (Kaplan & Stone, 2013). However, the landscape of both EMAs and EMIs has shifted significantly with the advent and relatively rapid dissemination of mobile devices. Now, technologically robust methodologies are being developed and studied within the emerging field of mobile health (mHealth).

Mobile devices provide promising new opportunities to develop both EMIs and EMAs that deliver personalized, intelligent, and real-time healthcare (Patrick et al., 2008; Riley et al., 2011). The World Health Organization broadly defines mHealth as any initiative that utilizes mobile and wireless technologies to support health objectives (Gaggioli & Riva, 2013). The first behavioral mHealth therapies that addressed addictive behaviors relied on short message service (SMS or text messaging) technology as a platform to conduct EMAs and deliver EMIs (see Newman et al., 2011, for a complete review). Of particular note is a randomized clinical trial (N = 1,705) that found nearly 30% of smokers who received regular and personalized text messages in the form of smoking cessation advice, support, and distraction quit after 6 weeks compared to only 13% of smokers in the control group without text messages (Rodgers et al., 2005). Similar results have been observed when providing SMS support to other behaviors such as alcohol use, substance use, obesity, schizophrenia, and depression (Cole-Lewis & Kershaw, 2010; Krishna, Boren, & Balas, 2009). Indeed, a recent survey of individuals enrolled in intensive outpatient substance abuse treatment found that 98% of respondents were interested in mobile phone support during and after treatment (Muench et al., 2013). More than 80% of respondents from this study also indicated that, if possible, they would use a mobile phone system to report lapses, send "help messages" during high-risk situations, and want their counselor/friends alerted if they felt at-risk for a relapse (Muench et al., 2013).

While SMS methodologies have been shown to be useful in promoting healthy behaviors, the technology is simple and arguably outdated. More recently, researchers and clinicians have shifted their focus to creating EMAs/EMIs on more powerful and Internet-enabled smartphone platforms (e.g., iOS or Android; Liu et al., 2011). To date, one of the more robust randomized clinical trial (N = 349) investigated the outcomes of supplementing treatment as usual for alcohol-dependent patients with a smartphone application (or "app") called A-CHESS (Gustafson et al., 2014). A-CHESS is a multifeature app that goes beyond SMS and includes functionality such as message boards, support group locator, relaxation techniques, learning materials, local events, news articles related to recovery, alert system when approaching risky locations, and weekly surveys to track progress. Results from the clinical trial using A-CHESS showed that after 8 months of intervention and 4 months of follow-up, patients who had access to the smartphone app had significantly fewer risky drinking days as compared to those receiving treatment as usual without the app. This study marks the first time, to our knowledge, that a smartphone app used to deliver both EMIs and EMAs has been shown to be clinically effective at potentially reducing the risks associated with an addictive behavior. Some researchers at the National Institutes of Health (NIH) are calling for more formalized research into the feasibility and efficacy of behavioral mHealth applications, much like A-CHESS, in order to establish best practices for this rapidly advancing technology (Kaplan & Stone, 2013). However, the increased complexity and cost to develop native apps for smartphones means fewer projects have been developed and even fewer studies have been conducted to assess the efficacy of mental health apps for smartphones (Weinstein et al., 2014).

Given the behavioral overlap between substance use disorders and PPG, as well as the success of other mHealth platforms for managing addictions and behaviors, we hypothesized that a multifeatured smartphone app for PPG could potentially lead to improved clinical outcomes (Newman et al., 2011; Potenza & Wareham, 2010). Carlbring & Smit (2008) developed an Internet-based computerized therapy for PPG that converted established cognitive-behavioral therapy (CBT) methods for PPG therapy into a computer-friendly format (Hodgins, 2004; Ladouceur & Lachance, 2007). The computerized CBT included various modules which were administered online and included PPG-related information, behavioral modification exercises, and follow-up assessments. Patient responses were analyzed by therapists and used to formulate positive feedback via weekly telephone calls and emails (Carlbring & Smit, 2008). After 8 weeks of minimal-contact, at-home therapy, those with PPG showed improvement in gambling behavior, anxiety, depression, and quality of life, which persisted through 36 months of follow-up as compared to control comparison subjects who did not receive the computerized therapy. These results suggest that digitized therapies for PPG may be effective and lead to positive outcomes, especially if they are integrated adequately into a patient's life. To that end, our research group has developed a smartphone app aimed at supplementing treatment as usual for those experiencing PPG. The application, called Advanced Behavioral Management for Gambling (ABMG), has been clinically rooted in our research group's manualized therapy for PPG and tailored for smartphones. Specifically, the ABMG mobile app uses EMIs designed specifically to help patients manage their gambling urges in real time through various interactive techniques. Moreover, we've incorporated novel EMAs into the app to gain insights on the behavioral and environmental aspects of a patient's gambling urges. We have simultaneously developed a web app which analyzes all data associated with a particular patient and presents various analyses to the clinician in the form of easy-to-read graphs. In this way, we can use ecologically valid data to inform therapeutic choices for each patient, making overall therapy more personalized and data driven.

This chapter mainly focuses on our research group's effort to develop and test the ABMG platform. Specifically, we discuss the technical development of our platform, including design and security, as well as the therapeutic basis for its content. Moreover, we outline the feasibility study we have designed to test the efficacy of our behavioral mHealth platform in a clinical setting. Last, we describe some of the challenges we have encountered while creating our application, as well as provide suggestions for researchers interested in developing their own behavioral mHealth applications.

Clinical Content, Technical Development, and Interface Design for ABMG

The clinical content of the ABMG platform has been derived from a self-help workbook our research group has jointly published with the Office of Problem Gambling in the California Department of Alcohol and Drug Programs (Fong & Rosenthal, 2010). The workbook was designed as a free resource for those seeking to treat or understand PPG and is used by providers enrolled in the state-supported treatment program for PPG located in California. There are five sections within the workbook that help those experiencing PPG to identify the extent of gambling problems, analyze the severity of the problem, provide behavioral modification techniques to resist urges, promote healthier alternative habits, and track progress toward recovery. Our goals with ABMG were to transform the workbook material into an interactive and Internet-enabled application that could be used alongside traditional therapy. We saw the urge management techniques, behavioral modification aspects, and progress tracking features of the workbook as most engaging and compatible for touchscreen devices. As such, we combined the urge management techniques with the behavioral modifications suggestions to create a dynamic EMI for PPG which is further augmented by tracking of recovery progress.

More specifically, ABMG allows individuals experiencing PPG to manage their urges in real time through six distinct modules. These modules focus on (1) reaching out to someone, (2) finding healthy alternative activities nearby, (3) finding nearby support group meetings, (4) guided mindfulness-based relaxation techniques used to deal with urges/addictions, (5) supporting notes/messages from a user's therapist, and (6) positive self-reminders and words of encouragement from a user's digital journal. Other therapeutic features of the app include (1) tracking physical health over the period of therapy, (2) monitoring recovery progress over time through easy-to-read analytics, and (3) recording journal entries regarding therapy progress to be used during trigger events. The technical foundation of ABMG was based on three facets of previous behavioral mHealth EMIs that have been shown to be effective: self-motivation, behavioral modification, and external support (Bickel, Christensen, & Marsch, 2011; Cohn et al., 2011; Gustafson et al., 2014; Kaplan & Stone, 2013; Marsch & Dallery, 2012).

In addition to mitigating urges for those with PPG, ABMG also benefits the clinician by providing ecologically valid analytics about his or her patients' urges not typically available in treatment as usual. A significant advantage of mHealth is the ecological validity of the data that can be collected from smartphone apps. However, a significant challenge is navigating the large amounts of data in order to personalize or inform therapies constructively. During the preplanning of ABMG, our development and clinical teams worked together to assess the quality of various data points that could be collected with the platform. From more than 80 different combinations of data points that could be analyzed, we selected 15 that our clinicians determined to be most informative for treating PPG. According to Smith et al. (2012), clinicians strongly prefer analytics on EMIs/EMAs data that are easy to read while still conveying important trends. Considering this, we simultaneously developed a web application for clinicians to access that automatically runs statistical analyses on select variables related to their patients. For example, clinicians can view charts and graphs that compare their patients' gambling urge frequency to the time of day or compare their patients' moods to their gambling urge intensity. We also have been implementing mapping functionality which charts where and when specific urges are occurring during the course of treatment, which may result in more holistic and data-driven therapeutic choices.

For the ABMG mobile app itself, we chose to develop on Apple's iOS platform. Data security is crucial for any mHealth application, particularly as it concerns the Health Insurance Portability and Affordability Act (HIPAA), and it has been suggested to be an important factor when patients determine acceptability and adoption (Gaggioli & Riva, 2013). While mHealth researchers could successfully develop secure apps for both iOS and Android, we ultimately selected iOS because it was targeted significantly less often by malicious software and security breaches compared to Android (Symantec Corporation, 2013). Moreover, iOS platforms natively encrypt data saved to the phone using high-security protocols that meet HIPAA requirements. However, to meet full HIPAA standards, this project utilized the services of a third-party vendor, TrueVault. TrueVault provides a HIPAA-secure platform to both transfer and store data from mobile and web apps. When the mobile app collects data regarding user activity (i.e., urge frequency), it is stored on a HIPAA-compliant remote server hosted by this vendor. These HIPAA-compliant servers are at the center of the ABMG platform and allow for effective and secure communication between the patient-facing mobile app and clinician-facing web app. By using this service, all transient data (data being transferred) can be sent using highly secure protocols and any static data (data saved to a local disk) can be encrypted to the highest standards set by the Department of Human Health Services for digital HIPAA data.

Final technical considerations for building the ABMG platform involved the user interface and graphic design. We've incorporated design suggestions from previous studies regarding mHealth EMIs/EMAs into the framework of the application by emphasizing (1) nonintrusive implementation, (2) multifeatured and layered functionality, (3) easy-to-read analytics about behavior, and (4) clearly communicated motivational feedback (Gustafson et al., 2014; Palmier-Claus et al., 2013; Smith et al., 2012). Utilizing the unique properties of smartphone touchscreens, we can get users engaged with specific tasks quickly while collecting rich data to be used by the therapist. Application design principles stay close to Apple's Human Interface Guidelines so they fits into a user's existing experiences on iOS (Apple, 2014). We created deep navigation by segmenting sections on a main menu that allow users to drill down into more specific areas that are actionable and therapeutic. Simplicity and functional minimalism were important to our design team as the main use case for the app will be in-the-moment urges that warrant rapid addressing.

Designing the format and implementation of EMAs required special consideration during development. Complex answer formats like Likert-type scales do not translate well on mobile devices, particularly as EMIs need to have very little hindrance to access therapeutic tools (Gustafson et al., 2014; Heron & Smyth, 2010; Smith et al., 2012). Smartphones are unique platforms that allow researchers to create assessments that take advantage of the rich display and touch features while not compromising the quality of the data collected. Specifically, we designed assessments for the application that take advantage of interactive sliders and dynamic images to gauge variables such as urge intensity, mood, and type of trigger. For example, we noted that during an average gambling trigger, users can get to actionable therapies after answering three questions that take approximately 5.5 seconds to complete. However, from this brief EMA, we collect six variables that are ecologically valid and informative to therapeutic decisions. We can accomplish this quick data collection through the use of automatic environmental data logging and direct user assessment while still being mindful of design standards established by Apple. During beta testing, these interactive methods of collecting data seemed to be more engaging and accurate than traditional paper methods, though our feasibility study will examine this possibility more closely.

Designing a Feasibility Study to Assess Acceptability, Limited-Efficacy, and Demand of mHealth Apps

Investigating the feasibility of the ABMG platform is crucial for determining potential efficacy. As such, this project will follow guidelines proposed by Bowen et al. (2009) with regards to the formulation of a feasibility study of factors relevant to the public health. Specifically, we will be studying (1) how patients and clinicians react to the ABMG platform (acceptability), (2) a small sample of those with PPGe using the platform (limited-efficacy testing), and (3) the actual use of the platform during therapy (demand). Participants in this study will be selected from the general population and must be 18 years or older, be clinically diagnosed as experiencing PPG via the Structured Clinical Interview for Pathological Gambling (SCI-PG; Grant et al., 2004), be seeking treatment, and own at least an iPhone 5 with an active data plan. Participants will be excluded from the study if they indicate any drug use; are taking medications for any psychiatric disorders; present clinically significant suicidality, depression, or anxiety as assessed by the Mini International Neuropsychiatric Interview (MINI; Lecrubier et al., 1997); or have any medical disorders that could lead to physical harm.

For the acceptability portion of the study, we have already recruited 20 participants with current PPG as well as 20 mental healthcare providers who specialized in treating PPG. The participants were asked to assess and give detailed feedback on the ABMG platform. All were given 45 minutes to use their respective platforms (i.e., those with PPG assessing the mobile app and providers assessing the web app). A 15-minute interview immediately proceeded the demo session wherein a researcher administered a quick questionnaire to gauge reactions to the features, design, and clarity of the platform. Afterward, all participant were able to discuss details of the platform, which was recorded and reviewed by a researcher for improving the software. Any "bugs" that were discovered during this time have been sent to our development team to fix in preparation for the next phase.

Results from the acceptability phase are encouraging and suggest that the ABMG platform can potentially be useful in mitigating problematic gambling behaviors. The entire sample of both those with PPG (n = 20, 100%) and providers (n = 20, 100%) reported that they would be interested in using the system during and after therapy. Nearly all of the PPG participants (n = 16, 80%) indicated they would use the mobile app daily as needed, while the remaining participants (n = 4, 20%) indicated they would use the app throughout the week as needed. In the provider sample, a majority (n = 14, 70%) reported they would use the web app a few times a week to check in on their patients, with the remaining sample (n = 6, 30%) reporting that they would use the app daily to track their patients' behaviors. Regarding the specific features, those with PPG rated the following functions as very useful: find nearby support groups (n = 20, 100%), reach out to a friend/therapist (n = 15, 60%), guided mindfulness techniques (n = 18, 90%), and journaling (n = 18, 90%). Similarly, providers reported that the behavioral analytics (n = 17, 85%) and messaging (n = 19, 95%) features of the web app were very useful. Overall, 90% (n = 18) of those with PPG and 95% (n = 19) of providers thought the ABMG platform was an improvement over existing methods of real-time urge management for gambling.

We are currently conducting limited efficacy testing to explore how ABMG will impact therapy sessions and clinical outcomes. For this portion, we are recruiting 10 PPG participants from the general population who have not previously been enrolled in gambling therapy for at least 6 months. To control for any clinical variability between providers, we have assigned one mental healthcare provider to all of the participants for the remainder of the trial. We plan to study the application using a cross-sectional design comparing two randomly assigned groups of those with PPG: those who receive treatment as usual (n = 5) and those who receive treatment as usual supplemented with ABMG (n = 5) for a period of 8 weeks. Considering previous research that suggests mHealth initiatives that act as an adjunct to treatment as usual seem to improve clinical outcomes, we hypothesize that those with PPG receiving ABMG support will show more improvement than controls (Carlbring & Smit, 2008; Gustafson et al., 2014; Reid et al., 2013; Smith et al., 2012). Specifically, as compared to those receiving only treatment as usual, we hypothesize that those with PPG receiving treatment supplemented by ABMG will show (1) decreased obsessive and compulsive thoughts/behaviors related to gambling, (2) decreased depression and anxiety related to gambling behaviors, and (3) diminished negative environmental impact due to gambling. The primary outcome measures for this portion of the study will be adapted from a recent clinical trial supported by the National Institute for Drug Abuse (NIDA) on PPG treatment and will include the pathological gambling adaption of the Yale-Brown Obsessive Compulsive Scale to gauge PPG severity (PG-YBOCS; Pallanti et al., 2005), the Sheehan Disability Scale to assess the environmental impact of gambling behavior (SDS; Leon et al., 1997), and the Hamilton Depression Rating Scale (HDRS; Hamilton, 1960) and the Hamilton Anxiety Rating Scale (HAM-A; Hamilton, 1959) to assess depression and anxiety, respectively. All primary outcome measures will be assessed pre-, mid-, and post-treatment, with follow-ups occurring at 1, 3, and 6 months after conclusion of the study.

The final portion of this feasibility study will be to assess the demand for the ABMG application during PPG therapy. To accomplish this, we are collecting data on how participants use the app by monitoring which screens they use, how often they use the ABMG app, and how long they spend on the app and the various screens. Comparing these data within the context of other clinical variables (e.g., problem gambling severity, gender, and recovery progress), we can investigate how any potential within-group differences affect app usage. Moreover, we will be able to identify any design elements that may inhibit or decrease app usage, which we can address in future versions of the application.

Future Directions and Challenges

The field of mHealth, and particularly behavioral mHealth, is still quite nascent, with much room to improve. As third-party technology develops, researchers and clinicians will have more tools at their disposal to build more features into their mHealth apps. For example, new in-app chat technologies allow developers to easily integrate a rich communication platform to create real-time chat and video between two parties (e.g., patient and provider) within their apps. Studies have shown that regular, real-time communication can contribute importantly to the efficacy of behavioral mHealth applications (Heron & Smyth, 2010; Kaplan & Stone, 2013). At the moment, this type of communications functionality needs to be individually developed for each mHealth platform, which costs significant time and money. However, turnkey solutions provided by new software companies lower the cost to implement these features in mHealth apps, making them potentially more effective. Rich video- and chat-enabled communications offer opportunities to run larger support groups on mobile devices that are running ABMG. We are currently working to implement real-time chat into future versions of ABMG to provide this level of communication.

Similar to virtual support groups, research suggests that social networks of users with similar diagnoses (e.g., pathological gambling) can improve the therapeutic outcomes of its members (Gustafson et al., 2014). Another feature being developed for ABMG is a social network which allows patients and clinicians across the entire ABMG platform to communicate with each other, send each other words of encouragement, and generally support each other while remaining semi-anonymous. Following suggestions by mHealth researchers and patients, we hope to include intelligent functionality that initiates a message to other members of the larger ABMG network, prompting words of encouragement or even an immediate, real-time communication during gambling urges (Muench et al., 2013). The social network can be incentivized for members who contribute the effort to help others during urges by awarding points, badges, and perhaps real-world rewards like discounts or coupons to local activities. In this way, we can further enhance the external support features of ABMG, which could lead to better outcomes.

A significant advantage of mHealth initiatives is the data generated by users of these platforms. This is the case with ABMG, where the data on ecologically assessed behaviors are used to inform a clinician on how to personalize therapies for each patient. However, the effectiveness of these data-driven therapies can be increased by the amount of varied data made available to the provider. As such, we are currently working with other mHealth innovators to tap into a larger reservoir of self-generated patient data. The Quantified Self movement has led to devices and software that allow users to track an array of variables such as exercise (e.g., Fitbit and Jawbone Up), sleep (e.g., Sleepio), food intake (e.g., Myfitnesspal), and even emotional states (EmotionTracker.fi). Currently, much of these data are stored on private databases, and sharing between apps and companies is sparse. But as mHealth matures, more companies are finding synergy in developing systems to allow access to data between platforms, which can improve outcomes for providers, patients, and software developers alike. Innovations such as Apple's Healthkit and Google

Health give mHealth developers access to a common bed of data shared by hundreds of apps, potentially allowing them to implement algorithms to detect trends in data over time and across millions of patients. Results from such large-scale analyses could lead to mHealth therapies that are more holistic and more effective and could generate novel research discoveries rooted in ecologically valid data from diverse health populations.

While mHealth applications and solutions are promising for improving healthcare, there are some challenges facing individuals innovating in this space. For example, during the creation and initial focus group testing of ABMG, one issue that we encountered was that of engagement and novelty. Since the therapeutic course of ABMG lasts for 12 weeks, the application needed to maintain the attention of our users for the entire period of time. To address this consideration, we included dynamic content into the application that adds novelty regularly (e.g., therapist messages, journaling, and reading material). Monitoring and quantifying user activity during the feasibility trial will give us better insights on engagement over the entire course of therapy and how we might improve it. This aspect of mHealth development is particularly important when working with a patient group that may be highly motivated by novelty and may have high dropout rates from therapy, such as those with PPG (Melville, Casey, & Kavanagh, 2007; Wulfert et al., 2006). In future versions of ABMG, we hope to include modules that are entirely dynamic (e.g., social networking, real-time communication, and live events/activities), thus generating novelty within the platform on a continual basis and potentially leading to sustained engagement throughout the course of therapy. It is crucial that mHealth innovators put emphasis on dynamic and novel content that complements their particular therapeutic goals in order to maintain their users' attention for the duration of therapy. A lack of dynamic and interactive content could impede the therapeutic efficacy of mHealth applications.

Another challenge of mHealth development involves regulatory bodies and healthcare policymakers. Again, due to the infancy of mHealth, many regulatory bodies are unfamiliar with the practices and language of mHealth therapies. For this project, receiving Institutional Review Board (IRB) approval required clear communication between our research group and various IRB members. The top concern from our IRB regarded HIPAA and patient data security. As most mHealth platforms will utilize smartphones, servers, and web browsers to varying degrees, the way in which data security is described needs to be clearly documented. For our platform, we utilized a third-party vendor to ensure HIPAA compliance for data storage and transfer. Because the vendor has taken rigorous steps to maintain continual HIPAA compliance, we needed to explain clearly how we utilized their service and how that service conferred HIPAA compliance to our platform. It is highly recommended that any new mHealth endeavor consider HIPAA compliance and data security during preplanning and before any development occurs. Building a mHealth application before conducting data security analysis will cost significant time and money should HIPAA compliance be required later on, particular if databases and processes have already been developed. In addition to IRBs, developers and researchers should be aware of how the US Food and Drug Administration (FDA) will approach behavioral mHealth therapies in the future. At the moment, the FDA has published a series of guidelines for behavioral mHealth applications that are suggested, but not currently required (US Food & Drug Administration, 2014). As more behavioral mHealth platforms solicit funding from various government agencies and become central parts of clinical trials, the FDA may move to establish stricter guidelines for any behavioral mHealth platform. Again, significant preplanning may help to ensure that both HIPAA compliance and any potential FDA requirements are integrated into any new behavioral mHealth framework.

Last, a unique challenge we faced for the ABMG platform was the popularity of social casino games on smartphones. A study that our research group conducted found that, as of December 2013, there were approximately 3,000 social casino games that have been downloaded at least 122 million times on US-based Android smartphones (Rahman et al., 2013). Because this analysis did not study social casino games on iOS smartphones, the actual total number of apps and downloads is likely higher. Due to the popularity of social casino games, there is concern that patients using ABMG may be triggered to gamble or play casino games by the mobile device itself, which would be contradictory to the therapeutic goals of ABMG. While social casino games on smartphones may not involve monetary wagering (due to legal reasons), some research would suggest that virtual currency is a close enough proxy to elicit excitability similar to real-world currency gambling (Griffiths, 2010, 2012; Griffiths & Parke, 2010). However, there are no formal studies on the possible influence of virtual currency–based social casino games may have on PPG behavior, though we plan to monitor external app usage closely during the ABMG feasibility trial to determine this more precisely.

Conclusion

Here we have outlined our particular approach for a novel behavioral mHealth platform to address PPG. We have discussed the clinical and technical foundations of our mHeatlh app, as well as our proposed feasibility study to test its efficacy. While clinical work on behavioral mHealth apps is still sparse, we have built the ABMG platform using current evidence and trends that have shown positive outcomes with respect to addressing similar behaviors. Internet-enabled mobile devices have already become integrated into the lives of millions of people, and this figure grows every year. This unprecedented access to a patient's environment opens new opportunities to administer more efficient healthcare. Mental healthcare is particularly receptive to technologically robust solutions and will continue to see innovation as mobile devices develop. As researchers, clinicians, and developers work together to improve the practice of mental healthcare, new software, devices, and platforms will be created that can positively impact behavioral health therapies. There are still many unanswered questions, challenges, and risks associated with this new frontier, but, with careful planning and thorough study, most of these issues will likely be resolved, and this likelihood may lead to smarter, more informed mental healthcare.

References

American Psychiatric Association. (2000). *Diagnostic and statistical manual of mental disorders DSM-IV-TR* (text version). Washington, DC: APA.

Apple. (2014). *iOS Human Interface Guidelines*. https://developer.apple.com/library/ios/documentation/userexperience/conceptual/mobilehig/

Barry, D. T., Stefanovics, E. A., Desai, R. A., & Potenza, M. N. (2011). Differences in the associations between gambling problem severity and psychiatric disorders among black and white adults: Findings from the National Epidemiologic Survey on Alcohol and Related Conditions. *American Journal on Addictions, 20*(1), 69–77.

Bickel, W. K., Christensen, D. R., & Marsch, L. A. (2011). A review of computer-based interventions used in the assessment, treatment, and research of drug addiction. *Substance Use and Misuse, 46*(1), 4–9.

Bowen, D. J., Kreuter, M., Spring, B., Cofta-Woerpel, L., Linnan, L., Weiner, D., . . . & Fernandez, M. (2009). How we design feasibility studies. *American Journal of Preventive Medicine, 36*(5), 452–7.

Carlbring, P., & Smit, F. (2008). Randomized trial of internet-delivered self-help with telephone support for pathological gamblers. *Journal of Consulting and Clinical Psychology, 76*(6), 1090–4.

Cohn, A. M., Hunter-Reel, D., Hagman, B. T., & Mitchell, J. (2011). Promoting behavior change from alcohol use through mobile technology: The future of ecological momentary assessment. *Alcoholism, Clinical and Experimental Research, 35*(12), 2209–15.

Cole-Lewis, H., & Kershaw, T. (2010). Text messaging as a tool for behavior change in disease prevention and management. *Epidemiologic Reviews, 32*(1), 56–69.

Csikszentmihalyi, M., & Hunter, J. (2003). Happiness in everyday life: The uses of experience sampling. *Journal of Happiness Studies, 4*(2), 185–99.

Csikszentmihalyi, M., & Larson, R. (1987). Validity and reliability of the experience-sampling method. *The Journal of Nervous and Mental Disease, 175*(9), 526–36.

Fong, T. W., & Rosenthal, R. J. (2010). *Freedom from problem gambling*. UCLA Gambling Studies Program and California Office of Problem Gambling.

Gaggioli, A., & Riva, G. (2013). From mobile mental health to mobile wellbeing: Opportunities and challenges. *Studies in Health Technology and Informatics, 184*, 141–7.

Grant, J. E., Steinberg, M. A., Kim, S. W., Rounsaville, B. J., & Potenza, M. N. (2004). Preliminary validity and reliability testing of a structured clinical interview for pathological gambling. *Psychiatry Research, 128*(1), 79–88.

Griffiths, M. D. (2010). Social networking: Gaming in social networking sites: A growing concern? *World Online Gambling Law Report, 9*(5), 12–3.

Griffiths, M. D. (2012). Gambling on Facebook: A cause for concern? *World Online Gambling Law Report, 11*(9), 10–11.

Griffiths, M. D., & Parke, J. (2010). Adolescent gambling on the internet: A review. *International Journal of Adolescent Medical Health, 22*(1), 59–75.

Gustafson, D. H., McTavish, F. M., Chih, M. Y., Atwood, A. K., Johnson, R. A., Boyle, M. G., . . . & Isham, A. (2014). A smartphone application to support recovery from alcoholism: A randomized clinical trial. *JAMA Psychiatry, 71*(5), 566–72.

Hamilton, M. (1959). The assessment of anxiety states by rating. *British Journal of Medical Psychology, 32*(1), 50–5.

Hamilton, M. (1960). A rating scale for depression, *Journal of Neurology, Neurosurgery, and Psychiatry, 23*(1), 56.

Heron, K. E., & Smyth, J. M. (2010). Ecological momentary interventions: Incorporating mobile technology into psychosocial and health behaviour treatments. *British Journal of Health Psychology, 15*(Pt 1), 1–39.

Hodgins, D. C. (2004). Using the NORC DSM screen for gambling problems as an outcome measure for pathological gambling: Psychometric evaluation. *Addictive Behaviors, 29*(8), 1685–90.

Kalichman, S., Stein, J. A., Malow, R., Averhart, C., Devieux, J., Jennings, T., . . . & Feaster, D. J. (2002). Predicting protected sexual behaviour using the Information-Motivation-Behaviour skills model among adolescent substance abusers in court-ordered treatment. *Psychology, Health & Medicine, 7*(3), 327–38.

Kaplan, R. M., & Stone, A. A. (2013). Bringing the laboratory and clinic to the community: Mobile technologies for health promotion and disease prevention. *Annual Review of Psychology, 64*, 471–98.

Kazantzis, N., Deane, F. P., & Ronan, K. R. (2000). Homework assignments in cognitive and behavioral therapy: A meta-analysis. *Clinical Psychology: Science and Practice, 7*(2), 189–202.

Krishna, S., Boren, S. A., & Balas, E. A. (2009). Healthcare via cell phones: A systematic review. *Telemedicine and e-Health, 15*(3), 231–40.

Ladouceur, R., & Lachance, S. (2007). *Overcoming your pathological gambling: Workbook*. New York: Oxford University Press.

Lecrubier, Y., Sheehan, D. V., Weiller, E., Amorim, P., Bonora, I., Sheehan, K. H., ... & Dunbar, G. C. (1997). The Mini International Neuropsychiatric Interview (MINI). A short diagnostic structured interview: Reliability and validity according to the CIDI. *European Psychiatry, 12*(5), 224–31.

Leon, A. C., Olfson, M., Portera, L., Farber, L., & Sheehan, D. V. (1997). Assessing psychiatric impairment in primary care with the Sheehan Disability Scale. *The International Journal of Psychiatry in Medicine, 27*(2), 93–105.

Liu, C., Zhu, Q., Holroyd, K. A., & Seng, E. K. (2011). Status and trends of mobile-health applications for iOS devices: A developer's perspective. *Journal of Systems and Software, 84*(11), 2022–33.

Lynch, W. J., Maciejewski, P. K., & Potenza, M. N. (2004). Psychiatric correlates of gambling in adolescents and young adults grouped by age at gambling onset. *Archives of General Psychiatry, 61*(11), 1116–22.

Marsch, L. A., & Dallery, J. (2012). Advances in the psychosocial treatment of addiction: The role of technology in the delivery of evidence-based psychosocial treatment. *Psychiatric Clinics of North America, 35*(2), 481–93.

Melville, K. M., Casey, L. M., & Kavanagh, D. J. (2007). Psychological treatment dropout among pathological gamblers. *Clinical Psychology Review, 27*(8), 944–58.

Muench, F., Weiss, R. A., Kuerbis, A., & Morgenstern, J. (2013). Developing a theory driven text messaging intervention for addiction care with user driven content. *Psychology and Addictive Behaviors, 27*(1), 315–21.

Newman, M. G., Szkodny, L. E., Llera, S. J., & Przeworski, A. (2011). A review of technology-assisted self-help and minimal contact therapies for drug and alcohol abuse and smoking addiction: Is human contact necessary for therapeutic efficacy? *Clinical Psychology Review, 31*(1), 178–86.

Pallanti, S., DeCaria, C. M., Grant, J. E., Urpe, M., & Hollander, E. (2005). Reliability and validity of the pathological gambling adaptation of the Yale-Brown Obsessive-Compulsive Scale (PG-YBOCS). *Journal of Gambling Studies, 21*(4), 431–3.

Palmier-Claus, J. E., Rogers, A., Ainsworth, J., Machin, M., Barrowclough, C., Laverty, L., ... & Lewis, S. W. (2013). Integrating mobile-phone based assessment for psychosis into people's everyday lives and clinical care: A qualitative study. *BMC Psychiatry, 13*, 34.

Patrick, K., Griswold, W. G., Raab, F., & Intille, S. S. (2008). Health and the mobile phone. *American Journal of Preventive Medicine, 35*(2), 177.

Petry, N. M., & Roll, J. M. (2001). A behavioral approach to understanding and treating pathological gambling. *Seminars in Clinical Neuropsychiatry, 6*(3), 177–83.

Potenza, M. N. (2001). The neurobiology of pathological gambling. *Seminars in Clinical Neuropsychiatry, 6*(3), 217–26.

Potenza, M. N., & Charney, D. S. (2001). Pathological gambling: A current perspective. *Seminars in Clinical Neuropsychiatry, 6*(3), 153–4.

Potenza, M. N., Kosten, T. R., & Rounsaville, B. J. (2001). Pathological gambling. *Journal of the American Medical Association, 286*(2), 141–4.

Potenza, M. N., & Wareham, J. D. (2010). Pathological gambling and substance use disorders. *American Journal of Drug and Alcohol Abuse, 36*(5), 242–7.

Potenza, M. N., Steinberg, M. A., Skudlarski, P., Fulbright, R. K., Lacadie, C. M., Wilber, M. K., ... & Wexler, B. E. (2003). Gambling urges in pathological gambling: A functional magnetic resonance imaging study. *Archives of General Psychiatry, 60*(8), 828–36.

Rahman, A. S., Rosenthal, R. J., Fink, A., Davtian, M., Abarbanel, B., Fong, T. W. (2013). Casino games on mobile devices: Tracking development and popularity trends among US players. Unpublished Manuscript..

Reid, S. C., Kauer, S. D., Hearps, S. J., Crooke, A. H., Khor, A. S., Sanci, L. A., & Patton, G. C. (2013). A mobile phone application for the assessment and management of youth mental health problems in primary care: Health service outcomes from a randomised controlled trial of mobiletype. *BMC Family Practice, 14*, 84.

Riley, W. T., Rivera, D. E., Atienza, A. A., Nilsen, W., Allison, S. M., & Mermelstein, R. (2011). Health behavior models in the age of mobile interventions: Are our theories up to the task? *Translational Behavioral Medicine, 1*(1), 53–71.

Rodgers, A., Corbett, T., Bramley, D., Riddell, T., Wills, M., Lin, R. B., & Jones, M. (2005). Do u smoke after txt? Results of a randomised trial of smoking cessation using mobile phone text messaging. *Tobacco Control, 14*(4), 255–61.

Shaffer, H. J., & Korn, D. A. (2002). Gambling and related mental disorders: A public health analysis. *Annual Review of Public Health, 23*, 171–212.

Smith, B., Harms, W. D., Burres, S., Korda, H., Rosen, H., & Davis, J. (2012). Enhancing behavioral health treatment and crisis management through mobile ecological momentary assessment and SMS messaging. *Health Informatics Journal, 18*(4), 294–308.

Smyth, J. M., & Stone, A. A. (2003). Ecological momentary assessment research in behavioral medicine. *Journal of Happiness Studies, 4*(1), 35–52.

Stone, A., Shiffman, S., Atienza, A., & Nebeling, L. (2007). *The science of real-time data capture*. New York: Oxford University Press

Symantec Corporation. (2013). *Internet security threat report 2013: Volume 18, from* https://scm.symantec.com/resources/istr18_en.pdf.

Toneatto, T., & Wang, J. J. (2009). Community treatment for problem gambling: Sex differences in outcome and process. *Community Mental Health Journal, 45*(6), 468–75.

US Food and Drug Administration. (2014). *Mobile medical applications.* http://www.fda.gov/MedicalDevices/ProductsandMedicalProcedures/ConnectedHealth/MobileMedicalApplications/ucm255978.htm

Weinstein, R. S., Lopez, A. M., Joseph, B. A., Erps, K. A., Holcomb, M., Barker, G. P., & Krupinski, E. A. (2014). Telemedicine, telehealth, and mobile health applications that work: Opportunities and barriers. *The American Journal of Medicine, 127*(3), 183–7.

Wulfert, E., Blanchard, E. B., Freidenberg, B. M., & Martell, R. S. (2006). Retaining pathological gamblers in cognitive behavior therapy through motivational enhancement: A pilot study. *Behavior Modification, 30*(3), 315–40.

PART 8

Treatment of Problematic Internet Use and Video Gaming

CHAPTER

38 Psychotherapeutic and Pharmacological Treatment for Problematic Digital Technology Use

Formulating Principles and Practice Guides from the Scientific and Professional Literature

David Faust, Marc N. Potenza, Charles Gaudet, *and* Kyle A. Faust

Abstract

This chapter focuses on the psychological treatment of problem Internet and digital technology use (PRIU), such as excessive gaming, and also briefly overviews pharmacological approaches. Forms of Internet and digital technology use that provide alternative vehicles for more specific problem or addictive behavior, such as excessive gambling or shopping, and which often seem to present with differing features, are not covered here [editors' comment: but rather addressed in other chapters of this book]. Although treatment research is still in an early stage of development, an accumulating body of literature involving a diverse range of presentations and populations and a variety of treatment strategies has often yielded positive and robust effect sizes. Hence, a relatively compelling justification can be provided for therapeutic intervention, especially when using treatments of demonstrated effectiveness with similar clients, when PRIU seems to be associated with significant malfunction or worsening of co-occurring conditions, and when trends suggest that problems are not remitting or are worsening. Beyond these broad conclusions, research on PRIU in general and treatment studies, although often considerably less complete than preferable, provide varying levels of guidance for tailoring or designing intervention in lines with client presentation. Hence, the chapter also covers various specific topics and possible guides for therapeutic planning and implementation.

Keywords: gaming, Internet addiction, cognitive-behavior therapy, Internet gaming disorder, digital technology, pathological Internet use

Demand for treatment, as opposed to justification and design of treatment, are distinguishable matters. In the domain of problematic Internet and digital technology (DT) use, it seems clear that there is considerable treatment demand (e.g., see King, Delfabbro, Griffiths, & Gradison, 2011; King et al., 2017). Hence, the latter part of the equation will be the focus here, not only in examining the general question of treatment justification, but also by considering more specific questions, such as how one might shape intervention in line with individual differences and clinical presentations.

As described herein, the scientific literature on treating excessive Internet and DT use, despite its somewhat nascent state, creates a relatively strong overall case for the merits of treatment. Furthermore, despite obvious limitations in the present body of knowledge, this same literature suggests a number of guides—or at least educated formulations—about specific or individualized treatment design. In the materials that follow, we will begin with certain foundational matters (e.g., the domains of excessive Internet and DT use that are the focus of this chapter; concerns about definitions and categorization).

We will then consider a series of applied questions, such as the type of treatments that have and have not garnered scientific support, evaluation of treatment need, and consideration of therapeutic options. Such discussion often necessitates extrapolation from more general literature on psychotherapeutic and pharmacological interventions for conditions or behaviors that may share common features with problematic Internet or DT use (e.g., certain impulse control disorders; excessive or compulsive behavioral patterns). One would prefer a larger body of literature examining when and to what extent such generalizations hold for DT use and maladaptive behavior, but that largely remains the subject of ongoing and future research.

Foundational Issues

Domain Addressed; Primary Versus Secondary Mechanisms

Given wide variations in Internet and DT activities and technologies, lumping them all together when considering problematic use may reduce clarity. Many uses of DT, for example, are productive and positive, and, among different types of problematic use, there is often considerable variation and discontinuity at psychological, biological, and social levels. For example, a highly disciplined individual who games professionally and achieves substantial fiscal reward and social recognition is likely to have little in common with someone who seems unable to resist the impulse to spend nearly everything he or she earns shopping online for luxury items. Furthermore, although partly artificial or fuzzy, a distinction can be made between problematic behaviors or disorders for which the Internet may serve as one of multiple possible vehicles for expression as opposed to those for which the Internet is primary. For example, pathological gambling does not require, and often is not limited to, the Internet, although the availability of online gambling can make the problem considerably worse, as might also be said for excessive shopping. In contrast, excessive participation in massively multiplayer online role-playing games (MMORPGs) did not exist before and cannot exist without the Internet, although other forms of video gaming existed prior to the Internet's introduction.

Hence, much of what follows will not address forms of problematic behaviors and maladjustment for which the Internet or DT use might be considered "secondary" or one among other potential avenues of expression (e.g., gambling, excessive shopping). Rather, we focus on problems for which the Internet or DT more routinely plays a primary role. It is not always easy to differentiate between DT uses that are productive, neutral, or detrimental overall. Focusing on the latter, however, potential examples that fall within the scope of this chapter include excessive or problem gaming, as well as extensive or excessive time spent on the Internet that appears linked to negative consequences, such as neglect of school work, social isolation, or worsening of psychological disorders.

Considering the enormous variation that can exist across the full range of Internet and DT use, narrowing down to these aforementioned subdomains may help to reduce the degree of heterogeneity and identify certain relatively common features. Also, there is a body of literature that covers this domain, whereas other literature, which we will not cover, is more specific to disorders in which the Internet or DT mainly serves as a medium of expression and arguably or typically is not a primary cause (e.g., excessive gambling). Additionally, when one considers excessive or problem Internet use and gaming in their various forms or modalities, including various types of DT, the total number of involved individuals on national and international levels is enormous. Although epidemiological studies have sometimes generated widely varying prevalence rates (due partly to differing criteria for identifying problematic Internet or digital gaming use), even by conservative estimates the total number of problematic users may extend into the millions or tens of millions (Kuss, Griffiths, Karila, & Billieux, 2014; see also Chapters 5 by Rumpf, 7 by Ko and Yen, and 9 by Hao and Cai).

Definitional and Classification Issues

We will not focus on conceptual complexities and debates engendered by the term "addiction." We will use more neutral terminology to address problem gaming and Internet use together: *problematic Internet use* (PRIU). (We have added the "R" between the "P" and the "I" to maintain a distinction with another commonly used term, "pathological Internet use.") When we are addressing problematic gaming specifically and not problem Internet use more broadly, we will simply make specific reference to problematic gaming or, as defined by the Diagnostic and Statistical Manual of Mental Disorders (DSM-5), *Internet gaming disorder* (IGD). Gaming disorder has been included in the eleventh revision of the International Classification of Diseases (ICD-11), classified together with gambling disorder as a disorder due to addictive behaviors.

Thus, our use of more neutral terminology is not meant to dismiss the potential extent and seriousness of excessive gaming or Internet use. Furthermore, this somewhat arbitrary selection of the descriptor "problematic" is viewed as a placeholder for now and until the scientific advances that are occurring provide clearer guidance or clarify taxonomic status. Additionally, although the same certainly could be said for addictions to substances, we would argue for the utility of a biopsychosocial perspective when considering PRIU, appraising its potential impact on adaptation, and designing and appraising interventions.

General Treatment Questions and Issues

We are now in a position to consider a series of applied or practical treatment questions and issues. We start with more general considerations, such as whether PRIU may require treatment and, assuming treatment is needed, whether scientific literature provides overall support for treatment efficacy. After progressing through these types of broad questions, we move on to more specific or individualized treatment issues, such as how one might determine if treatment is needed for a particular individual, evaluate PRIU and treatment progress, and select among alternative treatment options.

Should Excessive DT Use or PRIU Be Treated?

Various uses of DT or the Internet can be positive (establishing supportive social networks, increasing knowledge, enhancing skills, improving occupational performance, avoiding traffic jams) or more or less neutral (reading a newspaper article on the computer vs. borrowing someone else's hard copy). However, considerable literature has demonstrated an association or potential link between PRIU and a wide range of problem traits, behaviors, psychological states, and other types of concerning or adverse outcomes (Anderson, 2001; Beard, 2011; Delfabbro & King, 2015; Nakayama, Mihara, & Higuchi, 2017; Ko, Yen, Yen, Chen, & Chen, 2012; Moreno, Jelenchick, Cox, Young, & Christakis, 2011; Pontes, Kuss, & Griffiths, 2015; see also Chapters 7 by Ko and Yen and 9 by Hao and Cai). Adverse impacts range from minor to considerably worse and may include, for example, excessive nonproductive use of time, decreased school and work performance, the development or worsening of depression and anxiety, reduced social contact and social functioning, increased social anxiety, disrupted sleep, decreased physical activity and exercise, diminished family relationships, decreased communication among family members, exposure or contact with dangerous individuals or predators, substantial financial resources being spent on the Internet or digital gaming, and arguably increased propensities toward violence in subgroups of individuals.

The extent to which PRIU is a primary or contributing cause of new disorders or leads to worsening of disorders arising from other factors is frequently uncertain, but it is doubtful these varying forms of problematic adjustment are merely epiphenomena and unconnected to excessive DT use itself. A person with depression may spend time stamp collecting or cleaning the basement, but this does not establish that these activities caused the mood disorder. Likewise, although individuals with diverse problems, such as body dysmorphic disorder, spend time gaming, it would be illogical and often counterfactual to assume gaming is *necessarily* the primary cause or accelerator of any and all co-presenting difficulties. For example, long-term problems may predate involvement with gaming and apparently not change in relation to gaming activities.

It seems almost equally misplaced, however, to believe that excessive DT or Internet use makes little or no independent contribution across the board or rarely is an important contributing factor in its own right. For example, as noted, epidemiological studies show that many individuals spend large amounts of time playing DT games and using the Internet (Kuss et al., 2014; see also Chapters 5 by Rumpf, 7 by Ko and Yen, and 9 by Hao and Cai). Games and Internet sites are often designed to attract players and, through such mechanisms as intermittent reinforcement and creation of attractive stimuli, to foster increased usage. Although problematic use is not strictly equivalent to time spent gaming (King et al., 2011; Lee et al., 2014), individuals spending more and more time on gaming or the Internet are often spending less and less time on activities that could well be more conducive to mental and physical health and development. If nothing else, this represents lost opportunity costs.

In addition, research suggests that excessive or problematic Internet and DT use can and does contribute to maladjustment and may compound existing problems such as mood disorders, social isolation, and deficient school and occupational performance (e.g., Ko, Yen, Chen, Yeh, & Yen, 2009; King et al., 2011; Kraut et al., 1998; Lee et al. 2014). Excessive gaming and Internet use may also compromise physical conditioning and health.

For example, individuals who commonly participate in long gaming sessions may neglect their diets, curtail their exercise, and suffer from disrupted sleep or sleep deprivation.

Even if excessive Internet and DT use is associated with a range of adverse impacts, if such excesses are short-lived or only a "phase," there may be limited reason for concern and consequently limited need for treatment. However, although the scope of longitudinal research is limited, studies suggest that excessive or problem Internet and DT use and adverse impacts often persistent, with many players showing continuing or escalating adjustment problems over at least a year and perhaps considerably longer (Gentile et al., 2011; Ko et al., 2009; Kraut et al. 1998; Lam, 2014; Salmela-Aro, Upadyaya, Hakkarainen, Lonka, & Alho, 2017). Excessive gaming and Internet use can lead to behavioral patterns that perpetuate or worsen maladjustment, such as social isolation among youth, which in turn reduces opportunities to acquire social skills through direct personal interactions. Likewise, excessive use can lead to avoidance behaviors that temporarily reduce emotional distress or discomfort but that can compound problems or create new difficulties, the latter of which may in turn compromise functioning in a widening array of areas. For example, an individual with PRIU may choose to avoid real-life situations that increase anxiety, such as social events. In turn, reduction in social, academic, or occupational activities may lead to increased time gaming, reduced grades, increasingly negative self-beliefs, alienation from friends, and familial conflict.

Longitudinal studies, especially in relatively new areas of scientific endeavor, often create challenges. Consequently, although this work has provided valuable initial information, current limits in the overall volume and scope of longitudinal data on PRIU, and the almost inevitable methodological restrictions that accompany such initial efforts, leave various critical questions largely unresolved. Such ambiguities include, for example, the relative frequency of worsening as opposed to stable or improving course over time and whether, how often, and the extent to which excessive Internet or DT use creates or reflects maladjustment. In any case, one often finds significant maladjustment persisting over time. Developmental considerations are also important. Specific age groups can be impacted differently by exposure to varying Internet content (e.g., Internet pornography; American College of Pediatricians, 2016).

Given the very large number of individuals engaged in such activities as gaming and other forms of Internet use, then again, even if we conservatively estimate the prevalence of individuals with PRIU as falling at 1–2% based on epidemiological studies (Cheng & Li, 2014; Pontes et al., 2015; Kuss et al., 2014; see also Chapters 5 by Rumpf, 7 by Ko and Yen, and 9 by Hao and Cai), the total number of individuals with PRIU across the United States, Europe, and Asia alone runs into the millions or tens of millions. One might also keep in mind that PRIU is often only one type of excessive or problematic DT use.

Are Treatments of Demonstrated Benefit Available?

We probably need not make the case for the relative benefits of meta-analysis in comparison to subjective integration of results across studies or consideration of single studies, and thus we will start by emphasizing the former in addressing the broad question of treatment effectiveness. Subject to limitations and reservations to be discussed shortly, meta-analyses on treatment of PRIU generally provide strong support for overall treatment effectiveness (Chun, Shim, & Kim, 2017; Winkler, Dörsing, Rief, Shen, & Glombiewski, 2013; Yeun & Han, 2016). These meta-analyses show a predominance of what would usually be described as robust effect sizes, commonly reaching or exceeding the 1.00–1.99 range, depending on the variables being studied. For example, across 28 outcome variables, Winkler et al. (2013) reported effect sizes exceeding 1.00 on 12 of these variables, and 2.00 on 7 of them. In Yeun and Han's (2016) meta-analysis, effect sizes were modest to small for general level of self-control (mean = 0.29), but considerably greater for favorable changes on Internet addiction scales (mean = 1.19). Despite these apparently promising results, additional well-controlled studies are needed as analyses suggest that, for other conditions described as behavioral addictions (e.g., gambling disorder), initially robust effect sizes diminish in subsequent trials that adhere to more rigorous methodologies (see Bartley & Bloch, 2013).

Treatment studies often show moderate to substantial reductions in time spent using the Internet or other DT. Such shifts, if nothing else, may well lead to greater time spent on what are arguably more constructive activities, which, in the case of very high-level use, can be life-changing. Studies also often show statistically significant or marked reductions in symptoms or characteristics that may have a primary or secondary connection with PRIU, such as social isolation and interpersonal conflict with family members. One commonly finds reduction in associated or co-occurring problems, such as markedly negative self-appraisals or irrational self-beliefs, or in adverse mood or affective states, such as depression and anxiety. However, causal mechanisms often remain uncertain or obscure. For example, it may be uncertain whether diminished DT use itself was a substantial contributor to reduction in adverse psychological conditions or whether such positive changes stemmed mainly from the provision of interventions, such as cognitive-behavioral therapy (CBT) or targeted pharmacological agents, with established efficacy for treating co-occurring conditions frequently observed among individuals with high-level use. Learning approaches for altering negative self-beliefs, for example, may help someone reduce DT use, which in turn may lessen depression. In addition to or instead, such coping strategies might be generalized to thoughts and behaviors that perpetuate depressive mood.

Perhaps surprisingly, there is often little overlap in studies included in different meta-analyses in this area, in part due to different targeted populations and primary research interests. For example, the studies in Yeun and Han's (2016) meta-analysis primarily involved school children at or below the sixth-grade level, whereas Winkler et al.'s work (2013) focused mainly on individuals in their teens or 20s, but did include some older groups. Winkler et al. (2013) targeted studies on American and Chinese populations, whereas the other two meta-analyses targeted either studies involving South Korean adolescents (Chun et al., 2017) or studies published in English or Korean (Yeun & Han, 2016).

That predominantly high effect sizes were obtained across such diverse studies, individuals, and outcome variables provides some degree of consensual validation for the outcomes. These results also suggest that effective treatment is probably not confined to relatively narrow groups or a relatively small percentage of individuals with PRIU and, further, may well generalize beyond (or well beyond) the groups studied. There are also separate literature reviews (e.g., Kuss & Lopez-Fernandez, 2016), as opposed to meta-analyses, which discuss not only overlapping studies, but also research not included in meta-analytic work. It appears *unlikely* that most of these latter studies were excluded from meta-analyses due to methodological concerns or shortcomings and more likely that limits in overlap often result from differences in the groups of interest. Although such reviews lack the methodological rigor and precision of meta-analytic work, as authors tend to openly discuss, resultant conclusions seem to generally comport with those reported in meta-analytic studies.

As we later discuss, this body of literature on treatment outcome has various limits that call for caution in accepting the magnitude of reported treatment effects as necessarily reflecting the typical level of change in applied settings. However, even if effect sizes in clinical settings are often only half the magnitude of those commonly reported in studies, this would still provide strong justification for treatment because it would indicate that many individuals are making substantial treatment gains. Suppose, for example, effect sizes for a variable like amount of time spent in negative or nonproductive Internet use are not 2.0, but 1.0. This could still translate into a reduction in time spent on such activities from, say, 7 hours a day to 3.5 hours a day, or something akin to nearly half an average workday daily. Hence, despite the various questions about treatment—and especially the specifics of treatment—and despite limits in methodology that have to be carefully considered, explicated, and eventually surmounted, we would again state that research to date provides impressive support for the conclusion that treatment often is associated with substantial positive changes in PRIU. Of course, this favorable conclusion applies to variants of treatment that have been studied or studied more extensively, such as CBT, and which also tend to have established efficacy and effectiveness across a range of psychological conditions and disorders.

Established effectiveness across a range of disorders carries important advantages in treating individuals with PRIU. First, as noted, PRIU often presents with co-occurring conditions (Delfabbro & King, 2015; Kwon, 2011; Lee et al. 2014; Pontes et al., 2015) such as depression and anxiety. Hence, if one uses an intervention approach with established effectiveness in treating these co-presenting problems, this can prove helpful in its own right and may also have a secondary or additive impact in reducing PRIU. For example, if PRIU partly stems from social anxiety, decreased social anxiety may lead to reduced Internet use and more positive social relationships. Second, because core elements of PRIU may involve such domains as problematic habit formation and reduced impulse control, therapies with a proven track record for managing or decreasing such problems may well also diminish PRIU and adverse functional impacts.

As will be discussed, when it comes to more specific or refined questions, such as those involving which variations of treatment best suit different individuals and presentations or how different treatment approaches compare to one another, one often finds substantial gaps in scientific knowledge, at least at present. However, the meta-analyses and treatment outcome studies conducted to date provide a critical start and make a good case for the merits of intervention.

Broad Treatment Aims

For the types of PRIU under consideration in this chapter, as opposed, say, to such conditions or activities as problem gambling or texting while driving, treatment is often directed at harm reduction versus abstinence (Beard, 2011; Rowicka, 2016; Su, Fang, Miller, & Wang, 2011; Wölfing, Beutel, Dreier, & Müller, 2014). This is one area in which the emphasis sometimes placed on the treatment of substance abuse, especially with individuals who seem to lose self-control should they engage in even minimal use or who partake in dangerous practices, may be overextended. Although one can see how complete cessation of Internet or DT use might be called for among individuals with extreme PRIU at the onset of treatment, setting a goal of continuing nonparticipation, especially in Internet use, is often impractical and unlikely to succeed.

The Internet and DTs have infused so many aspects of everyday life that it is often difficult to function effectively or competitively without it, trends that are almost certain to expand and deepen further over time. For example, in many educational and work settings, an individual who does not use the Internet may not be able to conduct essential activities. Additionally, many Internet uses are positive, or facilitate productive or effective activity and social connectedness: for example, using a device equipped with a global positioning system (GPS) to find one's way out of a dangerous area one entered inadvertently, conducting a literature search or finding trustworthy informational sources when preparing a homework assignment or expanding personal knowledge, maintaining contact with loved ones in remote locations, or finding support groups that provide information and solace for individuals with rare conditions who cannot find other affected individuals in accessible locations. Although it is hard to argue that the pros overweigh the cons when it comes to such activities as tobacco use or intravenous drug use, Internet use is hardly so clear-cut, both because there are a considerable range of positive uses and because Internet activities are so varied, some being almost entirely positive and others carrying various balances of positive and negative impacts.

In addition, one has to question adopting therapeutic approaches that are likely to fail, especially when it seems unlikely that an all-or-none approach is necessary. A therapist who sets ideological and extreme expectations, especially without compelling reasons for doing so and which are unlikely to gain genuine client buy-in, is unlikely to achieve much success. Furthermore, with PRIU, one is often dealing with behavioral patterns for which change need not be complete or nearly complete for meaningful gains to be made—in contrast, say, to behavioral patterns in which almost any level of involvement may trigger excessive or dangerous behaviors or in which the behavior itself carries major risks. For example, an adolescent who reduces gaming activities from, say, 5 to 2–3 hours a day may garner various benefits such as improved school performance and greater involvement in physical activities. Hence, a harm reduction approach, as one sees incorporated in various treatment programs and strategies for PRIU (see later discussion), may be the overriding strategy of choice in the large majority of interventions.

Harm reduction approaches might incorporate two overriding principles. The first is to change the amount and type of Internet activity (e.g., gaming for IGD) and to shift activities and involvement in more constructive or positive directions. For example, one might aim to alter gaming involvement away from potentially more harmful or detrimental activities, such as games containing extremely violent content, reduce the total amount of time spent gaming, and try to redirect newly available free time in beneficial directions, such as increased participation in physical activities and social interactions. Specific approaches may well vary depending on individual differences in presentation and circumstances and the possible presence and mix of co-occurring problems.

The second principle is to recognize that many individuals enter treatment, especially youth forced by parents, with limited motivation to change. In such situations, expecting quick or immediate action may carry a considerable risk of failure and early client drop-out or poor compliance. Rather, in these circumstances, the initial goal may be to move the individual from the present position of giving minimal thought to the possible downside of current behavior and the potential benefits of change to increased consideration of these pros and cons. As Prochaska and colleagues have eloquently described and has been demonstrated by extensive research (see Prochaska & Prochaska, Chapter 30), moving an individual from a state of precontemplation to a state of contemplation may be viewed as a success or as a critical step forward in a progression that may well eventuate in critical behavioral changes. Thus, rather than expecting immediate movement from precontemplation to behavioral change, and perhaps viewing anything less than this as failure, movement through steps leading to behavioral change may be viewed as positive progress. Of course, some individuals will enter treatment with a stronger commitment to positive change than will others, and hence there may be reduced need for motivational messages and guidance, allowing the therapist to move more rapidly to implementation strategies.

Individual or Specific Treatment Issues: Evaluating Treatment Needs and Formulating Treatment Goals

Circumstances of Referral and Implications for Gathering Information

PRIU may be the primary reason for therapeutic referral or recognized early on as a significant treatment concern. In other cases, PRIU may not be identified for a considerable period of time or may be missed entirely. Given the latter possibilities, it would seem advisable to screen for PRIU routinely, especially among groups at increased risk (e.g., adolescents), given the frequency of occurrence and potential impacts on everyday adaptation and on co-presenting issues, such as social isolation and affective disorders.

Questionnaires designed to assess PRIU often emphasize concrete items addressing Internet and DT activities and functional consequences, rather than more abstract self-descriptions or labeling, probably for good reason. Questions requiring an individual to self-label as having problematic usage may be less effective than questions that address concrete activities and consequences. An example of the former might be a question like, "Do you believe your use of games has become excessive?" and of the latter, "Have there been times, or how often, have you had trouble waking up for school because you were up late playing games?"

Questions that address types of Internet and gaming activities, the amount of time spent on such activities, and concrete or specific consequences, such as average hours of sleep per night, performance at work or school, or frequency of arguments with others over use, may well lead to more useful information than more inferential questions addressing self-labeling, such as whether individuals identify themselves as problem users. There are various reasons that the latter type of items may show low yield: individuals simply may not view themselves as having a problem or may lack insight. Alternatively, especially in the case of youth referred by parents or other concerned individuals, such an admission may lead to efforts to restrict a highly valued activity. In the following section, we address the potential benefits of adding formal questionnaires for assessing Internet and DT use to other evaluative methods, such as unstructured intake interviews.

To state the obvious, underreporting may be much less of a concern with a self-referred individual who is motivated for treatment as opposed to a 12-year-old child brought (dragged) to treatment by a parent. At treatment onset or soon after, that child recognizes that efforts will be made to curtail his or her Internet/DT use, activities that may have become elevated above almost all else. Hence, despite even highly skillful questioning, youth may be anticipated to underreport their use—at times by a wide margin—and may deny any participation in various activities they engage in regularly or extensively. Defensive reporting may be difficult to detect or adjust for systematically to reach more accurate appraisals (see Faust, Faust, Baker, & Meyer, 2012). Consequently, we recommend the use of collateral informants when evaluating youths' Internet and DT use. Of course, parental report carries its own set of potential concerns, such as defensiveness, generational differences that result in misperception (including overperception) of problems, or limits in knowledge about their children's levels and types of use, including joint use with peers. However, despite these potential shortcomings, obtaining information from collateral sources may prove invaluable and may permit clinicians to uncover conflicting information and take steps to try to reach more accurate appraisals.

Methods of Assessment and Areas of Inquiry

Various questionnaires or scales have been developed to assess Internet use, DT use, and gaming, alone or in combination. Coverage, length, and format vary across these questionnaires, often due to such considerations as intended applications (clinical settings, research settings, or both), target interests, and, especially, conceptualization of PRIU. For example, some developers emphasize traditional models of addiction to substances, and others use criteria for gambling disorder. However, most place considerable reliance on one or another set of criteria from the DSM, including the proposed DSM-5 criteria for IGD as a condition meriting future study. Across the wide variety of questionnaires, only a relatively small subset have been subjected to multiple evaluative studies, with results often providing initial validation or encouraging results (for overviews and reviews and greater information on the content of questionnaires, see Faust, Faust, Meyer, & Cook, Chapter 14; King, Haagsma, Delfabbro, Gradisar, & Griffiths, 2013; Laconi, Rodgers, & Chabrol, 2014).

Given various practical circumstances, such as the rapidly changing and emerging state of science in the area of PRIU and related domains, these scales have understandable limitations or may be difficult to match to exact clinical purposes. For example, the breadth of content may be restricted, there may be little or no inquiry into changes or trends in use over time, potential positive uses or impacts may be disregarded, tendencies toward under- or overreporting are frequently not assessed, and relatively basic psychometric properties, such as analysis of dimensions or factor structure, may be lacking. Additionally, given differences in questionnaire content, measurement design, and, if available, thresholds or cutoff points for identifying problematic use, those identified as having adaptive difficulties can vary considerably depending on the questionnaire selected. One anticipates future developments in which comprehensive assessment methods become available that have been investigated thoroughly, may be tailored in accord to pertinent sociodemographic factors, provide options or branching procedures that allow thorough coverage of specific areas or DT activities of potential interest, and rest on well-corroborated theoretical models or theories with high construct validity.

In balance, despite these limitations, when one considers the promising results obtained for a number of these questionnaires, their advantages in providing a structured method of information gathering, and the possibility of comparing results to normative or reference samples, it seems prudent to use one or more such measures when evaluating for PRIU. These questionnaires may provide valuable adjuncts to other forms of information gathering and may help in appraising whether treatment is needed and in designing certain aspects of treatment. At the same time, given their limits, in particular what is often relatively narrow content coverage, it seems wise to supplement questionnaires with more comprehensive information gathering.

Supplemental information gathering will differ depending on what questionnaires are used given variation in questionnaire content. Hence, although we will provide some suggestions for areas of coverage, some of these may not be needed if adequate inquiry is already included in the questionnaire or questionnaires selected. It is also worth noting that leading experts have often taken primary roles in questionnaire design. Hence, whether or not one uses questionnaires, there may be much to learn by gathering and examining a number of leading measures. Doing so may increase awareness of various content areas and methods of inquiry, which may be incorporated into one's intake or evaluative procedures.

Due to their intended purposes, many questionnaires for appraising PRIU do not cover possible co-occurring conditions that may require treatment in their own right or complicate treatment of PRIU, such as anxiety disorders, depression and other mood disorders, social avoidance and social skill deficits, or attention-deficit/hyperactivity disorder (ADHD). Hence, as with almost any other intake procedure, possible adaptive difficulties, especially those that show association with PRIU, should be thoroughly covered, with consideration given to supplementing interview procedures with well-validated and targeted measures (e.g., a depression inventory).

As already discussed, determining time spent on the Internet or using DTs is important but insufficient in appraising PRIU. For example, an individual may spend many hours a day in a work setting using DTs to accomplish productive tasks, and other individuals may spend considerable time on recreational uses with minimal negative impact. As follows, it often helps to inquire about varying types of uses, purposes of use, and time spent on those activities. It also may be mistaken to do too much lumping (e.g., to consider all gaming activities as essentially equivalent). Rather, for example, one may inquire in some detail about types of games being played, including whether specific content is age appropriate. A 7-year-old and an 18-year-old may both spend about 5 hours a day playing games. However, if the 7-year-old spends most of this time playing games involving explicit violence and comes to identify strongly with aggressors, the impact may be very different compared to an 18-year-old who rarely engages in these types of gaming activities. When inquiring about specifics, one might also ask about whether gaming involves isolated or solo activities as opposed to group participation, the latter of which may promote social connectedness or perhaps relational skill development.

It may also be important to cover potential positive aspects of DT use. An adolescent, for example, who is mainly or solely questioned about potential negative aspects may quickly assume, perhaps correctly, that the therapist is biased against DT use or gaming. Imagine asking someone who may be heavily committed to some form of activity, such as watching sports on TV, question after question about potential adverse effects. Such an approach is considerably less likely to enhance rapport than diminish it. The Internet and DTs may be used for recreation; for a temporary, healthy escape from the stresses and strains of everyday life; as a mechanism for learning or a means for facilitating school work; as a way to connect with other individuals in healthy or positive ways and to gain social support and sound advice; or as a substitute or replacement for more dangerous or potentially damaging activities. Obtaining more thorough and balanced information about Internet and DT use may not only help build the therapeutic relationship and convey a more informed and empathic position, but also may prove extremely useful in guiding harm reduction strategies. Broad familiarity with the client's range and balance of negative and positive uses and varying types of DT activities may greatly assist in identifying activities that are not too difficult to alter in more positive directions.

Evaluation or intake interviews might also cover trends over time, such as consistent versus increasing participation in Internet use, or shifts in types of gaming activities. Especially among youth, family factors usually should be explored, as well as broader social relations, for almost all individuals. For example, one may find high levels of use among parents, parents who make little or no effort to monitor or control their children's use, or high levels of family conflict. Family conflict may make DT use an especially attractive mechanism for avoidance or escape. Parents may also be motivated to limit or control their children's use but lack effective approaches or strategies. For both adolescents and adults, Internet use may provide a major means for connecting with other individuals and, depending on patterns and types of use, may promote or impede the formation of healthy interpersonal relationships.

Arguably, it is of foremost importance to inquire into the potential impact of DT use on everyday functioning and the capacity to meet life demands. Again, although time spent on Internet activities is a critical variable, how that time is spent and how it impacts everyday life is often more important as some individuals, despite spending a great deal of time on the Internet, seem to experience negligible ill impacts. Some areas of inquiry may include school and work function; mood, affect, and general psychological adjustment; preoccupation and potential obsessive thought stimulated by or related to DT use; impulse control in general and when engaged in DT activities; and various health and related factors, such as diet, exercise, and sleep. In general, rather than asking about self-labeling or categorization (e.g., "Do you believe you have a problem controlling your DT use?"), specific or concrete questions about activities and functioning may yield more accurate and informative results (e.g., "How many hours of sleep do you average each night?" "Are there times you continue gaming beyond the amount of time you originally planned?" (If yes) "How often each week does this occur?").

Appraising motivation and readiness to change may help in adjusting interventions accordingly. For example, an individual who has not seriously considered the possibility or potential advantages of behavioral alteration may respond poorly to direct and immediate efforts to initiate action steps. If the therapist instead fosters consideration of the pros and cons of behavioral alterations, it may move the client closer to initiating behavioral change (see Prochaska & Prochaska, Chapter 30). A few simple questions may yield important insights into level or stage of readiness to implement strategies for altering PRIU. Such questions may include whether the client is in treatment mainly because of coercion versus choice, whether he or she has made prior attempts to change behavior, and what, if any, thinking has been directed toward the potential pros and cons of behavioral change.

Determining If Treatment Is Indicated or Justified

Appraising the need for treatment often results in more ambiguous outcomes than we would like given gaps in current knowledge and the variety of potentially relevant factors meriting consideration. For example, if assessment methods and prediction of likely changes over time without treatment versus with treatment were more advanced, we would be able to reach better-informed conclusions. However, the extant literature can provide helpful guidance. For example, it seems relatively clear that serious negative consequences may occur, especially in cases of extreme PRIU; that many individuals may persist in maladaptive PRIU for relatively long periods of time, and certainly long enough to compromise functional adaptation and psychological status; and that a considerable percentage of individuals may benefit from treatment. There is also good reason to believe that if individuals with a variety of primary psychological problems, such as social avoidance, excessive anxiety, or depressed mood, engage in extreme DT use or certain forms of DT use, such psychological problems may well worsen. Hence, even a person who has become involved in therapeutic treatment due to primary problems or challenges in other areas may also benefit from interventions aimed at PRIU as well.

When deciding whether or not to proceed with treatment, one might clearly prefer the use of formal diagnostic categories to assist in determinations, or at least an established set of multidimensional criteria tied rigorously to outcome or prognosis. However, the present state of knowledge and methodology might thwart such efforts. For example, variations among conceptualizations, proposed diagnostic criteria, questionnaires, and thresholds (if available) for distinguishing the presence or absence of disorder can create considerable uncertainty. Under such circumstances, the rationale or dividing line for identifying someone as needing treatment may come down to the level of functional consequences and to trends that may have been exhibited toward persistent or worsening problems.

With a thorough intake and assessment, the evaluator should usually be able to draw reasonably sound conclusions about the level of negative impact, motivation and readiness for change, and whether treatment stands a reasonable likelihood of helping. With individuals "forced" into treatment, however, defensive responding may obscure status, and here judicious use of collateral sources or information should be strongly considered. If in doubt, one may use an initial treatment session or two as a means for further information gathering or appraisal of treatment needs or readiness, or one may instead schedule a follow-up meeting to see how the individual is progressing.

Tailoring Treatment, Treatment Guides, and Treatment Targets

Beyond the general question of whether treatment tends to impact PRIU favorably, studies often yield limited precise information about treatment specifics and may not have such important methodological features as carefully controlled structures and assessment of fidelity of therapist-delivered treatments (King et al., 2012, 2017). Studies are lacking in which all variables but one or a few are held constant or controlled in order to compare differing treatment approaches. More often, if comparisons are made, contrasting interventions differ across multiple dimensions, such as theoretical orientation, treatment duration, and populations under consideration. Developing refined knowledge about treatment specifics commonly requires extended, well-funded, and large-scale efforts. Hence, it seems unreasonable to criticize those who have undertaken initial, valuable studies on treatment for not having delivered something that cannot be realistically expected at this stage of research. At the same time, given these limits, much of what might be said about treatment specifics should be considered cautiously and might rest primarily on educated guesswork or more conjecture than one would prefer.

Theoretical Orientation and Therapeutic Approach

Within the domain of PRIU, CBT and variations of CBT tailored to presenting problems with DT use and interventions that include CBT approaches as a major component of treatment have the largest body of supportive studies (Bai & Fan, 2007; Cao, Su, & Gao, 2007; Du, Jiang, & Vance, 2010; Lanjun, 2009; Li & Dai, 2009; Liu et al., 2015; Orzack, Voluse, Wolf, & Hennen, 2006; Rong, Zhi, & Yong, 2005; Young, 2007, 2009, 2013). It is also the case, however, that CBT is the most studied treatment (Winkler et al., 2013). Thus, the amount of supportive literature should not be equated with the demonstration of greater efficacy, a distinct matter that, as noted, requires further research.

Specific adaptations or tailoring of CBT-based treatments to comport with PRIU and clinical presentations have sometimes varied widely (although the same can often be said about the use of CBT in general or its application to varying symptoms and clinical needs). For example, some approaches start by targeting behavioral change and others by emphasizing problematic beliefs or assumptions. Length of proposed treatment, emphasis on individual versus group treatment, adjunct treatment components, and other particulars may also differ.

Whether and the extent to which specific treatment modifications, recommended progression of intervention goals, use of adjunct treatment approaches, and other such variations impact outcome also remain largely matters requiring further study. Thus, steadfast assertions about such treatment specifics may rest less on science than on impressionistic evidence or even elements of dogmatism. Fortunately, various thoughtful reviews and discussions of treatment guides appear in the literature, a number of which extend beyond approaches emphasizing CBT (e.g., see Delfabbro & King, 2015; King, Delfabbro, Griffiths, & Gradisar, 2012; Pontes et al., 2015; Rowicka, 2016; also Chapter 9 by Hao and Cai). For example, Delfabbro and King (2015) provide an informative discussion of maladaptive beliefs and treatment considerations particular to problem gaming, Pontes et al. (2015) review steps and stages in implementing CBT-based approaches and limits in the scientific literature, and King et al. (2012) offer a carefully developed summary of clinical practices and guides.

Providing a few examples of treatment approaches may help to convey a more concrete sense of intervention methods. Young (2011) has developed a specialized form of CBT for Internet Addiction (CBT-IA). Young's CBT-IA is designed for individual treatment and consists of three phases across 12 weekly sessions: behavior therapy, cognitive therapy, and harm reduction therapy (HRT). The first phase, behavior therapy, is tailored to gradually reduce time spent online. Cognitive therapy then engages the individual in an exploration of distorted thought patterns that contribute to excessive Internet use. To conclude, harm reduction aims to address coexisting issues that may contribute to excessive Internet use, such as maladaptive coping strategies leading to compulsive use.

In one study, Young (2013) investigated the utility of CBT-IA in 128 male and female adults, aged 22–56 (with mean age not reported). Self-reported problematic Internet use behaviors included such activities as pornography viewing, gaming, chats, shopping, and gambling. The Internet Addiction Diagnostic Questionnaire (IADQ; Young, 2009) and an outcome checklist were used to measure treatment results. Pre- and post-treatment ratings showed statistically significant improvements, which seemed to persist over a 6-month follow-up. Unfortunately, effect sizes were not reported, and the study also lacked a control or comparison group.

Wölfing, Beutel, Dreier, and Muller (2014; see also Woelfing, Muller, Dreier, & Beutel, Chapter 39) provide a detailed description and initial outcome data on their variant of CBT-based intervention for PRIU. Their study involved 42 male adults, after excluding individuals with severe co-occurring conditions. Treatment consisted of 15 group and 8 individual outpatient sessions. General treatment goals focused on harm reduction as opposed to cessation of all Internet use. Initial status and outcome were assessed using multiple measures and structured interviews, including a questionnaire designed specifically to measure PRIU or Internet addiction. The group sessions were divided into three phases: an early phase, which emphasized psychoeducation and the formulation of mutual therapy goals; a middle phase, which focused on interventions to promote more positive Internet use; and a final or termination phase, which emphasized such topics as relapse prevention. Individual therapy sessions varied in relation to specific client needs and problem areas but primarily addressed reduction of problematic DT and Internet use. For example, sessions commonly covered familial conflicts, other social and relationship problems, and their connection with excessive or problem use patterns. Outcome data indicated large, positive effect sizes, with changes seen in such areas as time spent on the Internet, work performance, and level of social conflict. This study also lacked a control or comparison group but, like Young's work, provided important scientific beginnings in the development and appraisal of CBT-based approaches.

A variety of other treatment approaches and hybrid or combined treatment approaches have been used, such as acceptance and commitment therapy (ACT), reality therapy, medications, and combinations of these and other approaches (for an overview, see Nakayama et al., 2017). To the extent that these various interventions have been studied, outcomes, as previously described, have generally been favorable or highly favorable (see Chun et al. 2017; Winkler et al., 2013; Yeun & Han, 2016), although effects sizes reported in such early studies may decrease as subsequent studies are conducted due to such factors as potential publication bias.

Some examples of research on varied treatment approaches can also be provided. Twohig and Crosby (2010) assessed ACT in treating individuals with problematic Internet pornography viewing. In their study, six adult males participated in eight 1.5 hour sessions of ACT targeting their pornography use. Treatment outcomes were assessed across various scales and measures, although a major emphasis was placed on self-reported level of Internet pornography viewing. The study yielded a self-reported reduction of 85% at the conclusion of treatment, which remained at a similar level (83%)

at 3-month follow-up. As with much other intervention research in PRIU, the study did not include control or comparison groups, thereby hampering the ability to evaluate the relative efficacy of differing treatments.

Zhang et al. (2016a) provided a craving behavioral intervention involving components of CBT- and mindfulness-based training to men with IGD. When compared to a test-retest group, this intervention led to significantly greater reductions in time gaming, craving, and scores on Internet addiction measures. Furthermore, changes in functional brain activation to gaming cues and in resting-state functional connectivity were observed from before to after treatment that differed from test-retest results (Zhang et al., 2016a, 2016b). The findings indicate that brain functional connectivity patterns involving regions previously implicated in craving, memory, and motor function may be impacted by this intervention, suggesting possible brain mechanisms underlying behavioral change in men with IGD. The extent to which these findings generalize to other groups (e.g., women) and other forms of PRIU warrants additional study.

Studies also suggest that group therapy may offer an efficient and effective alternative to individual treatment (Bai & Fan, 2007; Cao et al., 2007; Du et al., 2010; Liu et al., 2015). To again provide a concrete exemplar, Liu et al. (2015) evaluated multifamily group therapy for adolescents. The study sample consisted of 46 adolescents, aged 12–18, and 46 of their parents, aged 35–46. Based on participation availability, 21 families received the intervention and 25 families served as controls. The intervention consisted of two, 2-hour sessions each week, across 3 consecutive weeks. The sessions included such topics as parent–adolescent communication skills training, parent–adolescent communication practices on Internet addiction, parent–adolescent relationship building skills training, associations between psychological needs and Internet use, and the formation of appropriate and healthy expectations for the family system. Several measures were used to assess status before treatment, at the completion of treatment, and at 3-months follow-up. Although effect sizes were not reported, the intervention group showed statistically significant and favorable differences from the control group across all post-intervention measures. Notably, at 3 months post-intervention, when examining results on a questionnaire used to identify PRIU or Internet addiction, 87% of control group members exceeded the specified cut-point in comparison to only 11% of the treated adolescents.

Although also of considerable importance, especially given a potential impact that could well equal or exceed individual and group therapy, we will not cover public education and population-based initiatives. We refer interested readers to other sources (e.g., Kwon, 2011; Nakayama et al., 2017; Vondráčková & Gabrhelík, 2016; see also Chapter 9 by Hao and Cai).

Despite the increasing body of outcome research, limits in specific knowledge or clear information on the relative benefits of different treatment options and approaches may create quandaries for treatment providers trying to design interventions in the most informed way possible. Hence, although far from ideal, we offer two potential guidelines, one that is probably obvious and another that might not be so evident. First, all else being equal, and especially if co-occurring conditions are present with clear treatment choices or methods of established differential effectiveness, one should favor treatments with stronger or broader scientific support. Second, given various treatments with similar levels of general support, one might wish to review inclusion and exclusion criteria used across studies. One may find that some or all of the supportive research for one approach as opposed to other potential approaches involves individuals who have little in common with one's client. For example, the client in question may differ in age, patterns of use, type of use, and presence or absence of co-occurring conditions from nearly all or even all individuals in the studies of interest. Hence, in general, the closer the match between one's client and the individuals in the outcome studies, especially on key variables, the more the chances of achieving maximum treatment benefits are likely to increase. An approach that works for an adolescent boy using the Internet to bully others or who constantly texts while driving may have no sensible connection to treatment approaches for DT use involving, say, IGD. There is wide variation in DT use, potential associated positive and negative impacts, possible co-occurring problems, and other characteristics, and here even a quick check on inclusionary and exclusionary criteria in studies may yield important information on level of potential match or mismatch.

Pharmacological Interventions

Relatively few pharmacological trials have been conducted for PRIU. Given co-occurrences between IGD and depression and bupropion's effects in reducing craving for gaming in individuals with IGD (operationalized or defined as excessive online gaming) (Han, Hwang, & Renshaw, 2010), bupropion was tested in a placebo-controlled fashion in 50 men with IGD (again operationalized or defined as excessive online gaming) and major depression (Han & Renshaw, 2012). All subjects received an educational interventional platform. Bupropion was superior to placebo in reducing measures of Internet addiction, time gaming, and depression. The reductions in gaming persisted longer than the reductions in depression. A subsequent study of 119 adolescents with IGD found that both bupropion and escitalopram (another medication with an indication for depression, albeit with a different mechanism of action than bupropion) found that both medications were superior to no medication in reducing measures of Internet addiction, depression, and ADHD (Song et al. 2016). However, bupropion was superior to escitalopram in reducing impulsivity and improving attention (Han et al., 2009).

The medication-related decrease in both psychiatric domains is consistent with findings in other behavioral addictions, notably gambling disorder. In people with gambling disorder, medications targeting a co-occurring disorder have been found to associate with improvements in both the co-occurring and gambling domains, with preliminary treatment algorithms based on presence and absence of specific co-occurring disorders having been proposed (Bullock & Potenza, 2012).

Other forms of PRIU warrant consideration as treatments for these behaviors but may differ in part based on the activity being performed on the Internet. Several case reports have described possible pharmacological interventions for PRIU involving pornography viewing. One study found that in three open-label cases paroxetine was associated with decreases in anxiety and pornography viewing but also with the emergence of problematic sexual behaviors in other domains. As such, caution is noted when using paroxetine (and possibly other serotonin reuptake inhibitors) in treating individuals with PRIU related to pornography viewing, and the importance of assessing offline behaviors in conjunction with online behaviors is evident. In a separate case report, an individual with PRIU related to viewing of pornography entered treatment, and, while CBT was associated with reduced pornography viewing, cravings concurrently increased (Kraus, Meshberg-Cohen, Martino, Quinones, & Potenza, 2015). Given naltrexone's effects on reducing craving in substance use and gambling disorders, open-label naltrexone was initiated and naltrexone treatment was associated with a reduction in craving and maintenance in reduction of pornography viewing. Additional studies are needed to evaluate the efficacy and tolerability of naltrexone in helping individuals with PRIU relating to pornography viewing and perhaps other behaviors.

Additional Therapeutic Issues and Considerations

Finally, we wish to briefly discuss a number of additional issues in the design and implementation of treatment, again having to depend more than we would prefer on general knowledge about therapeutic processes as opposed to particularized knowledge about PRIU. We look forward to increasing yields from outcome studies and reduced need to depend on such partial knowledge and extrapolation.

EVALUATE READINESS FOR CHANGE AND ACT ACCORDINGLY

Prior to a serious commitment to change or even consideration of the possibility, movement in that direction among individuals experiencing significant PRIU and detrimental impacts can be viewed as a positive outcome or as progression in a favorable direction. For example, approaches that utilize motivational interviewing (Miller & Rollnick, 2012) may not elicit immediate action, but may move the individual closer to that point and eventuate in substantial behavioral change and improvement. Tailoring intervention in relation to readiness to change may bolster therapeutic outcomes (see Prochaska & Prochaska, Chapter 30).

CONSIDER POSSIBLE CO-OCCURRING DISORDERS ON "BOTH SIDES OF THE EQUATION"

There can be a tendency to overlook PRIU when individuals are referred for other problems or to not evaluate this possibility at all. There can also be a tendency to give insufficient attention to co-presenting problems when PRIU is the focus of referral. Given the frequency of PRIU and the growing role of DTs in everyday life, increasing numbers of individuals may be prone to developing PRIU and experiencing significant or even severe consequences. We suggest that in most routine intakes, at least some screening questions or a brief questionnaire addressing potential PRIU be given serious consideration. Furthermore, given the potential for compounding or undesirable synergistic impacts across problem domains, overlooking potential co-occurring concerns, especially those that tend to be associated with PRIU, may diminish or impede therapeutic success.

ASPECTS OF CAUSAL ANALYSIS MAY BE CHALLENGING, AT BEST, BUT SOMETIMES MAY MAKE LITTLE DIFFERENCE

Determining what caused what when it comes to a mixture of PRIU and co-occurring problems may introduce a complex weave of intersecting and obscure causal factors that are not well understood at present, particularly given the relatively limited number of longitudinal studies and the rapidly changing DT environment. At times, identifying and disentangling potential causative factors is of great benefit (e.g., learning that endocrine dysfunction, rather than mood disorder, plays a key role in lethargy). However, many other times, either because it just cannot be done or because it minimally impacts treatment choices, one may have to or can proceed despite causative ambiguities. For example, medications may reduce symptoms of depression even when causal mechanisms vary or are not well understood (which is not to overlook the improvements that can be gained in immediate or long-term management when causal understanding improves). Similarly, trying to tease out whether PRIU was a primary or secondary cause of one or another disorder may be largely speculative yet make little difference, at least at the onset of treatment or when designing initial intervention steps.

We would suggest the conservative assumption that PRIU and co-occurring problems may interact to make one another worse. Hence, inroads on one or the other should be helpful not only in addressing that particular problem, but also in reducing other symptoms or problems. One implication is that, all else being equal, one might not worry so much about the area in which therapeutic efforts might start as opposed to selecting an area in which treatment resistance is likely to be lower and benefits more likely to be achieved—and achieved in relatively short order. There are, however, likely to be exceptions. For example, PRIU may have reached a level of almost complete dominance over a person's life, resulting in major failure in multiple domains such as school, work, and social relations. Also, some individuals may be particularly susceptible to the impact of excessive gaming or may be engaging in dangerous or destructive online activities. Obviously, in such cases, all else is not equal and such behaviors may need to be given top priority and immediate attention.

TREATMENT INTENSITY, DURATION, AND SETTING

There are an insufficient number of treatment studies that directly compare efficacy in relation to "dosage," such as the frequency or number of treatment sessions, the duration of treatment, the forms or varieties of intervention provided (e.g., individual, group, both), or the treatment setting. Rather, one has more or less a conglomeration of studies across which multiple variables often differ, such as duration of treatment, type of treatment, and treatment setting, thus making it very hard to isolate the impact of such variations. One might consider the position of an investigator studying and designing an intervention, especially in the relatively early stages of research. Such research often occurs in applied settings in which clinicians have a previous track record of responding to the needs of clients with PRIU and significant functional consequences. A natural tendency may involve designing interventions that seem most likely to achieve the needed impact, rather than to conduct systematic exploration of the minimal intervention that may be needed to achieve therapeutic progress. Hence, although one could form the impression that all of the components and hours of service were essential in achieving obtained benefits, one of course does not really know what the outcome would have been had the total therapeutic package been reduced. In this context, brief interventions warrant examination, as well as studies into the natural histories of different forms of PRIU.

Although two meta-analyses suggest an association between treatment length and effect sizes (Chun et al., 2017; Yeun & Han, 2016), the paucity of studies formally varying and comparing parameters related to intensity, duration, and modality largely limits one to impressionistic judgments about relationships between standing along such dimensions and treatment outcomes. We would note that some studies that seem to provide considerably less intense, broad-based, or lengthy intervention do report impressive improvements (e.g., Twohig & Crosby, 2010). It is understood that some providers have carefully designed treatment protocols that are organized and delivered as a whole and arguably could be compromised if disaggregated. However, when feasible, and perhaps especially when PRIU is a secondary treatment focus or seems to have had no more than mild to moderate psychological or functional consequences, one might start with less intensive or lengthy therapeutic interventions. For example, one might start with 3–4 sessions of CBT-based treatment and then appraise outcome. Additional services and forms of intervention can then be provided if needed or if one finds on follow-up that problems have reemerged or worsened. Providing no more (but no less) than what appears needed conserves resources and may extend treatment availability and accessibility, which are often important considerations (see later discussion for the possible extension of services by using DT-based interventions).

Finally, although there may well be sufficient rationale for residential treatment in extreme cases, we recommend against so-called boot camps that use punitive approaches or corporal punishment as these may do more harm than good and have been associated with a few reports of resultant death (see Hao & Cai, Chapter 9). These boot camp or paramilitary approaches are to be distinguished from appropriate residential services that may emphasize self-discipline or outdoor activities but use constructive therapeutic methods (see Nakayama et al., 2017).

LANGUAGE, CULTURE, INDIVIDUAL DIFFERENCES

Individuals with PRIU are remarkably diverse, as Internet use now spans much of the world population with a reach that is growing daily. Individuals with PRIU cover nearly the full spectrum of humanity, cutting across country of origin, socioeconomic status, cultural background, and race and ethnicity, and it certainly may defy common stereotypes. Although treatment research has often involved varying populations, there is very limited discussion about the ways in which interventions designed for one or certain groups of individuals might need to be modified for other groups of individuals. For example, the potential need to translate and adapt assessment methods and intervention guides often does not seem to have been given the attention it merits. Furthermore, public health initiatives and interventions that incorporate governmental agencies and institutions may need to be modified considerably across countries and forms of government.

Although this is much too vast a topic to cover in detail here, we would urge increased consideration of diversity in conducting studies when appraising potential extension or generalization of findings, performing assessments of PRIU, designing measures, and developing and implementing interventions. General literature on diversity may provide some assistance when particularized knowledge is lacking. For excellent sources on adapting evaluation and testing methods across cultures, see Hambleton, Merenda, and Spielberger (2005) and reports prepared by and available through the International Test Commission (www.intestcom.org). For a discussion of DT and cultural considerations, see Mena, Cook, Faust, Faust, and Holt (Chapter 32).

USING ONLINE TREATMENT TO TREAT PRIU

Although, in general, there is growing acceptance of teletherapy and associated approaches, there has been some controversy about using the Internet or DT to treat PRIU. For example, such an approach has sometimes been compared to treating an individual with substance abuse problems with substances. We believe this may be extrapolating addiction models too far when considering varying forms of PRIU, such as problematic gaming. For example, various forms of Internet or DT use can be primarily or almost exclusively positive. A second and related point is that the Internet and DT are often essential for performing various everyday life activities and meeting important responsibilities, such as completing homework or work assignments. For these and other reasons, a goal of treatment is often harm reduction, not abstinence. The former often stands a much greater chance of success than the latter and thus is arguably the more efficacious approach overall. To the extent that the ratio of negative to positive uses is shifted in the favorable direction, benefits are likely to result. Of course, exceptions may involve highly destructive activities that can have grave consequences even if performed infrequently or occasionally, such as gambling for high stakes or becoming involved in activities that could create exposure to sexual predators. Third, preliminary studies examining the use of the Internet and DT to treat PRIU have generated promising results (e.g., Su et al., 2011). Creating and developing Internet-based treatment approaches could greatly increase treatment availability by reducing cost and eliminating a variety of physical barriers such as remote locations and reduced mobility. Thus, even if somewhat less efficacious or suitable for only a subgroup of presentations and problems, the capacity to provide benefits to many individuals who otherwise may have to forgo treatment is a very attractive feature.

References

American College of Pediatricians. (2016, June). *The impact of pornography on children.* https://www.acpeds.org/wordpress/wp-content/uploads/6.28.16_The-Impact-of-Pornography-on-Children-updated-with-sex-trafficking.pdf

Anderson, K. J. (2001). Internet use among college students: An exploratory study. *Journal of American College Health, 50*, 21–6.

Bai, Y., & Fan, F. M. (2007). The effects of group counseling on internet-dependent college students. *Chinese Mental Health Journal, 21*, 247–50.

Bartley, C. A., & Bloch, M. H. (2013). Meta-analysis: Pharmacological treatment of pathological gambling. *Expert Review of Neurotherapeutics, 13*, 887–94.

Beard, K. W. (2011). Working with adolescents addicted to the Internet. In K. S. Young & C. N. de Abreu (Eds.), *Internet addiction: A handbook and guide to evaluation and treatment* (pp. 173–89). Hoboken, NJ: Wiley.

Bullock, S. A., & Potenza, M. N. (2012). Pathological gambling: Neuropsychopharmacology and treatment. *Current Psychopharmacology, 1*, 67–85.

Cao, F.-L., Su, L.-Y., & Gao, X.-P. (2007). Control study of group psychotherapy on middle school students with internet overuse. *Chinese Mental Health Journal, 21*, 346–9.

Cheng, C. & Li, A. Y. (2014). Internet addiction prevalence and quality of (real) life: A meta-analysis of 31 nations across seven world regions. *Cyberpsychology, Behavior, and Social Networking, 17*, 755–60.

Chun, J., Shim, H., & Kim, S. (2017). A meta-analysis of treatment interventions for Internet addiction among Korean adolescents. *Cyberpsychology, Behavior, and Social Networking, 20*, 225–31.

Delfabbro, P., & King, D. (2015). On finding the C in CBT: The challenges of applying gambling-related cognitive approaches to video-gaming. *Journal of Gambling Studies, 31*, 315–29.

Du, Y.-S., Jiang, W., & Vance, A. (2010). Longer term effect of randomized, controlled group cognitive behavioural therapy for internet addiction in adolescent students in Shanghai. *The Australian and New Zealand Journal of Psychiatry, 44*, 129–34.

Faust, K. A., Faust, D., Baker, A. M., & Meyer, J. F. (2012). Refining video game use questionnaires for research and clinical application: Detection of problematic response sets. *International Journal of Mental Health and Addiction, 10*, 936–47.

Gentile, D. A., Choo, H., Liau, A., Sim, T., Li, D., Fung, D., & Khoo, A. (2011). Pathological video game use among youths: A two-year longitudinal study. *Pediatrics, 127*, e319–29.

Hambleton, R. K., Merenda, P. F., & Spielberger, C. D. (Eds.). (2005). *Adapting educational and psychological tests for cross-cultural assessment.* Mahwah, NJ: Erlbaum.

Han, D. H., Hwang, J. W., & Renshaw, P. F. (2010). Bupropion sustained release treatment decreases craving for video games and cue-induced brain activity in patients with Internet video game addiction. *Experimental and Clinical Psychopharmacology, 18*, 297–304.

Han, D. H., Less, Y. S., Na, C., Ahn, J. Y., Chung, U. S., Daniels, M. A.,...Renshaw, P. F. (2009). The effect of methylphenidate on Internet video game play in children with attention-deficit/hyperactivity disorder. *Comprehensive Psychiatry, 50*, 251–6.

Han, D. H., & Renshaw, P. F. (2012). Bupropion in the treatment of problematic online game play in patients with major depressive disorder. *Journal of Psychopharmacology, 26*, 689–96.

King, D. L., Delfabbro, P. H., Griffiths, M. D., & Gradisar, M. (2011). Assessing clinical trials of internet addiction treatment: A systematic review and CONSORT evaluation. *Clinical Psychology Review, 31*, 1110–16.

King, D. L., Delfabbro, P. H., Griffiths, M. D., & Gradisar, M. (2012). Cognitive-behavioral approaches to outpatient treatment of Internet addiction in children and adolescents. *Journal of Clinical Psychology, 68*, 1185–95.

King, D. L., Delfabbro, P. H., Wu, A. M. S., Doh, Y. Y., Kuss, D. J., Pallesen, S.,...Sakuma, H. (2017). Treatment of Internet gaming disorder: An international systematic review and CONSORT evaluation. *Clinical Psychology Review, 54*, 123–33.

King, D. L., Haagsma, M. C., Delfabbro, P. H., Gradisar, M., & Griffiths, M. D. (2013). Toward a consensus definition of pathological video-gaming: A systematic review of psychometric assessment tools. *Clinical Psychology Review, 33*, 331–42.

Ko, C. H., Yen, J. Y., Chen, C. S., Yeh, Y. C., & Yen, C. F. (2009). Predictive values of psychiatric symptoms for Internet addiction in adolescents. *Archives of Pediatrics and Adolescent Medicine, 163*, 937–43.

Ko, C. H., Yen, J. Y., Yen, C. F., Chen, C. S., & Chen, C. C. (2012). The association between Internet addiction and psychiatric disorder: A review of the literature. *European Psychiatry, 27*, 1–8.

Kraus, S. W., Meshberg-Cohen, S., Martino, S., Quinones, L. J., & Potenza, M. N. (2015). Treatment of compulsive pornography use with naltrexone: A case report. *The American Journal of Psychiatry, 172*, 1260–1.

Kraut, R., Patterson, M., Lundmark, V., Kiesler, S., Mukophadhyay, T., & Scherlis, W. (1998). Internet paradox: A social technology that reduces social involvement and psychological well-being. *American Psychologist, 53*, 1017–31.

Kuss, D. J., Griffiths, M. D., Karila, L., & Billieux, J. (2014). Internet addiction: A systematic review of epidemiological research for the last decade. *Current Pharmaceutical Design, 20*, 4026–52.

Kuss, D. J., & Lopez-Fernandez, O. (2016). Internet addiction and problematic internet use: A systematic review of clinical research. *World Journal of Psychiatry, 6*, 143–76.

Kwon, J. H. (2011). Toward the Prevention of Adolescent Internet Addiction. In K. S. Young & C. N. de Abreu (Eds.), *Internet addiction: A handbook and guide to evaluation and treatment* (pp. 223–43). Hoboken, NJ: Wiley.

Laconi, S., Rodgers, R. F., & Chabrol, H. (2014). The measurement of Internet addiction: A critical review of existing scales and their psychometric properties. *Computers in Human Behavior, 41*, 190–202.

Lam, L. T. (2014). Internet gaming addiction, problematic use of the Internet, and sleep problems: A systematic review. *Current Psychiatry Reports, 16*, 1–9.

Lanjun, Z. (2009). The applications of group mental therapy and sports exercise prescriptions in the intervention of internet addiction disorder. *Psychological Science (China), 32*, 738–41.

Lee, J., Hwang, J. Y., Park, S. M., Jung, H. Y., Choi, S. W., Kim, D. J.,...Choi, J. S. (2014). Differential resting-state EEG patterns associated with comorbid depression in Internet addiction. *Progress in Neuro-Psychopharmacology and Biological Psychiatry, 50*, 21–6.

Li, G., & Dai, X.-Y. (2009). Control study of cognitive–behavior therapy in adolescents with internet addiction disorder. *Chinese Mental Health Journal, 23*, 457–70.

Liu, Q. X., Fang, X. Y., Yan, N., Zhou, Z. K., Yuan, X. J., Lan, J., & Liu, C. Y. (2015). Multi-family group therapy for adolescent Internet addiction: Exploring the underlying mechanisms. *Addictive Behaviors, 42*, 1–8.

Miller, W. R., & Rollnick, S. (2012). *Motivational interviewing: Helping people change* (3rd ed.). New York: Guilford.

Moreno, M. A., Jelenchick, L., Cox, E., Young, H., & Christakis, D. A. (2011). Problematic Internet use among US youth: A systematic review. *Archives of Pediatrics and Adolescent Medicine, 165*, 797–805.

Nakayama, H., Mihara, S., & Higuchi, S. (2017). Treatment and risk factors for Internet use disorders. *Psychiatry and Clinical Neurosciences, 71*, 492–505.

Orzack, M. H., Voluse, A. C., Wolf, D., & Hennen, J. (2006). An ongoing study of group treatment for men involved in problematic internet-enabled sexual behavior. *Cyberpsychology & Behavior, 9*, 348–60.

Pontes, H. M., Kuss, D. J., & Griffiths, M. D. (2015). Clinical psychology of Internet addiction: A review of its conceptualization, prevalence, neuronal processes, and implications for treatment. *Neuroscience & Neuroeconomics, 4*, 11–23.

Rong, Y., Zhi, S., & Yong, Z. (2005). Comprehensive intervention on internet addiction of middle school students. *Chinese Mental Health Journal, 19*, 457–9.

Rowicka, M. (2016). Internet addiction treatment. In B. Lelonek-Kuleta & J. Chwaszcz (Eds.), *Gambling and Internet addictions: Epidemiology and treatment* (pp. 55–64). Natanaelum Association Institute for Psychoprevention and Psychotherapy.

Salmela-Aro, K., Upadyaya, K., Hakkarainen, K., Lonka, K., & Alho, K. (2017). The dark side of Internet use: Two longitudinal studies of excessive Internet use, depressive symptoms, school burnout and engagement among Finnish early and late adolescents. *Journal of Youth and Adolescence, 46*, 343–57.

Song, J., Park, J. H., Han, D. H., Roh, S., Son, J. H., Choi, T. Y., . . . Lee, Y. S. (2016). Comparative study of the effects of bupropion and escitalopram on Internet gaming disorder. *Psychiatry and Clinical Neurosciences, 70*, 527–35.

Su, W., Fang, X., Miller, J. K., & Wang, Y. (2011). Internet-based intervention for the treatment of online addiction for college students in China: A pilot study of the Healthy Online Self-Helping Center. *Cyberpsychology, Behavior, and Social Networking, 14*, 497–503.

Twohig, M. P., & Crosby, J. M. (2010). Acceptance and commitment therapy as a treatment for problematic internet pornography viewing. *Behavior Therapy, 41*, 285–95.

Vondráčková, P., & Gabrhelík, R. (2016). Prevention of Internet addiction: A systematic review. *Journal of Behavioral Addictions, 5*, 568–79.

Winkler, A., Dörsing, B., Rief, W., Shen, Y., & Glombiewski, J. A. (2013). Treatment of internet addiction: A meta-analysis. *Clinical Psychology Review, 33*, 317–29.

Wölfling, K., Beutel, M. E., Dreier, M., & Müller, K. W. (2014). Treatment outcomes in patients with Internet addiction: A clinical pilot study on the effects of a cognitive-behavioral therapy program. *BioMed Research International, 2014*, 1–8.

Yeun, Y. R., & Han, S. J. (2016). Effects of psychosocial interventions for school-aged children's internet addiction, self-control and self-esteem: Meta-analysis. *Healthcare Informatics Research, 22*, 217–30.

Young, K. S. (2007). Cognitive behavior therapy with internet addicts: Treatment outcomes and implications. *Cyberpsychology & Behavior, 10*, 671–9.

Young, K. S. (2009). Internet addiction: Diagnosis and treatment considerations. *Journal of Contemporary Psychotherapy, 39*, 241–6.

Young, K. S. (2011). CBT-IA: The first treatment model to address Internet addiction. *Journal of Cognitive Therapy, 25*, 304–12.

Young, K. S. (2013). Treatment outcomes using CBT-IA with Internet-addicted patients. *Journal of Behavioral Addictions, 2*, 209–15.

Zhang, J. T., Yao, Y. W., Potenza, M. N., Xia, C. C., Lan, J., Liu, L., . . . Fang, X. Y. (2016a). Effects of craving behavioral intervention on neural substrates of cue-induced craving in Internet gaming disorder. *Neuroimage: Clinical, 12*, 591–9.

Zhang, J. T., Yao, Y. W., Potenza, M. N., Xia, C. C., Liu, L., Lan, J., . . . Fang, X. Y. (2016b) Altered resting-state neural activity and changes following a craving behavioral intervention for Internet gaming disorder. *Scientific Reports, 6*, 28109 (PMC4933876).

CHAPTER

39 Internet Addiction and Internet Gaming Disorder

A Cognitive-Behavioral Psychotherapeutic Approach

Klaus Wölfling, Kai W. Müller, Michael Dreier, *and* Manfred E. Beutel

Abstract

Several forms of excessive pathological Internet use, such as Internet addiction (IA), Internet gaming disorder (IGD), or gaming disorder (GD) are perceived as public health concerns. IGD was included in the *Diagnostic and Statistical Manual of Mental Disorders* (DSM-5) as a research diagnosis and recently GD was announced for the International Classification of Disease (ICD-11). IA represents a variety of excessive and unregulated consumption of video games, social networking, chat rooms, use of online pornography, online gambling, or the aimless gathering and research of information. The outpatient treatment program Short-Term Treatment of Internet and Computer Game Addiction (STICA) aims to reduce psychosocial burden and foster abstinence of the former problematic behavioral pattern. The outpatient program consists of 15 group and up to 8 individual sessions lasting 4 months. The cognitive-behavioral psychotherapeutic rational for paradigmatic sessions, as well as the consequent phases, is delineated and working materials are described in this chapter. The therapy contract, weekly protocols, and a subjective model of IA, as well as its individual development and the development of media education, are especially highlighted. Recently, the program was proofed in a multicenter randomized controlled trial regarding its efficacy.

Keywords: Internet addiction, Internet gaming disorder, gaming disorder, cognitive-behavioral therapy, STICA

Introduction

The classification and diagnosis of Internet addiction (IA) is widely discussed. Formally, a research diagnosis referring to online gaming is defined as Internet gaming disorder (IGD) in the *Diagnostic and Statistical Manual of Mental Disorders* (DSM-5). However, this classification merely covers pathological online gaming behavior. Before its inclusion in the diagnostic manual, salience, mood modification, tolerance, withdrawal symptoms, conflict, and relapse were suggested as diagnostic criteria of IA (Griffiths, 2000). *Salience* refers to increased attention toward an excessive behavior, as the addicted individual is constantly emotionally and cognitively involved with the addiction. *Mood modification* refers to an addictive behavior being used to regulate current mood status, to reduce anxiety and loneliness, or to enhance mood. The addicted individual spends increasingly more time online or plays more frequently to be satisfied (*tolerance*) and shows physical and cognitive withdrawal symptoms (sleeplessness, sweating, restlessness, etc.) when the computer game is unavailable (*withdrawal*). *Conflict* refers to conflict with social contacts or in occupational/academic settings as a result of an excessive behavior. Last, *relapse* refers to an inability for an addicted individual to successfully quit the excessive behavior for longer than a short period of time. With increasing preoccupation, education and/or employment suffer, social contacts (parents or partners) are reduced, and social tension increases (Young, 2004).

The recent implementation of IGD in the DSM-5 Appendix Section 3 is a logical consequence of the evidence provided (American Psychiatric Association [APA], 2013). Nonetheless, IGD represents a limited approach because there are a broad range of online addictive behaviors (e.g., excessive use of social networking sites [SNS], online gambling, and online pornography). The World Health Organization might follow the APA approach of classifying pathological online behavior in the cluster of Behavioral Addictions, and GD was implemented in the subsection "Disorders Due to Addictive Behaviours" of the ICD-11 in 2019 (WHO, 2019). The general approach of Behavioral Addictions would also allow for the classification of other patterns of pathological online use.

IGD is commonly reported to be associated with psychosocial burden resulting in sleep-disturbance that may lead to depression (Lam, 2014). Depression, anxiety, and general negative mood are more common in pathological than in nonpathological gamers (Müller, Beutel, & Wölfling, 2014). Furthermore, low self-efficacy is associated with high amounts of IA with respective to IGD symptoms (Wölfling, Beutel, Dreier, & Müller, 2014).

Increasing psychosocial stress, burden, and symptom severity indicate a significant need for treatment of those subjects suffering from IA/IGD. Cognitive-behavioral therapy (CBT) has been shown to be the most effective treatment for these groups (Winkler, Dörsing, Rief, Shen, & Glombiewski, 2013). Subjects suffering from IA/IGD significantly benefited from CBT treatment, and psychosocial burden could be significantly reduced in a pilot study for IA/IGD (Wölfling et al., 2014).

Current Delineated Psychotherapeutic Approaches

At present, research in efficacy of treatment programs in IA lacks strong scientific support. Winkler and colleagues (2013) published the first meta-analysis on therapy effects in patients suffering from IA/IGD. Their review included 16 therapy studies that encompassed cognitive-behavioral approaches, multimodal therapy, and psychopharmacotherapy. Results revealed that any treatment strategy analyzed had significant effects on the symptoms of IA/IGD, with comparably high effect sizes. CBT yielded higher effects than other psychological approaches, especially regarding the reduction of associated depressive symptoms. Furthermore, medication-based approaches (e.g., antidepressant treatment) turned out to have significant effects on IA/IGD. These results show potential value in these IA/IGD treatments, particularly CBT therapy combined with medication-based approaches. Based on these findings, this chapter describes a potential CBT intervention that has been developed specifically to treat IA/IGD. An international systematic review and CONSORT evaluation of different treatment types (CBT, pharmacological treatment, multimodal counseling, and combined treatment approaches) revealed CBT as most effective (King et al., 2017).

Detailed Description of a Manualized CBT Program

In the Outpatient Clinic for Behavioural Addictions, in Mainz, Germany, patients seeking treatment for IA behavior undergo an intense phase of diagnostics before the start of treatment. The diagnostic process includes aspects of the IA itself (e.g., type of addiction, severity, negative repercussions), differential diagnosis, an evaluation of psychosocial functioning and motivation to change, and the gathering of biographical information regarding the IA behavior (e.g., phases of abstinence).

Regarding symptoms of IA, it is recommended that self-report measures and clinical expert ratings be combined. A number of questionnaires addressing IA have been published in the past few years. One of the most commonly used self-reports is Young's Internet Addiction Test (IAT; Young, 1999). Other examples are the Compulsive Internet Use Scale (CIUS; Meerkerk, van den Eijnden, Vermulst, & Garretsen, 2009), the Chen Internet Addiction Test (CIAS; Ko et al., 2005), or the Scale for the Assessment of Internet and Computer game Addiction (AICA-S; Wölfling, Müller, & Beutel 2010; Müller, Beutel & Wölfling, 2014). A common feature of these self-report scales is their relation to DSM criteria for pathological gambling and substance-related disorders. Most of these measures include aspects of tolerance, withdrawal, continuation of use despite negative consequences, loss of control, and emotion regulation. Some also take into consideration *craving*, a motivational state leading to a dominant urge to go online. Although craving has not been defined as a specific diagnostic criteria for IGD in the DSM-5, a recent study on diagnostic accuracy of the criteria for IA concluded that craving adds diagnostic validity (Ko et al., 2014). Some researchers have challenged these various measures due to their potential lack of clinical validity (Beard & Wolf, 2001). Indeed, there are few studies examining the diagnostic accuracy of these self-reports by comparing them with external clinical criteria (e.g., diagnostic interviews; Müller et al., 2014).

To minimize confounding effects related to self-report measures and to enhance the clinical validity of the diagnosis of IA/IGD, it is recommended that one may conduct an additional standardized clinical interview with the patient. Unfortunately, at present, there are few formal diagnostic interviews available for IA/IGD, and their clinical validity has been investigated only at explorative levels. For example, Wölfling and colleagues (Wölfling et al., 2012) developed a clinical interview related to the Scale for the Assessment of Internet and Computer Game Addiction (AICA-S; Wölfling et al., 2010). This clinical expert rating, the Checklist for the Assessment of Internet and Computer Game Addiction (AICA-C), encompasses six core criteria for IA: preoccupation, tolerance, loss of control, withdrawal, continued use despite negative repercussions, and loss of interests. Each criterion is operationalized with specific anamnestic questions; answers are rated on 5-point Likert scales. A comparison of results from the AICA-C with the independent diagnostic judgments of trained psychologists in 141 patients presenting for IA/IGD demonstrated good diagnostic accuracy, with a sensitivity of 85.1% and a specificity of 87.5% (Wölfling et al., 2012). In Eastern Asia, Ko and colleagues (2005) developed the DC-IA, which is a similar expert rating with promising diagnostic validity (Ko et al., 2005).

Clinical and epidemiological research have repeatedly demonstrated that IA and IGD are accompanied by high rates of comorbid disorders (Morrison & Gore, 2010; Wölfling, Beutel, Koch, Dickenhorst, & Müller, 2013a). This has sometimes led to the premature conclusion that IA/IGD cannot be perceived as a unique diagnostic entity but rather as a consequence of an underlying mental disease, like affective or anxiety disorders. However, this point of view has proved insufficient as research has shown that these enhanced rates of comorbid disorders, typically manifesting in depressive episodes or anxiety, can also develop as a secondary consequence caused by IA (Ko et al., 2014).

In clinical practice, it is important to address potential comorbid disorders in patients with IA. To select an optimal treatment setting for these patients, a careful exploration of other mental problems is indicated. Likewise, depressive symptoms that were observable before the start of treatment might increase through therapeutic progress (e.g., reduced online behavior or abstinence) and thus might lead to the decomposition of a patient who has used the Internet as a means of coping with depression. Thus, depressive symptoms should be given special consideration during the therapy progress. In the following, a brief delineation of the manualized Short-Term Treatment for Internet and Computer Game Addiction (STICA; ClinicalTrials.gov Identifier: NCT01434589) is presented (Wölfling, Jo, Bengesser, Beutel, & Müller, 2013).

Short-Term Treatment of Internet and Computer Game Addiction (STICA): A Manualized CBT Approach

This short-term CBT program for patients with Internet and computer game addiction aims at treating patients of at least 17 years of age who meet criteria for an IA/IGD. In addition to the main therapy goal of abstinence, the program aims at facilitating an understanding of the concept, recognizing the triggers of addictive behavior, developing useful alternative strategies, and increasing patients' self-esteem and self-regulation. The basis of these interventions lies in those learning processes crucial to the development and maintenance of addictive behaviors. IA/IGD can be seen as learned dysfunctional behaviors where learning occurs based on biological, genetic, and evolutionary conditions. In line with this understanding, facets of the disorder can also be unlearned. Thus, repeated processes of learning are focused on, particularly the reduction of pathological habits (abstinence), the weakening of neural associations (exposition training), and the (re-)activation of missing or alternative behavior patterns (e.g., functional coping strategies).

Therapy Structure

The program was developed and tested in clinical practice at the Outpatient Clinic for Behavioural Addictions, in Mainz, Germany (Wölfling, et al., 2013). It is conceptualized as an outpatient therapy program consisting of 15 sessions of group therapy (duration of 100 minutes each) and ideally 8 sessions of individual therapy (duration of 50 minutes each). Group sessions are conducted on a weekly basis, whereas individual sessions are conducted fortnightly. The frequency of both group and individual sessions may be adapted at the discretion of the therapist (e.g., with an increase of frequency in case of critical developments and a reduction and phasing out at the end of therapy). Therapy groups are guided by a medical or psychological psychotherapist and include 8–10 patients.

GROUP SESSIONS

In group sessions, the therapy program includes psychoeducative components as well as specific change-oriented strategies based on CBT. Aside from the first group session that serves the purpose of mutual acquaintance and motivation of the patients for abstinence, the structure of the group sessions remains the same. Each group session begins with a welcome and a review of the previous session, followed by an abstinence round with a duration of approximately 30 minutes. Here, positive changes are reinforced, and resources are activated. Priority is always given to handling relapses. Afterward, the specific topic of the session is addressed for approximately 50 minutes (see Table 39.1 for an overview) in which a topic is introduced and worked on using discussions, worksheets, and exercises. Last, conclusions are drawn. The group sessions can be subsumed under three main phases: early, middle, and termination phases.

- *Sessions 1–3, the early phase*: Main focus is on psychoeducation and reaching agreement on therapy goals. Psychoeducative knowledge on the mechanisms of addiction is imparted, and individual models of the development and maintenance of the addiction, as well as therapy goals, are elaborated. The three group sessions are accompanied by one individual therapy session.
- *Sessions 4–12, the middle phase:* Main focus is on psychotherapeutic interventions to facilitate functional Internet use. Interventions include the functional analysis of addictive behavior (diary keeping), skills training (e.g., coping strategies, social skills), and promotion of social interaction and communication, as well as exposition training. The group sessions are accompanied by six fortnightly individual sessions.
- *Sessions 13–15, the termination phase*: Main focus is on the termination of the therapy program and relapse prevention. Treatment tools are transferred to daily life, functional computer and Internet use is facilitated, and tools that prevent relapse are elaborated.

Please consult Table 39.1 for an overview of session topics.

INDIVIDUAL SESSIONS

In individual sessions, the main focus of the therapy lies in the reduction of excessive or addictive computer and Internet use by therapy participants. Not all aspects that affect the individual patient in group therapy can be appropriately and elaborately discussed in the group setting. Up to eight individual sessions offer the possibility to work on these matters. Exemplary, topics include performance and motivational deficits and conflicts with family, peer, or romantic relationships. These topics are often connected to the addictive behavior and thus not only can these matters be addressed in more detail in individual sessions, but the therapist can also motivate the patient to present this in the group to allow for the sharing of similar experiences. Furthermore, these individual sessions offer the possibility to include relatives in the therapeutic process.

Characteristics of Treatment

Most patients report rather strained relationships with relatives and peers, often characterized by neglect or devaluation. Thus, social interactions with other members of the group, as well as with the therapist, are essential as corrective relationship experiences because facilitation of interpersonal skills is a major concern of this therapy. Furthermore, it is important that the therapist has a basic knowledge of computer games, social networks, etc. Therapists should also be familiar with some connected vocabulary to signal competence in this special field. However, specific, game-related questions are not taboo for the therapist since they signal interest and offer the patient an opportunity to take over the expert role. Social inhibition or general fears and distrust are all serious obstacles in therapy. In contrast to their behavior in the virtual setting, many patients are reluctant to show exploration behavior in the real world out of fear of rejection or failure. Especially at the beginning of group therapy, patients often seek limited and guarded interaction with other patients. It is therefore an important concern of the therapist to facilitate interaction and cohesion in the group.

Since orientation toward an immediate need satisfaction is a crucial part of addictive behavior, intensive motivational work and a continuous clarification of the short- and long-term costs and benefits of the problem behavior, as well as a focus on the real instead of the virtual environment, are all quite valuable.

A prevalent topic in the treatment of computer and Internet addiction is the patient's wish for controlled gaming, chatting, etc. The therapist must be decisive in taking this wish seriously and clarifying the motives behind it. From a therapeutic perspective, it has to be made clear that abstinence is, from a prognostic standpoint, the best strategy and includes fewer relapses. Additionally, tendencies for an addiction to shift to other Internet activities have to be attended to carefully.

Table 39.1 Overview of group sessions

Session and topic	Content
1. Familiarization, therapy contract, and goals	- Presentation of therapy program - Acquaintance and introduction round - Discussion of a first abstinence attempt for the upcoming week - Identification of individual therapy goals and development of a therapy contract for each patient - Self-observation using week protocols
2. Triggers and maintaining factors of addictive behavior	- Abstinence round: evaluation of abstinence attempt - Analysis of week protocols - Development of the vicious circle model
3. Resources and alternative strategies	- Abstinence round - Collection of alternative strategies - Search for and documentation of resources using the flip chart (model learning)
4. Psychoeducation	- Abstinence round - Psychoeducation with comparison of behavior addiction and substance addiction/gambling addiction - Cost-benefit analysis of addictive behavior and abstinence
5. Generation of individual development models	- Abstinence round - Development of the TRIAS model: introduction with example (e.g., depression) - Development of individual models of disorder
6. Development of individual SORC-schemes I	- Abstinence round - Introduction of SORC schemes (SORC: stimulus, organism, reaction, consequences): individual micro-analyses using weekly protocols - Emotion-regulative factors of addictive behavior
7. Development of individual SORC-schemes II	- Abstinence round - In-depth individual micro-analyses using weekly protocols - Cost-benefit analysis of dysfunctional behavior
8. Exposition with reaction prevention	- Abstinence round - Exposition with reaction prevention - Preparation regarding possible increased craving and relapse possibility; emergency cards - Discussion of possible changes in group hierarchy due to the exposition
9. Approval and self-esteem	- Abstinence round - Approval and self-esteem: psychoeducation regarding self-esteem and self-efficacy
10. Development and media affinity	- Abstinence round - Elaboration on biographical development and media affinity and the connection to psychological characteristics

Session and topic	Content
11. Development and media affinity	- Abstinence round - Continuation of development and media affinity
12. Relapse prevention	- Abstinence round - Relapse prevention: imagination and anticipation of a relapse, possible relapse situations and triggers
13. Continued elaboration	- Abstinence round - Continued elaboration
14. Continued elaboration	- Abstinence round - Continued elaboration
15. Therapy termination	- Reflection of therapy success and changes through abstinence

Exemplary Session

THERAPY CONTRACT AND WEEK PROTOCOLS (SESSION 1)

Apart from getting to know each other, one aim of the first session is to give a brief overview of the therapy program. Furthermore, the patients should become motivated to attempt abstinence during the following week and to conduct a first self-observation using weekly protocols. Individual therapy objectives are formulated and a binding therapy contract is made.

Important functions of the therapist in the process of getting to know each other are

- To integrate all of the patients into the peer group
- To prevent the exclusion of patients, as well as preventing single patient's tendencies to isolate themselves
- To support the patients' capability to build social relationships
- To establish a pleasant and honest group atmosphere

Moreover, in the first therapy session the patients are strongly recommended to completely dispense with using the PC during the following 6 weeks. In previous therapies, there have been good experiences with this procedure. As the wish for controlled gaming, chatting, etc. may arise, it should be repeatedly signaled that abstinence is, from a prognostic standpoint, the most advantageous coping strategy and is accompanied by less relapses in the long run.

When individual therapy objectives are framed, attention should be paid that objectives be realistic, specific, positive, and attainable. Thus, objectives like "I will never again use the PC" are not sensible. A better objective would be "I will carry out university tasks in the library using the university PC for literature research."

To facilitate self-observation during the week of attempting to be abstinent, patients write down their experienced craving to be online as well as their specific online behavior as part of a weekly protocol. While observing and documenting the automatized behavior, current external and internal triggering conditions of dysfunctional PC use, addiction-specific assumptions, and permission-giving thoughts are identified. Taking a meta-level perspective enables a distancing from one's own behavior, and thereby a strengthening of self-control is achieved. When observing situations in which patients have a strong desire yet are able to prevent the dysfunctional behavior, the patients' self-efficacy expectations are strengthened. This also helps them identify helpful strategies for dealing with desire. Patients frequently report that simply performing the task to document their online behavior leads to a reduction of their Internet use (Figure 39.1).

SUBJECTIVE MODEL OF INTERNET ADDICTION AND ITS INDIVIDUAL DEVELOPMENT: TRIAS (SESSION 5)

In this session, patients work out an individual model of development (the TRIAS model) of their addiction problem in order to gain a better understanding of the influencing factors. With the help of the TRIAS model (describing the interplay between the characteristics of the patient, the environment, and the addictive behavior), patients are sensitized for deficient physiological-biological characteristics (e.g., the presence of attention deficit hyperactivity

date/ situation	thoughts What did you think in this situation?	feelings What did you feelin this situation?	Physical sensation What did you physically perceive?	strength of desire after the game (from 0 to 100)	behavior Which behaviors did you carry out instead of computer gaming?	Computer game use or behavior close to computer gaming Did you play on the computer? If so, how long and where?

Figure 39.1 Weekly protocol.

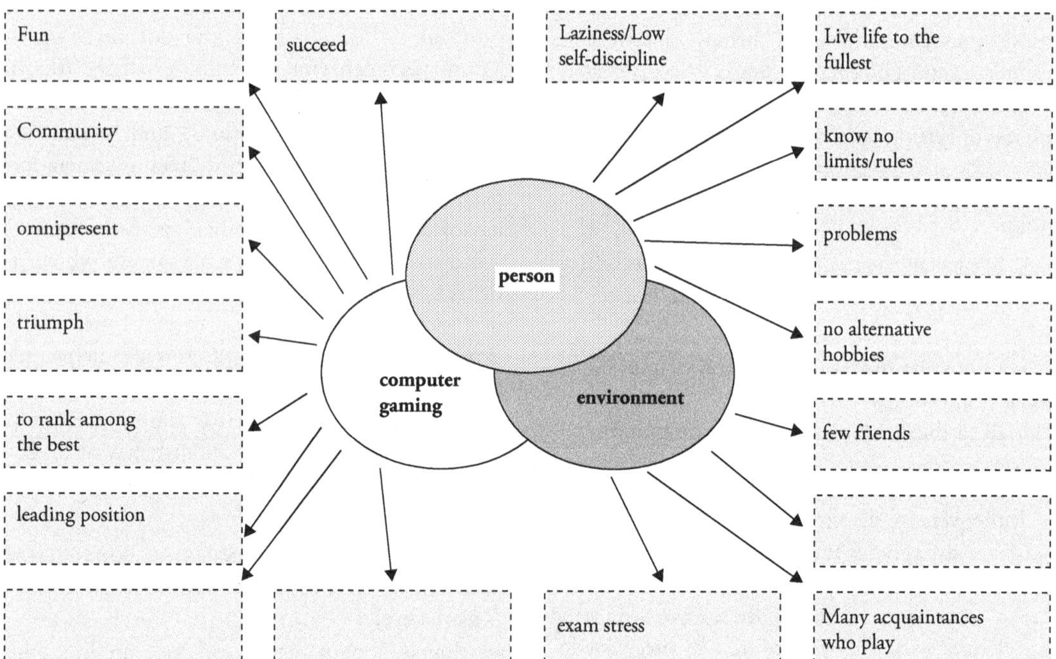

Figure 39.2 Adapted individual TRIAS-model.

disorder [ADHD]) that may be compensated for by a dysfunctional media use behavior, which in some circumstances existed since childhood.

Generally, it is helpful for patients to learn that the development and especially the maintenance of addictive behavior is a complex process which is multifactorially conditioned. Accordingly, it is not about analyzing "the one reason" for their addiction, but rather the disclosure of different influencing factors and their interactions. For illustration,

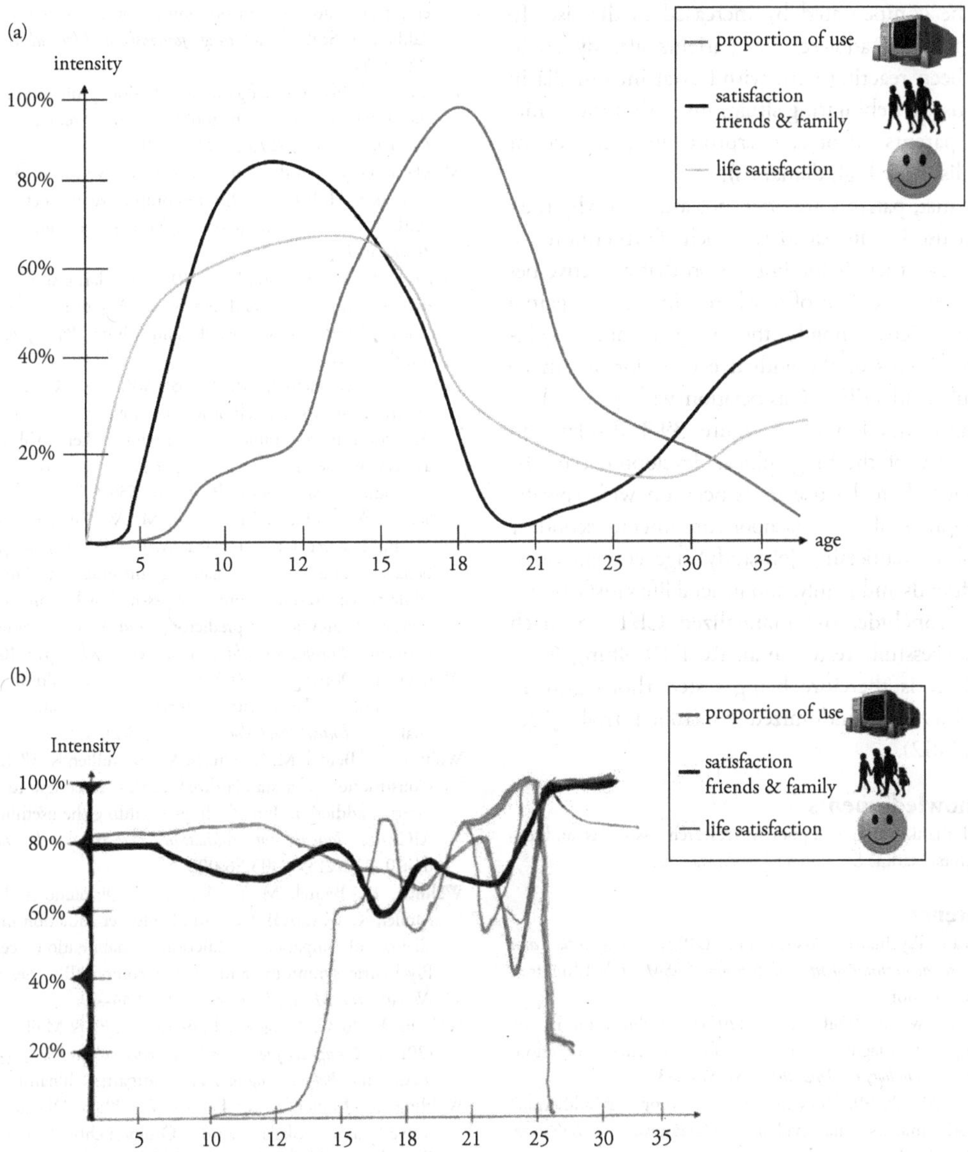

Figure 39.3 Example of development and media use (a) and individual development and media use of a patient (b).

the TRIAS model based on Kielholz and Ladewig (1973) can be used in a form that has been adapted for online gaming/Internet addiction. The model points out different conditions that can play an important role in the development of an online gaming addiction. Aspects of the person (e.g., genetic and neurobiological conditions, personality traits, psychological difficulties, perception, and management of stress), of the environment (e.g., problematic family situations; strains at school, job, or leisure time; lacking relationships; and social resources), and of the computer (e.g., availability, possibility for a flattering self-presentation, quick and easy success) are considered as the main influencing factors (Figure 39.2).

DEVELOPMENT AND MEDIA EDUCATION (SESSION 10)

Patients' media usage behavior is frequently associated with life events or biographical developments, general life satisfaction, and contentedness in social relationships. In the tenth session, patients ideally develop an understanding for the change of their PC behavior across the life span.

An example of a change across the life span is moving out from the family home after finishing school. This change may lead to less life satisfaction because it is accompanied by requirements for autonomy, as well as potential difficulties in socializing within a new environment. Decreased life satisfaction may be compensated by increased media use. In childhood or adolescence, patients already could have been reacting with withdrawal into media in response to debilitating situations within the family (e.g., parents' divorce, overprotection, neglect, or unrealistically high demands).

At first, patients are often not aware of why their media use has increased so much. Furthermore, in some cases there is the impression that addictive behavior emerged "out of nowhere." In order to gain a deeper understanding for the emergence and individual conditions of the addictive behavior, it can be helpful to identify the association with precise biographical development. Figure 39.3 displays an exemplary of the biographical development of the intensity of media use in association with specific developmental stages (school enrollment, secondary school, apprenticeship, job/study), age, contentedness with friends and family, and general life satisfaction.

To conclude, the manualized CBT approach was successfully tested in an RCT (Wölfling et al., 2019). It is therefore being tested thoroughly in a multicenter randomized controlled trial (Jäger et al., 2012).

Acknowledgments

Special thanks to our supportive research assistants and co-translators: Nadine Schabinger and Anita Kusay.

References

American Psychiatric Association. (2013). *Diagnostic and statistical manual of mental disorders (DSM 5)*. Washington, DC: Author.

Beard, K. W., & Wolf, E. M. (2001). Modification in the proposed diagnostic criteria for Internet addiction. *CyberPsychology & Behavior*, *4*(3), 377–83.

Griffiths, M. (2000). Does Internet and computer "addiction" exist? Some case study evidence. *CyberPsychology & Behavior*, *3*(2), 211–8.

Jäger, S., Müller, K. W., Ruckes, C., Wittig, T., Batra, A., Musalek, M.,... Beutel, M. E. (2012). Effects of a manualized Short-term Treatment of Internet and Computer game Addiction (STICA): Study protocol for a prospective randomised controlled multicentre trial. *Trials*, *13*(43). doi:10.1186/1745-6215-13-43

Kielholz, P., & Ladewig, D. (1973). *Die Abhängigkeit von Drogen*. München: Deutscher Taschenbuch Verlag.

King, D. L., Delfabbro, P. H., Wu, A. M., Doh, Y. Y., Kuss, D. J., Pallesen, S.,,... Sakuma, H. (2017). Treatment of Internet gaming disorder: An international systematic review and CONSORT evaluation. *Clinical Psychology Review*, *54*, 123–33.

Ko, C. H., Yen, J. Y., Chen, S. H., Wang, P. W., Chen, C. S., & Yen, C. F. (2014). Evaluation of the diagnostic criteria of Internet gaming disorder in the DSM-5 among young adults in Taiwan. *Journal of Psychiatric Research*, *53*, 103–10.

Ko, C. H., Yen J. Y., Yen C. F., Chen C. C., Yen C. N., & Chen S. H. (2005). Screening for Internet addiction: An empirical study on cut-off points for the Chen Internet Addiction Scale. *Kaohsiung Journal of Medical Sciences*, *21*(12), 545–51.

Lam, L. T. (2014). Internet gaming addiction, problematic use of the Internet, and sleep problems: A systematic review. *Current Psychiatry Reports*, *16*(4), 1–9.

Meerkerk, G. J., van den Eijnden, J. J. M., Vermulst, A. A., & Garretsen, H. F. L. (2009). The compulsive internet use scale (CIUS). Some psychometric properties. *Cyberpsychology & Behavior*, *12*(1), 1–6.

Morrison, C. M., & Gore, H. (2010). The relationship between excessive internet use and depression: A questionnaire-based study of 1,319 young people and adults. *Psychopathology*, *43*(2), 121–6.

Müller, K. W., Beutel, M. E., & Wölfling, K. (2014). A contribution to the clinical characterization of Internet Addiction in a sample of treatment seekers: Validity of assessment, severity of psychopathology and type of co-morbidity. *Comprehensive Psychiatry*, *55*(4), 770–7.

Müller, K. W., Janikian, M., Dreier, M., Wölfling, K., Beutel, M. E., Tzavara, C.,... Tsitsika, A. (2014). Regular gaming behavior and internet gaming disorder in European adolescents: Results from a cross-national representative survey of prevalence, predictors, and psychopathological correlates. *European Child & Adolescent Psychiatry*, 1–10.

Winkler, A., Dörsing, B., Rief, W., Shen, Y., & Glombiewski, J. A. (2013). Treatment of Internet addiction: A meta-analysis. *Clinical Psychology Review*, *33*(2), 317–29.

Wölfling, K., Beutel, M. E., Dreier, M., & Müller, K. W. (2012). Construction of a standardized clinical interview to assess internet addiction: First findings regarding the usefulness of AICA-C. *Journal of Addiction Research and Therapy*. doi:10.4172/2155–6105.S6-003

Wölfling, K., Beutel, M. E., Koch, A., Dickenhorst, U., & Müller, K. W. (2013). Comorbid Internet addiction in male clients of inpatient addiction rehabilitation centres: Psychiatric symptoms and mental comorbidity. *Journal of Nervous and Mental Disease*, *201*(11), 934–40.

Wölfling, K., Jo, C., Bengesser, I., Beutel, M. E., & Müller, K. W. (2013). *Computerspiel- und Internetsucht—Ein kognitiv-behaviorales Behandlungsmanual*. Stuttgart: Kohlhammer.

Wölfling, K., Müller, K., & Beutel, M. (2010). Diagnostische testverfahren: Skala zum Onlinesuchtverhalten bei Erwachsenen (OSVe-S). In D. Mücken, A. Teske, F. Rehbein, & B. te Wildt (Eds.), *Prävention, diagnostik und therapie von computerspielabhängigkeit* (pp. 212–5). Lengerich: Pabst Science Publishers.

Wölfling, K., Müller, K. W., Dreier, M., & Ruckes, C., Deuster, O., Batra, A.,... Hanke, S., Beutel, M. E. (2019). Efficacy of short-term treatment of internet and computer game addiction: a randomized clinical trial. *JAMA psychiatry*. *76*(10), 1018–1025.

World Health Organization, WHO (2019). The ICD-11 classification of mental and behavioral disorders: Diagnostic criteria for research. Geneva, Switzerland: World Health Organization.

Young, K. S. (1999). Internet addiction: Symptoms, evaluation and treatment. In L. Vande-Creek & T. Jackson (Eds.), *Innovations in clinical practice: A source book*. Sarasota, FL: Professional Resource Press.

Young, K. S. (2004). Internet addiction. A new clinical phenomenon and its consequences. *American Behavioral Scientist*, *48*(4), 402–15.

CHAPTER

40 Future Directions

Marc N. Potenza, Kyle A. Faust, *and* David Faust

Abstract

As digital technology development continues to expand, both its positive and negative applications have also grown. As such, it is essential to continue gathering data on the many types of digital technologies, their overall effects, and their impact on public health. The World Health Organization's inclusion of Gaming Disorder in the eleventh edition of the International Classification of Disease (ICD-11) indicates that some of the problematic effects of gaming are similar to those of substance-use disorders and gambling. Certain behaviors easily engaged in via the internet may also lead to compulsive levels of use in certain users, such as shopping or pornography use. In contrast, digital technologies can also lead to improvements in and wider accessibility to mental health treatments. Furthermore, various types of digital technologies can also lead to benefits such as increased productivity or social functioning. By more effectively understanding the impacts of all types of digital technologies, we can aim to maximize their benefits while minimizing or preventing their negative impacts.

Keywords: digital technologies, public health, World Health Organization, gaming disorder, benefits

The considerable changes witnessed over the past several decades in the area of digital technology development are likely to continue and create both predictable and unanticipated outcomes and consequences. Currently, society is in some ways "playing catch-up" with respect to measuring and understanding the impact of various forms of digital technologies, their usage, and their impacts on mental health. Recently emerging digital phenomena like eSports and games with "loot boxes" or "loot crates" have gained considerable popularity and may blur boundaries between gaming and gambling activities. With advances in augmented reality and virtual reality likely to make significant advances in the coming years, it is important to gather information relating to the prevalence of specific types and patterns of digital technology usage and their impacts on public health.

Given such developments, experts from around the globe have been convening in association with the World Health Organization (WHO) to understand and address potential concerns relating to Internet use. In the first meeting, held in 2014 in Tokyo, discussions focused on the legitimacy of possible concerns relating to types and patterns of internet use. In the second meeting in 2015, in Seoul, discussions focused on defining potentially problematic forms or types of internet use and identifying a related research agenda. In the third meeting in 2016, in Hong Kong, discussions focused on how specific international jurisdictions were addressing Internet use. At this meeting, proposed definitions for gaming and gambling disorder that had been discussed in the Seoul meeting were discussed further as beta draft versions of these conditions for consideration in the eleventh edition of the International Classification of Diseases (ICD-11). At meetings in Istanbul in 2017 and Changsha in 2018, these topics were discussed further as the criteria for gambling disorder and gaming disorder in the ICD-11 were released in June 2018. The criteria for both disorders include online and offline specifiers and the disorders are classified as "Disorders Due to Addictive Behaviors," grouping them together with substance-use disorders. This grouping of gambling and gaming disorders together with substance-use disorders shares similarities with respect to how gambling and gaming disorders were considered in the process of generating the fifth edition of the *Diagnostic and Statistical Manual of Mental Disorders* (DSM-5), with the exception that gaming disorder is listed as a fully recognized condition in the ICD-11 (American Psychiatric Association, 2013). Additionally, proposed definitions for hazardous gaming and hazardous gambling were discussed at the meetings and included in the ICD-11 as released in 2018. These proposed elements in the ICD-11 were officially approved at a World Health Assembly meeting in May, 2019. A subsequent WHO-related meeting in Abu Dhabi in November of 2019 continued work related to gambling and gaming behaviors and disorders, with a focus on developing screening and diagnostic instruments to assess ICD-11 constructs related to gambling and gaming. Data from field-testing trials have helped move the ICD-11 process forward in an empirically supported manner, and will continue to provide important information so that improved policy, prevention and treatment efforts may be developed and employed.

As research into the domain of Internet-related behaviors continues to mature, it is hoped that additional entities will be considered with respect to their potential negative health impacts. For example, problems relating to certain behaviors conducted on the internet (shopping, social networking, pornography viewing) do not have related diagnostic entities in DSM-5, and they do not officially appear in the ICD-11. One possible approach to helping individuals with problems in these areas might be to consider the diagnostic code of "other specified disorders due to addictive behaviors." Currently, there is little information in the ICD-11 as to which entities might be defined by this construct, and this remains an area of important future investigation and discussion.

It should also be noted that, with respect to problematic pornography viewing, criteria for compulsive sexual behavior disorder have been included in the ICD-11, with the condition classified as an impulse-control disorder. This inclusion differs from the exclusion of hypersexual disorder in the DSM-5 (American Psychiatric Association, 2013). Although individuals appear to be experiencing problems relating to internet use in non-gambling and non-gaming domains, individual views on these topics vary. For example, in the recent documentary *Addicted to Porn: Chasing the Cardboard Butterfly* (see http://www.imdb.com/title/tt5946552/plotsummary?ref_=tt_ov_pl, accessed October 17, 2017) researchers express differing views on pornography. How pornography is considered may have significant public health impact given that pornography viewing has expanded substantially in the era of the internet, likely due to specific aspects of the internet (relating to anonymity, affordability, and availability; Kor, Fogel, Reid, & Potenza, 2013). Perhaps even more concerning is the impact that widespread pornography use may be having in educating youth about sexual behaviors. The documentary mentions that the average age of onset of pornography viewing is 10 years, with researchers describing that young viewers are being instructed in sexual education by the pornography that they watch. In an era where sexual harassment and abuse are increasingly making headlines and many young men are encountering erectile dysfunction which they attribute to viewing pornography, understanding the developmental impact that pornography viewing at young ages may have appears imperative. Similarly, there is a need for research into other areas in which use of digital technologies may impair mental health. Unfortunately, for such research in the United States to move forward in a significant and timely fashion, the National Institutes of Health will need to provide more support than it has in recent years to address how digital technologies may be harming the general public (Potenza, 2015; Potenza et al., 2018). Additionally, other stakeholders (e.g., internet providers, generators of internet content) should also support research and interventions in these areas.

Although certain types and patterns of digital technology use can be detrimental to individuals' mental health, it is also important to be mindful of the many potential ways that digital technologies may enhance mental health and functioning. Many people can increase productivity, satisfaction, or functioning in social and entertainment domains, as well as in the workplace and other domains, given advances in digital technologies. Additionally, and as detailed in this book, prevention and treatment efforts in multiple areas of mental health may be promoted and advanced through the use of digital technologies. As digital technologies continue to develop and become more widely intertwined, integrated, and assimilated into different facets of life, we should not overlook the potential for both positive and negative impacts. In this process, we should continue to collect information that will be helpful in promoting public health in general and mental health and psychological well-being in particular.

References

American Psychiatric Association. (2013). *Diagnostic and statistical manual of mental disorders* (5th ed). Washington, DC: Author.

Kor, A., Fogel, Y., Reid, R., & Potenza, M. N. (2013). Should hypersexual disorder be classified as an addiction? *Sexual Addiction Compulsivity, 20*, 27–47.

Potenza, M. N. (2015). Behavioural addictions matter. *Nature, 522*, S62.

Potenza, M. N., Higuchi, S., & Brand, M. (2018) Call for research into a wider range of behavioural addictions. *Nature, 555*, 30.

INDEX

Note: Figures and tables are indicated by an italic "*f*" and "*t*" respectively, following the page number.

B

C

D

E

F

G

O

P

Q

R

Z